Radiology in the Management of Cancer

Radiology in the Management of Cancer

Edited by

R. J. Johnson
Senior Lecturer in Diagnostic Radiology, University of
Manchester; Consultant Radiologist, Christie Hospital and
Holt Radium Institute, Manchester, UK

B. Eddleston
Director of Diagnostic Radiology, Christie Hospital and Holt
Radium Institute, Manchester, UK

R. D. Hunter
Director of Radiotherapy, Christie Hospital and Holt
Radium Institute, Manchester, UK

CHURCHILL LIVINGSTONE
EDINBURGH LONDON MELBOURNE AND NEW YORK 1990

CHURCHILL LIVINGSTONE
Medical Division of Longman Group UK Limited

Distributed in the United States of America by
Churchill Livingstone Inc., 1560 Broadway, New York,
N.Y. 10036, and by associated companies, branches
and representatives throughout the world.

First Edition 1990

ISBN 0 443 037329

British Library Cataloguing in Publication Data
Radiology in the management of cancer.
1. Man. Cancer. Radiotherapy
I. Johnson, R. J. II. Eddleston, B. II. Hunter, R. D.
616.99′40642

Library of Congress Cataloging in Publication Data
Radiology in the management of cancer / edited by R. J.
  Johnson, B. Eddleston, R. D. Hunter. — 1st ed.
        p. cm
    1. Cancer — Diagnosis. 2. Diagnostic imaging.
    3. Tumors — Classification. I. Johnson, R. J. (Richard
      Joseph) II. Eddleston, B. (Brain) III. Hunter, R. D.
    [DNLM: 1. Neoplasms — diagnosis.
    2. Neoplasms — radiography.
    3. Neoplasms — therapy, QZ 241 R1293]
    RC270.3.D53R33 1990
    616.99′40757 — dc20
    DNLM/DLC
    for Library of Congress   89–24030
                                                   CIP

Produced by Longman Singapore Publishers (Pte) Ltd.
Printed in Singapore

Preface

In the last twenty years there has been an enormous increase in the range of imaging techniques available to investigate the patient with cancer. New techniques like radioisotope imaging, ultrasound, X-ray computed tomography and magnetic resonance imaging have often been developed by specialist groups who have assessed their value in patients with benign or malignant tumours. These techniques are then employed in other departments or offered on a restricted basis to colleagues. The effect is a patchy introduction and further development without analysis of their relative value. Some may have limited application in common diseases or only be useful in rare tumours and confusion can arise about the role and value of these newer techniques.

The result is that patients are sometimes referred for oncological opinion without having had simple investigations on which major treatment decisions can be made. In other situations they may have been subjected to inappropriate investigations, incomplete studies which need to be repeated or multiple unnecessary investigations. This creates extra work, wastes finite resources and may delay treatment. The patient with cancer should have the relevant investigations carried out as quickly and efficiently as possible. Different techniques are appropriate in initial assessment, staging, monitoring the response to treatment and in the management of relapse. This requires the radiologist to understand the particular relevance of all techniques to the patient's management, at any time in the course of their illness.

This book aims to improve understanding of the role radiology has to play in the management of cancer. It is not a standard textbook illustrating the radiological appearances of cancer and only limited space is given to the role of radiology in the initial diagnosis. The main thrust of the text relates to the integration and limitations of available imaging modalities in staging patients and assessing the response to treatment or the complications of therapy. In addition to the chapters on tumours at specific sites there are chapters dealing with radioisotope and magnetic resonance imaging and one on the use of radiology in radiotherapy treatment planning.

Whilst primarily intended for Radiologists and Oncologists the text should also be of value to all clinicians who treat patients suffering from cancer.

Manchester, 1990
R.J.J
B.E.
R.D.H

Acknowledgements

The editors would like to acknowledge the help and advice of colleagues at the Christie Hospital, Saint Mary's Hospital and at the Paterson Institute of Cancer Research. Particular mention should be given to Professors Victor Tindall and Alwyn Smith, Drs C H Buckley, R Yule, N Thatcher and Michael Moore.

We would also like to thank Miss Michelle Robinson for her secretarial work and Mr S F Griffin for his photographic expertise.

Contributors

F. G. Adams FRCR
Consultant Radiologist, Western Infirmary,
Glasgow, UK

Judith E. Adams MB BS LRCP FRCR
Senior Lecturer, Department of Diagnostic
Radiology, University of Manchester; Honorary
Consultant Radiologist, Manchester Royal
Infirmary, UK

Jonathan J. K. Best MSc MB ChB FRCP MRCP
FRCR DMRD
Forbes Professor and Head, Department of
Medical Radiology, University of Edinburgh;
Honorary Consultant in Diagnostic Radiology,
The Royal Infirmary, Edinburgh, UK

J. Beynon MS FRCS
Senior Surgical Registrar, Department of
Surgery, University Hospital of Wales, Cardiff,
UK

Keith E. Britton MD MSc FRCP MA MB BChir
MRCS
Consultant Physician and Consultant in charge
of Nuclear Medicine, St. Bartholomew's
Hospital, London, UK

P. J. Cadman BM FRCR
Consultant Radiologist, Wycombe General
Hospital, High Wycombe, UK

C. R. Chapple BSc FRCS
Senior Urological Registrar, The Middlesex
Hospital, London, UK

Brian Eddleston MB ChB FRCR FFR DMRD
Director of Diagnostic Radiology, Christie
Hospital and Holt Radium Institute,
Manchester, UK

Wellesley St. Clair Forbes MA MB BCh DRCOG
DMRD FRCR
Lecturer, Department of Diagnostic Radiology,
University of Manchester; Consultant
Radiologist, Hope Hospital, Salford,
Manchester, UK

Phillip Gishen MB BCh(Rand) DMRD FRCR
Consultant Radiologist, King's College Hospital,
London, UK

I. H. Gravelle BSc MB ChB FRCPE FRCR DMRD
Clinical Teacher, University of Wales College of
Medicine, Cardiff; Senior Consultant
Radiologist, University Hospital of Wales,
Cardiff, UK

R. D. Hunter FRCPE FRCR
Director of Radiotherapy, Christie Hospital and
Holt Radium Institute, Manchester, UK

Janet E. Husband MRCP FRCR
Director of the Cancer Research Campaign
Radiology Research Group; Consultant
Radiologist, The Royal Marsden Hospital,
Sutton and London, UK

W. D. Jeans MB BS DMRD FRCR
Reader in Radiodiagnosis, University of Bristol;
Honorary Consultant Radiologist, Bristol Royal
Infirmary, UK

Jeremy P. R. Jenkins MB ChB MRCP DMRD FRCR
Senior Lecturer in Diagnostic Radiology,
University of Manchester; Honorary Consultant
Radiologist, Withington Hospital, Manchester,
UK

R. J. Johnson BSc MRCP FRCR
Senior Lecturer in Diagnostic Radiology,
University of Manchester; Consultant
Radiologist, Christie Hospital and Holt Radium
Institute, Manchester, UK

Robert Jones DMRD FRCR
Honorary Tutor, Department of Medical
Radiology, University of Edinburgh; Consultant
Radiologist, Pilgrim Hospital, Boston, UK

R. K. Levick MB BCh FRCP M FRCR FFR DMRD
Honorary Clinical Lecturer in Paediatric
Radiology, University of Sheffield; Consultant
Radiologist, Sheffield Children's Hospital, UK

Derrick F. Martin MRCP FRCR MB ChB
Lecturer in Radiology, University of
Manchester; Honorary Consultant Radiologist,
Withington Hospital, Manchester, UK

N. J. McC. Mortensen MD FRCS
Consultant Surgeon, John Radcliffe Hospital,
Oxford, UK

D. J. Nolan MD MRCP FRCR
Consultant Radiologist, John Radcliffe Hospital,
Oxford, UK

D. Rickards FRCR FFRDSA
Consultant Uroradiologist, The Middlesex
Hospital, London, UK

Elizabeth H. Sawicka MA MD MRCP
Consultant Thoracic and General Physician,
Bromley Hospital, London, UK

I. W. Turnbull BSc MB ChB FRCR DMRD
Consultant Neuroradiologist, North Manchester
General Hospital, Manchester, UK

J. Virjee MB ChB FRCR
Consultant Radiologist, Bristol Royal Infirmary,
UK

Contents

1. Nuclear medicine

K. E. Britton

INTRODUCTION

Imaging using the techniques of conventional radiology, computed tomography (CT) and ultrasound shows the structural changes which occur with tumour growth. The techniques show the site, size, shape, density, space occupation and what the presence and effects of metastases look like in other tissues. Nuclear medicine techniques depend on the emission of gamma rays arising from the nuclei of atoms from within a patient who has received a particular radiopharmaceutical. They show how the presence of the tumour or metastasis affects one or other of the metabolic functions of the organ or system under study.

Nuclear medicine is thus pertinent to the assessment of the patient with cancer, not to its primary diagnosis. The question 'Has this patient a renal tumour?' is appropriately answered by the structural techniques of ultrasound and radiology, whereas the question 'How much renal function will the patient lose as a result of nephrectomy?' is the province of nuclear medicine. Nevertheless, alteration of function may be an exquisitely sensitive, if not very specific way of detecting the presence of metastases; an example is the widespread use of the whole body 'bone scan'.

A new approach in nuclear medicine is to demonstrate the presence of cancer more specifically, not by its position or dimensions, but by tissue characterization: firstly through the identification of the presence of tumour associated antigens, and secondly through a tumour's receptor binding status. The oncogene/anti-oncogene hypothesis of cancer indicates that there are specific deoxyribonucleic acid chains in cancer tissue which alter its growth characteristics. The

hope is that specific oncoproteins related to these gene alterations will be identified so that cancer tissue characterization may be performed by in vivo imaging using radiolabelled antibodies specific to such oncoprotein antigens. This technique, termed radioimmunoscintigraphy, has a long way to progress before meeting this requirement. It also holds out the hope for specific unsealed source radiotherapy and chemotherapy by the binding of alpha or beta particle emitting radionuclides or cellular toxins to the antibody to target them to the malignant tissue. Experimental work in this field is under way.

The presence on cancer cells of receptors for active molecules is well recognized. The most encouraging recent development in this approach is the use of the noradrenaline analogue *meta*-iodobenzyl guanidine, MIBG, which is taken up by the neurosecretory granules of many neural crest tumours, particularly benign and malignant phaeochromocytoma and neuroblastoma where its use in both staging and therapy is being exploited.

MATERIALS AND EQUIPMENT

Radiopharmaceuticals

It is often difficult for the diagnostic radiologist, who is used to receiving contrast material sterile, pyrogen free and conveniently packaged in an ampoule, to appreciate the recent complexity in providing routine radiopharmaceuticals for nuclear medicine. For the UK the combined requirements of the Medicines Act, the Administration of Radioactive Substances Advisory Committee (ARSAC) and the Ionising Radiations Regulations, make the production and dispensing of radiopharmaceuticals, particularly when distributed to more than one department, a matter for the professional radiopharmacist and a highly trained technical staff.

Dispensing demands a fully aseptic technique in a positive pressure room by a gowned, masked and capped technician taking the necessary precautions against radiation hazard and calculating and measuring the appropriate activity for the time of administration. To meet the logistics of having the right patient at the right time so that activity is not wasted by decay, the nuclear medicine department should have its own designated porter.

Most routine work is undertaken using ^{99m}Tc technetium. It has a halflife of six hours and a gamma ray energy of 0.140 MeV, which is ideal for the modern gamma camera. Each morning technetium is 'milked' from its parent ^{99}Mo molybdenum 'cow' – a sterile lead-encased generator containing ^{99}Mo bound to a solid matrix from which its daughter decay product ^{99m}Tc is eluted using a saline solution into a shielded sterile ampoule. After determining the activity in an ionization chamber, appropriate aliquots of the ^{99m}Tc pertechnetate solution are added to sterile ampoules of the various 'kit' preparations following the manufacturer's instructions: MDP (methyldiphosphonate) for bone imaging; DTPA (diethylene triamine penta-acetate) for kidney and brain studies; HMPAO (hexamethylpropylene amine oxime) for brain and white cell labelling; tin colloid for liver Kupffer cell uptake; microspheres for lung or nanocolloids for marrow imaging etc. Some materials may be bought in ready prepared such as ^{131}I-MIBG (*meta*-iodobenzyl guanidine). Many have been synthesized and radiolabelled in the radiopharmacy before becoming commercially available, such as ^{123}I-MIBG for imaging neuroblastoma. The radiolabelling of monoclonal antibodies with ^{123}I (halflife 13 h, gamma ray energy 0.159 MeV) or ^{111}In indium (halflife 67.4 h, gamma ray energies 0.171 and 0.250 MeV) is another example.

The gamma camera computer system

The technical problems consist essentially of determining the quantity and distribution of radioactivity in an organ or tissue under study at a particular time and of measuring how this changes with time. When a radionuclide such as ^{99m}Tc is combined in a radiopharmaceutical and distributed in the tissues after intravenous injection, its gamma rays penetrate the body. Some interact with the tissue and are scattered, travelling with a lower energy at different angles (Compton scattering), others pass through and may be detected by their interaction with the camera's crystal of sodium iodide, which contains a small proportion of thallium impurity. Flashes of light are emitted, which pass from the crystal to a light sensitive photomultiplier tube, so they are detected as pulses of electricity in this 'scintillation detector'. A gamma camera consists of a single large crystal, for example, 37 cm in diameter and 1 cm thick, to which is applied a large array of photomultiplier tubes, 37 or more. In front of the face of the camera is fixed a lead sheet (collimator) 4 cm thick, in which many thousands of parallel holes reduce the entry of gamma rays other than those travelling perpendicular to the face of the detector. The design of the collimator depends on the energy of the gamma rays emitted by the radionuclide; the higher the gamma ray energy, the thicker must be the lead septa around each hole to prevent their penetration by gamma rays coming in at an angle. The more lead there is in the collimator, the lower the sensitivity of the camera. A 'low energy' collimator is used for ^{99m}Tc and ^{123}I, whereas a heavier 'medium energy' collimator must be used for ^{111}In and ^{131}I.

Beyond the photomultiplier tube is an analyser which may be set so that only pulses equivalent to the original energy of the gamma rays are registered; thus the scattered lower energy gamma rays are not recorded. This is achieved by setting a 'window' of e.g. 20% around the photopeak, which represents the particular energy of unscattered gamma rays. This allows the acceptance of gamma ray energies 10% higher and lower than that from the particular radionuclide in use. ^{111}In has two important gamma rays of different energies so two photopeaks have to be chosen in this 'pulseheight analyser' when imaging with ^{111}In-labelled compounds. Checking that the correct collimator is being used, and the setting of the photopeak(s) are important initial steps before imaging is undertaken.

A complex electronic network determines the position at which each gamma ray struck the crystal and this is displayed as a dot on a cathode ray tube. The number of gamma rays detected determines the brightness of the display. The distribution of dots may be viewed using a 'persistance' scope, which is used to check the positioning of the gamma camera over the patient. Once this is decided the image recording is made. The distribution of gamma rays may be summed on transparent film to give the conventional image of scan. In addition, this distribution is transferred electronically on line through an interface directly into the computer, where it is stored in a matrix of picture elements (pixels), usually a 128×128 matrix, for display in black and white or colour on a visual display unit (VDU). Sophisticated data manipulation is undertaken and, depending on the nature of the programs, includes, for example, region of interest (ROI), selection, image translation and rotation and image comparison or subtraction.

Single photon emission computed tomography (SPECT)

Single photon emission computed tomography (SPECT) is a technique for reconstructing sections through the body of the distribution of uptake from the collection of all the data from a region by rotating the gamma camera full circle around the patient. The filtered back projection computer algorithm which performs the reconstruction is complex and similar to that used for X-ray computed tomography (CT), although SPECT predated CT by over ten years. The sections are usually transverse axial, but coronal and sagittal sections may be reconstructed. The advantage is the increased contrast of the target in the plane of the section and particularly the ability to separate objects from in front of and behind the target, e.g. the bladder from a pelvic tumour, which may overlap on a conventional view. Another practical advantage is the ability to quantitate the amount of activity in a region of the transverse section, for example, for dosimetry; however, this is much more difficult than expected. Errors occur due to less than perfect rotation and linearity of response of the camera, Poisson's statistical noise, algorithm

noise, artefacts due to overlapping tissue activities, the partial volume effect, patient and organ movement and difficulties in correcting for tissue attenuation. Accuracy is thereby considerably reduced and the anatomical relationships of tissues and target may be difficult to visualize and to interpret. SPECT sections, once created, cannot be repositioned. The technique is a potentially useful adjunct to, but not a substitute for, planar imaging.

Positron emission tomography (PET)

This technique is designed to image radiopharmaceuticals labelled with a positron-emitting radionuclide. The annihilation of a positron gives two 511 keV gamma photons which travel in opposite directions. PET uses a ring of opposing detectors and the technique of coincidence counting to determine positional information. The advantage is that the net attenuation of the gamma ray pair is independent of the location of their source and constant. Thus attenuation correction can be made accurately using data from a transmission measurement taken from an external radiation source before imaging commences. This means that quantification with PET is much more accurate than with SPECT and resolution has been made greater by improved detector development. Only the elements of life, carbon, nitrogen and oxygen, have positron-emitting radionuclides. Thus PET is the key to precise physiology and most advances have been in the quantitative characterization of a variety of neuroreceptors in the brain. The disadvantage is that these have very short halflives (^{11}C, 20 min; ^{13}N, 11 min; ^{15}O, 2 min), making the radiochemistry and radiopharmacy complex. Even though the cyclotrons for producing these radionuclides have been automated and reduced in size to fit into a room 19×22 feet, the capital cost of a PET, hot cell, cyclotron complex is of the order of two million pounds with staff and revenue costs of about a quarter of a million per year. In oncology, the main application has been in the grading of the malignancy of brain tumours (Di Chiro et al 1984) and the demonstration of viable brain tumour recurrences (La France et al 1986).

BONE IMAGING

Introduction

The use of whole body bone imaging in the management of patients with cancer is well documented (McNeil 1984). The osteoblastic response to the presence of a bone metastasis increases the blood flow to and the metabolic activity of the bone at the site of invasion and thus the uptake of bone-seeking radiopharmaceuticals such as ^{99m}Tc technetium-labelled methyldiphosphonate (MDP) is increased at the site. Multiple unevenly distributed focal areas of increased uptake with an emphasis on the axial skeleton are the typical features of bone metastases (Fig. 1.1a and b). Whereas a metastasis may need to cause a more than 30% loss of bone in a vertebra for it to be evident on a plain radiograph, a very small metabolically provocative metastasis may be easily detectable by radionuclide imaging. It is necessary to understand that size is *not* the main criterion for detectability; a radioactive pinhead in the body would be visualized if it were sufficiently radioactive. It would appear as a spot apparently two centimetres across due to the limitations of resolution of the gamma camera. Conversely, a larger tumour causing no reaction in the surrounding bone may not be detected at all. As a generalization, tumours of tissues to which the bone is accustomed, i.e. the cells of bone marrow, cause much less reaction than tumours of tissues external to the skeleton. Hodgkin's and non-Hodgkin's lymphomata and myeloma are therefore best imaged using a conventional radiographic skeletal survey when investigating such patients for bone involvement, whereas for all adenocarcinoma the bone scan is a more sensitive and cost-effective method of detecting bone metastases before treatment. Metabolic activity, occasionally after an initial 'flare', typically decreases with successful treatment and so positive lesions on the bone scan become less evident and may disappear, whereas the skeletal radiograph may become more evident with treatment. As the cells in a previously undetected site of bone metastasis die, they are replaced by fibrous tissue and often calcify, thereby becoming more radiologically evident. In patients with adenocarcinomatous metastases to bone, the radiologically positive, bone scan nega-

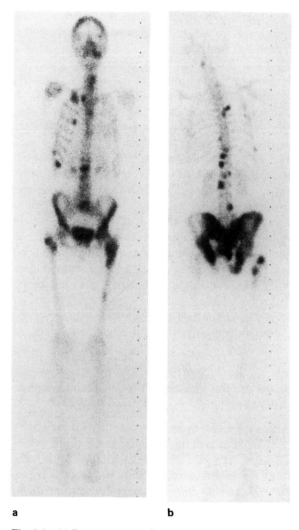

a   b

Fig. 1.1   (a) Bone metastases from breast carcinoma. An anterior view of the whole body bone scan shows multiple focal areas of increased uptake in the skull, sternum, ribs, spine, pelvis and proximal femora, a typical distribution. (b) Bone metastases from prostatic carcinoma. A posterior view of the whole body bone scan shows multiple focal areas of increased uptake in the spine, pelvis, proximal right femur and some ribs, a typical distribution.

tive finding usually indicates a patient who has received chemotherapy or radiotherapy previously. Focal loss of normal bone uptake may also be a feature of some bone metastases (Fig. 1.2).

Bone-imaging is undertaken 2–3 hours after the intravenous injection of 600 MBq (15 mCi) ^{99m}Tc methyldiphosphonate, MDP, or equivalent radiopharmaceutical. During the period before

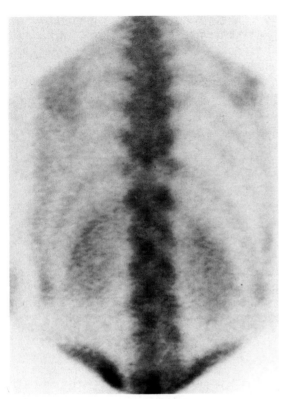

Fig. 1.2 Bone metastases from bronchial carcinoma. A posterior view of the thoraco-lumbar spine showing a focal defect in the eleventh thoracic vertebra. [67]Gallium scan was positive at this site, and bone biopsy confirmed metastasis.

region of the right shoulder as compared to the left in a right-handed patient and increased uptake in one or both sternoclavicular joints is often noted. These normal or common findings are not to be confused with metastatic disease. The lack of specificity means that a single focal area of increased uptake in a bone such as a vertebra or rib should not be considered as evidence of a metastasis and a local radiograph will usually help determine the nature of the lesion if it is due to a benign cause. In infants and children the epiphysiseal plates, the sites of bone growth, show high symmetrical uptake.

Bone imaging in specific cancers

Breast cancer

The incidence of a positive bone scan indicating metastasis at the time of presentation in stage I and stage II breast cancer is low, probably under 5%. When radical surgery to the breast was regularly undertaken, it was crucial to avoid such operations on anyone with a possibility of metastatic disease and therefore logical to undertake a bone scan before such surgery was contemplated in all patients with a clinical diagnosis of breast cancer. The less radical surgical approach and the lower incidence of bone metastases than previously thought has altered this rationale. It should be performed if there are symptoms referable to the axial skeleton, if there is locally advanced disease or if a 'base line' is required for follow-up purposes and prognosis. There is general agreement that a bone scan is essential in patients with stage III disease where the incidence of bone metastases is between 15 and 40%, and in stage IV disease (McKillop 1987).

A bone scan will typically be performed before commencing chemotherapy or undertaking local radiotherapy (Kunkler et al 1985). How frequently should the scan be repeated? Either an 'active' approach is pursued with regular bone scanning at six-monthly intervals, or a 'passive' approach is adopted with bone scanning being performed on some clinical indication, usually axial skeleton pain. The incidence of bone metastases is about five times greater in those scanned using a passive approach than an active one (Derimanov 1987) but

imaging the patient should be encouraged to have a high fluid intake since increased renal clearance of the ^{99m}Tc MDP improves bone image contrast. The bladder must be emptied before imaging starts in order to improve the view of the pubic bones and should be emptied again after the imaging has been completed to reduce the small gonadal radiation dose. Some workers advise giving 400 mg potassium perchlorate orally at the time of the injection to reduce thyroid and stomach uptake of any free ^{99m}Tc pertechnetate, but adequate radiopharmaceutical preparation and quality control should obviate the need for this.

The lack of specificity of the bone scan must be remembered. The simple bunion at the base of the big toe will show as a focal area of increased activity, as will the commonly found increased osteophytosis around the fifth lumbar vertebra, and osteoarthritis of the knee, hip and base of the thumb in the elderly. The increased uptake in the

the conversion rates of 2% to 10% per year in stage III suggest an active approach is appropriate if early treatment is to be instituted. The average time for appearance of bone metastases in a stage II patient who goes on to develop them is 51 months, and in stage III, 32 months (Derimanov 1987). The typical sites are the vertebral column and pelvis. Due to the limitation of the field of view of the gamma camera the arms and hands are often omitted on a routine whole body bone scan and so a particular request should be made if the upper limbs are thought to be involved.

The assessment of the effects of therapy may be undertaken by serial bone scanning at three-monthly intervals provided that certain pre-cautions in interpretation are taken. In the first three months after instituting effective therapy for bone metastases the 'flare' phenomenon may sometimes be seen where the scan shows more active uptake at the sites of known metastases and additionally small 'new' metastases may appear due to their increased metabolic activity in response to effective treatment. Such a finding should not be interpreted as progression of disease, and many avoid performing the next bone scan until at least four months after starting therapy. Loss of previously demonstrated metastases may be taken as a sign of regression but reduction in activity of known metastases, even after allowing for different photographic settings, is a less reliable indicator of response. Many semiquantitative approaches have been tried but none has been found reliable in practice because of the variability of the biological response to treatment.

Genito-urinary cancer

Prostatic cancer has so frequently metastasized to bone at presentation (5% in stage I, 10% in stage II and 20% in stage III) that a bone scan is indicated on diagnosis, and regular follow-up at three to six-monthly intervals during chemotherapy or hormonal treatment is usual. The so-called 'super scan' is where there is a high bone uptake with a rather uniform appearance which may occur due to wide involvement of the vertebral column, but usually small asymmetries in uptake, particularly in the ribs, point to the diagnosis of prostatic metastases rather than active metabolic bone dis-ease. Bladder and renal abnormalities are frequently demonstrated but should not be over-interpreted (Mlodkowska et al 1985). In particular, 'hot spots' in calyces, minor pelvic retention and minor differences in relative uptake should be ignored, but clear severe pelvic retention or hydroureter should be further investigated. The absence of part of one kidney may be due to renal tumour. Bone scanning is more sensitive than the serum acid or alkaline phosphatase measurement in demonstrating bone involvement (Merrick et al 1985). A negative bone scan in patients at presen-tation and particularly a negative bone scan at two years are good prognostic signs; the conversion rate is approximately 10% per year. A bone scan should also be performed in patients demonstrated to have renal cancer since the incidence of skeletal involvement is high. However, in uterine, cervical, testicular and ovarian cancers bone scanning should not be routinely undertaken.

Lung cancer

Since the surgical treatment of primary lung can-cer is a major procedure, the bone scan is required in the initial evaluation. In this way the 5–20% of patients who will have bone metastases will be demonstrated and surgery can be avoided (McNeil et al 1977). An 'active' follow-up is not usually undertaken and the 'passive' approach is usual. A positive bone scan is associated with a significantly reduced survival (Merrick & Merrick 1986). The peri-osteal reaction of hypertrophic pulmonary os-teoarthropathy, in forearms and legs, shows up dramatically on the bone scan and should not be misinterpreted.

Primary bone tumours

Primary osteosarcoma gives the typical 'inverted fir tree' appearance of high uptake at the expanded end of a long bone, and demonstrates the extent of the disease (Fig. 1.3). However, increased activity in the involved and related bones as com-pared to the contralateral side are evidence of generally increased vascularity 'in sympathy' and should not be taken to indicate extension of the tumour. A bone scan is useful in the assessment of the extent of the tumour and in detecting

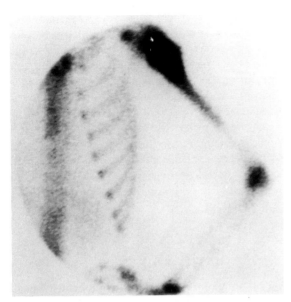

Fig. 1.3 Primary osteosarcoma of the humerus. An anterior view of the left upper chest and humerus showing an area of uniform and intense uptake in the head and proximal shaft extending outside the line of the normal bone, a typical distribution. Note the 'active' elbow joint 'in sympathy'.

synchronous or metastatic tumours. Although there are case reports of chest metastases being seen only on the bone scan and not on the chest X-ray, this is rare. Chondrosarcoma in a long bone typically gives a rather irregular pattern with local soft tissue activity, focal areas of increased uptake and focal defects (McLean & Murray 1984). The bone scan cannot be used to decide whether a lesion is benign or malignant, but high and/or irregularly increased uptake and increased vascularity are features more typical of malignant disease.

Paget's disease may provide difficulties in the presence of multiple metastases, but the characteristic uniformity of the hemipelvis, or long bone involvement and the 'trilobed' appearance of the vertebra with Paget's disease involving the spine as well (unusual for metastases), should help in the differentiation.

Bone imaging in other tumours

Neuroblastoma, primary and soft tissue metastases will often take up the bone imaging agent as well as bone metastases. Local involvement of bone may be demonstrable in the context of malignant tumours of the head and neck, particularly those of the eye, the maxillary sinus and the parotid. SPECT may be very useful in this context. Focally increased uptake local to the site is characteristic of meningioma and may demonstrate more widespread involvement than the skull X-ray. No help is given, however, in the evaluation of pituitary adenoma. In parenthesis it should be noted that many vascular or calcifying cerebral tumours and recent cerebral infarcts take up the bone imaging agents. Bone scanning should be performed in thyroid cancer in conjunction with ^{131}I surveys.

In conclusion, bone imaging is an essential service for the management of many cancer patients, having a higher sensitivity but lower specificity in the detection of metastases, and being cheaper and giving a lower radiation dose than conventional skeletal radiology.

ADRENAL CORTICAL IMAGING

The adrenal cortex is functionally at least two organs: the outer cortex producing the minerocorticoid aldosterone and the inner cortex producing the glucocorticoid cortisol.

Primary hyperaldosteronism is associated with Conn's syndrome of hypertension and hypokalaemia and may be due to hyperplasia, which may be micronodular, macronodular or adenoma. Adenocarcinoma is very rare. The prime reason for imaging is to lateralize the adenoma once the clinical, biochemical and endocrinological diagnosis has been confirmed. Using ^{75}Se selenocholesterol, the findings in a unilateral adenoma are an increased uptake than normal in the gland with adenoma and a normal uptake in the contralateral gland (normal range 0.07–0.3% of the injected dose). In bilateral macronodular hyperplasia, uptake in both glands is increased above normal but some overlap with the normal range may occur (Shapiro et al 1981).

A quantitative approach is essential since adrenal depth varies from person to person and on each side so a planar image may cause a false interpretation whereby a gland closer to the skin surface may be mistaken for a gland that has increased uptake. Adrenal depth is therefore determined approximately from true lateral images of a prior ^{99m}Tc DTPA renal study (Britton et al 1979a), then 10 MBq (250 μCi) of ^{75}Se seleno-cholesterol are injected and imaging is carried out 7 and 14 days later. The correction factor for attenuation at different depths determined from a phantom study is used to obtain the true count rate from the adrenal. The adrenal count rate is also corrected for tissue background activity using a circumferential background region of interest and the uptake is expressed as a percentage of the activity administered (Hawkins et al 1980).

When ^{131}I norcholesterol is used some authorities recommend dexamethasone suppression, so that only aldosteronomas are seen (Seabold et al 1976). However, a normal result is no image at all and early imaging at 3–4 days is necessary since 'dexamethasone escape' occurs at about 5 days. At these early stages, tissue background, liver, biliary and gut uptake are high, making for difficulties in interpretation. The combination of X-ray CT and ^{75}Se selenocholesterol imaging should make the diagnosis of a functioning aldosteronoma in the majority of cases, thereby avoiding the need for the potentially difficult and traumatic technique of adrenal venous sampling.

Many hypertensive patients are now having X-ray CT of the adrenals and an enlargement may be shown. It is essential to use a functional technique to demonstrate that such masses are functionally significant through adrenal radionuclide imaging (radiolabelled cholesterol and radio-iodine-labelled *meta*-iodobenzyl guanidine (MIBG) before invasive investigations or surgery are contemplated.

Secondary hyperaldosteronism and Barrter's syndrome usually show bilaterally increased adrenocortical uptake.

In confirmed Cushing's syndrome due to adenoma, the production of cortisol suppresses pituitary adrenocorticotrophic hormone, ACTH, so that the normal adrenal is *not* visualized. The adenoma has high uptake and is easily lateralized. In bilateral hyperplasia one or both adrenals have uptake which is above the normal range and usually asymmetrical. The visualization of both adrenals indicates hyperplasia even if uptake on one side is not increased. The cause of hyperplasia, a pituitary adenoma or ectopic ACTH production, cannot be determined. After the previous practice of bilateral subtotal adrenalectomy, the adrenal remnant grows under continued ACTH stimulation and can be lateralized and demonstrated to be the cause of recurrent Cushing's syndrome in such patients using ^{75}Se selenocholesterol. Adrenal cortical carcinoma, however, even when producing excess glucocorticoids does not usually take up ^{75}Se selenocholesterol. Congenital adrenal hyperplasia causes markedly increased uptake by both glands.

HYPERPARATHYROIDISM

The first requirement is a combined clinical, biochemical and endocrinological diagnosis of hyperparathyroidism. The difficulties in demonstrating adenoma or hyperplasia before surgery are well known. Thallium ^{201}Tl is the latest non-specific radiopharmaceutical to be used for localization of adenoma based on its increased uptake at sites of increased flow and metabolism. Since it is also taken up by thyroid tissue and particularly by thyroid adenoma, care must be exercized in interpreting the results of imaging and of any subtraction technique. Normal parathyroids are not seen, hyperplastic glands are identified in about 50% and adenoma in about 85% of cases. The smallest adenomas detectable are generally over 400 mg, and benign and malignant tumours are not distinguishable (Young et al 1983, Gimlette & Taylor 1985, Gimlette et al 1986, Blake et al 1986).

The subtraction technique used at St Bartholomew's Hospital is given in Appendix 1 (page 456).

THE PANCREAS

The pancreas is well visualized using ^{75}Se selenomethionine (SM) when a composite liver pancreas scan has a conventional liver colloid scan subtracted from it (Kaplan et al 1966).

The problem of tumour identification is that one

is seeking a defect of uptake in an organ whose normal variation in position and thickness makes interpretation difficult (Cotton et al 1978). If a pancreatic tumour is found using X-ray CT or ultrasound, the SM scan will show the extent of normally functioning tissue: the more normal the image, the more likely the tumour operability. After a Whipples operation, an SM scan will show if the pancreatic remnant is functioning.

THE RETICULO-ENDOTHELIAL SYSTEM

Liver, spleen and bone marrow

Imaging of deposits in the liver, spleen and bone marrow is undertaken using the phagocyte properties of the cells of the reticulo-endothelial system in these organs. For the conventional liver colloid scan, ^{99m}Tc-labelled tin colloid with a particle size of 2–4 microns is used which is appropriate for the Kupffer cells. At least four views are taken: anterior with a costal margin flexible lead strip marker; anterior, right lateral and posterior views with additional views; right posterior oblique, standing and supine views; left lateral and left posterior oblique for the spleen where appropriate. SPECT increases the accuracy of detection of small deep deposits (Khan et al 1981, Brendal et al 1984). The presence of a metastasis is demonstrated by a focal defect or defects in one or more views at sites away from regions of high normal variation: the gall bladder fossa, the porta hepatis and the exit of the hepatic veins superiorly (Lunia et al 1975). Well circumscribed defects are typical of gastro-intestinal metastases, including carcinoid, whereas those from breast or lung tend to be smaller with less distinct margins (Sears et al 1975). Focal defects in the liver scan are not specific as to aetiology, for an area of decreased or absent Kupffer cell function has many causes including cyst, abscess, congenital abnormalities and areas of liver necrosis or fibrous replacement in hepatitis or cirrhosis, and its routine use in the evaluation of possible metastases has given way to ultrasound which is more specific. However, ultrasound may miss liver metastases in some circumstances particularly when air in the bowel

or lung prevents an adequate view, or if the lesion is isoechoic. In colorectal and stomach cancer a combined use of ultrasound and the liver colloid scan has been recommended to maximize tumour detection (Taylor et al 1977, Clarke et al 1986).

The liver colloid scan has been modified to attempt the early detection of gastro-intestinal metastases in the following way. Liver metastases derive their blood supply almost exclusively from the hepatic artery and it has been demonstrated by Leveson et al (1983) that the hepatic to total liver blood flow ratio increases with such metastases before focal defects are detectable. Since an intravenous bolus arrives about five seconds before that travelling to and returning from the gut and spleen by the portal vein, the hepatic artery contribution can be obtained by careful analysis of the early part of the activity–time curve from a region of interest over the liver. The choice of the region of interest is performed retrospectively after viewing all the dynamic images so that areas of overlap with lung, kidney and spleen are excluded. A typical arterial curve is obtained from a region of interest over the left kidney where it is free of overlap from the spleen and a typical portal venous curve is obtained from the spleen. These curves are used to help define the time limits of the arterial and portal venous phases of the hepatic activity–time curve, in techniques developed by different authors (Fleming et al 1981, Wraight et al 1982). The normal hepatic artery to total liver blood flow ratio as a percentage is less than 30%. Definite metastases are present when the percentage exceeds 45% with a borderline range below this. 50% of patients with colorectal cancer with a value over 45% with normal liver colloid scan and liver ultrasound at that time developed overt liver metastases within six months of follow-up (Gough et al 1985).

Hepatoma shows a vascular blush during dynamic scintigraphy followed by a defect in the colloid scan. This may be contrasted with the increased uptake of ^{67}Ga gallium citrate scan in hepatoma, but many liver metastases also take up gallium. Neither the liver scan nor the spleen scan are reliable in determining involvement of these organs in Hodgkin's disease (Lipton et al 1972, Silverman et al 1972, Ell et al 1975). Spleen scanning with denatured labelled red cells is only required when looking for splenunculi.

^{67}Ga gallium

^{67}Ga gallium citrate scanning has a long track record of use in lymphoma (Hoffer 1978), but has never been sufficiently specific nor reliable to come into routine use. Whole body imaging at the time of staging of Hodgkin's disease will show focally increased uptake only in a percentage of the involved nodes present. The demonstration of uptake in previously normal nodes on follow-up indicates progression. Use of the whole body longitudinal section scanner or SPECT with coronal sections is advantageous for the reliable demonstration of para-aortic nodes, particularly under the left lobe of the liver which normally takes up gallium (Turner et al 1978). This technique also aids the interpretation of abdominal images since gallium is excreted by the large bowel. ^{67}Ga with ultrasound may have a rôle prior to staging laparotomy (White et al 1984). ^{111}In bleomycin which is not bowel-excreted had a brief vogue as an alternative agent. In the chest, focal uptake of ^{67}Ga in the mediastinum may help to elucidate the nature of a mediastinal mass, for example in distinguishing recurrence from post-therapy fibrosis, but it cannot differentiate between a soft tissue metastasis, an involved lymph node or a site of infection. A negative gallium scan does not exclude active disease. Use of high dose ^{67}Ga is advocated by some to overcome the inherent disadvantages of ^{67}Ga as an imaging agent (Anderson et al 1983). ^{67}Ga is no longer routinely used in oncology and is only applicable in a highly selected lymphoma population. Imaging of lymphoma by radio-immunoscintigraphy using lymphoma specific monoclonal antibodies is under development (see subsequent section).

Bone marrow imaging is being used more frequently due to the introduction of ^{99m}Tc-labelled nanocolloids. This provides a method of demonstrating bone scan negative metastases as focal defects in the marrow distribution in the skull, vertebral column, ribs and pelvis. In this way previously undetected metastases from carcinoma of the breast and lung are being revealed. The technique is not specific since fat infiltration and non-malignant conditions will cause defects. Marrow imaging also has a rôle in patients with therapy-induced bone marrow suppression to determine the presence of islets of functioning marrow from which recovery can occur.

Lymphoscintigraphy

Conventional lymphoscintigraphy relies on the uptake of an appropriate radiolabelled colloid injected subcutaneously into a region of skin drained by the lymph node group under evaluation. Visual evidence of uptake by the nodes is taken to indicate their normality and filling defects or lack of uptake to indicate involvement. Although it may be appreciated that in principle it is neither a very sensitive nor a very specific technique because lack of visualization may be due to absence of a normal node, previous damage to a node or non-malignant as well as malignant infiltration, nevertheless it has benefit in certain defined contexts where it is more accurate than clinical examination or biopsy studies. Most work has been done in visualizing lymph node involvement in the internal mammary chain and axillary group in patients with breast cancer, where it has been of value in staging the disease (Ege 1980, Osborne et al 1983, Ege & Clark 1985, Mazzeo et al 1986). The detection of metastatic involvement of the axillary nodes in breast cancer is of great prognostic importance (Fisher et al 1983). Clinical examination of the axillary nodes is prone to error in the assessment of the presence or absence of metastases: 38% of nodes with metastases were clinically negative and 37% of nodes without metastases were called clinically positive in one study (Cutler et al 1970). In another study axillary node biopsy showed that due to sampling error 42% of nodes with metastases were biopsy negative, and that only 24% of nodes with metastases were correctly identified (Davies et al 1980). The technique is of some benefit in evaluating the internal iliac chain after peri-anal injection of colloid in patients with seminoma (Kaplan 1983) but has not found favour in the routine evaluation of other pelvic malignant disease, or melanoma.

Technique and results

The size of the colloid particles used for lympho-scintigraphy ranges from 10–50 nm (Lennart et al 1983). Most work has been performed using ^{99m}Tc antimony sulphide colloid which replaced ^{198}Au gold colloid. More recently ^{99m}Tc rhenium sulphide colloid and ^{99m}Tc nanocolloidal albumin which are more stable and more rapidly diffusible have been used. For the internal mammary chain single sub-xiphisternal or bilateral subcostal injections each of 20 MBq (500 uCi) in less than 0.3 ml colloid are given directly into the posterior rectus sheath at the insertion of the diaphragm (Ege 1983). For the axillary nodes a sub-areolar injection for each breast is used (Mazzeo et al 1986). Images are obtained with a gamma camera placed over the appropriate region at 40–60 min for the axillary group using nanocolloidal albumin and at 2.5–3 h for the internal mammary chain using antimony sulphide colloid.

Injection technique is important and at least one node needs to be visualized to confirm this. For the intercostal chain, the ipsilateral side to the tumour is injected first and imaged at 3 h and if the result is difficult to interpret, the contralateral side is injected and imaging repeated 3 h later. For axillary nodes both breasts are injected within a minute. Interpretation of both techniques depends on demonstrating symmetry or acceptable asymmetry of uptake for normality and unacceptable asymmetry or absence of uptake for an abnormal result. A recent study of axillary node lymphoscintigraphy showed a remarkable sensitivity of 80% and a specificity of 100% when compared with the subsequent histological findings (Mazzeo et al 1986). Ege (1980) showed in a group of 243 women that a normal internal mammary study was associated with a 34% overall incidence of recurrence of breast cancer whereas a positive study was associated with a 67% recurrence rate indicating a value in prognosis.

Dosimetry is of the order of 27 mGy/MBq (100 rads/mCi) for the rectus sheath injection site (Brunskill 1983) and this local absorbed dose is an important concern and the limiting factor when perlymphatic unsealed source radiotherapy is attempted at whatever site.

Radio-immunolymphoscintigraphy should show sites of positive lymph node involvement directly where conventional scintigraphy shows no node, provided that lymphatic obstruction does not prevent access. This technique is under evaluation at present in breast cancer (Pateisky et al 1985) and after intra-operative injection in cervical cancer (Gitsch et al 1984). This approach using a peri-anal or per-rectal mucosal injection may be rewarding in staging the internal iliopelvic chain of lymph nodes in pelvic cancers in the future.

CEREBRAL TUMOURS

Conventional ^{99m}Tc pertechnetate or diethylene triamine penta-acetate (DTPA) brain imaging is an accurate way of excluding primary brain tumours and metastases (Boucher & Sears 1980) and has a rôle in evaluating such patients in centres without X-ray CT facilities. It is not cost-effective to screen patients with cancer for brain metastases by imaging and should be done only when there are specific neurological symptoms or signs. Occasionally the confused, agitated patient may be more easily assessed by radionuclide imaging than by X-ray CT since it is easier to restrain the patient.

SPECT increases the sensitivity of the technique, can distinguish tumours with cystic changes from those without, and may help in pituitary tumours (Britton and Shapiro 1981). Small vascular meningiomas take up ^{201}Tl thallium avidly and this may occasionally aid their identification (Ancri et al 1978).

^{99m}Tc hexamethyl propylene amine oxime (HMPAO) rapidly crosses the blood brain barrier and here tumours show as defects in uptake against the distribution of this agent in the grey matter on SPECT. However, if such tumours are initiating epileptic episodes, focally increased uptake is seen during an attack.

Undifferentiated tumours are usually more aggressive and more metabolically active than differentiated tumours: the glycolytic pathway in particular is active. Work with a positron-emitting radionuclide-labelled glucose derivative ^{18}F fluorodeoxyglucose (FDG) can demonstrate such tumours. Brain tumours have been graded in malignancy by the degree of uptake of FDG (Di Chiro et al 1984). An alternative approach is the use of ^{11}C methionine, where the greater the degree of amino acid uptake, the more malignant is the tumour (Muller et al 1986). ^{11}C methionine is also able to demonstrate whether a lesion seen on X-ray CT or magnetic resonance imaging (MRI) post-radiotherapy for a primary or metastatic brain tumour is due to viable tumour or just post-therapy gliosis (La France et al 1986).

RENAL TUMOURS

If a patient presents with haematuria, finding the location of a tumour is not the province of nuclear medicine, but the question of how much renal function the patient will lose through nephrectomy can only be answered by a renal radionuclide study. The contribution of each kidney to total uptake is measured during a ^{99m}Tc DTPA study. 400 MBq (10mCi) is injected intravenously into a well-hydrated patient reclining back against the gamma camera. Serial images are made while the data is also fed on-line to the computer for analysis. The relative uptake by each kidney is measured after allowing 90 s for mixing and during the time before any activity first leaves a kidney – normally 2–5 min. During the first 30 s a vascular tumour site may show a blush of activity which may persist for a short time followed by a defect in the parenchymal distribution of uptake (O'Reilly et al 1986). The technique is not very reliable in distinguising benign from malignant space-occupying lesions.

Obstructive nephropathy, as may occur with a ureteric tumour, may be demonstrated by the prolongation of the transit of ^{99m}Tc DTPA through the parenchyma due to the resistance to outflow. This is measured as the parenchymal transit time index, PTTI (Britton et al 1979b). The response to frusemide may also be helpful (O'Reilly et al 1986, Britton et al 1987).

In children ^{99m}Tc dimercapto succinate (DMSA) is preferred since the image is taken three hours after the injection and can be repeated if the child moves. Any space-occupying lesion, scar or infarct will cause a defect. In adults, uptake of DMSA will demonstrate a pseudotumour which has caused calyceal distortion on the intravenous urogram (Corty et al 1975, O'Reilly et al 1986).

RADIO-IMMUNOSCINTIGRAPHY

Radio-immunoscintigraphy is the name given to the technique of imaging using radionuclide-labelled antibodies. This approach has been mainly applied to the demonstration of malignant disease but it has other uses, for example, in the demonstration of acute myocardial infarction with an ^{111}In indium-labelled antimyosin monoclonal antibody fragment.

Four factors are required for radio-immuno-scintigraphy: an antibody as specific as possible for a cell surface antigen of the cancer; a radiolabel to give the best signal with a halflife appropriate to the kinetics of antibody uptake by the tumour; a radiolabelling method with the necessary quality control to give a reagent suitable for human use while maintaining the full immunoreactivity of the antibody; and an imaging system optimized for the detection of the radionuclide and suitable for the region under study. For radioimmunotherapy there are two additional requirements: an estimate of the therapeutic ratio of uptake by the target to that of the most critical non-target organ; and an estimate of the absorbed dose delivered to the tumour, to the critical non-target organ, to the bone marrow and to the whole body.

Three different approaches to the development of antibodies for labelling have been made. They are to develop antibodies against circulating components, against surface components present in cancer cells, and against normal cell components which are hidden or remote from blood. The disadvantage of using circulating components such as carcinoembryonic antigen (CEA) and human choriogonadotrophin (HCG) is that, in addition to their low specificity, some part of any injected antibody may be taken up in the blood and prevented from reaching the tumour. The possibility of reactions to immune complex formation arises. The antigen, therefore, should preferably be fixed to the cell surface and be an integral part of that surface – the second approach. However, such cancer-specific antigens are not known and there is the possibility that they might be lost if there were de-differentiation of the tumour. The third approach is to use an antigen that is a constituent of the normal cell, but one that is not normally exposed to blood – for example, a component of an epithelial surface lining. Only with the excessive growth and the architectural disruption that characterize malignant change would such an epithelial surface antigen be exposed in quantity to blood and therefore be able to take up the labelled antibody.

The production of antibody has undergone a revolution which has made progress in this field rapid. The conventional method of production is to inject an extract of tissue containing the antigen into an appropriate animal and by repeating this injection, for example at weekly intervals, to boost the immune response. This response consists of the production of stimulated lymphocytes and a whole range of antibodies varying in immunoglobulin class, avidity and specificity. Such a mixture of antibodies is termed 'polyclonal' as it comes from a variety of immune cells.

Kohler & Milstein (1975) demonstrated a technique for isolating and culturing individual immune cells produced in such a response so that each cell becomes the head of a family, or clone, of similar offspring. Normally such a clone would reproduce but die out soon. The trick was to impart immortality to such immune cells through their fusion with a line of myeloma cells from the same animal, initially the mouse. The hybridoma cell resulting from the fusion of the myeloma and the immune cells was shown to produce one particular antibody of one class and one specificity, called a 'monoclonal' antibody. Then, by a process of screening and selection, the clone producing the most suitable monoclonal antibody in terms of avidity or specificity is selected and cultured. The result is a continuous production of a single species of antibody of homogenous quality and definable characteristics in potentially unlimited amounts. The search is on for monoclonal antibodies with the specificity and avidity required for individual cancer detection.

In order to demonstrate the localization of the antibody in vivo, an appropriate radioactive label is required. The choice of label depends on the physical properties of available radionuclides and their suitability for labelling antibodies. A disadvantage of ^{131}I is that it produces beta rays responsible for 80% of the radiation attributable to this radionuclide. The long halflife of eight days also means that only a relatively small amount of activity can be given, since the radiation dose is related to the product of the activity given and the halflife. The high energy penetrates the thin crystal of the modern gamma camera and so the efficiency of count collection is poor. However, the ready availability, cheapness and ease of labelling with ^{131}I used to commend it as the label with which new studies are commenced. On the other hand, ^{123}I has an energy level ideal for the gamma camera, while its short halflife allows a count rate which is about 100 times that of ^{131}I for the same administered radioactivity. Its availability in Europe, however, is limited to twice weekly and in lower concentrations than ^{131}I. It is also costly. For labelling, added carrier-stable iodine is necessary to push the reaction to completion, and so synthesis of the labelled antibody is a little more difficult than with ^{131}I. The labelling of antibody with iodine has been a standard procedure for decades, and ^{125}I-labelled antibody is the cornerstone of the in vitro radio-immunoassay procedures for the measurement of hormones. The chloramine T and iodogen techniques are the most frequently used, the latter being the milder of the two methods. The essential requirement is to label the antibody at a site far away from the active centre so as not to affect its immunospecificity. To this end, a 1:1 iodine:antibody molar ratio is recommended.

The use of iodine-labelled antibody has some disadvantages. The patient must be loaded with stable iodine, usually in the form of potassium iodide 60 mg b.d. from the day before and for three days after the study with ^{123}I and for two weeks after with ^{131}I. The in vivo metabolism of iodine-labelled antibody is relatively rapid, and about 20% free iodine is liberated in 24 h. However, it is evident from animal studies that the iodine label attached to antibody bound to tumour does not become detached and it is the unbound labelled antibody that is metabolized. Thus it does matter whether the iodine is bound or free in blood or tissues other than the cancer, as it all contributes to the background 'noise' against which the signal from the cancer target is to be determined.

The energy of ^{111}In is well suited to the gamma camera fitted with a medium energy collimator. Its longer halflife gives it commercial potential in its distribution and allows imaging over a few days. The labelling procedure requires the use of bifunctional chelate, one end of which binds the indium while the other binds the protein. The cyclic anhydride diethylene triamine penta-acetate (DTPA) is a satisfactory chelate for this purpose (Hnatowich et al 1983). Antibody labelled with ^{111}In is less rapidly metabolized in the body – about 5% per 24 h – than radio-iodine-labelled antibody. However, a higher than expected liver uptake of the ^{111}In-labelled antibody may be seen, and ^{111}In-labelled antibody fragments (Fab[1])$_2$ are trapped in the kidney with ^{111}In retained in the tubules, unlike [123]I (Fab[1])$_2$ fragments which are metabolized with the iodine released into the urine.

Technetium ^{99m}Tc appeared to have two major disadvantages. It was particularly difficult to label biologically active proteins so that they remained stable in vivo for 24 h, and its short halflife of six hours was thought to mean that too little activity was present at the time of maximum antibody uptake, which is between 12 and 24 h, but its use in labelling anti-melanoma antibody (Fab[1])$_2$ fragments has been successful and clinically efficacious (Siccardi et al 1986) (Fig. 1.4). The Schwarz technique has now solved the problem of labelling antibodies with ^{99m}Tc in a manner that is stable in vivo.

The key requirements for the monoclonal antibody are specificity and avidity. The higher the specificity, the more labelled antibody will be on the tumour, provided that there are sufficient antigenic sites available, and – conversely – the lower the non-target background will be. Even more important is the avidity of the antibody, not only in terms of its initial binding strength to the surface antigen but in its staying power when attached to the antigen. An adequate residence time is essential if delayed imaging is to be undertaken.

There are two imaging strategies for radio-immunoscintigraphy. The first is to image early, at a time of maximum uptake of the labelled antibody, which is between 4 and 24 h, using a short halflife, high count rate radionuclide label to give maximum sensitivity. However, the higher

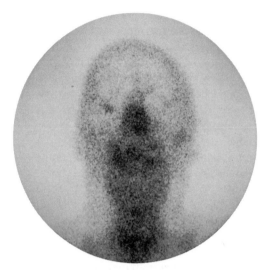

Fig. 1.4 Ocular melanoma. Radio-immunoscintigraphy of the anterior skull at six hours after injection of ^{99m}Tc-labelled (Fab[1])$_2$ fragment of a monoclonal antibody against a high molecular weight melonoma antigen. Focal uptake in the right eye is evident at the site of melanoma confirmed surgically. (Courtesy Dr J. Bomanji)

normal tissue activity may require correction using a background subtraction or target enhancement technique. This used to be performed by injecting a blood pool agent and subtracting its distribution from that of the labelled antibody (Goldenberg et al 1980). There are major theoretical and practical problems attributable to the different gamma ray energies of the blood background agent (for example, ^{99m}Tc) and the antibody label (for example, ^{131}I) (Ott et al 1983). An alternative approach is to subtract an early static image, taken perhaps at 10 min, from later images, such as 4 and 24 h. This requires accurate patient and image repositioning techniques and the use of change detection algorithms to recognize and test for significant differences between the early, mainly blood pool image and the late image which contains the sites of uptake of the labelled antibody (Granowska et al 1983). The alternative is to use SPECT to separate target uptake from other tissues. The second approach is to image late, using a longer-lived radionuclide such as [131]I. Since labelled antibody fixed to the tumour keeps up its signal strength while the other tissue and blood background noise is falling away due to metabolism and loss with time, the target to non-target ratio improves with time after peak uptake. However, the total count rate with ^{131}I is relatively low, and so statistical noise may obscure the image. The first approach, using ^{99m}Tc, ^{123}I or ^{111}In, is gaining favour because 'counts count in nuclear medicine'. More than half the 'noise' in an image is due to the signal: the lower the count rate, the disproportionately higher the noise due to the square root relationship between the two (Britton & Granowska 1987).

An example of the radiolabelling of a monoclonal antibody, the imaging technique and the results is given with reference to the imaging of ovarian cancer and its metastases (Granowska et al 1984, 1986). Human milk fat globule (HMFG) is a large molecular weight glycoprotein found in the epithelial surface lining of the breast. It is also present in the crypts of the colon and the internal surface lining of ovarian follicles, thus it is not normally exposed to blood. The antigen was first determined by injecting delipidated human milk into a mouse. For the hybridoma technique, a mouse cell line called NSI is fused with the spleen cells of a mouse which has previously received an initial injection of delipidated human milk followed by a tissue culture of normal milk epithelial cells. The resulting lymphocyte hybrids are cultured and the clone giving the antibody with highest specificity and avidity selected by screening. Its antibody to HMFG is highly purified to free it of other protein and any potential viral contamination resulting in a homogenous immunoglobulin, class IgG1, for labelling.

The iodogen technique is used for labelling. Iodogen tubes are prepared by dissolving iodogen in dichloromethane to make iodogen solution, which is evaporated to dryness at 37°C in sterile polypropylene tubes. Iodogen reagent is then-coated on the inside of the tube, which can be stored at 5°C for six months without loss of reactivity. Synthesis of ^{123}I HMFG occurs by mixing 10 mCi pure ^{123}I, the antibody (0.5 mg in 1 ml 10^{-5} mol/l citrate buffer pH 6) and potassium iodide (4×10^{-4} mol/l solution), in that order, in the iodogen tube. The pH is adjusted to 8.5 and the mixture left at room temperature for 10 min with gentle shaking. The mixture is decanted onto a Sephadex G50 filtration column in a 20 ml syringe prewashed with 1% human serum albumin in phosphate buffered saline. The eluate is collected in 1 ml fractions and their activities determined. The active fraction is sterilized using a micropore filter.

After prior skin testing has been shown to be negative, 80–120 MBq (2–3 mCi) ^{123}I HMFG is injected intravenously with the patient supine under the gamma camera, which is positioned anteriorly over the lower abdomen and pelvis. Dynamic studies are recorded directly into the computer for the first 10 min, 4 h and 24 h, anteriorly and posteriorly of the whole of the abdomen, together with scans of three markers on bony landmarks. These are required for the patient repositioning and computer aided repositioning of the static images, later to be superimposed for proportional background subtraction and target enhancement, using change detection algorithms if necessary (Granowska et al 1987). On many occasions the images on the standard transparent films are sufficient. The patient goes for surgery following a 22 h scan and the tumour and/or metastases are excised. Between 2 and 3% of the injected activity is usually found in the tumour mass (Fig. 1.5).

The technique of radio-immunoscintigraphy of malignancies is developing rapidly. Over 15 malignancies and their metastases can be imaged by means of this technique, including melanoma, neuroblastoma, and colonic, ovarian and thyroid carcinoma – and with less reliability, malignant breast and lung lesions and glioma. The sensitivity of radio-immunoscintigraphy in ovarian and colorectal cancers and melanoma is between 75% and 95% but with lower specificities at present. The crucial requirement when introducing a new technique of imaging is to define the clinical circumstances under which it should be able to contribute to clinical management if successful: relevant diagnostic tests are those whose results alter clinical management. However, many diagnostic tests are undertaken in relation to a particular clinical problem and this strict criterion of a successful test is yet to be met by radio-immunoscintigraphy.

The tumour specificity and avidity of currently available monoclonal antibodies is still much less than optimal. Until these qualities are improved, their adoption for routine diagnostic imaging and the promising work on their targeting of

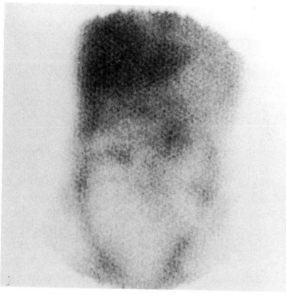 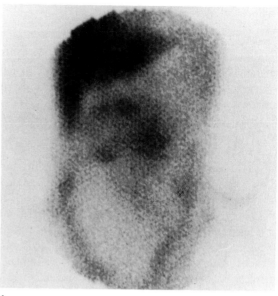

a   b

Fig. 1.5 Abdominal recurrences of ovarian cancer. Radio-immunoscintigraphy with ^{111}In indium-labelled whole monoclonal antibody HMFG2 against human milk fat globule protein. (a) Anterior abdominal image at 22 h. (b) Anterior abdominal image at 76 h. Both show multiple focal areas of increased uptake in the upper abdomen confirmed at second look laparotomy. Note the relatively increased tumour, bowel and liver uptake on the later image. (Courtesy Dr M. Granowska)

therapeutic doses of radionuclides or immuno-toxins to cancers will be retarded. Nevertheless, the work is in its early stages and when the results of prospective studies already underway are available with existing antibodies, the present clinical indications will be better defined. However, a number of generalizations about the technique in the management of malignant disease may be made.

1. The technique is not designed to be applicable as a screening test of well people for cancer. The lack of specificity of the currently available antibodies, the need to administer radioactivity and a compound which is immunogenic mitigate against this.

2. The technique might have a rôle in the evaluation of patients picked up as a result of a screening procedure such as confirmation of breast cancer after mammography or confirmation that a pelvic mass found by ultrasonography is malignant. However, present antibodies are insufficiently specific.

3. The technique might have a rôle in imaging patients in whom serum analysis has shown tumour associated markers by using a radio-labelled antibody to the same marker. This approach has potential but it is yet to be demonstrated that it would be more effective than conventional radiology, ultrasound or X-ray CT in this context. It is also recognized that tumour markers may not appear in the patient's serum even when there is positive uptake of the radiolabelled antibody by the tumour. Present circulating tumour markers are also not cancer specific.

4. The technique has a rôle in primary staging of known cancer, e.g. biopsy positive colonic carcinoma, as the specificity of uptake is not such a problem since the diagnosis of cancer is made. The high sensitivity of radio-immunoscintigraphy is then of benefit with the potential to show uptake in lymph nodes and liver metastases as examples. For this, computer analysis of the data using serial or other subtraction techniques, kinetic analysis or SPECT may be essential to demonstrate a negative whereas transparent film images may be sufficient to show a positive.

5. The prime rôle for radio-immunoscinti-graphy is in the re-evaluation of the patient after primary cancer surgery and/or chemotherapy. Is the mass in the pelvis fibrosis due to previous surgery or a tumour recurrence? Labelled monoclonal antibody should be able to distinguish between these two. This information is essential to the management of abdominal and head and neck tumours. Has the chemotherapy been successful or can a second look operation be avoided? Again these are crucial management decisions in patients with genito-urinary and gastro-intestinal tumours and lymphomata which should be answerable by this technique with computer analysis of the data as above.

6. The technique has a rôle in screening for unsuspected metastases, for example, recurrences in bone marrow in patients with previous cancer who have completed their treatment.

7. The technique has a rôle in assessing the feasibility of intraperitoneal, intrapleural, intrapericardial or endolymphatic therapy with monoclonal antibody either radioactively labelled, e.g. with ^{131}I, [114m]In or an alpha particle emitter, or with an immunotoxin.

In conclusion, the promise of radio-immuno-localization of cancer is clear. Benefits will come from careful selection of clinical indications wherein the patient management will be affected by the results of study.

RECEPTOR-RELATED IMAGING

A characteristic of all cells is the presence of surface receptors specific to a range of biologically important compounds including hormones and transmitter substances, but different tissues contain different selections of receptors. Such receptors are present in differentiated malignant tissues to differing degrees and may influence treatment, for example, the oestrogen receptors. Although not at all specific to malignant tissue, they can be used to demonstrate the presence of malignant tissue in a site remote from its origin, that is in a tissue not possessing such a receptor. In benign tumours and well differentiated malignant tumours, an increase in receptor concentration may be used to demonstrate the abnormality even

in its normal environment, for example ^{18}F-labelled oestrogens are reported to demonstrate local breast carcinoma using PET (Welch personal communication).

Most work has been done on the noradrenaline analogue, *meta*-iodobenzyl guanidine (MIBG) which we have shown is taken up in proportion to the number of neurosecretory granules present in the tumour (Bomanji et al 1987a). Thus phaeochromocytoma and neuroblastoma which usually have abundant granules show high uptake whereas other neural crest tumours, medullary carcinoma of thyroid and carcinoid tumours show very variable and often absent uptake.

MIBG was initially labelled with [131]I (Wieland et al 1980) and more recently with [123]I (Horne et al 1984) which gives excellent images. ^{123}I-MIBG routinely demonstrates the normal adrenal medullae whereas these are seen only in 15% of cases using ^{131}I-MIBG because of the poorer counting statistics (Shapiro et al 1985). A quantitative measure of the percentage uptake of the administered dose of ^{123}I-MIBG helps to determine the normality of adrenal uptake (0.01–0.2%, Bomanji et al 1987b). Phaeochromocytomata show uptakes in the range of 0.5–2% and widespread metastases of neuroblastoma may take up almost 40% of the administered activity. The absence of a rise in plasma or urinary metabolites of noradrenaline does not mean lack of uptake of MIBG, because its uptake depends on the storage capacity not the secretion of noradrenaline by the tissue. Consequently other competing compounds must be excluded and stopped at least three days before imaging is undertaken. These include antidepressants of the reserpine series and many sympathomeinectic drugs, particularly the constituents of nose drops and sprays, e.g. phenylephrine, which the patient will not consider as a drug.

The patient is further prepared by being given potassium iodide 60 mg from the day before the injection and for a further three days. After an injection of at least 80 MBq ^{123}I-MIBG intravenously over 30 s, imaging is performed at 10 min to give the blood and tissue background image, at 4 h and at 22 h. Normal uptakes in the salivary glands (absent if denervated), lacrimal glands, liver, heart, adrenal medullae, renal and urinary tract, and to a lesser extent lung, spleen, and occasionally in the gastro-intestinal tract are seen. Uptake in phaeochromocytoma or neuroblastoma shows up usually at 4 h and clearly by 22 h. Metastases in liver, lung or bone are usually clear on planar images in spite of the normal tissue background. Quantitation of uptake for dosimetry may be performed with ^{123}I-MIBG but to obtain the tissue halflife of retention, use of ^{131}I-MIBG is preferred when therapy with ^{131}I-MIBG is considered. No immediate untoward effects of diagnostic doses on blood pressure or pulse have been noted. Therapy doses are usually infused over 60 min in 5% dextrose solution; again no immediate side-effects have been noted. An advantage of ^{123}I-MIBG over X-ray CT in the location of phaeochromocytoma is that the whole torso from neck to thigh can be surveyed in a single image using a whole body 'bone scanning' facility, and this approach is important in confirming that an adrenal-related mass seen with X-ray CT is functionally active. Imaging with ^{123}I-MIBG is becoming an essential part of the staging of neuroblastoma.

RADIONUCLIDE THERAPY

The contribution of nuclear medicine to the therapy of cancer is becoming increasingly important in other tumours in addition to its established rôle in the treatment of metastases from thyroid cancer. This is because of the potential for targeting unsealed source radiotherapy specifically to the sites of tumour recurrence without the need to irradiate the whole field potentially involved by tumour as for external beam therapy. Three mechanisms of specifically enhanced uptake are used: metabolic function such as iodide trapping by the thyroid, ^{32}P uptake in polycythaemia, and strontium and phosphate derivative accumulation at sites of new bone formation; antibody surface antigen interaction through the use of radio-labelled monoclonal antibodies; and receptor binding such as the uptake of MIBG by tissues derived from the neural crest. It should be appreciated, however, that such enhancement of tumour uptake of the therapeutic radiopharmaceutical may be heterogenous, varying between different parts of the tumour and in different patients.

Thyroid cancer

The use of ^{131}I for therapy is well established and forms a model for the newer radionuclide-based therapy of other malignancies. Diagnosis depends on the clinical examination of the thyroid and its regional lymphatic drainage after the discovery by the patient of a lump in the neck. The detection of a solitary nodule in the thyroid leads to a final diagnosis of thyroid cancer in 1 in 20 of the general population or 1 in 5 of the hospital population in the UK. A radionuclide thyroid scan with 80–160 MBq of ^{99m}Tc pertechnetate will demonstrate that it is not a solitary nodule in 45% and a toxic nodule with suppression of other normal thyroid tissues in 3%. In a few cases, a so-called 'warm' nodule will be seen where there is a focal area of increased activity greater than in the surrounding thyroid. Such cases are usually due to an adenoma but such appearances may be due to a very vascular malignant tumour with sufficient frequency that repetition of the scan with [123]I (or ^{131}I) is always indicated. A nodule that is 'hot' with pertechnetate and 'cold' with iodine is often malignant. In the residual 50% of solitary nodules, radionuclide thyroid imaging cannot distinguish benign from malignant and attempts to use other radiopharmaceuticals such as ^{67}Ga and ^{201}Tl are insufficiently discriminating to be worthwhile. Ultrasound is required to show the 15% of simple cysts and with widespread availability of ultrasound, some recommend that it should precede thyroid radionuclide imaging to exclude these patients whose simple cysts may be aspirated (Belcher et al 1984). The residuum of solitary nodules need fine needle aspiration biopsy, the cytological findings determining the need for surgery. Some recommend surgery for all residual solitary nodules with frozen section to determine the degree of radical surgery. Once thyroid cancer is demonstrated histologically, total thyroidectomy is often the best approach if it is practical. It is necessary to spare the parathyroid glands and recurrent laryngeal nerve. Since metastases of papillary and follicular cancer take up iodine less avidly than normal thyroid tissue it is essential that the function of the residual thyroid tissue left after surgery is totally ablated. In order to determine the size of this remnant, a thyroid scan with 10–40 MBq (0.2–1.0 mCi) of ^{131}I is performed about two weeks after surgery.

The patient with a small remnant receives 3 GBq (80 mCi) [131]I therapy as a single capsule. For this the patient has to be isolated in a properly designed side ward with a self-contained shower and toilet. The floors, walls and ceiling have to be covered with a non-porous material coved at the junctions so that any spill can be easily cleaned. The patient uses disposable eating utensils and money is set aside by the patient before therapy to allow the purchase of newspapers etc. Linen is preferably disposable. The patient should shower at least twice a day since ^{131}I is secreted in sweat. Visitors are not allowed on the first day, and children under 12 and pregnant women not at all. Visitors should be a metre from the patient when visiting is allowed. The door of the ward must have a proper radiation sign, the name of the patient, the time and amount administered and nursing instructions. Nursing should be kept to the minimum. The main problem for the patient is the isolation experienced with this regime and preparatory counselling is essential. [131]I should not be given to incontinent patients and urine should not be collected but passed normally into the toilet. On the fourth and usually last day of a patient's stay, a whole body profile using a whole body counter and/or a neck and whole body scan for possible thyroid metastases is made and the residual dose is evaluated. Patients may travel home by public transport with less than 400 MBq (10 mCi) and by private transport or ambulance with less than 800 MBq (20 mCi) in the UK (NRPB 1988). The linen is bagged, monitored and removed to the decay store until it is at a level acceptable to be sent to the laundry. Waste is monitored and stored if necessary and the room is monitored and cleaned. If the patient has a large thyroid remnant then two ^{131}I doses of 1.5 GBq (40 mCi), one month apart, are advised to reduce the likelihood of radiation induced swelling of the thyroid at 2–3 days after administration.

After the ablation dose the patient is treated with tri-iodothyronine, T_3, 20 μg three times daily and a serum check is made to show that thyroid stimulating hormone (TSH) is suppressed fully, since some metastases have a thyrotrophic response. After three months T_3 is stopped for four days, the patient is admitted to hospital and investigated with routine blood tests, chest X-ray, bone scan and serum thyroglobulin. On the eighth day after stopping T_3, 80 mg thyrotrophin releasing hormone (TRH) is given orally to enhance possible iodine uptake and two hours later a test dose of 40–200 MBq (1–5 mCi) [131]I is given. Four days after this a whole body profile and/or neck and whole body scan is undertaken. The amount of uptake at any site is measured. If the scan is equivocal a further profile or set of images is taken three days later. In our practice negative scan enters the patient into the follow-up regime with attendances at 6, 6, 12, 12, 24 and 24 months later where the same regime is repeated. No recurrence at seven years is considered a cure. If the scan is positive and the abnormal site of uptake is confirmed clinically or radiologically the patient may receive a therapy dose. Note that a raised serum thyroglobulin is suggestive of metastases but does not replace the requirement for the ^{131}I assessment which is essential to guide therapy.

The therapy dose is usually 6 GBq (160 mCi) [131]I and with this dose for a typical uptake of 0.2% of administered dose 10 000 rads (cGy) would be delivered. If, however, uptake is high, particularly with pulmonary metastases, pulmonary fibrosis is probable or if cord compression is possible, then a lower dose of 3 GBq (80 mCi) is preferred and dexamethasone cover may be required. After the therapy dose which requires the patient to be isolated as above for a week, a set of images are taken at one week to show the full distribution of functioning metastases. Up to a total of 6 × 6 GBq (160 mCi) doses may be prescribed over a period of time. Platelet depression may occur and recovery may be slower after each dose. The prescription of a further therapy dose is determined by a positive test dose scan at the appropriate follow-up period, the regime of which starts again after each therapy dose.

Therapy for other cancers

There is a long history of using intracavity injections

of radionuclides for therapeutic purposes, for example in malignant pleural effusions and malignant ascites, with ^{198}Au gold colloid or ^{32}P phosphorus. Some responses have been noted but the techniques are messy and non-specific and proved no better than instillation of conventional cytotherapeutic agents. The development of radio-immunoscintigraphy with labelled monoclonal antibodies has shown the localization by imaging of over fifteen different types of cancer and the potential goal of specific targetting for imaging purposes has led to the enthusiastic evaluation of antibodies labelled with beta emitters for therapy. The problems are still considerable. The antibodies are against tumour associated and not tumour specific antigen, so the uptake by normal tissues for any therapeutic approach is a major drawback. The percentage uptake of the administered dose by the tumour is very small, usually less than 1% depending on tumour size, and between 0.01–0.0001% per gram. For thyroid cancer an uptake in metastases of over 0.5% and preferably over 1% of the administered ^{131}I is usually considered necessary to justify therapy. Thus, the therapeutic ratios for intravenously administered ^{131}I-labelled monoclonal antibody are low and cannot yet be used to justify the intravenous route for ^{131}I-labelled monoclonal antibody therapy. Some lymphomata and childhood neuroblastoma are exceptions. Uptakes of up to 7% of intravenously administered ^{131}I-UJ13A antineural crest antibody have been demonstrated in neuroblastoma (Goldman et al 1984). Thus, to avoid the unnecessary irradiation of normal tissues the intravenous route should be avoided for therapy at present.

Intracavity therapy is the alternative. Intraperitoneal therapy with ^{131}I-labelled HMFG2 or H17E2 for ovarian cancer presenting as peritoneal seedlings with ascites after full conventional chemotherapy has been applied is being evaluated (Hammersmith Oncology Group 1984). Initial enthusiasm is being tempered with findings that uptake of non-specific antibody may sometimes be similar although ratios of specific to non-specific antibody uptake of 2:1 to 10:1 are more usual. The critical test of making a comparison with the earlier non-specific agents such as ^{198}Au has not yet been performed. Similar approaches have been made to malignant pleural or pericardial effusions and malignant meningitis. In colon cancer the treatment of liver metastases by intra-arterial infusion of ^{131}I-antiCEA is under study (Delaloye et al 1985) as well as intraperitoneal administration of ^{131}I labelling of the anticolon membrane antibody, AUAI, for peritoneal spread with ascites. ^{131}I-antiferritin is being assessed for therapy in hepatoma (Order 1982). For glioma, introduction of labelled ^{131}I-UJ13A via the cerebrospinal fluid has been described (Richardson et al 1985) and ^{131}I-H17E2 given by intra-arterial infusion is being undertaken (Hooker et al 1985). Work is in progress on alternative beta emitters ^{90}Y yttrium (Hnatowich et al 1985) and ^{109}Pd palladium (Fawwaz et al 1984) for antibody labelling. The perlymphatic route is also being considered for cancer therapy and specific direct injection of ^{32}P chromic phosphate under stereotactic control for the brain or ultrasound control for liver tumours has been proposed (Beierwaltes 1985, Taasan et al 1985). The incorporation of alpha particle emitters, e.g. ^{211}At astatine (halflife 7.2 h, α 5.87 MeV decaying to ^{211}Po, halflife 0.52 sec, α 7.45 MeV) for greater therapeutic effect is also suggested (Bloomer et al 1984), but this requires homogenous uptake by the malignancy. Beta emitters with longer ranges allow for some heterogeneity of tumour cell uptake (Humm 1986).

All these approaches attempt to improve the therapeutic ratio of specific to non-specific uptake and increase the amount of specific uptake, so an adequate irradiation dose is achieved. Since the smaller the tumour, the greater the proportion of specific to non-specific uptake of monoclonal antibody, and conversely the larger the tumour the more non-specific uptake predominates due to blood supply, capillary permeability, proportionally greater diffusion area and extracellular fluid volume, and necrotic or cystic parts, the aim should be to sterilize the small tumour deposits (less than 2 cm diameter) and not to attempt to tackle the clinically and radiologically evident larger masses. The problem of determining accurate dosimetry remains, however, considerable.

The receptor binding approach has been the most successful of the new therapies to date. The binding and storage of ^{131}I MIBG in presynaptic sympathetic nerve terminals has led to the success-

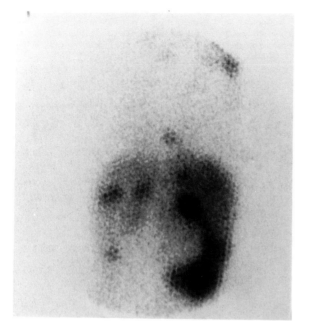
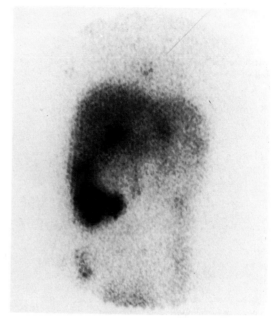

Fig. 1.6 Neuroblastoma. Imaging one week after an ^{131}I MIBG 2.5 GBq (100 mCi) therapy dose in a four-year-old child with stage IV neuroblastoma. Left: Posterior view of chest and abdomen. Right: Anterior view of abdomen. Multiple focal areas of increased uptake in the abdomen, liver and chest are seen, a typical distribution. Note that the high energy of ^{131}I gives a 'collimator pattern' to the areas of high activity. 6% of the injected activity is calculated to be in tumour tissue giving an absorbed radiation dose of approximately 6000 rads (60 Gy).

ful palliation of symptoms, reduction of tumour size, and correction of chemical markers in some patients with malignant phaeochromocytoma (Sisson et al 1984) and particularly in childhood neuroblastoma (Shapiro & Fischer 1985). In the latter, ^{131}I MIBG therapy is still given as the last resort and given the current responses, it is hoped that such therapy may be instituted earlier in the clinical course. Here is a specific therapeutic approach with high tumour uptake (up to 40% of the administered dose has been recorded) with great potential for the future (Fig. 1.6).

The palliation of bone metastases particularly those of prostatic cancer using unsealed source radionuclide therapy is again under consideration.

Therapeutic doses of radiation may be delivered locally by ^{89}Sr strontium in some cases (Silberstein & Williams 1985) or by ^{32}P or ^{131}I-labelled diphosphonate derivatives (Eisenhut et al 1985). These may be helpful in the control of bone pain when all other active therapies have been exhausted.

The special expertise of the properly trained and qualified nuclear medicine practitioner in the understanding of the clinical indications, the problems of administration and the radiation dosimetry and safety aspects of the therapeutic application of unsealed sources of radionuclides places nuclear medicine at the forefront of this exciting new approach to the treatment of cancer.

REFERENCES

Ancri D, Basset J-Y, Leuchampt Y et al 1978 Diagnosis of cerebral lesions by thallium-201. Radiology 128: 417–422

Anderson K C, Leonard R C F, Canellos G P, Skarin A T, Kaplan W D 1983 High dose gallium imaging in lymphoma. American Journal of Medicine 75: 327–331

Beierwaltes W H 1985 Horizons in radionuclide therapy: 1985 update. Journal of Nuclear Medicine 26: 421–427

Belcher E H, Britton K E, Nemec J et al 1984 The optimization of nuclear medicine procedures for the diagnosis and management of thyroid disorders in developing countries. Nuclear Medicine Communications 5: 339–351

Blake G M, Percival R C, Kavis J A 1986 Thallium pertechnetate subtraction scintigraphy: a quantitative comparison between adenomatous and hyperplastic parathyroid glands. European Journal of Nuclear Medicine 12: 31–36

Bloomer W D, McLaughlin W H, Lambrecht R M et al 1984 ^{211}At radiolabelled therapy: further observations with radiocolloids of ^{32}P, ^{165}Dy and ^{90}Y. International Journal of Radiation Oncology and Biological Physics 10: 341–348

Bomanji J, Flatman W D, Horne T et al 1987a Quantitation of meta(^{123}I)-iodobenzyl guanidine uptake by normal adrenal medulla. Journal of Nuclear Medicine 28: 319–324

Bomanji J, Flatman W D, Horne T et al 1987b Uptake of ^{123}I meta-iodobenzyl guanidine by phaeochromocytomas, other paragangliomas and neuroblastomas, a histopathological comparison. Journal of Nuclear Medicine 28: 973–978

Boucher B J, Sears R 1980 A summary of the results of radio-isotope brain scans on a large series of patients. British Journal of Radiology 53: 1174–1176

Brendal A J, Leccia F, Drouillard J et al 1984 Single photon emission computed tomography (SPECT), planar scintigraphy, and transmission computed tomography: a comparison of accuracy in diagnosing focal hepatic disease. Radiology 153: 527–532

Britton K E, Shapiro B 1981 Single photon emission tomography of the pituitary. Journal of the Royal Society of Medicine 74: 667–669

Britton K E, Granowska M 1987 Experience with ^{123}I labelled antibodies. In: Srivastava S R (ed) Radiolabelled monoclonal antibodies for imaging and therapy — Potential problems and prospects, NATO Advanced Scientific Institute, Barga, July 1986. Plenum Press, New York

Britton K E, Shapiro B, Hawkins L A 1979a Emission tomography for adrenal imaging. Nuclear Medicine Communications 1: 37–40

Britton K E, Nimmon C C, Whitfield H N et al 1979b Obstructive nephropathy, successful evaluation with radionuclides. Lancet 1: 905–907

Britton K E, Nawaz M K, Whitfield H N et al 1987 Obstructive nephropathy: comparison between parenchymal transit time index and frusemide diuresis. British Journal of Urology 59: 127–132

Brunskill M J 1983 Radiation dose estimates for interstitial radiocolloid lymphoscintigraphy. Seminars in Nuclear Medicine 13: 20–25

Carroll M J, Bomanji J, Britton K E Unpublished data

Clarke D P, Cosgrove D O, McCready V R 1986 Radionuclide imaging for liver malignancy and its relationship to other hepatic investigation. Clinics in Oncology 5: 159–181

Corty A T, Short M D, O'Connoll M A 1975 The diagnosis of renal pseudotumours. British Journal of Urology 47: 495–498

Cotton P B, Britton K E, Hazra D K et al 1978 Is pancreatic isotope scanning worthwhile? British Medical Journal 1: 282–283

Cutler S J, Axtell L M, Schottenfeld D, Farrow J H 1970 Clinical assessment of lymph nodes in carcinoma of the breast. Surgery, Gynaecology and Obstetrics 131: 41–52

Davies G C, Mills R R, Hayward J L 1980 Assessment of axillary lymph node status. Annals of Surgery 192: 148–151

Delaloye B, Bischof-Delaloye A, Volant J C et al 1985 First approach to therapy of liver metastases in colorectal carcinoma by intrahepatically infused ^{131}I labelled monoclonal anti-CEA antibodies. European Journal of Nuclear Medicine 11: A11

Derimanov S G 1987 For or against bone scintigraphy of patients with breast cancer. Nuclear Medicine Communications 8: 79–86

Di Chiro G, Brooks R A, Patronas N J et al 1984 Issues in the in vivo measurement of glucose metabolism of human central nervous system tumours. Annals of Neurology 15 (suppl): S138–S146

Ege G N 1980 Internal mammary lymphoscintigraphy in the conservative surgical management of breast carcinoma. Clinical Radiology 31: 559–563

Ege G N 1983 Lymphoscintigraphy — techniques and application in the management of breast carcinoma. Seminars in Nuclear Medicine 13: 26–34

Ege G N, Clark R M 1985 Internal mammary lymphoscintigraphy in the conservative management of breast carcinoma: an update and recommendations for a new TMN staging. Clinical Radiology 36: 469–472

Eisenhut M, Berberich R, Kimmig B, Oberhausen E 1985 ^{131}I labelled diphosphonates for palliative treatment of bone metastases II Preliminary clinical results with iodine-131 BDP3. Journal of Nuclear Medicine 27: 1255–1261

Ell P J, Britton K E, Farrer Brown G et al 1975 An assessment of the value of spleen scanning in the staging of Hodgkin's disease. British Journal of Radiology 48: 590–593

Fawwaz R A, Wang T S T, Srivastava S C et al 1984 Potential of palladium-109 labelled antimelanoma monoclonal antibody for tumour therapy. Journal of Nuclear Medicine 25: 796–799

Fisher B, Bauer M, Wickerham D L, Redmond C K, Fisher E 1983 Relation of number of positive axillary nodes to the prognosis of patient with primary breast cancer. Cancer 52: 1551–1557

Fleming J S, Humphries N L M, Karran S J, Goddard B A, Ackery D M 1981 In vivo assessment of hepatic arterial and portovenous components in liver perfusion. Journal of Nuclear Medicine 22: 18–21

Gimlette T M D, Taylor W H 1985 Localisation of enlarged parathyroid glands by thallium-201 and technetium-99m subtraction imaging. Clinical Nuclear Medicine 10: 235–239

Gimlette T M D, Brownless S M, Taylor W H et al 1986 Limits to parathyroid imaging with thallium-201 confirmed by tissue uptake and phantom studies. Journal of Nuclear Medicine 27: 1262–1265

Gitsch E, Phillipp K, Pateisky N 1984 Intra-operative lymph scintigraphy during radical surgery for cervical cancer. Journal of Nuclear Medicine 25: 486–489

Goldenberg D M, Kim E E, Deland F H, Bennett S, Primus F J 1980 Radio-immunodetection of cancer with radioactive antibodies to carcino-embryonic antigen. Cancer Research 40: 2984–2992

Goldman A, Vivian G, Gordon I, Pritchard J, Kemshead J T 1984 Immunolocalisation of neuroblastoma using radiolabelled monoclonal antibody UJ13A. Journal of Paediatrics 105: 252–256

Gough M J, Leveson S H, Wiggins P A, Giles G R, Parkin A, Robinson P J 1985 Improved staging of colorectal cancer by dynamic hepatic perfusion scintigraphy. British Journal of Surgery 72 (suppl): S120–S120

Granowska M, Britton K E, Shepherd J 1983 The detection

of ovarian cancer using ^{123}I monoclonal antibody. Radiobiologie Radiotherapie (Berlin) 25: 153–160.

Granowska M, Shepherd J, Britton K E et al 1984 Ovarian cancer: Diagnosis using ^{123}I monoclonal antibody in comparison with surgical findings. Nuclear Medicine Communications 5: 485–499

Granowska M, Britton K E, Shepherd J H et al 1986 A prospective study of ^{123}I-labelled monoclonal antibody imaging in ovarian cancer. Journal of Clinical Oncology 4: 730–736

Granowska M, Britton K E, Crowther M, Nimmon C C, Slevin M, Shepherd J 1987 Kinetic analysis with probability mapping in radio-immunoscintigraphy. In: Srivastava S R (ed) Radiolabelled monoclonal antibodies for imaging and therapy — Potential, problems and prospects. NATO Advanced Scientific Institute, Barga, July 1986. Plenum Press, New York.

Hammersmith Oncology Group 1984 Antibody guided irradiation of malignant lesions. Lancet 1: 1441–1443

Hawkins L A, Britton K E, Shapiro B 1980 Selenium 75-selenomethyl cholesterol: a new agent for quantitative functional scintigraphy of the adrenals. British Journal of Radiology 53: 883–889

Hnatowich D J, Layne W W, Childs R L et al 1983 Radioactive labelling of antibody: a simple and efficient method. Science 220: 613–615

Hnatowich D J, Virzi F, Doherty P W 1985 DTPA coupled antibodies labelled with yttrium-90. Journal of Nuclear Medicine 26: 503–509

Hoffer P B 1978 The utility of [67]gallium in tumour imaging: a comment on the final reports of the co-operative study group. Journal of Nuclear Medicine 19: 1082–1084

Hooker G, Snook D, Pickering D et al 1985 Antibody guided irradiation of brain gliomas. European Journal of Nuclear Medicine 11: A11

Horne T, Hawkins L A, Britton K E, Granowska M, Bouloux P, Besser G M 1984 Imaging of phaeochromocytoma and adrenal medulla with ^{123}I meta-iodobenzyl guanidine. Nuclear Medicine Communications 5: 763–768

Humm J L 1986 Dosimetric aspects of radiolabelled antibodies for tumour therapy. Journal of Nuclear Medicine 27: 1490–1497

Kaplan W D 1983 Iliopelvic lymphoscintigraphy. Seminars in Nuclear Medicine 13: 9–19

Kaplan E, En-Porath M, Fink S, Clayton G D, Jacobson B 1966 Elimination of liver interference from the selenomethionine pancreas scan. Journal of Nuclear Medicine 7: 807–809

Khan O, Ell P J, Jarritt P H et al 1981 Comparison between emission and transmission computed tomography of the liver. British Medical Journal 282: 1212–1214

Kohler G, Milstein C 1975 Continuous cultures of fused cells secreting antibody of proven defined specificity. Nature 256: 495–497

Kunkler I H, Merrick M V, Roger A 1985 Bone scintigraphy in breast cancer — a nine year follow-up. Clinical Radiology 36: 279–282

La France N D, Links J, Williams D et al 1986 [11]C Methionine and ^{18}F deoxyglucose (FDG) in the post-operative management of patients with brain tumours with positron emission tomography. Nuklearmedizin 25: A26

Lennart B, Sven-Erik S, Persson B R R 1983 Particle sizing and biokinetics of interstitial lymphoscintigraphic agents. Seminars in Nuclear Medicine 13: 9–19

Leveson S H, Wiggins P A, Nasim T A 1983 Improved detection of hepatic metastases by the use of dynamic flow scintigraphy. British Journal of Cancer 47: 719–721

Lipton M J, De Nardo G L, Silverman S et al 1972 Evaluation of the liver and spleen in Hodgkin's disease I. The value of hepatic scintigraphy. American Journal of Medicine 52: 356–361

Lunia S, Parthasarathy K L, Baksh S et al 1975 An evaluation of ^{99m}Tc-sulfur colloid liver scintiscans and their usefulness in metastatic workup: a review of 1424 studies. Journal of Nuclear Medicine 16: 62–65

Mazzeo F, Accurso A, Petrella G et al 1986 Pre-operative axillary lymphoscintigraphy in breast cancer: experience with sub-areolar injection of ^{99m}Tc nanocolloidal albumin. Nuclear Medicine Communications 7: 5–16

McLean R G, Murray I P C 1984 Radionuclide scanning and chondrosarcoma: reports of two cases. Nuclear Medicine Communications 5: 711–719

McKillop J H 1987 Bone scanning in metastatic disease. In: Fogleman I (ed) Bone scanning in clinical practice. Springer Verlag, Berlin, pp 41–67

McNeil B J 1984 Value of bone scanning in neoplastic disease. Seminars in Nuclear Medicine 14: 277–286

McNeil B J, Collins J J, Adelstein S J 1977 Rationale for seeking occult metastases in patients with bronchial cancer. Surgery, Gynaecology and Obstetrics 144: 389–393

Merrick M V, Merrick J M 1986 Bone scintigraphy in lung cancer: a reappraisal. British Journal of Radiology 59: 1185–1194

Merrick M V, Ding C L, Chisholm G D 1985 The prognostic significance of alkaline phosphatase and bone scintigraphy in carcinoma of the prostate. British Journal of Urology 57: 715–720

Mlodkowska E, Nawaz K H, Carroll M J, Nimmon C C, Britton K E 1985 Comparison of ^{99m}Tc MDP static and dynamic methods of obstructive nephropathy detection using transit time analysis as a reference: pilot study. Nuclear Medicine Communications 5: 397–410

Muller J A, Scholeser O, Meyer C J, Gaab M R, Becker H, Hundeshagen H 1986 Grading brain tumours by ^{11}C-methyl methionine positron emission tomography. Nuklearmedizin 25: A26

NRPB 1988 Guidance noted for the protection of persons against ionising radiations arising from medical and dental use. HMSO, London, p 57

Order S E 1982 Monoclonal antibodies: potential role in radiation therapy and oncology. International Journal of Radiation Oncology and Biological Physics 8: 1193–1201

O'Reilly P H, Shields R A, Testa H J 1986 Nuclear medicine in urology and nephrology, 2nd edn. Butterworth, London, pp 91–125

Osborne M P, Payne J H, Richardson V J, McCready V R, Ryman B E 1983 The pre-operative detection of axillary lymph node metastases in breast cancer by isotope imaging. British Journal of Surgery 70: 141–144

Ott R J, Grey L J, Zivanovic M A et al 1983 The limitations of the dual radionuclide subtraction technique for the external detection of tumours by radio-iodine labelled antibodies. British Journal of Radiology 56: 101–108

Pateisky N, Philip K, Skodler D, Burchell J 1985 Radio-immunoscintigraphy of the lymphatic system versus intravenous application of tumour associated monoclonal antibodies: indications and clinical usefulness in the management of cancer patients. In: Cox P, Donato L, Britton K E (eds) Immunoscintigraphy, Monographs in Nuclear Medicine vol I. Gordon & Breach, London, pp 371–374

Richardson R B, Davies A G, Bourne S, Kemshead J T, Coakham H B 1985 Antibody guided radiolocalisation and radiotherapy of primary brain tumours. Nuclear Medicine Communications 6: 598

Seabold J E, Cohen E L, Beierwaltes W H et al 1976 Adrenal imaging with ^{131}I-19-iodocholesterol in the diagnostic evaluation of patients with aldosteronism. Journal of Clinical Endocrinology and Metabolism 42: 41–51

Sears H F, Gerber F H, Sturtz D L et al 1975 Liver scan and carcinoma of the breast. Surgery, Gynecology and Obstetrics 140: 409–411

Shapiro B, Fischer M 1985 Workshop on ^{131}I meta-iodobenzyl guanidine. Nuclear Medicine Communications 6: 179–186

Shapiro B, Britton K E, Hawkins L A et al 1981 Clinical experience with ^{75}Se selenomethylcholesterol adrenal imaging. Clinical Endocrinology 15: 19–27

Shapiro B, Copp J E, Sisson J C, Eyre P L, Wallis J, Beierwaltes W H 1985 Iodine-131 meta-iodobenzyl guanidine for the locating of suspected phaeochromocytoma experience in 400 cases. Journal of Nuclear Medicine 26: 576–585

Siccardi A G, Buraggi G L, Callegaro L et al 1986 Multicentre study of immunoscintigraphy with radiolabelled monoclonal antibodies in patients with melanoma. Cancer Research 46: 4817–4822

Silberstein E B, Williams C 1985 Strontium-89 therapy for the pain of osseous metastases. Journal of Nuclear Medicine 26: 345–348

Silverman S, De Nardo G L, Glastein E et al 1972 Evaluation of the liver and spleen in Hodgkin's disease II. The value of spleen scintigraphy. American Journal of Medicine 52: 362–366

Sisson J C, Shapiro B, Beierwaltes W H et al 1984 Radiopharmaceutical treatment of malignant phaeochromocytoma. Journal of Nuclear Medicine 24: 197–206

Taasan V, Shapiro B, Taren J A et al 1985 Phosphorus-32 therapy of cystic grade IV astrocytomas: technique and preliminary application. Journal of Nuclear Medicine 26: 1335–1338

Taylor K J W, Sullivan D, Rosenfield A T et al 1977 Gray scale ultrasound and isotope scanning: complementary techniques for imaging the liver. American Journal of Roentgenology 128: 277–281

Turner D A, Fordham E W, Ali A, Slayton R E 1978 Gallium-67 imaging in the management of Hodgkin's disease and other malignant lymphomas. Seminars in Nuclear Medicine 8: 205–218

White L, Miller J H, Reid B S 1984 Pre-operative ultrasound and gallium-67 evaluation of abdominal non-Hodgkin's lymphoma. American Journal of Diseases of Children 138: 740–745

Wieland D M, Wu J, Brown L E, Mangner T J, Swanson D P, Beierwaltes W H 1980 Radiolabelled adrenergic neuron-blocking agents: adrenomedullary imaging with ^{131}I iodobenzyl guanidine. Journal of Nuclear Medicine 21: 349–353

Wraight E P, Barber R W, Ritson A 1982 Relative hepatic arterial and portal flow in liver scintigraphy. Nuclear Medicine Communications 3: 273–279

Young A E, Gaunt J I, Croft D N et al 1983 Location of parathyroid adenomas by thallium-201 and technetium-99m subtraction scanning. British Medical Journal 286: 1384–1386

2. Magnetic resonance imaging in oncology

J. P. R. Jenkins

Magnetic resonance imaging (MRI) is an established diagnostic technique which initially demonstrated its clinical value and efficacy in the evaluation of the central nervous system. Further experience has extended its clinical rôle to the assessment of the spine, pelvis and musculoskeletal system where it has, in certain centres, become the imaging method of choice. MRI has particular advantages including a very high soft tissue contrast resolution and discrimination, an ability to image in any plane, an absence of bone and some metal artefacts in the resultant image, and the use of non-ionizing radiation. Artefacts from respiration, cardiac motion and bowel peristalsis degrade images of the thorax and abdomen when conventional scanning techniques are used. These motion artefacts can be much reduced by the use of faster scanning techniques. Disadvantages include high cost, limited availability especially in the UK, relatively long data acquisition times (in the order of minutes), relatively poor bone and calcium detail, and claustrophobic effects.

In an effort to overcome some of these disadvantages and extend further the range of MRI, advances have been, and are currently being, made. Technological progress has been rapid over the last few years with the introduction of contrast agents, new hardware designs (e.g. in magnet and surface coil technology) and software developments (e.g. new pulse sequences and data processing), which require further evaluation. Thus the precise role of MRI in oncology has yet to be determined.

This review sets out some of the technical aspects, current status and future perspectives of magnetic resonance (MR) in the assessment of patients with cancer.

TECHNICAL ASPECTS

Equipment

MRI systems require the following (as arranged in Fig. 2.1): magnet; radio-frequency (RF) transmitter and receiver coils; gradient coils; and computer, display unit and digital storage facilities. An important consequence of such complex instrumentation is the need to check regularly and optimize the various components such as gradients and RF pulses to maintain temporal resolution.

Magnet

A key component of any MRI system is the presence of a relatively stable and homogeneous static magnetic field. This is provided by one of two main types of magnet design – a permanent magnet or an electromagnet. Permanent magnets consist of blocks of magnetized or magnetizable material which, when assembled, produce a magnet with north and south poles separated by an air gap of sufficient size for imaging. Electromagnets use electric current to generate the magnetic field and consist of two main types, resistive or superconducting. Each type of magnet has its advantages and disadvantages (McFarland & Rosen 1986). The single most costly item of manufacture for an MR system is the magnet, making up about a third of the total cost, and new low cost designs are currently being developed.

The static magnetic field strength for MRI systems ranges from 0.02 to 2 T*. There is no

---

*Magnetic field strength is measured in tesla (T) (SI unit) or gauss (G). One tesla = 10 000 gauss or 10 kilogauss. The earth's magnetic field strength varies with position but is approximately 0.05 mT or 0.5 G.

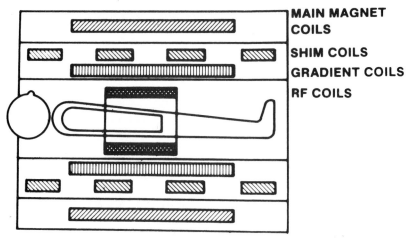

MAIN MAGNET
COILS
SHIM COILS
GRADIENT COILS
RF COILS

Fig. 2.1   Longitudinal section through an MR magnet system with the patient positioned in the body coil for scanning the abdomen. (Reproduced from Sutton D (1987) Textbook of radiology and imaging (4th edn.), Churchill Livingstone.)

consensus at present as to the optimum field strength for MRI although Hoult et al (1986) proposed a medium-field strength (0.5–1 T) as representing the best compromize when imaging time was of major importance. Experience has shown that diagnostic images can be produced by low- to medium-fields (0.06–0.5 T) as well as by high-field (1–2 T) systems. Each has its advantages and disadvantages with the most important aspect being the stability and homogeneity of the field. If spectroscopy or imaging of nuclei other than protons is required then a high-field system is necessary.

Radio-frequency coils

There are two main types of radio-frequency (RF) coils used, either saddle-shaped or solenoid, depending on the type of magnet and its field orientation. The basic RF coil surrounds the part of the patient to be examined in order to transmit and receive RF signals to and from the patient. This produces the appropriate signal data from which images can be produced. Large body coils and smaller diameter head coils are commonly used. Surface and close-coupled receiver coils, which are simply circular loops, are of smaller diameter and more closely applied to the patient. These improve the signal-to-noise ratio over a limited field of view allowing thinner sections to be obtained, with resultant improvement in

spatial resolution and soft tissue discrimination. In addition, motion artefacts outside the field of view of the surface coil, e.g. respiratory and cardiac motion artefacts across the dorso-lumbar spine, are significantly reduced.

Gradient coils

Gradient coils are used to spatially encode information in the MR signal by modifying the static magnetic field for short periods (typically a few milliseconds). This gradient system allows sections of tissue in any plane, as well as within the plane of section, to be identified from the magnetized volume. There are three sets of gradient coils (termed X, Y and Z) which are orientated in the three orthogonal directions. Gradient field strengths are only a few percent of the main magnetic field. During data acquisition the gradients are rapidly switched on and off and this produces mechanical noise as the RF coils move in response to the changing fields. This is the noise associated with an MRI system. More rapid gradient switching, especially during multisection acquisition or fast scanning techniques, can be especially loud.

Computer, display unit and digital storage facilities

These facilities are similar to those employed in

CT. The signal data obtained is amplified, filtered, digitized and processed by computer for image reconstruction and display on a viewing console. The digital data can be stored onto magnetic tape, optical or floppy disc, or a hard copy can be made.

Physical principles of MR

The basic physics of MR is discussed in greater detail elsewhere (Smith 1985, Jenkins & Isherwood 1987a, Stark & Bradley 1988). In outline, atomic nuclei with an odd number of protons or neutrons (e.g. hydrogen (^{1}H), sodium (^{23}Na), phosphorus (^{31}P), carbon (^{13}C) and fluorine (^{19}F) possess an intrinsic spin. Since the nucleus is positively charged it generates a small magnetic field and behaves like a small bar magnet. In the absence of an external magnetic field these nuclei are randomly orientated but when placed within the static magnetic field they tend to align along the direction of that field. Application of an RF pulse (i.e. an oscillating magnetic field) can induce resonance of particular sets of nuclei. The required frequency of the RF pulse is determined by the strength of the static magnetic field and the particular nucleus under investigation. Resonance refers to a change in the alignment and thus energy level of the nuclei in the main magnetic field. The energy absorbed during this transition to a higher energy state is subsequently released to the environment when the RF pulse is turned off as the nuclei relax back to equilibrium and a lower energy state. The release of energy can be recorded as an electrical signal providing data from which digital images can be derived. Such an image is usually constructed using a mathematical process called two-dimensional Fourier transform (2DFT). MRI is, therefore, an emission technique compared with CT which uses a transmission method for encoding electron density of tissue by X-ray beam attenuation.

The hydrogen nucleus, i.e. the proton, is the one most suitable for conventional imaging, being most abundant in the human body and yielding the strongest MR signal compared with other spinning nuclei. The MR signal is derived mainly from protons in water and lipids, with the former in the majority. Protons in proteins, DNA and solid structures such as cortical bone do not contribute significantly to the resultant MR signal.

MR tissue parameters

Unlike CT which has a fixed grey scale dependent upon the linear attenuation coefficient based on the electron density of tissue, the MR signal is a more complex interplay of at least ten tissue parameters (Bydder 1988a). The strength (amplitude) of the signal depends not only on the number of measurable or mobile protons ('proton' or 'spin density') in the tissues but also on the relaxation times, blood flow, chemical shift effects, magnetic susceptibility, diffusion, perfusion and RF absorption. Thus in MRI there are multiple tissue parameters which provide a complex input into the MR signal and resultant image. It is the RF pulse sequence selected which determines the MR image dependence or weighting on the different tissue parameters (Table 2.1).

Two relaxation times are described termed T_1 and T_2. The T_1 (otherwise known as 'spin-lattice' or 'longitudinal') relaxation time is a term used to describe the return of protons towards equilibrium following application and then removal of the RF pulse. T_2 (otherwise called 'spin-spin' or 'transverse') relaxation time is used to describe the associated loss of coherence or phase between individual protons immediately following the RF pulse. Both relaxation times are exponential time constants which are only indirectly interrelated. The T_1 value is always greater than its T_2 and in the majority of tissues is an order of magnitude

Table 2.1 Main RF pulse sequences with their major signal intensity weighting

RF pulse sequences	Image weighting
Partial saturation recovery (PSR) (gradient echo)	T_1 Proton density Phase-contrast
Spin echo (SE)	
Short TR/short TE	T_1
Long TR/long TE	T_2
Long TR/short TE	Proton density
Inversion recovery (IR)	
Medium to long TI	T_1
Short TI ('STIR')	$T_1 + T_2$

greater (e.g. grey matter at 0.26 T has a T_1 value of 750 ms compared with a T_2 of 70 ms). The relaxation times of tissues are much shorter than those of pure water which has equivalent T_1 and T_2 values of approximately three seconds. In order to explain this difference it is postulated that water, when in close proximity to biological macromolecules (such as protein and cell membranes), become 'bound' (Fullerton et al 1982). The motion of bound water is restricted thus shortening its T_1. The fraction not bound is termed 'free' or 'bulk' water which relaxes more slowly and has a longer T_1. An equilibrium exists between the free and bound water fractions and it is probably this that is altered in certain pathological conditions. Variations in the macro-molecular structure in tissues will result in differences in their water binding characteristics. Thus it is assumed that the elevation in the T_1 and T_2 values in tumours and other pathologies, relative to normal tissue, is due to a reduced binding of water with increase in the free water component. Relaxation times vary with magnetic field strength, the imaging instrument and the method used for their measurement. Although there is debate as to the optimum method of measuring in vivo relaxation times, they have the potential to characterize normal and pathological tissues (vide infra).

Pulse sequences and image interpretation

A variety of RF pulse sequences can be used to generate an image with the most commonly used sequences termed partial saturation recovery (PSR), inversion recovery (IR) and spin echo (SE) (Fig. 2.2). For each RF pulse sequence there are a number of operation- or machine-dependent factors, viz. echo time (TE), inversion time (TI), and repetition time (TR), any one of which can be varied with profound effect on image grey scale and contrast. Different RF pulse sequences provide different weighting in the received signal to the various tissue parameters (Table 2.1). A high signal intensity, using typical sequences, is observed from tissues with an increased proton density, a short T_1 or a prolonged T_2. A low MR signal is produced by tissues with the opposite parameters. Most lesions have a long T_1 and long

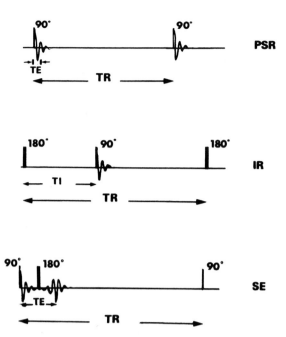

Fig. 2.2 Three standard pulse sequences: partial saturation recovery (PSR), inversion recovery (IR) and spin echo (SE) with appropriate RF pulses, signal data and timing parameters. TE = echo time; TI = inversion time in the IR sequence; TR = repetition time. By convention the RF pulse sequence is abbreviated as follows: PSR TR/TE, IR TR/TI, and SE TR/TE (timings are quoted in milliseconds).

T_2 and appear low and high signal on T_1-weighted (T_1W) and T_2-weighted (T_2W) sequences res-pectively. The MR signal relating to flowing blood is a complex interplay of many factors, with turbulent and fast-flowing (arterial) blood providing little or no signal whereas static or slow-moving (venous) blood can give a high signal.

An RF pulse sequence with its defined timing parameters needs to be repeated a number of times (typically 256), each with a new gradient increment in order to produce an image matrix of 256×256. Each gradient increment can be repeated to provide two or more signal excitations, which are then averaged in order to improve the signal-to-noise ratio. The overall scanning time per sequence can be calculated by multiplying the TR of the sequence by the number of gradient increments and signal excitations used. The data for a single section MR image, using typical sequences, can take 2–8 min to collect. Much of this time is non-productive allowing tissue relaxation processes to occur before re-excitation. Efficient use can be made of this relaxation period by exciting protons in adjacent sections, thus obtaining sufficient data to image 4–16 contiguous sections in the same time it would take to image one or two sections. Such multisection imaging significantly reduces patient scanning time.

PSR, IR and short TR/short TE SE sequences can provide varying T_1W scans with T_2W images from long TR/long TE SE sequences (Table 2.1). Efficient use can be made of the relaxation period (long TR) in the T_2W SE sequences by adding pulse timings to the sequence to produce multi-echo scans, i.e. separate images at different TE values. The heaviest T_1W image is obtained by using the IR sequence but can take significantly (up to four times) longer to perform than either of the other T_1W sequences. The short inversion time IR (STIR) sequence provides additive T_1 and T_2 contrast together with cancellation of the signal from fat (Bydder & Young 1985, Dwyer et al 1988). It is especially useful in delineating tumour as a high signal contrasted against a low signal from fat, marrow or muscle. It has, however, a low signal-to-noise ratio and is prone to artefacts.

There are particular advantages in using the PSR sequence, in low-to-medium field strength units, in the evaluation of the central nervous system and musculoskeletal system. These include T_1, blood flow and chemical shift information, rapid acquisition with multisection capability and sensitivity to changes in magnetic susceptibility*. The PSR sequence uses a gradient echo rather than a spin echo for image production and one consequence is that changes in magnetic susceptibility are more readily identified compared with SE sequences. This is an advantage overcoming an earlier limitation of MRI in that blood degradation products (deoxy-haemoglobin and haemosiderin), formed secondary to haemorrhage, have a strong magnetic

susceptibility and are more readily demonstrated. An important consequence of such sensitivity when using gradient echoes is unwanted artefacts due to alteration in magnetic susceptibility which normally exist at some disparate tissue interfaces (i.e. between soft tissues and bone or air as in the air sinuses, mastoids and bowel) and near ferromagnetic implants. Chemical shift effects occur due to a change in the MR behaviour of protons relating to differences in the chemical environment between protons attached to carbon in a lipid molecule and those bound to oxygen as in water. This difference can be exploited in chemical shift imaging to produce separate water and lipid or composite ('phase-contrast') images using the PSR sequence (Bydder 1988b). Another problem with gradient echo sequences is the appearance of an artificial low signal intensity border at fat/water interfaces (more pronounced at high field) due to a chemical shift effect which should not be confused with an anatomical structure. Further use of gradient echos is described in the section on fast scanning techniques. It should be noted that not all MRI systems at present have the capability to implement the IR or PSR sequences.

In addition, it is important to understand that there are a variety of common, subtle and sometimes unusual artefacts noted in the MR images, recognition of which is important to allow correct interpretation (Stark & Bradley 1988).

Fast scanning techniques

Many acronyms are ascribed to individual RF pulse sequences which are generically gradient echoes with low flip angles, i.e. pulse angles $< 90°$. Image contrast depends on the specific 'flip' angle chosen and T_1W or T_2W images can thus be produced. Such rapid imaging is not only efficient in patient scanning time but helps to minimize physiological motion artefacts allowing dynamic scanning and MR angiography studies to be performed. Dynamic scanning combined with gadolinium-DTPA allows assessment of tissue perfusion.

Echo-planar imaging is another approach to rapid scanning providing very rapid real time images of the brain or body within seconds (Crooks et al 1988).

---

*The term 'magnetic susceptibility' of a tissue can be used to describe the magnetization induced in that tissue by the applied magnetic field. In general there are both diamagnetic and paramagnetic contributions to tissue susceptibility, the diamagnetic contribution tending to reduce the local field and the paramagnetic increasing it.

Safety aspects of MRI

These are discussed in more detail elsewhere (Jenkins & Isherwood 1987b; Stark & Bradley 1988). Using currently available instrumentation MRI is a safe procedure as long as the safety guidelines are followed. Of primary concern for the patient and operator is the presence of ferromagnetic metallic objects. MRI should not be performed on patients with cardiac pacemakers or intracranial aneurysm clips and caution must be exercised in patients with embedded shrapnel or pacemaker wires.

MR contrast agents

There are two main groups of MR contrast agents, termed paramagnetic and superparamagnetic, which have been used in clinical studies so far (Stark & Bradley 1988). Both affect local tissue magnetic susceptibility. The paramagnetic agents shorten T_1 producing increased signal on T_1W images (positive contrast) whereas superparamagnetic agents shorten T_2 leading to a signal void on all sequences (negative contrast). Both types of agents have been administered intravenously and orally. Gadolinium-DTPA, a paramagnetic agent, was the first one used in clinical practice (Laniado et al 1984). It is a safe, effective agent providing information on the extracellular compartment. The integrity of the blood–brain barrier can be assessed as well as the vascularity of tumours. The use of fast scanning techniques combined with these agents can provide information on tissue perfusion. Other contrast agents are currently being developed and assessed (Lauffer 1988). The linking of monoclonal antibodies to paramagnetic contrast agents, although a theoretically attractive approach to tumour imaging, has been unsuccessful. This is due to an insufficient number of tumour target sites available to allow sufficient concentration of paramagnetic agents to be achieved.

MRI IN CHILDHOOD ONCOLOGY

The advantages of MRI have particular relevance to the study of infants and children when compared with other imaging techniques. Ultra-sound, although a good initial non-invasive screening investigation, has limitations including an inability to define the full extent of some abdominal and pelvic lesions due to overlying bone or bowel gas. CT is technically more difficult in children, requiring oral and intravenous contrast media administration for the assessment of abdominal and pelvic mass lesions. The poorly developed fat planes, compared with adults, makes definition of boundaries between different structures and the extent of lesions difficult to define precisely. In the study of paediatric spinal disorders, water-soluble contrast myelography, with its attendant risks and morbidity, is also technically difficult to perform. MRI combines the multiplanar and non-invasive facilities of ultrasound with a higher soft tissue contrast discrimination compared with CT and/or CT myelography. Children under 6–8 years can be safely sedated and monitored within the tunnel of the magnet.

In the paediatric age group a different spectrum of disease occurs compared with adults with emphasis on congenital lesions, different tumour types and a much lower incidence of metastases. Children vary markedly in size requiring surface coils of different sizes in order to obtain high resolution thin section MR scans. The normal neonatal and infant brain, relative to that of an adult, has longer T_1 and T_2 values which, together with the lack of myelination, makes oedema and mass effect more difficult to define. Thus the RF pulse sequences and techniques used in adults are not necessarily optimal when evaluating childhood pathology. The clinical utility of MRI in the assessment of tumours in this age group will be discussed in more detail in the appropriate sections below.

CENTRAL NERVOUS SYSTEM (CNS)

In a relatively short time since the first head image in 1980 (Hawkes et al 1980), MRI has had a major impact on imaging strategies in the CNS especially in the evaluation of the temporal lobes, posterior fossa, cranio-cervical junction and spine. This has occurred by virtue of its ability to demonstrate and discriminate between normal and abnormal tissues in multiple planes without bony artefacts. The cranio-cervical junction is a watershed area particularly difficult to image satisfactorily on CT or myelography.

Brain

MRI displays all the gross anatomy of the brain including surface features, grey/white matter differentiation, deep grey nuclei, brain stem, individual cranial nerves and cerebrospinal (CSF) spaces (Daniels et al 1987). The coronal plane is useful for demonstrating lesions in the cerebellum, temporal lobes or convexity. Sagittal plane imaging most clearly depicts midline structures including brain stem, corpus callosum, pituitary gland and infundibulum, aqueduct and foramen magnum. In the brain there is exquisite grey and white matter separation, especially with IR images, allowing the process of normal myelination to be accurately assessed (Barkovich et al 1988). Grey matter, relative to white matter, has a longer T_1 and T_2 appearing lower and higher signal on T_1W and T_2W images respectively. Cerebrospinal fluid has a very long T_1 and T_2, similar to water, and can be readily distinguished.

A thorough knowledge of the normal changes which occur in the brain with age is important before 'abnormal' findings can be correctly interpreted. Patchy white matter lesions called 'unidentified bright objects' (UBOs) (high signals on T_2W images) have been noted in 20–30% of neurologically asymptomatic healthy elderly subjects. They are associated with loss of brain parenchyma and increased tissue water caused by a spectrum of histological changes (Drayer 1988). Thus foci of high signal on T_2W images in the elderly patient require careful interpretation and do not necessarily indicate sinister pathology.

MRI is more sensitive to the detection and display of the majority of intracranial lesions when compared with CT (Brant-Zawadzki 1988, Hyman & Gorey 1988). The high sensitivity of MRI in the detection of most intracranial tumours, with the exception of meningiomas, is related to its ability to detect minor degrees of brain oedema particularly on T_2W images. A good protocol technique, using both T_1W and T_2W sequences, is required for optimal detection and delineation of pathological processes. T_1W sequences demon-strate good morphological detail, whereas T_2W sequences are more sensitive to the demonstration of pathological processes. Cystic and solid lesions can be differentiated. T_2W images are unhelpful, however, in the majority of cases in separating tumour from peritumoral oedema (Fig. 2.3). The STIR sequence is useful for accentuating lesions with long T_1/long T_2 and for cancelling the signal from fat which is of major importance when studying lesions of the optic nerve. Vascular structures and lesions can be demonstrated, especially with gradient echo sequences, without the need for contrast medium administration. Precise localization of peripheral brain tumours into the extra- or intra-axial compartment has important implications in treatment planning and prognosis and can be more easily demonstrated by MRI than CT (Curnes 1987).

Accurate planning of stereotactic neurosurgery or radiotherapy can be achieved by MRI but requires precise spatial information. Geometric artefacts from a variety of sources can produce significant spatial distortions of MR images which, although not affecting clinical diagnosis, need to be corrected in order to provide images with accurate spatial information (Schad et al 1987). MRI is superior to CT in delineating the position of the brain stem and optic chiasm and tracts relative to tumour, and together with direct sagittal and coronal scanning is considered useful in planning treatment.

The inability to detect intracranial calcification with the same degree of certainty as with CT is a significant disadvantage. Its presence and morphological appearance is important in specific tumour diagnoses. On MR the presence of calcification can only be inferred by identification of focal areas of signal void (Oot et al 1986). This is a non-specific finding which can also be produced by flowing blood and thus misinterpreted.

It is the use of a paramagnetic contrast agent (gadolinium-DTPA) which has overcome some of the early limitations and extended the clinical utility of MRI in the brain (Stack et al 1988a). The integrity of the blood–brain barrier can be assessed and lesions with an active blood supply, e.g. meningiomas and leptomeningeal tumour, demonstrated. An intact blood-brain barrier,

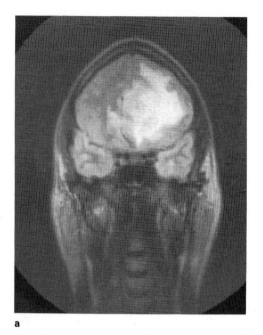

a

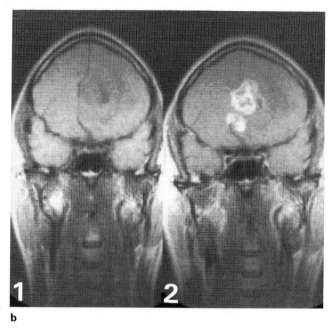

b

Fig. 2.3 Astrocytoma grade IV. (a) coronal pre-Gd-DTPA T_2W (SE 2000/80) image demonstrating a mass lesion with extensive oedema. The tumour cannot be distinguished from oedema. (b) coronal (1) pre- and (2) post-Gd-DTPA T_1W (SE 560/26) images of the same patient demonstrating clear delineation of tumour and tumoral cysts on enhanced scan. (Reproduced with permission from Neuroradiology 1988, 30: 145–154).

which is composed of a network of capillaries with tight endothelial junctions, prevents water and contrast agents from leaving vessels and passing into the extracellular space. A number of intracranial pathologies including tumours can disrupt the blood–brain barrier producing extravasation of contrast into the lesion leading to focal signal enhancement on T_1W images. Using a stereotactic biopsy technique in patients with brain tumours, Earnest et al (1988) correlated regions of contrast enhancement, demonstrated on post-gadolinium-DTPA MR scans, with areas of malignant neovascularity and endothelial proliferation within solid tumour. It is important to note, however, that margins of enhancement demonstrated only the most damaged part of the blood–brain barrier and did not necessarily correlate with the full extent of tumour.

Intracerebral tumours

Most tumours, whether primary or secondary, demonstrate a non-specific increase in T_1 and T_2 producing low and high signal on T_1W and T_2W images respectively. More structural detail is recognized within tumours on MRI than with CT but there remains difficulty in separating tumour from vasogenic oedema without paramagnetic tracer enhancement (Fig. 2.3). Primary brain tumours tend to be solitary whereas the hallmark of metastatic tumours is multiplicity of lesions. It may be difficult on CT to demonstrate contiguity of a lesion showing apparent unconnected multiple foci of enhancement which on MR images can be readily appreciated to be solitary. Small brain stem gliomas can be visualized due to abnormal signal and mass effect, as well as their relationship to adjacent structures. Intrinsic lesions in the cerebellum can be differentiated from ependymomas within the fourth ventricle. In the diagnosis of CNS lymphoma, MRI detects more areas of abnormality than CT, allowing the disease process to be more accurately monitored during treatment.

Gadolinium-DTPA has proved unreliable in identifying tumour margin in low grade gliomas (Stack et al 1988a). Although slow growing low-grade lesions with relatively intact blood–brain barrier demonstrated far less enhancement than rapidly growing high-grade tumours, precise tumour grading with gadolinium-DTPA was not possible. Enhancement characteristics following gadolinium-DTPA may, however, prove helpful in biopsy guidance towards the most viable part of the tumour.

Intraparenchymal metastases are more clearly demonstrated with additional lesions identified compared with contrast-enhanced CT. Contrast-enhanced CT, however, more clearly demonstrates leptomeningeal metastases compared with non-enhanced MRI (Krol et al 1988). With the use of gadolinium-DTPA more lesions can be identified and leptomeningeal spread clearly depicted. Haemorrhage can be demonstrated in primary intracranial tumours but is much more commonly seen in metastases. Certain CNS metastases, including those from malignant melanoma, choriocarcinoma, carcinoma of the kidney, bronchus or thyroid, have a tendency to haemorrhage and this can be clearly demonstrated as a high signal (short T_1) on T_1W images. Intracranial melanoma metastases can also appear high signal on T_1W images due to the presence of melanin which in itself is paramagnetic (Atlas et al 1987a).

Large intracranial vessels associated with haemorrhage suggests an arteriovenous malformation or a very vascular tumour such as an haemangioblastoma. These can be differentiated by the use of gadolinium-DTPA (Stack et al 1988a). The distinction between non-neoplastic intracerebral haematoma and haemorrhagic intracerebral malignant lesions can be made from the different signal intensity patterns (Atlas et al 1987b). MR images of haemorrhagic intracerebral malignancies showed notable signal heterogeneity, often with identifiable non-haemorrhagic tissue corresponding to tumour, and pronounced or persistent oedema. These appearances were not found with non-neoplastic haematomas.

Radiation change and residual/recurrent tumour

A high occurrence of clinically asymptomatic signal intensity alterations in MR brain studies of patients treated previously by surgery and/or radiotherapy appears to limit the diagnostic value of this technique in differentiating post-treatment change from tumour. Contrast-enhanced CT has been considered of more value than non-enhanced MRI in assessing these patients (Oot et al 1988). Changes secondary to radiotherapy, such as oedema, ischaemia, demyelination and necrosis, can produce prolongation of relaxation times which can be shown as a non-specific high signal on T_2W images (Tsuruda et al 1987). Radiation-induced abnormality is characterized by symmetrical high signal foci in the periventricular white matter with relative sparing of the posterior fossa, basal ganglia and internal capsules. The effect is more marked in older patients.

Lampert and Davis (1964) separated the clinical effects of cranial irradiation into acute, early-delayed and late-delayed. The acute effects, which occur during the course of the irradiation, are thought to be due to vasogenic oedema from damage to capillary endothelium leading to breakdown of the blood–brain barrier. Early-delayed effects occurring a few weeks to a few months after irradiation are in keeping with axonal demyelination and are thought to be reversible. Late-delayed effects occurring months to years later and considered due to radiation necrosis may be demonstrated on CT or MRI as a mass lesion with surrounding oedema associated with breakdown of the blood–brain barrier. In an animal study of brain radiation injury, Hecht-Leavitt et al (1987) suggested that gadolinium-DTPA may be helpful in separating necrosis from demyelination and oedema. Radiation necrosis enhanced following gadolinium-DTPA with no change noted in areas of demyelination or oedema. Thus contrast enhancement following gadolinium-DTPA in radiation necrosis may well be indistinguishable from that of recurrent tumour (Earnest et al 1988) (Fig. 2.4). Following radiotherapy, in addition to any reduction in tumour mass and oedema, a return to a more normal signal in the area of abnormality has been noted. It is uncertain at present whether this represents true remission.

In a study of paediatric patients after brain tumour resection, Bird et al (1988) demonstrated that the use of gadolinium-DTPA significantly improved the identification of residual/recurrent tumour with differentiation from postoperative change. The interval between surgery and MRI was important, as differentiation could not be

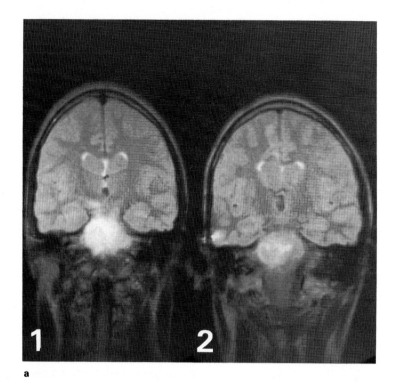

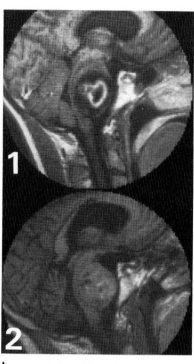

a

b

Fig. 2.4   Brain stem glioma (1) before and (2) six months after radiotherapy. (a) coronal T_2W (SE 2000/80) images (1) preradiotherapy demonstrating a mass lesion with oedema in the pons; (2) postradiotherapy showing reduction in signal intensity and oedema. (b) sagittal post-Gd-DTPA T_1W (IR 2060/500) images (1) preradiotherapy image showing well-defined enhancement indicating tumour with surrounding non-enhanced oedema; (2) postradiotherapy scan shows a less intense and more diffuse enhancement with little surrounding oedema in keeping with radiation change.

reliably made on gadolinium-DTPA enhanced scans in the early (1–2 months) postoperative period. During the first few months following surgery a hypervascular scar was formed at the resection site and, being devoid of a blood–brain barrier, was enhanced following gadolinium-DTPA. Gliosis and microcystic encephalomalacia (hypovascular scar) which developed after about six months showed no enhancement and was recognized as ill-defined areas of high signal on T_2W images (Hesselink & Press 1988).

Extracerebral tumours

Meningioma is the commonest benign intracranial tumour and early MR studies have shown CT to be more accurate in the diagnosis of these tumours. This low sensitivity in the detection of meningiomas by MRI is due to a lack of contrast between tumour and adjacent brain and an inability to detect calcification. The use of gadolinium-DTPA makes these tumours much more readily demonstrable due to consistent intense homogeneous enhancement on T_1W images, thus overcoming this earlier limitation (Stack et al 1988a) (Fig. 2.5). Multiplanar imaging and tumour enhancement characteristics allow detection of en plaque meningiomas and dural extension which can be difficult to demonstrate on CT. Indeed, the pre- and post-gadolinium-DTPA appearances of these tumours on MRI are characteristic and can be used to differentiate meningioma from most other intracranial and intraspinal tumours.

Acoustic neuromas (Schwannomas) typically have homogeneous low signal on T_1W and heterogeneous high signal on T_2W images. Large lesions can be easily recognized and often differentiated from meningiomas by morphological appearance and demonstration of an intrameatal

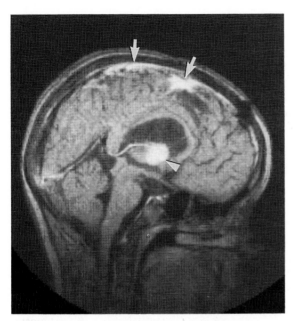

Fig. 2.5 Patient with neurofibromatosis showing an enhanced III ventricle meningioma (arrowhead) on a sagittal post-Gd-DTPA PSR (500/18) scan. There is also abnormal enhancement within the interhemispheric fissure and over the dura (straight arrows) due to a recurrent second meningioma.

portion. Small neuromas confined to the internal meatus are poorly demonstrated on unenhanced MR scans. Gadolinium-DTPA increased the sensitivity in detection of acoustic neuromas including small intrameatal tumours (Stack et al 1988b). Uniform intense enhancement, similar to meningioma, was noted with clearer margination and relationship to adjacent structures compared with non-enhanced MR scans. The intrameatal portion of large acoustic neuromas was more clearly delineated. Cystic degeneration of tumour could be differentiated from associated arachnoid cyst by rim enhancement of the tumoral cyst wall following gadolinium-DTPA. The combination of intravenous gadolinium-DTPA and fast imaging techniques (dynamic MR studies) has indicated characteristic time courses of contrast enhancement enabling differentiation between meningiomas and neuromas (Felix et al 1988).

MRI evaluation of the sella and juxtasellar region requires the use of thin (3 mm) section high resolution scanning (Daniels & Haughton 1987). The extent of large pituitary adenomas can be well shown on coronal and sagittal MRI. Solid adenomas have a signal intensity similar to that of brain on T_1W and T_2W images. Cystic and necrotic areas within the tumour are characterized by having a signal intensity approached that of CSF. Haemorrhage, producing a high signal on T_1W images, can be easily appreciated on MR but not on CT. Any suprasellar extension can be demonstrated together with its relation to the optic chiasm. In a study of 26 large pituitary tumours with suprasellar extension, 16 tumours were markedly constricted at the diaphragma sellae on sagittal MRI (Mikhael & Ciric 1988). The importance of recognizing this appearance is that a transphenoidal surgical approach did not allow total removal. In addition, significant problems occurred in some patients as the remaining suprasellar portion of the tumour rapidly increased in size following surgery from postoperative haemorrhage or oedema.

Coronal MR scanning can visualize the carotid syphon. This can obviate the need for angiography to rule out an intrasellar aneurysm which on contrast-enhanced CT can mimic a pituitary tumour. In a prospective study of 30 patients undergoing surgery for pituitary tumour, MRI revealed a sensitivity for predicting cavernous sinus invasion of only 55% (Scotti et al 1988). The reason was that the medial dural reflection (pituitary capsule) could not be identified on MR although dural infiltration by pituitary microadenomas was frequently found on pathological review. The lateral dural margin of the cavernous sinus could be recognized as a discrete low intensity line. Unilateral carotid encasement within the cavernous sinus adjacent to a pituitary tumour was found to be an infrequent but specific sign predicting infiltration. Pituitary microadenomas (less than 10 mm) can be demonstrated on T_1W images as a focal low intensity area within the pituitary. Following gadolinium-DTPA serial T_1W images displayed early enhancement of the normal pituitary gland and delayed enhancement of the microadenomas (Dwyer et al 1987). The rôle of gadolinium-DTPA in the assessment of microadenomas and cavernous sinus invasion has yet to be determined.

Craniopharyngiomas may be cystic, often with high cholesterol content, or solid containing calcium. They differ from most sella and juxtasellar lesions in that their diagnosis depends to a large extent on the detection of calcification, in which CT is superior to MRI. In a study of 20 patients with craniopharyngioma, Pusey et al (1987) noted that, although CT was superior to MR in detection of calcification, the identification of the presence and extent of the tumour was better on MR. There was a wide range of appearances on the T_1W images in keeping with variable histological pattern. Areas of short T_1 may reflect the presence of high cholesterol content or methaemoglobin. MR and CT were found to be complementary with CT being more specific in establishing the diagnosis of craniopharyngioma and MR preferred in the evaluation of tumour extent for presurgical and radiation planning.

Chordomas involving the clivus and adjacent structures can be well delineated on sagittal and coronal T_1W images (Oot et al 1988). Similar appearances, however, can occur with metastatic involvement of the clivus. Pineal tumours (pinealomas, teratomas and gliomas) are well shown but not differentiated.

Orbital and ocular MRI

The MRI evaluation of orbital and ocular lesions has improved since the introduction of thin (3–5 mm) section high resolution surface coil imaging providing spatial resolution comparable to the latest generation of CT scanners (Zimmerman & Bilaniuk 1988a). Significant MR image degradation due to eye movement remains a major problem. CT and ultrasound are established techniques in the evaluation of ocular and orbital disease respectively and comparative studies with MRI are required.

A variety of ocular tumours, the majority being primary uveal melanomas, have been studied using thin section high resolution MRI and CT (Peyster et al 1988). All tumours were visualized by MRI but only 88% were shown on CT. There was sufficient variation in signal intensity between different tumours on MRI to allow some separation. Gholkar et al (1988) reported a case of plexiform trigeminal neurofibroma which extended into the orbit and the use of gadolinium-DTPA was assessed. Distinction of

the intraorbital part of the tumour from orbital fatty tissue was made more difficult post-gadolinium-DTPA due to the increase in signal intensity within the tumour. Thus the role of gadolinium-DTPA in orbital lesions may be limited but needs to be assessed in the evaluation of ocular pathology.

Phakomatoses

The phakomatoses include neurofibromatosis, tuberous sclerosis and von Hippel–Lindau syndrome and the CNS manifestations on MRI have been the subject of a recent review (Braffman et al 1988). All three phakomatoses have an increased incidence of tumours which in the case of neurofibromatosis and von Hippel–Lindau syndrome are characteristically multiple (Fig. 2.5). MRI can significantly contribute to the diagnostic evaluation providing an opportunity for early detection of tumours and subsequent improved management and prognosis. Although clinical stigmata are usually diagnostic, when clinical features are not yet apparent or forme fruste cases occur the diagnosis may depend on radiological assessment. Indeed, a definitive diagnosis is important for prognostic reasons and for genetic counselling of patients and relatives.

The high sensitivity in the detection of the various CNS tumours, especially with the use of gadolinium-DTPA, and the lack of ionizing radiation makes MRI an attractive screening technique in view of the multiple examinations recommended in patients in this group (Jennings & Gaines 1988).

SPINE

MRI has had a major impact on spinal imaging but further research is required in the assessment of new techniques and developments including 3D-imaging and contrast media (Haughton 1988). The advantages over other imaging techniques include an impressive image quality, a multiplanar facility and negligible risk. Surface coil imaging has provided much improved spatial resolution with reduction in artefacts from respiratory and cardiac motion. Significant CSF flow artefacts can occur particularly in the cervical region which, however, can be reduced by using a combination of CSF-gating and gradient echo techniques (Enzmann & Rubin 1988).

The spinal cord, including the conus, cauda equina and nerve roots, can be directly and routinely demonstrated on both T_1W and PSR sequences. The surrounding CSF within the spinal canal provides a low signal whilst epidural fat and veins give a high signal. Neural tissue is delineated as an intermediate signal. On heavily T_2W images a high signal is obtained from CSF (due to its very long T_2) producing an MR myelographic effect. High resolution surface coil imaging, particularly with gradient echo sequences, can demonstrate grey/white matter differentiation (Czervionke & Daniels 1988).

Spinal tumours

Intramedullary, intradural-extramedullary and extradural tumours can be differentiated and MRI provides more information than myelography and CT (Jenkins et al 1988a, Zimmerman & Bilaniuk 1988b, Isherwood et al 1989). Most spinal tumours produce a non-specific prolongation in T_1 and T_2 compared with neural tissue, and can be distinguished from surrounding CSF on moderate T_2W images. The extent and location of tumours and their appearance can be fully evaluated particularly with the use of gadolinium-DTPA. More lesions are demonstrated with increased conspicuity compared with non-enhanced MR scans and other imaging techniques (Jenkins et al 1988a, Sze 1988). Normal spinal cord and nerve roots do not enhance following gadolinium-DTPA due to an intact blood–brain barrier in the intradural space.

The majority of intramedullary tumours are gliomas, mainly ependymomas or astrocytomas, with the remainder including oligodendrogliomas, haemangioblastomas and metastases. MRI cannot distinguish between ependymomas and astrocytomas. These tumours show irregular expansion of the cord usually over several vertebral segments which can be well demonstrated on sagittal imaging (Fig. 2.6). Differentiation of cystic from solid components of intramedullary tumours can be made in the majority of cases, but

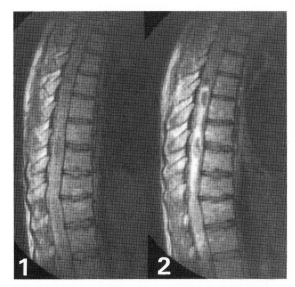

Fig. 2.6 Low grade glioma on sagittal T_1W (SE 700/40) (1) pre- and (2) post-Gd-DTPA images through the dorsal spine demonstrating enhancement of a partially cystic tumour. (Reproduced with permission from Clinical Radiology, 1989 (in press).)

ambiguity can occur when cysts contain proteinaceous fluid simulating solid components on MRI (Goy et al 1986). Both tumoral cysts and tumour-associated syrinxes can occur and can be differentiated using gadolinium-DTPA (Jenkins et al 1988a). In tumoral cysts early enhancement of the cyst wall with late enhancement within the cyst was observed with no abnormal enhancement noted in syrinxes. Late postradiation necrosis of the cord, which shows delayed patchy enhancement within myelomalacic areas, can be differentiated from recurrent tumour with gadolinium-DTPA. Haemangioblastomas are found in association with von Hippel–Lindau syndrome and following gadolinium-DTPA show characteristic marked enhancement. MR, particularly with gadolinium-DTPA, appears to be the optimum method for demonstrating intramedullary metastases.

The two most common intradural-extramedullary tumours, meningiomas and neurofibromas/Schwannomas, can usually be differentiated by signal intensity appearances. While large meningiomas and neurofibromas/Schwannomas can be demonstrated and differentiated in the majority of cases, small intradural-extramedullary tumours and leptomeningeal tumour infiltration may go undetected (Sze 1988). Intradural-extramedullary metastases are not as well demonstrated on non-enhanced MRI compared with water-soluble myelography with or without CT. The administration of gadolinium-DTPA overcomes this limitation, allowing more lesions of smaller size to be demonstrated compared with other imaging techniques (Jenkins et al 1988a, Sze 1988) (Fig. 2.7). Leptomeningeal tumour infiltration shows increasing enhancement and is better demonstrated on delayed post-gadolinium-DTPA scans. En plaque leukaemia and lymphomatous infiltration can be detected as a non-specific enhancing diffuse enlargement of the cauda equina.

Extradural tumours in the adult population are mainly metastases in the vertebral body and epidural space. MRI can demonstrate bony change and soft tissue extent including cord compression or involvement due to extradural tumour. Replacement of marrow by plasmacytoma or multiple myeloma can be well shown on T_1W images as a non-specific intermediate signal contrasted by a high signal from surrounding uninvolved marrow. Tumours in the paediatric age group include neuroblastomas and ganglioneuromas which can infiltrate spinal structures. The soft tissue extent, bone involvement and cord compression from such tumours can be well demonstrated on MRI (vide infra). Following gadolinium-DTPA, the paraspinal soft tissue component of the extradural tumour enhances and is well delineated, but bone involvement can be less conspicuous. This is found particularly in patients following radiotherapy where the replacement of normal marrow by fat within the radiation field predominates. The low signal intensity tumour (long T_1) enhances following gadolinium-DTPA and becomes isointense with marrow on T_1W images. The PSR sequence has been found to be particularly useful in this situation with enhancing tumour contrasted against low signal vertebral marrow (Jenkins et al 1988a) (Fig. 2.8).

EXTRACRANIAL HEAD AND NECK

The primary rôle of imaging in head and neck tumours is to define the extent of disease as this

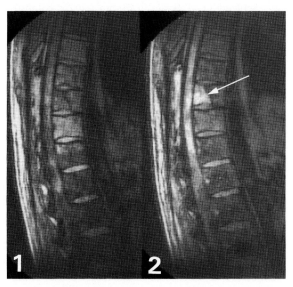

Fig. 2.8 Metastatic carcinoma involving D9 vertebral body with intramedullary metastases following laminectomy and palliative radiotherapy. Sagittal PSR (500/18) scans (1) pre- and (2) post-Gd-DTPA. The spinal metastasis (arrowed) and intramedullary lesions can only be demonstrated on the post-Gd-DTPA scan. The uninvolved marrow shows an increased signal due to fatty replacement from previous radiotherapy making the spinal metastases less conspicuous on the unenhanced scan.

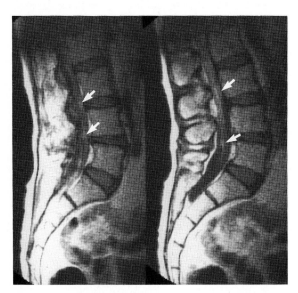

Fig. 2.7 Intradural drop metastases (arrowed) on spinal nerve roots on contiguous sagittal T_1W (SE 600/40) post-Gd-DTPA scans.

information is important in determining management and treatment. MRI, even at an early stage of development, is the imaging method of choice in the assessment of the majority of extracranial head and neck lesions (Lufkin & Hanafee 1988, Rafto & Gefter 1988). The advantages of MRI include a higher soft tissue contrast resolution and discrimination than can be achieved with CT, an ability to demonstrate head and neck vessels without the need for intravenous contrast medium, a multiplanar facility, and the absence of artefact from dental amalgam or beam hardening which degrades CT scans. The use of surface coils has improved the resolution particularly for small structures within the larynx. Whilst dental amalgam causes no problem, significant local artefact occurs with ferromagnetic dental appliances and surgical clips, although the extent of artefact is much reduced compared with CT scans of the same area (Hinshaw et al 1988).

T_1W images are useful in defining contrast between tumour and adjacent fat/mucosa with T_2W images providing information on tumour infiltration of muscle. MRI has significant advantages over CT for planning radiation therapy for the head and neck including improved delineation of tumour extension, ability to image in any plane without changing patient position and a lack of artefact from the immobilization cast (Toonkel et al 1988). A new needle for MR-guided aspiration cytology of the head and neck has been described and can be used with the fast gradient echo technique. Early studies have indicated a potential role for gadolinium-DTPA in the study of head and neck tumours (Jenkins et al 1988b).

Paranasal sinuses

MRI not only clearly defines extent but can differentiate paranasal tumours from inflammatory tissue on the basis of their signal intensity appearances on T_2W images (Som et al 1988a) (Fig. 2.9). The majority (90–95%) of these tumours have an intermediate signal on T_2W images, whereas inflammatory disease, characterized by interstitial oedema, serous fluid and mucus secretion, has a high signal. Similar high signals are noted with polyps, retention cysts and

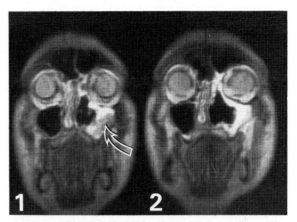

Fig. 2.9   Coronal T_2W (SE 2000/80) images (1) pre- and (2) postradiotherapy. In (1) the recurrent tumour (arrowed) can be delineated as an intermediate signal separate from surrounding inflammatory tissue (high signal). Follow-up examination six months postradiotherapy (2) indicates resolution of tumour with residual inflammatory tissue.

mucocoeles. The remaining 5–10% of sinonasal tumours include adenoidcystic carcinomas and mucoserous minor salivary gland tumours. The importance of differentiating tumour from adjacent inflammatory tissue is in providing more accurate staging, thus allowing more precise treatment in terms of extent and size of radiation portals. Areas of much reduced signal within areas of high signal on T_2W images usually represents fibrosis, calcification, bone, mycetoma or haemorrhage rather than tumour.

Following radiotherapy or chemotherapy MRI can be used to assess response and allow differentiation of recurrent or residual tumour and inflammatory disease. Problems arise in differentiating postoperative mature fibrosis (low signal) which when mixed with inflammatory disease produces an intermediate signal similar to that from recurrent tumour. Primary bone tumours are more accurately defined and extent determined by CT. Bone involvement by paranasal tumours is more easily defined on CT although erosion of the bony sinuses can be defined on MR by loss of the normal low signal cortical bone. Extension outside the sinuses is more accurately determined by MRI allowing differentiation between tumour and muscle/fat to be made with a high degree of precision. Assessment of skull base infiltration and

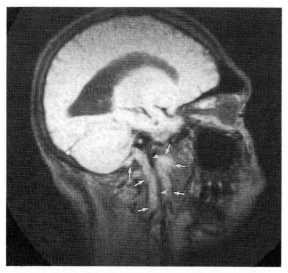

Fig. 2.10 Nasopharyngeal carcinoma (straight arrows) on parasagittal PSR (500/18) scan. The tumour is surrounding the carotid artery (arrowheads) and has infiltrated through the jugular foramen into the intracranial cavity.

intracranial extension is more clearly defined by MR particularly using sagittal and coronal planes with gadolinium-DTPA (Lloyd et al 1987, Jenkins et al 1988b). Angiofibromas have a rich vascular bed and can be diagnosed by the demonstration of flow void channels within the stroma of low–intermediate signal on T_1W and T_2W images.

Nasopharynx

Confines of the nasopharynx are well demonstrated on multiplanar imaging. Normal mucosa give a high signal on T_2W images contrasting with an intermediate signal from underlying muscle. A significant limitation with the use of gadolinium-DTPA is the intense enhancement of the mucosal tissue which can obscure any contrast difference between it and the tumour. Nasopharyngeal carcinomas tend to infiltrate submucosally into and through the skull base (Teresi et al 1987) (Fig. 2.10). MRI can be helpful in demonstrating the presence of an undisclosed primary in the nasopharynx in a patient with a solitary enlarged metastatic neck node (Lufkin & Hanafee 1988).

Salivary glands

In the evaluation of clinically suspected parotid masses MRI is able to site accurately the location of the tumour either intrinsic or extrinsic to the parotid. Although this distinction can be made on CT, by demonstrating a fat plane separation between the deep lobe of the parotid and parapharyngeal space, it is more clearly defined on MRI. More detail of the internal structure of the tumour is evident on MRI. By using surface coils the facial nerve can be directly visualized and small- and medium-sized masses can be sited superficial or deep to this nerve.

Salivary tumours have long T_2 and are better shown on T_2W images. MRI is unable to specify tumour type and although an indistinct tumour margin suggests malignancy, this is not a consistent finding. Also, focal calcification (a finding suggestive of a pleomorphic adenoma) and cystic necrosis (indicating a malignant tumour) were not seen on MRI in the series reported by Som et al (1988b). These findings were better shown on CT thus providing more clinically relevant information.

Tongue and oropharynx

Tongue and tonsillar fossa tumours, although well shown on MRI, can be overestimated on T_2W images due to surrounding oedema. Superficial spreading tumours may not be detected even with gadolinium-DTPA (Vogl et al 1988). The use of gadolinium-DTPA more accurately demonstrates the size, depth of invasion and spread across the midline compared with non-enhanced scans and CT. Although there is some loss of image detail due to swallowing, MRI provides superior soft tissue detail in the evaluation of the tongue and oropharynx compared with CT (Lufkin & Hanafee 1988).

Parapharyngeal space

Paragangliomas (glomus tumours) are slow-growing hypervascular tumours originally reported as having a characteristic 'salt and pepper' appearance on T_2W images due to a high signal from slow-flowing blood and tumour interspersed with serpentine areas of signal void (Olsen et al 1986). Som et al (1987) demonstrated that other vascular lesions in the parapharyngeal space can produce a similar appearance including renal and thyroid metastases and venous haemangiomas. Small paragangliomas (less than 1.5 cm) have uniformly intense appearance on T_2W images. Other parapharyngeal lesions, including salivary gland tumours, neurogenic tumours, lymphoma and sarcoma are hypovascular with relatively homogeneous signal intensity. The majority of lesions within the parapharyngeal space have an intermediate signal on T_1W and a relatively high signal on T_2W images. Som et al (1988b) have indicated that the three main extraparotid tumours – glomus tumour, neurofibroma and minor salivary gland tumour – can be differentiated on MR. The glomus tumour had a different signal intensity appearance from the other two tumours. Although neuromas were indistinguishable from salivary gland tumours they displaced the internal carotid artery anteriorly whereas salivary gland tumours displaced the artery posteriorly. This artery is better demonstrated on MR than on CT.

Larynx

MRI shows superior soft tissue discrimination defining deep infiltration and full extent of laryngeal tumour compared with CT. T_1W images maximize contrast between tumour (intermediate signal) and surrounding normal tissue (high signal). Macroscopic cartilage invasion with early invasion of cartilage can be detected by intermediate signal intensity on T_1W images (Castelijns et al 1987). Motion artefact due to chronic respiratory disease, however, produced non-diagnostic scans in 16% of patients. Coronal and sagittal scans can visualize the intrinsic laryngeal muscles which are important in recognizing subtle tumour extension. Any associated lymphadenopathy can be demonstrated using similar criteria as in CT. Limitations in imaging the larynx include an absence of mucosal detail and an inability to detect microscopic spread of tumour and to differentiate between inflammation, oedema, haemorrhage or tumour. Although at an early stage of development, MRI is the imaging method of choice in defining the extent of laryngeal disease.

Thyroid

The thyroid gland has a signal intensity slightly greater than muscle on T_1W and a much more intense signal on T_2W images. MRI can detect focal (4–5 mm) or diffuse lesions within the thyroid but is unable to differentiate between benign nodules and focal carcinoma. Haemorrhagic degeneration which is more suggestive of an adenoma can be defined on MRI. Surrounding infiltration from carcinoma is also well shown. MRI has been shown to be helpful in patients who have undergone previous thyroidectomy for carcinoma in distinguishing between recurrent/residual tumour and chronic fibrosis (Auffermann et al 1988). Tumour appeared low and high signal on T_1W and T_2W images respectively whereas chronic fibrosis appeared low signal on both. MRI is able to demonstrate a pseudocapsule which is a fibrous structure forming a boundary between tumour and normal thyroid tissues. Noma et al (1988) by relating the appearance of this pseudocapsule have demonstrated characteristic patterns helpful in differentiating benign and malignant disease.

MUSCULOSKELETAL SYSTEM

Since the first MR image of a wrist was reported by Hinshaw et al (1977) the applications of MRI in the musculoskeletal system have gained wide acceptance and importance (Sartoris & Resnick 1987, Ehman et al 1988). Its use in the evaluation of musculoskeletal disease is, in terms of ranking, second to brain imaging in many MR units. Technical advances including the development of surface coils, higher resolution 3-dimensional gradient echo techniques and paramagnetic contrast agents have brought about rapid improvement.

There is good delineation of the fascial planes, subcutaneous fat, vessels, nerves, ligaments, tendons and muscles on both T_1W and PSR sequences. The joint capsule, cartilage, ligaments, menisci and growth plates are well distinguished. The major tissues in the extremities are muscle and fat. Muscle has a very short T_2 and appears low signal on T_2W images enabling distinction to be made between most mass lesions and muscle. Fat in adipose tissues and fatty marrow has a very short T_1, appearing high signal on T_1W and PSR images and providing good contrast between mass lesions and fat. Compact bone gives no signal on all sequences. The neurovascular bundles in the extremities can be routinely visualized using surface coil imaging.

Primary bone and soft tissue tumours

The preservation of life and limb function are the two important aims in the treatment of most malignant musculoskeletal tumours. The improved contrast resolution associated with the multiplanar facility of MRI allows the intra- and extraosseous extent of bone and soft tissue tumours to be more clearly and accurately defined compared with plain radiographs and CT (Vanel et al 1987, Ehman et al 1988). Displacement and involvement of adjacent neurovascular structures by soft tissue tumours can be accurately assessed (Fig. 2.11a). In a primary bone tumour, MRI is superior to CT in demonstrating not only its intraosseous extent

(including the presence or absence of 'skip' lesions), but also in assessing the integrity of the growth plate, joint space and adjacent tissues. Gillespy et al (1988) studied 17 patients with osteosarcoma of an extremity comparing the accuracy of preoperative CT and MRI in measurement of intraosseous tumour extent with macroslides of surgical specimens. MRI was more accurate than CT with an average of 2–5 mm difference between the macroslide and MRI measurements (for CT the difference was 17 mm).

Most tumours and other soft tissue masses have long T_1 and long T_2 relaxation times, appearing as low or high signal on T_1W or T_2W images respectively. T_1W images demonstrate high contrast between tumour and fat or marrow and are useful in the evaluation of intraosseous extent of tumour. T_2W images provide high contrast between tumour and muscle or blood vessels in which there is rapid blood flow (Fig. 2.11). The PSR sequence is useful in delineating tumour and adjacent blood vessels, together with intraosseous extent, providing a higher soft tissue contrast within bone than either T_1W or T_2W sequences (Fig. 2.12). A similar effect is also noted when using STIR where

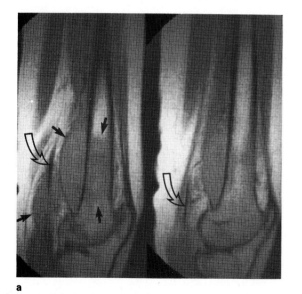 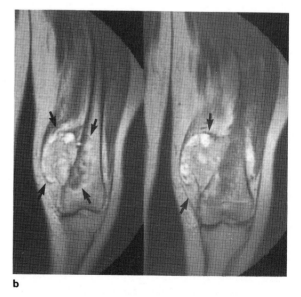

a   **b**

Fig. 2.11   Osteosarcoma in a lower femur on contiguous (a) sagittal T_1W (SE 1100/26) and (b) coronal T_2W (SE 2000/80) images. The extent of the tumour within bone and soft tissues (straight arrows) is clearly delineated. The popliteal artery (curved open arrow) is displaced by the extraosseous mass. (Reproduced from Galasko C S B, Isherwood I (eds) 1989 Imaging techniques in orthopaedics, Springer-Verlag, Berlin.

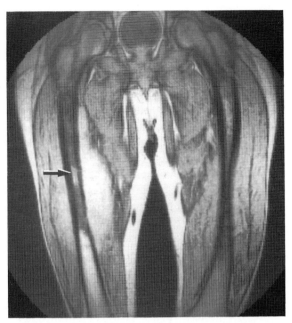

Fig. 2.12 Malignant lymphoma on coronal PSR (500/18) image. The tumour is of high signal and is infiltrating along the medial shaft of the femur into the marrow cavity (arrowed). There is a lower signal from adjacent marrow due to oedema/hyperaemia.

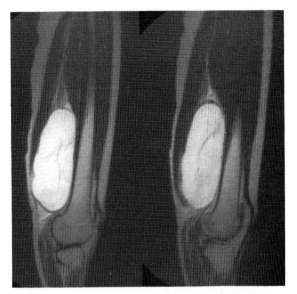

Fig. 2.13 Liposarcoma on contiguous sagittal T_2W (SE 2000/80) images. The tumour has a relatively homogeneous signal, different in signal intensity to that of surrounding fat. It appears well marginated with a low intensity rim.

the signals from T_1 and T_2 are summated (Dwyer et al 1988). In addition to using different pulse sequences, more than one imaging plane is required in order to evaluate accurately the extent, especially the peripheral margins, of a tumour.

In general, there are no specific characteristics on MRI which distinguish a malignant from a benign tumour, or tumour from other pathology such as infection. Similar morphological criteria hold as for CT. Whether a lesion is well demarcated from or infiltrating adjacent tissues is not a reliable indicator of malignancy (Levine et al 1987) (Fig. 2.13). Malignant and benign tumours usually overlap in signal intensity and Pettersson et al (1988) have found T_1 and T_2 measurements to be of limited value for histological characterization. Most malignant lesions exhibit homogeneous and heterogeneous signal intensity on T_1W and T_2W images respectively. Homogeneity in signal intensity is often seen with benign soft tissue tumours but some, particularly neurofibromas and haemangiomas, have heterogeneous signal intensity on T_2W images. Intramuscular haemangiomas have a

consistent MR appearance in the majority of cases, with a high signal on T_1W and T_2W images associated with focal muscle atrophy (Yuh et al 1987). On T_2W images small lesions (<2 cm) appeared homogeneous and well defined; larger haemangiomas consisted of dilated tortuous vascular channels enabling a preoperative diagnosis to be made. Cohen et al (1988) have noted that the MR appearance and configuration of cartilage lesions vary depending on the presence of a hyaline matrix. Osteochondromas, enchondromas and chondrosarcomas have a distinctive homogeneous high signal intensity in a defined lobular pattern on T_2W images corresponding to areas of hyaline cartilage matrix. Other cartilage lesions including chondromas and clear cell chondrosarcoma were isointense or hypointense compared with muscle on all sequences, due to the presence of a much more cellular stroma and less mature chondroid matrix. These latter tumours could not be differentiated from non-cartilage tumours. Calcification strongly suggestive of cartilage matrix on plain radiographs could not be consistently identified on MRI.

Although lipomas (short T_1, long T_2) have a characteristic MR appearance, appearing as high signal on both T_1W and T_2W images, Petasnick et al (1986) noted no differences in signal intensity in the majority (six out of seven) of benign and malignant fatty tumours (Fig. 2.13). One exception was a liposarcoma, which had very little fatty element on subsequent histological review. Similar signal intensity changes to fat have been noted in intramuscular haemorrhage and haematomas, and from haemorrhage within tumour, thus making these pathologies difficult to distinguish on MR signal intensity appearances alone. The use of phase-contrast imaging is likely to overcome this limitation. Areas of necrosis and cystic change are characterized by prolonged T_1 and T_2 values, giving very low or high signals on T_1W or T_2W images respectively. In aneurysmal bone cysts a distinctive appearance has been reported in which the cysts demonstrate fluid levels containing blood of various ages (Hudson et al 1985).

Both benign and malignant fibrous tumours have been noted to have low signal on all sequences, in keeping with a low proton density related to abundant collagen and marked acellularity within the tumour (Sundaram et al 1987). Aggressive fibromatosis (desmoid tumour) differs in that the majority have signal intensity greater than muscle on T_2W images and slightly higher on T_1W images. These tumours have irregular margins infiltrating along the neurovascular bundle and are particularly difficult to define on CT.

In the assessment of tumour recurrence in the postoperative patient metallic surgical clips or prostheses produce only minimal localized artefact on the MR image and diagnostic scans can often be obtained. There are some metallic implants, however, which are ferromagnetic, producing significant MR image artefact. Irregular metal objects such as screws and the screw ends of Harrington rods can produce similar problems. As with CT, problems can arise in interpretation of MR images in separating tumour from radiation therapy and early postoperative change, due to oedema, infection or acute haemorrhage, although some discrimination can be made. Vanel et al (1987) have observed that if a low signal intensity lesion (scar tissue) was seen on T_2W images in a patient with primary malignant musculoskeletal tumour who had undergone radiation therapy or surgery, the patient most likely did not have active tumour.

However, if a high signal lesion was seen after such a patient had undergone surgery, the patient probably had active tumour. In the presence of a high signal on T_2W images in those who had undergone radiation therapy there was difficulty in differentiating active tumour from radiation-induced inflammatory reaction.

The main limitations of MRI in assessment of bone and soft tissue tumours include the inability to grade tumours accurately and separate viable tumour, necrosis and surrounding oedema. Early results have indicated that by using gadolinium-DTPA with rapid acquisition gradient echo sequences these limitations may be overcome (Reiser et al 1988). In malignant tumours early signal increase was more rapid and intense compared with benign lesions. Viable tumour could be differentiated from necrosis and surrounding oedema — a distinction which could not be made on conventional T_1W post-gadolinium-DTPA scans. Although early recurrence following surgery could not be differentiated from postoperative change, late recurrence using gadolinium-DTPA could, however, be defined. Plain radiography or CT remain superior in the detection of calcification, periosteal reaction, fractures or gas formation. CT is the imaging method of choice in determining the presence or absence of pulmonary metastases, with radionuclide bone scanning being used in the identification of bone metastases.

Bone marrow imaging

MRI is ideally suited for studying bone marrow due to a high inherent soft tissue contrast resolution, a high sensitivity in detection of disease and an absence of streak artefacts from cortical bone (Sartoris & Resnick 1987, Vogler & Murphy 1988). T_1W and T_2W sequences have been commonly used for bone marrow imaging to date but the use of STIR, phase-contrast and gradient echo images have particular advantages (Vogler & Murphy 1988).

There is an age-related change in the relative proportions of fatty and haemopoeitic marrow within cancellous bone. Young children have a more extensive distribution of haemopoeitic marrow compared with adults and this is reflected in lower marrow signals on T_1W and PSR images in the appendicular skeleton and spine (Vogler & Murphy 1988). With increasing age the haemopoeitic marrow gradually recedes from the appendicular skeleton, being replaced in part by fatty marrow which can be demonstrated as a high signal on T_1W and PSR images. The largest red marrow fractions reside in the axial skeleton (particularly the lumbar spine), pelvis and proximal femora.

Multiple myeloma, metastases, leukaemia and lymphoma produce focal or generalized infiltration of bone marrow leading to non-specific prolongation of relaxation times. Difficulty has been noted in assessment of focal as opposed to more diffuse disease. In a preliminary study of nine adult patients with acute leukaemia, Thomsen et al (1987) have shown that measured T_1 values of vertebral body marrow were significantly ($p<0.01$) prolonged in patients compared with normal control. Following chemotherapy, T_1 values decreased towards the reference range in those who underwent remission but remained prolonged in those who did not. Similar findings have been observed in children. These results indicate an important and clinically useful area of progress in the assessment of disease and monitoring treatment with MRI.

Irradiation of marrow or chemotherapy can result in ablation of haemopoietic active tissue which is subsequently replaced by fatty marrow. This change can be visualized on MRI by diffuse increase in signal (short T_1) on T_1W and particularly PSR images of vertebral bodies allowing the radiation portal to be sharply defined (Fig. 2.7).

ABDOMEN AND RETROPERITONEUM

There are several factors limiting the clinical utility of MRI in the abdomen including significant motion artefacts from breathing, bowel peristalsis and cardiac and blood vessel pulsation, and reduced signal-to-noise ratio especially with the longer data acquisition sequences (IR and T_2W). Advances in MRI technology with the development of new pulse sequences, including fast scanning techniques, and MR contrast agents are likely to have a significant impact (Laniado et al 1988).

Liver

The normal liver has a homogeneous intermediate signal with a shorter T_1 and T_2 than spleen. On T_1W images it is difficult to distinguish bile ducts and hepatic arteries at the porta hepatis. On T_2W images the bile ducts (long T_2) show a high signal (Kressel 1988). The vascular anatomy can be clearly visualized due to the high contrast provided by flowing blood. An optimal technique is of paramount importance in achieving sufficient image contrast in the liver in order to detect disease (Kressel 1988, Wittenberg et al 1988, Glazer 1988).

Controversy exists over the use of CT or MRI as the method of choice for staging the extent of abdominal disease in patients with known or suspected cancer. Stark et al (1987) and Chezmar et al (1988) showed MRI to be a more sensitive technique compared with CT (dynamic plus delayed contrast-enhanced CT) in the detection of liver metastases. The former group recommended MRI as a screening technique whereas the latter suggested CT. The reason for this discrepancy is that Chezmar et al (1988) placed more emphasis on the inability of MRI to demonstrate extrahepatic lesions in adjacent organs which occur in approximately 12% of patients at risk from liver metastases. This limitation is due to difficulty in distinguishing extrahepatic tumour from adjacent bowel and should therefore be overcome with the introduction of a suitable bowel contrast agent. Liver metastases show a variable signal intensity appearance, typically low and high signal on T_1W and T_2W images respectively. Haemangiomas appear sharply marginated with low signal on T_1W and have a characteristic very high signal on T_2W images (Wittenberg et al 1988). This allows distinction between haemangioma and malignant lesions in the majority of patients. Hypovascular metastases, as from colon carcinoma, could be distinguished from haemangioma more frequently than could hypervascular endocrine metastases from islet cell tumor, carcinoid and phaeochromocytoma (Glazer 1988). Regenerating liver nodules appear low signal on T_2W images and can be differentiated from malignant lesions in patients with cirrhosis.

Several studies have indicated that hepatocellular carcinoma can be distinguished from other tumours in the liver based on the present of a pseudocapsule in around a third of cases (Itoh et al 1987, Glazer 1988). Lesions less than 2 cm in diameter were not visualized. Hepatoblastoma, a common malignant hepatic tumour in children, can be well demonstrated on MRI. In cholangio-carcinoma Dooms et al (1986) noted minimal contrast difference between tumour and liver in approximately half the cases studied (four out of nine) indicating some difficulty in identifying this tumour. Involvement of liver by lymphoma could not be detected in the majority of cases and in only one out of thirteen patients with histologically-proven lymphomatous involvement did MRI demonstrate a focal abnormality (Weinreb et al 1984). Measurements of relaxation times have been unhelpful in aiding the detection of liver involvement by lymphoma due in part to significant motion artefact during the time scale of the data collection.

A number of exogenous intravenous MR contrast agents have been studied in the liver indicating a potential future rôle. Gadolinium-DTPA combined with rapid gradient echo sequences (performed during a breath hold) have demonstrated hepatic blood flow and tissue perfusion (Hamm et al 1987). Ferrite, an iron oxide, localizes in reticulo-endothelial cells resulting in improved contrast between normal liver and hepatic metastases (Stark et al 1988).

Spleen

The spleen has a longer T_1 and T_2 compared with the liver. A consequence of this is that there is little contrast between focal tumours (metastases or lymphoma) and normal spleen using T_1W and T_2W sequences. Improvement in sensitivity in detection of focal lesions in the spleen has been demonstrated using fast gradient echo sequences (Hess et al 1988). An iron oxide MR contrast agent administered to 18 patients with splenic metastases allowed enhanced detection of disease (Weissleder et al 1988). The importance of the detection of splenic metastases is that it allows more accurate tumour staging.

Pancreas

The pancreas has a similar signal intensity to liver on T_2W images and slightly lower intensity on T_1W images. Retroperitoneal fat, when present, aids demarcation of the margin of the pancreas from adjacent bowel. The major abdominal vessels can be routinely visualized. Improvement in image quality and definition has been achieved by using an antiperistaltic agent together with gaseous distension of the stomach and duodenum.

Pancreatic carcinomas over 2 cm in diameter produce a focal increase in relaxation times and can be demonstrated using similar morphological criteria as for CT (Jenkins et al 1987, Tscholakoff

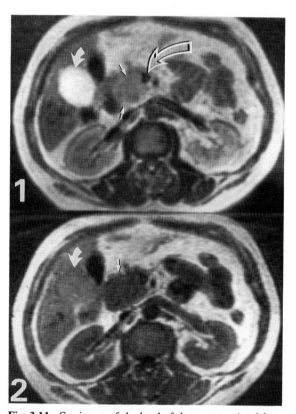

Fig. 2.14 Carcinoma of the head of the pancreas (straight arrows) on (1) intermediate T_2W (SE 1000/60) and (2) T_1W (IR2080/500) images. There is encasement of the superior mesenteric vein (curved open arrow). The signal from the gall bladder contents (curved solid arrow) is related to the relatively short T_1/long T_2 from concentrated bile in a fasted patient. (Reproduced with permission from British Journal of Radiology 1987, 60: 333–341.)

et al 1987). Local extension, biliary obstruction and involvement of major vessels can be demonstrated (Fig. 2.14). Areas of necrosis within tumour demonstrate very long T_1/long T_2 indistinguishable from inflammatory pseudocyst. Islet cell tumours have much longer relaxation time values than adenocarcinoma. Measurements of relaxation times have been unhelpful in discriminating pancreatic tumour from other disease processes (Jenkins et al 1987). At the present time CT provides greater sensitivity for detection of small pancreatic tumours and in the demonstration of small pancreatic calcifications.

Adrenal glands

The transverse plane is the most useful for demonstrating normal-sized adrenals with coronal or sagittal scans helpful in determining the relationship of a large adrenal mass to surrounding structures. A normal adrenal gland has a similar signal intensity to liver on T_1W and T_2W images. Both adrenals can be identified on T_1W images as a low signal contrasting with the high signal from surrounding fat. The cortex and medulla of the adrenal gland cannot be distinguished.

Adrenocortical carcinomas, although rare, are aggressive tumours tending to be large at presentation and thus easily demonstrated. They have a non-specific heterogenous low and high signal relative to liver on T_1W and T_2W images respectively. Liver and bone metastases have similar signal intensity changes to the primary lesion. Involvement of surrounding soft tissues and vascular structures is well demonstrated on MR. In a case report of an adrenal carcinoma extending into the inferior vena cava, the tumour thrombus showed similar enhancement characteristics as the primary lesion following gadolinium-DTPA, allowing separation from non-tumour thrombus (Falke et al 1988). Adrenal metastases can be demonstrated but not distinguished from other mass lesions except on clinical grounds.

Phaeochromocytoma is the commonest tumour of the adrenal medulla and once the diagnosis is suspected the rôle of imaging is to site the tumour. These tumours usually arise in the adrenal gland and can be multiple. They are slightly hypointense and markedly hyperintense relative to liver on T_1W and T_2W images respectively. The markedly high signal on T_2W images is characteristic but can occur in metastatic lesions and other adrenal tumours (Baker et al 1987). The majority of adrenal adenomas are isointense with normal adrenal gland on moderate T_2W images and can usually be differentiated from phaeochromocytomas.

Neuroblastoma is one of the most common solid tumours in childhood usually presenting as an abdominal mass arising from the adrenal gland. Coronal T_1W images allow precise siting of tumour origin (Fig. 2.15). Its extent including any intraspinal component can be demonstrated, obviating the need for more invasive techniques such as water-soluble contrast myelography (Dietrich et al 1987). Neuroblastoma can be differentiated from Wilm's tumour on coronal or sagittal T_1W images. The superior depiction of vascular anatomy and tumour extent on multiplanar imaging allows MR assessment of tumour resectability to be more clearly demonstrated compared with other procedures. MRI can clearly show tumour

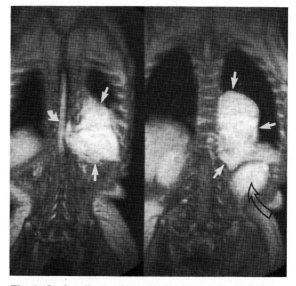

Fig. 2.15 Ganglioneuroblastoma in a three-year-old boy on coronal PSR (520/18) images. The extent of the large left paravertebral mass (straight arrows) is clearly delineated. There is extradural extension but the spinal cord (curved solid arrow) is separated from the tumour, as is the left kidney (curved open arrow).

encasement around major vessels thus making the lesion non-resectable.

Kidneys

On T_1W images the renal cortex and medulla can be distinguished due to the longer relaxation times of the latter. A linear low signal intensity artefact due to chemical shift misregistration (see page 29) can be seen between the renal cortex, or a peripherally located renal cyst, and perinephric fat and should not be misinterpreted as a normal structure.

Renal carcinomas greater than 3 cm in diameter can be readily demonstrated as a low and high signal on T_1W and T_2W images respectively (Hricak et al 1988a). Lesions less than 3 cm in diameter, however, appear isointense with surrounding parenchyma and can be difficult to detect except on the basis of deformity of the renal outline or disruption of the corticomedullary junction. The inability to detect small tumours limits the use of MRI, and is probably related to image degradation from motion artefact coupled with a poor signal-to-noise ratio obtained with body coil imaging (Quint et al 1988). MRI can provide clinically useful information in staging a known renal carcinoma with regard to extrarenal spread and tumour invasion of adjacent vascular structures. The accuracy of MRI staging is, however, only slightly greater than on CT (Glazer 1988). Large retroperitoneal nodes can be identified but distinction between reactive and malignant infiltration cannot be made.

Simple renal cysts have very prolonged relaxation times and appear as very low and high signal on T_1W and T_2W images respectively. They display similar morphological characteristics as on CT, appearing homogeneous in internal structure without a perceptible wall or mural nodules. Reliance cannot be made, however, on signal intensity appearances in distinguishing benign from malignant cysts. The presence of haemorrhage within a renal cyst changes the relaxation times, making it difficult to distinguish from a solid renal tumour. Cystic tumours can have identical MR characteristics to a simple cyst (Glazer 1988, Quint et al 1988). It is hoped, with the development of motion artefact suppression techniques, improved spatial resolution and the use of MR contrast agents, that the presence of a wall, septae and mural nodules in cystic tumour will be more clearly defined. Small foci of calcification, clearly identified on CT, cannot be detected on MRI, limiting its rôle in evaluating cystic renal lesions.

The site of origin and extent of a Wilm's tumour, the most common solid intra-abdominal neoplasm in children, can be defined on MRI with clear separation from other mass lesions, e.g. neuroblastoma. MRI, particularly with sagittal and coronal T_1W images, is superior to CT and ultrasound in the diagnosis and definition of extent of these tumours and can be used for monitoring the response to treatment. Other renal mass lesions in children, such as leukaemia or lymphoma infiltration, can also be demonstrated. The MR appearance of angiomyolipoma depends on the relative tissue composition of the tumour. The majority contain fat which produces characteristic high signals on T_1W and T_2W images which can be differentiated from haemorrhagic lesions by phase-contrast imaging. Renal metastases have a variable signal intensity appearance, being generally similar to that of the primary tumour. Transitional cell carcinoma can be defined as a filling defect within a dilated collecting system of different signal intensity to urine.

Retroperitoneum

Normal sized retroperitoneal and pelvic lymph nodes can be visualized. Metastatic involvement of normal sized nodes cannot be detected and tumour infiltration of enlarged nodes cannot be differentiated from reactive hyperplasia or inflammation.

The normal psoas muscle can be well visualized as can tumour infiltration on coronal T_2W images (Lee & Glazer 1986). Tumour infiltration cannot, however, be differentiated from psoas inflammation or abscess on MR appearances alone. Primary retroperitoneal tumours, usually sarcomas, are often large at presentation and the site of origin can be more clearly defined than on CT. The MR appearances of soft tissue sarcomas are detailed in the musculoskeletal section.

PELVIS

MRI is ideally suited for the evaluation of the pelvis. The advantages over other imaging techniques include a high soft tissue contrast discrimination including demonstration of vascular structures and bone marrow, imaging in multiple planes with little motion artefacts and no requirement for a full bladder (Fishman-Javitt et al 1988, Heiken & Lee 1988). These factors together with the absence of ionizing radiation are particularly useful in the assessment of paediatric pathology (Dietrich & Kangarloo 1987). Current problems include limited spatial resolution and lack of a satisfactory oral or rectal contrast agent in order to delineate the bowel. Both limitations are the subject of current research with improved spatial resolution achieved by new surface coil developments including endorectal and endovaginal RF coils for high resolution scanning.

T_1W images in the coronal or transverse plane are used for identifying lymphadenopathy and extension of tumour into adjacent pelvic fat (Fig. 2.16(1)). Lymph nodes can be differentiated from adjacent vasculature without requiring a contrast medium. T_2W images demonstrate the bladder musculature, zonal anatomy of the cervix, uterus and prostate, and detect tumour. MR has been found useful in the assessment of size and response to treatment of a variety of pelvic tumours.

Bladder

The bladder wall appears low signal on T_1W and T_2W images, whereas urine has a low and high signal respectively (Fig. 2.16). Bladder musculature can thus be demonstrated as a low signal band on T_2W images surrounded by high signal urine and perivesical fat. It is important to recognize that a chemical shift artefact (see page 29) can occur between the water protons of the bladder muscle and adjacent fat protons. This can produce a low signal intensity line at one edge of the bladder mimicking muscular hypertrophy, with a high signal intensity band opposite which can be mistaken for bladder wall invasion (Heiken & Lee 1988).

MRI can detect bladder carcinomas greater than 1.5 cm in diameter (Koelbel et al 1988). Assessment requires the use of optimal imaging planes, depending on the site of the tumour, and appropriate RF pulse sequences. Lesions involving the lateral wall of the bladder can be imaged using coronal and transverse planes; those involving the dome or base require sagittal or coronal scanning. T_1W images delineate the intravesical component and tumour extension into the perivesical fat. The presence or absence or ureteric obstruction and pelvic lymphadenopathy can also be assessed. T_2W images are necessary for demonstrating infiltration into the bladder wall and adjacent organs. Involvement of adjacent organs not only produces alteration in size and contour as in CT, but also changes in signal intensity. Bladder tumours involving only mucosa and submucosa cannot be differentiated from those with superficial muscle invasion (Heiken & Lee 1988). There is current debate as to whether distinction between early and late deep muscle involvement can be made, although in some respects this distinction is artificial. The important question is whether sufficient bladder muscle is present deep to tumour for endoscopic resection to be performed. The ability to obtain this information preoperatively might make some T3 lesions, at present treated by radiotherapy, amenable to endoscopic resection.

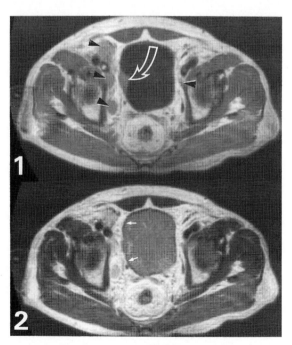

Fig. 2.16 Bladder carcinoma (T3bN) on transverse (1) intermediate T_1W (SE 1000/26) and (2) comparative T_2W (SE 1500/80) images. The tumour (curved arrow) has extended through the bladder wall which appears low signal (short arrows) in (2). The associated pelvic lymphadenopathy (arrowheads) is clearly seen in (1).

The histological grade and stage of tumour at presentation are important criteria in the survival of patients with bladder carcinoma. MRI appears to be at least as accurate (approaching 85%) a staging procedure as CT, although it is more accurate in the detection of local spread (Heiken & Lee 1988, Fishman-Javitt et al 1988). The use of a double surface coil can provide improved resolution relative to body coil imaging, resulting in more accurate staging of bladder carcinoma (Barentsz et al 1988).

Muscle hypertrophy of the bladder wall produces thickening but no change in signal intensity and can be differentiated from tumour. Oedema and inflammation of the wall, secondary to treatment, alters signal intensity and cannot be discriminated from tumour.

Cervix and uterus

Sagittal T_2W scans clearly display anatomy and relationships between the uterus, cervix, vagina, bladder and rectum (Fig. 2.17a). Transverse T_1W images of the cervix demonstrate paracervical and parametrial tissues although these can be optimally displayed using oblique plane imaging at right angles to the long axis of the cervix (Fig. 2.17b). On T_2W images three distinct areas are demonstrated within the uterus. There is a hyperintense central zone, which represents the endometrium combined with secretions within the endometrial canal, and an outer area of medium signal due to myometrium. Between the two is a low signal junctional zone representing the inner layer of compressed myometrium. In premenarchal and postmenopausal women, and including those on oral contraceptives, this junctional zone may not be identified. Changes in size and signal intensity of the three zones in the uterus occurs during menstruation. The cervix has two distinct layers — an inner hyperintense central zone representing the cervical mucus and epithelium with

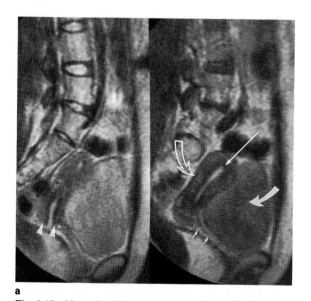

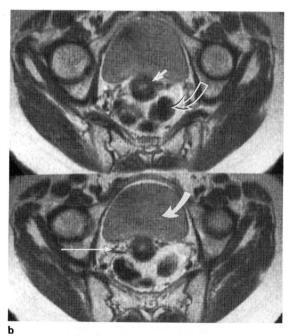

a

b

Fig. 2.17   Normal pelvic anatomy on contiguous T_2W images – (a) sagittal SE 3000/60 and (b) oblique SE 1500/80.
(a) Uterus (curved open arrow) and bladder (curved closed arrow) can be identified. In the uterus note the low signal junctional zone (long straight arrow) between the high signal endometrial zone and the intermediate signal from myometrium. The low signal anterior and posterior cervical lips (arrowheads) project into the vaginal fornices. High signal in vaginal canal (short straight arrows) is due to epithelium and secretions.
(b) The cervical stroma (short straight arrow), with high signal central zone, can be clearly demarcated from the high signal parametrial fat. Note position of rectum (curved open arrow), bladder (curved closed arrow) and parametrial vessels (long straight arrow).

a peripheral low intensity stroma similar to the uterine junctional zone. The vagina can be identified as a high signal central region of mucus and epithelium surrounded by a low signal intensity wall. A tampon in situ is useful for display of the vaginal walls.

Cervical carcinoma is better demonstrated on MR relative to CT and usually appears as high signal on T_2W images contrasting against the low signal cervical stroma (Lee 1988) (Fig. 2.18). The cervix may be enlarged and can obstruct the endometrial canal distending the uterus with retained secretion. Extent into the parametria, on T_1W transverse or oblique scans, is identified as a medium signal tumour breaching the low signal stromal wall into high signal pelvic fat (Fig. 2.19). Sagittal T_2W scans can be used to assess tumour extension into the lower uterine segment, vagina, bladder or rectum. There is difficulty on MR in discriminating infiltration of the vaginal wall from tumour occupying the upper vagina.

The volume and extent of disease at the time of diagnosis have important prognostic implications in cervical carcinoma. After histological diagnosis has been made accurate staging is critical in order

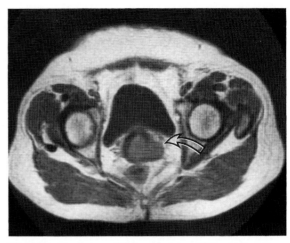

Fig. 2.19 Carcinoma of the cervix (stage IIb) on transverse T_1W (SE 820/40) image. The tumour (intermediate signal) has infiltrated through the left cervical stromal wall (low signal) into the parametrium (arrowed).

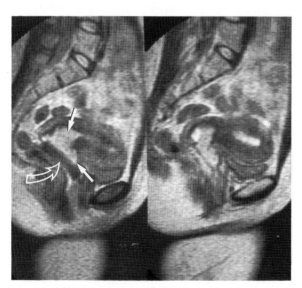

Fig. 2.18 Carcinoma of the cervix on contiguous sagittal T_2W (SE 1500/80) images. The cervical tumour (arrowed) is shown as a high signal expanding the cervix and extending into the upper vagina. The low signal cervical stromal wall can still be identified surrounding the tumour. Tampon (curved arrow) in situ.

to optimize treatment. Demonstration of parametrial infiltration (IIb–IVb using the FIGO classification) often precludes surgery and treatment is by radiotherapy. The clinical staging error rate can be 23% in patients with stage IIb disease and up to 64% with stage IIIb tumour (Hricak et al 1988b, Lee 1988). Limitations in the clinical assessment include inaccurate assessment of size of endophytic tumour and corpus extension together with evaluation of the parametria, pelvic side walls and lymphadenopathy.

Hricak et al (1988b) demonstrated in 57 patients with cervical carcinoma that MRI accurately staged the disease in 81%. MR measurements of tumour size, which has important prognostic implications, showed agreement with histological review in 70% of cases studied. The remainder were overestimated in size, in the majority of cases probably due to surrounding oedema. The accuracy of MRI in demonstrating the extent of tumour invasion to the pelvic side wall was 95%, with similar accuracy in demonstrating bladder involvement. MRI can be of particular value in detecting concomitant disease, e.g. uterine leiomyoma, and is an excellent method for assessing pregnant patients with cervical carcinoma without risk to the fetus. Significant overlap in measured T_1 values has been noted between normal cervix and those with tumour replacement.

Reduction in measured T_1 values has been demonstrated in cervical carcinomas following radiotherapy (Santoni et al 1987).

Endometrial carcinoma is best demonstrated on sagittal T_2W images and shows a variable appearance with low to high signal relative to surrounding endometrium. Abnormality within the endometrial cavity was demonstrated in 43 out of 51 (84%) patients with endometrial carcinoma (Hricak et al 1987a). No abnormality in signal intensity was noted in the remaining seven where the tumour was only 1–3 cm in diameter. Endometrial carcinoma cannot be differentiated from blood clot or adenomatous hyperplasia, indicating that histological review is essential. Difficulty has been observed in assessing myometrial invasion since the entire junctional zone may not be visible in some healthy postmenopausal women.

Staging of endometrial carcinoma, including assessment of site and depth of myometrial invasion, is important in defining appropriate treatment. The overall accuracy of MRI in staging endometrial carcinoma was 92% (Hricak et al 1987a). There was an 82% accuracy in demonstrating depth of myometrial invasion, best shown on T_2W images. Extrauterine extension, adnexal and peritoneal metastases were poorly detected.

MRI has been used to evaluate gestational trophoblastic tumours which are hypervascular masses with heterogeneous signal intensity, distorting normal uterine anatomy. The MR appearances of leiomyosarcoma have not allowed separation from leiomyomas.

Ovary

Normal sized ovaries can be demonstrated most easily on either transverse or coronal scans. They appear low–medium signal on T_1W images, and high signal (greater than fat) on T_2W sequences. Benign ovarian cysts tend to be small (less than 3 cm in diameter) and well marginated with low and very high signals on T_1W and T_2W images respectively. In the presence of haemorrhage the cysts have high signal on T_1W sequences similar to some endometriomas or ovarian teratomas.

Cystadenoma and cystadenocarcinoma cannot be distinguished unless lymphadenopathy, ascites or metastases are evident suggesting malignancy. Signal appearances vary depending on the amounts of solid and cystic components present. CT is more accurate in staging ovarian carcinoma and more sensitive in the detection of mesenteric and serosal metastases and abdominal lymphadenopathy compared with MRI (Fishman-Javitt et al 1988). Metastases to the ovaries (Krükenberg tumours) cannot be distinguished on signal intensity appearances from primary ovarian tumours.

Rectum

Although MRI can identify primary rectal carcinoma when invasion into perirectal fat or adjacent organs has occurred, it is unable to assess the extent of bowel wall infiltration in early disease. In assessment of patients previously treated for rectal carcinoma, a local soft tissue mass could be due to either recurrent tumour or post-treatment fibrosis. These can be difficult to differentiate and studies with MRI have indicated that it is a sensitive technique with the capability of separating recurrent tumour from post-treatment change (Johnson et al 1987, Krestin et al 1988). Johnson et al (1987), using a multipoint method for relaxation time measurements, have demonstrated that there was a highly significant ($p<0.001$) difference in the measured T_1 values for recurrent tumour compared with biopsy-proven chronic fibrosis. Measured T_2 values did not provide any discriminating value. Krestin et al (1988), however, observed in the majority (28 out of 35) of patients studied that the signal intensity appearance on T_2W images was useful in this separation. A low signal was noted from chronic scar tissue with recurrent tumour demonstrating a higher signal on T_2W images. Similar findings of signal intensity differences on T_2W images have been useful in distinguishing other pelvic tumours from chronic fibrosis (Ebner et al 1988). Difficulty in MR assessment was encountered in patients with metallic surgical clips in situ which produce susceptibility artefact leading to heterogeneity in signal of the soft tissue mass (Krestin et al 1988). Early bone infiltration of the sacrum from recurrent tumour can be easily demonstrated on sagittal PSR or moderate T_2W images.

Prostate

The normal prostate has a homogeneous low–intermediate signal on T_1W images. Zonal anatomy can be depicted using thin section T_2W sections with a low signal central zone and higher signal peripheral zone. This distinction is age-related, consistently seen in young men but probably not demonstrable in the elderly population (Hricak et al 1987b). The transitional and central zones, however, cannot be distinguished and the prostatic capsule is not usually visualized. A thin rim of higher signal on T_2W images anterolateral to the peripheral zone can be recognized in the majority of cases, corresponding to the periprostatic venous plexus. The urethra is shown as a high signal. A low intensity line representing Denonvilliers' fascia can be observed on sagittal sections separating prostate from rectum.

MRI has proved unreliable in the detection and diagnosis of prostatic carcinoma. Although initial work indicated that prostatic carcinoma could be differentiated on signal intensity appearances from prostatic hypertrophy, this has not been borne out in later studies (Heiken & Lee 1988). A normal appearing prostate on MR does not exclude presence of a tumour and inhomogeneity of the gland is a common non-specific finding. In addition, benign prostatic hypertrophy, prostatitis and carcinoma often occur concurrently.

Differences exist as to the signal intensity appearance of prostatic cancer. On low–medium (0.04–0.6 T) field systems prostatic carcinoma is usually recognized as an area of high signal on T_2W images. Using a high (1.5 T) field system the tumour has a low signal surrounded by hyperintense peripheral zone (Heiken & Lee 1988, Bezzi et al 1988).

MRI has a useful rôle in staging known disease. Recent studies have indicated MRI staging accuracy of 83–89% relative to 65% for CT (Hricak 1988, Heiken & Lee 1988). Tumour volume can be measured providing important prognostic information and can be used to monitor treatment (Bezzi et al 1988, Hricak 1988). The accuracy of MR volume measurements, however, has not yet been compared with histological data. Periprostatic tumour infiltration is best demonstrated on T_1W images as a low signal within high signal pelvic fat. Disruption of the periprostatic venous plexus, thought by some to be an indicator of extraglandular infiltration, appears to be an unreliable sign (Phillips et al 1987). Extension of tumour into the seminal vesicles can be identified by an abnormally low signal on T_2W images in addition to any enlargement produced. Detection of lymph node involvement remains difficult.

Relaxation time measurements have been reported as demonstrating no significant differences between benign prostatic hypertrophy and prostatic carcinoma groups (Kjaer et al 1987). Using a more advanced form of image analysis, based on measured relaxation time data, Prendergast et al (1987) were able to demonstrate an 88% (14 out of 16 patients with biopsy-proven prostatic disease) correct classification into either benign hypertrophy or prostatic carcinoma group. This indicates that more advanced forms of analysis are required to obtain the full potential value from relaxation time measurements.

THORAX

MRI of the thorax is limited by cardiac and respiratory motion artefacts resulting in poor spatial and contrast resolution (Gefter 1988, Stark & Bradley 1988). The ease of implementation of ECG-gating allows cardiac motion and flow-related artefacts to be successfully reduced. Resultant images show improved visualization of cardiac structures and great vessels and MRI offers particular advantages in the study of cardiovascular disease (Jenkins & Isherwood 1987b). Respiratory gating techniques are time consuming and not entirely reliable. Use of fast scanning techniques can allow scans to be obtained within a breath hold and provide blood flow information. An advantage of MR over non-enhanced CT is the inherent contrast resolution between soft tissues and vascular structures. Extent of lymphoma in the mediastinum and carcinoma can be well visualized on coronal and sagittal T_1W scans but equivalent information can be obtained on contrast-enhanced CT. Low signal from chronic fibrosis can be differentiated from intermediate signal of recurrent lymphoma or tumour. Lymph node size remains the sole criterion for detection of malignant mediastinal lymphadenopathy and

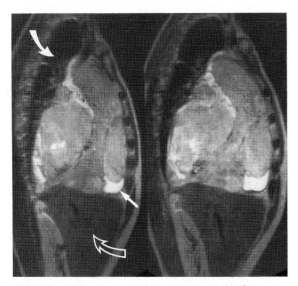

Fig. 2.20 Large pleural fibrosarcoma compressing lung (curved closed arrow) on contiguous sagittal T_2W (SE 1660/80) images. The liver (curved open arrow) is not infiltrated (this was difficult to determine on CT), and neither is the anterior chest wall. There is an associated anterior pleural effusion (straight arrow).

MR provides equivalent information relative to CT. At present anatomical detail of lung parenchyma is limited with MRI, and CT is the procedure of choice in assessing the presence or absence of lung metastases. Large lesions, however, can be more easily assessed with MRI relative to CT, as can the assessment of vascular, chest wall or brachial plexus involvement (Fig. 2.20). The brachial plexus can be well visualized on coronal MR scans even without the use of surface coils.

The ease of performance and wider availability of CT makes it the procedure of choice in assessment of most tumours of the thorax. Use of faster scanning techniques coupled with an MR perfusion agent may well exceed the information gained from contrast-enhanced CT offering a potential rôle for MRI.

MAGNETIC RESONANCE SPECTROSCOPY (MRS)

A detailed review of MRS is outside the scope of this chapter and is given elsewhere (Evanochko et al 1984, Stark & Bradley 1988). In vivo MRS is at an early stage of development with important clinical potential in oncology, particularly in monitoring the effects of treatment (Segebarth et al 1987, Semmler et al 1988). Preliminary results indicate that the presence of CNS tumours may be reflected in the MR spectra of CSF (Koschorek et al 1988). Intense debate occurred following a recent report of a blood test for cancer. Fossel et al (1986) proposed that water-suppressed MRS of plasma from patients could aid in the detection of cancer with a high degree of accuracy. Other workers have subsequently been unable to confirm these findings.

Differences between analytical MRS where the sample is small, uniform (homogeneous) and non-mobile as opposed to clinical MRS where the 'sample' is large, heterogeneous and mobile are important to appreciate in understanding the problems inherent in in vivo MRS.

CONCLUSION

It is important to emphasize that not all current MR systems are at the same stage in development and that their performance can vary widely. The present and future areas of development are listed below and are currently being assessed (Margulis & Crooks 1988, Bydder 1988a):

1. Surface coil imaging
2. Fast scanning techniques
3. Motion artefact suppressing techniques
4. New RF pulse sequences
5. MR contrast agents
6. Tissue characterization
7. Blood flow imaging and measurements in vivo
8. Volume (3-dimensional) imaging
9. Other nuclei imaged (e.g. sodium ^{23}Na, carbon ^{13}C, fluorine ^{19}F)
10. Human (proton ^{1}H and phosphorus ^{31}P) spectroscopy in vivo.

MR in terms of imaging and spectroscopy has tremendous potential in oncological practice which has yet to be fully realized.

REFERENCES

Atlas S W, Grossman R I, Gomori J M et al 1987a MR imaging of intracranial metastatic melanoma. Journal of Computer Assisted Tomography 11: 577–582

Atlas S W, Grossman R I, Gomori J M, Hackney D B, Goldberg H I, Zimmerman R A, Bilaniuk L T 1987b Hemorrhagic intracranial malignant neoplasms: spin-echo MR imaging. Radiology 164: 71–77

Auffermann W, Clark O H, Thurnher S, Galante M, Higgins C B 1988 Recurrent thyroid carcinoma: characteristics on MR images. Radiology 168: 753–757

Baker M E, Spritzer C, Blinder R, Herfkens R J, Leight G S, Dunnick N R 1987 Benign adrenal lesions mimicking malignancy on MR imaging: report of two cases. Radiology 163: 669–671

Barentsz J O, Lemmens J A M, Ruijs S H J et al 1988 Carcinoma of the urinary bladder: MR imaging with a double surface coil. American Journal of Roentgenology 151: 107–112

Barkovich A J, Kjos B O, Jackson D E, Norman D 1988 Normal maturation of the neonatal and infant brain: MR imaging at 1.5 T. Radiology 166: 173–180

Bezzi M, Kressel H Y, Allen K S et al 1988 Prostatic carcinoma: staging with MR imaging at 1.5 T. Radiology 169: 339–346

Bird C R, Drayer B P, Medina M, Rekate H L, Flom R A, Hodak J A 1988 Gd-DTPA-enhanced MR imaging in pediatric patients after brain tumor resection. Radiology 169: 123–126

Braffman B H, Bilaniuk L T, Zimmerman R A 1988 The central nervous system manifestations of the phakomatoses on MR. Radiologic Clinics of North America 26: 773–800

Brant-Zawadzki M 1988 MR imaging of the brain. Radiology 166: 1–10

Bydder G M 1988a Magnetic resonance imaging: present status and future perspectives. British Journal of Radiology 61: 889–897

Bydder G M 1988b Clinical use of the partial saturation and saturation recovery sequences. In: Kressel H Y (ed) Magnetic resonance annual. Raven Press, New York, pp 245–270

Bydder G M, Young I R 1985 MRI: clinical use of the inversion recovery sequence. Journal of Computer Assisted Tomography 9: 659–675

Castelijns J A, Gerritsen G J, Kaiser M C et al 1987 Invasion of laryngeal cartilage by cancer: comparison of CT and MR imaging. Radiology 166: 199–206

Chezmar J L, Rumancik W M, Megibow A J, Hulnick D H, Nelson R C, Bernardino M E 1988 Liver and abdominal screening in patients with cancer: CT versus MR imaging. Radiology 168: 43–47

Cohen E K, Kressel H Y, Frank T S et al 1988 Hyaline cartilage-origin bone and soft-tissue neoplasms: MR appearance and histologic correlation. Radiology 167: 477–481

Crooks L E, Arakawa M, Hylton N M et al 1988 Echo-planar pediatric imager. Radiology 166: 157–163

Curnes J T 1987 MR imaging of peripheral intracranial neoplasms: extra-axial vs intra-axial masses. Journal of Computer Assisted Tomography 11: 932–937

Czervionke L F, Daniels D L 1988 Cervical spine anatomy and pathologic processes: application of new MR imaging techniques. Radiologic Clinics of North America 26: 921–947

Daniels D L, Haughton V M 1987 Magnetic resonance imaging of the sella and temporal bone. In: Kressel H Y (ed) Magnetic resonance annual. Raven Press, New York, pp 1–47

Daniels D L, Haughton V M, Naidich T P 1987 Cranial and spinal magnetic resonance imaging. Raven Press, New York

Dietrich R B, Kangarloo H 1987 Pelvic abnormalities in children: assessment with MR imaging. Radiology 163: 367–372

Dietrich R B, Kangarloo H, Lenarsky C, Feig S A 1987 Neuroblastoma: the role of MR imaging. American Journal of Roentgenology 148: 937–942

Dooms G C, Kerlan R K, Hricak H et al 1986 Cholangiocarcinoma imaging by MR. Radiology 159: 89–94

Drayer B P 1988 Imaging of the aging brain part I. Normal findings. Radiology 166: 785–796

Dwyer A J, Frank J A, Doppman J L et al 1987 Pituitary adenomas in patients with Cushing disease: initial experience with Gd-DTPA-enhanced MR imaging. Radiology 163: 421–426

Dwyer A J, Frank J A, Sank V J, Reinig J W, Hickey A M, Doppman J L 1988 Short-TI inversion-recovery pulse sequence: analysis and initial experience in cancer imaging. Radiology 168: 827–836

Earnest IV F, Kelly P J, Scheithauer B W et al 1988 Cerebral astrocytomas: histopathologic correlation of MR and CT contrast enhancement with stereotactic biopsy. Radiology 166: 823–827

Ebner F, Kressel H Y, Mintz M C et al 1988 Tumour recurrence versus fibrosis in the female pelvis: differentiation with MR imaging at 1.5 T. Radiology 166: 330–340

Ehman R L, Berquist T H, McLeod R A 1988 MR imaging of the musculoskeletal system: A 5-year appraisal. Radiology 166: 313–320

Enzmann D R, Rubin J B 1988 Cervical spine: MR imaging with a partial flip angle, gradient-refocused pulse sequence. Radiology 166: 473–478

Evanochko W T, Ng T C, Glickson J D 1984 Application of in vivo NMR spectroscopy to cancer. Magnetic Resonance in Medicine 1: 508–534

Falke T H M, Peetoom J J, de Roos A, van de Velde C J H, Mazer M 1988 Gadolinium-DTPA enhanced MR imaging of intravenous extension of adrenocortical carcinoma. Journal of Computer Assisted Tomography 12: 331–334

Felix R, Schorner W, Sander B, Henkes H Bittner 1988 Contrast-enhanced MR brain studies: clinical experience with Gd-DTPA over four years. Diagnostic Imaging International (suppl) November: 13–15

Fishman-Javitt M C, Lovecchio J L, Stein H L 1988 Imaging strategies for MRI of the pelvis. Radiologic Clinics of North America 26: 633–651

Fossel E T, Carr J M, McDonagh J 1986 Detection of malignant tumours. Water-suppressed proton nuclear magnetic resonance spectroscopy of plasma. New England Journal of Medicine 315: 1369–1376

Fullerton G D, Potter J L, Dornbluth N C 1982 NMR relaxation of protons in tissues and other macromolecular water solutions. Magnetic Resonance Imaging 1: 209–228

Gefter W B 1988 Chest applications of magnetic resonance imaging: an update. Radiologic Clinics of North America 26: 573–588

Gholkar A, Stack J P, Isherwood I 1988 Case report: plexiform trigeminal neurofibroma. Clinical Radiology 39: 313–315

Gillespy III T, Manfrini M, Ruggieri P, Spanier S S, Pettersson H, Springfield D S 1988 Staging of intraosseous extent of osteosarcoma: correlation of preoperative CT and MR imaging with pathologic macroslides. Radiology 167: 765–767

Glazer G M 1988 MR imaging of the liver, kidneys, and adrenal glands. Radiology 166: 303–312

Goy A M C, Pinto R S, Raghavendra B N, Epstein F J, Kricheff I I 1986 Intramedullary spinal cord tumors: MR imaging, with emphasis on associated cysts. Radiology 161: 381–386

Hamm B, Wolf K-J, Felix R 1987 Conventional and rapid MR imaging of the liver with Gd-DTPA. Radiology 164: 313–320

Haughton V M 1988 MR imaging of the spine. Radiology 166: 297–301

Hawkes R C, Holland G N, Moore W S, Worthington B S 1980 NMR tomography of the brain: a preliminary clinical assessment with demonstration of pathology. Journal of Computer Assisted Tomography 4: 577–586

Hecht-Leavitt C, Grossman R I, Curran W J et al 1987 MR of brain radiation injury: experimental studies in cats. American Journal of Neuroradiology 8: 427–430

Heiken J P, Lee J K T 1988 MR imaging of the pelvis. Radiology 166: 11–16

Hess C F, Griebel J, Schmiedl U, Kurtz B, Koelbel G, Jaehde E 1988 Focal lesions of the spleen: preliminary results with fast MR imaging at 1.5 T. Journal of Computer Assisted Tomography 12: 569–574

Hesselink J R, Press G A 1988 MR contrast enhancement of intracranial lesions with Gd-DTPA. Radiologic Clinics of North America 26: 873–887

Hinshaw W S, Bottomley P A, Holland G N 1977 Radiographic thin-section image of the human wrist by nuclear magnetic resonance. Nature 270: 722–723

Hinshaw D B, Holshouser B A, Engstrom H I M, Tjan A H L, Christiansen E L, Catelli W F 1988 Dental material artefacts on MR images. Radiology 166: 777–779

Hoult D I, Chen C-N, Sank V J 1986 The field dependence of NMR imaging. II: Arguments concerning an optimal field strength. Magnetic Resonance in Medicine 3: 730–746

Hricak H 1988 Imaging prostate carcinoma. Radiology 169: 569–571

Hricak H, Stern J L, Fisher M R, Shapeero L G, Winkler M L, Lacey C G 1987a Endometrial carcinoma staging by MR imaging. Radiology 162: 297–305

Hricak H, Dooms G C, McNeal J E et al 1987b MR imaging of the prostate gland: normal anatomy. American Journal of Roentgenology 148: 51–58

Hricak H, Thoeni R F, Carroll P R, Demas B E, Marotti M, Tanagho E A 1988a Detection and staging of renal neoplasms: a reassessment of MR imaging. Radiology 166: 643–649

Hricak H, Lacey C G, Sandles L G, Chang Y C F, Winkler M L, Stern J L 1988b Invasive cervical carcinoma:

comparison of MR imaging and surgical findings. Radiology 166: 623–631

Hudson T M, Hamlin D J, Enneking W F, Pettersson H 1985 Magnetic resonance imaging of bone and soft tissue tumours: early experience in 31 patients compared with computed tomography. Skeletal Radiology 13: 134–146

Hyman R A, Gorey M T 1988 Imaging strategies for MR of the spine. Radiologic Clinics of North America 26: 505–533

Isherwood I, Hawnaur J M, Jenkins J P R 1989 Gadolinium-DTPA in magnetic resonance imaging of spinal tumours and angiomas. In: Imaging of brain metabolism and spinal cord in conventional neuroradiology. Springer-Verlag, Berlin, pp 77–86

Itoh K, Nishimura K, Togashi K et al 1987 Hepatocellular carcinoma: MR imaging. Radiology 164: 21–25

Jenkins J P R, Isherwood I 1987a Magnetic resonance imaging – technical aspects, CNS and spine. In: Sutton D (ed) A textbook of radiology and imaging, 4th edn. Churchill Livingstone, Edinburgh, pp 1654–1690

Jenkins J P R, Isherwood I 1987b Magnetic resonance imaging of the heart: a review. In: Rowlands D J (ed) Recent advances in cardiology. Churchill Livingstone, Edinburgh, 10: 219–247

Jenkins J P R, Braganza J M, Hickey D S, Isherwood I, Machin M 1987 Quantitative tissue characterisation in pancreatic disease using magnetic resonance imaging. British Journal of Radiology 60: 333–341

Jenkins J P R, Gholkar A, Antoun N M, Stack J P, Isherwood I 1988a Gd-DTPA as a contrast agent in MRI of the spine. Diagnostic Imaging International (suppl) November: 24–25

Jenkins J P R, Gholkar A, Johnson R J, Isherwood I 1988b Magnetic resonance imaging of head and neck tumours: comparison with CT. In: Proceedings of 7th SMRM, San Francisco (Society of Magnetic Resonance in Medicine, Berkeley) p 716

Jennings C M, Gaines P A 1988 The abdominal manifestation of von Hippel–Lindau disease and a radiological screening protocol for an affected family. Clinical Radiology 39: 363–367

Johnson R J, Jenkins J P R, Isherwood I, James R D, Schofield P F 1987 Quantitative magnetic resonance imaging in rectal carcinoma. British Journal of Radiology 60: 761–764

Kjaer L, Thomsen C, Iversen P, Henriksen O 1987 In vivo estimation of relaxation processes in benign hyperplasia and carcinoma of the prostate gland by magnetic resonance imaging. Magnetic Resonance Imaging 5: 23–30

Koelbel G, Schmiedi U, Griebel J, Hess C F, Kueper K 1988 MR imaging of urinary bladder neoplasms. Journal of Computer Assisted Tomography 12: 98–103

Koschorek F, Gremmel H, Stelten J, Offermann W, Leibfritz D 1988 Cerebrospinal fluid: detection of tumors and disk herniations with MR spectroscopy. Radiology 167: 813–816

Kressel H Y 1988 Strategies for magnetic resonance imaging of focal liver disease. Radiologic Clinics of North America 26: 607–615

Krestin G P, Steinbrich W, Friedmann G 1988 Recurrent rectal cancer: diagnosis with MR imaging versus CT. Radiology 168: 307–311

Krol G, Sze G, Malkin M, Walker R 1988 MR of cranial and spinal meningeal carcinomatosis: comprison with CT and myelography. American Journal of Roentgenology 151: 583–588

Lampert P W, Davis R L 1964 Delayed effects of radiation on the human central nervous system: 'early' and 'late' delayed reactions. Neurology 14: 912–917

Laniado M, Weinmann H J, Schörner W, Felix R, Speck U 1984 First use of Gd-DTPA/dimeglumine in man. Physiological Chemistry and Physics and Medical NMR 16: 157–165

Laniado M, Kornmesser W, Hamm B, Clauss W, Weinmann H-J, Felix R 1988 MR imaging of the gastrointestinal tract: value of Gd-DTPA. American Journal of Roentgenology 150: 817–821

Lauffer R B 1988 Preclinical studies of new MRI contrast agents. Diagnostic Imaging International (suppl) November: 10–12

Lee J K T 1988 The rôle of MR imaging in staging of cervical carcinoma. Radiology 166: 895–896

Lee J K T, Glazer H S 1986 Psoas muscle disorders: MR imaging. Radiology 160: 683–687

Levine E, Huntrakoon M, Wetzel L H 1987 Malignant nerve-sheath neoplasms in neurofibromatosis: distinction from benign tumors by using imaging techniques. American Journal of Roentgenology 149: 1059–1064

Lloyd G A S, Lund V J, Phelps P D, Howard D J 1987 Magnetic resonance imaging in the evaluation of nose and paranasal sinus disease. British Journal of Radiology 60: 957–968

Lufkin R, Hanafee W 1988 MRI of the head and neck. Magnetic Resonance Imaging 6: 69–88

McFarland E W, Rosen B R 1986 NMR instrumentation and hardware available at present and in the future. Cardiovascular and Interventional Radiology 8: 238–250

Margulis A R, Crooks L E 1988 Present and future status of MR imaging. American Journal of Roentgenology 150: 487–492

Mikhael M A, Ciric I S 1988 MR imaging of pituitary tumors before and after surgical and/or medical treatment. Journal of Computer Assisted Tomography 12: 441–445

Noma S, Kanaoka M, Minami S et al 1988 Thyroid masses: MR imaging and pathological correlation. Radiology 168: 759–764

Olsen W L, Dillon W P, Kelly W M, Normal D, Brant-Zawadzki M, Newton T H 1986 MR imaging of paragangliomas. American Journal of Roentgenology 148: 201–204

Oot R F, New P F J, Pile-Spellman J, Rosen B R, Shoukimas G M, Davis K R 1986 The detection of intracranial calcifications by MR. American Journal of Neuroradiology 7: 801–809

Oot R F, Melville G E, New P F J et al 1988 The role of MR and CT in evaluating clival chordomas and chondrosarcomas. American Journal of Roentgenology 151: 567–575

Petasnick J P, Turner D A, Charters J R, Gitelis S, Zacharias C E 1986 Soft-tissue masses of the locomotor system: comparison of MR with CT. Radiology 160: 125–133

Pettersson H, Slone R M, Spanier S, Gillespy III T, Fitzsimmons J R, Scott K N 1988 Musculoskeletal tumours: T_1 and T_2 relaxation times. Radiology 167: 783–785

Peyster R G, Augsburger J J, Shields J A, Hershey B L, Eagle R Jr, Haskin M E 1988 Intraocular tumors:

evaluation with MR imaging. Radiology 168: 773–779

Phillips M E, Kressel H Y, Spritzer C E et al 1987 Prostatic disorders: MR imaging at 1.5 T. Radiology 164: 386–392

Prendergast D J, Hickey D S, Jenkins J P R, Isherwood I 1987 Increased potential for tissue discrimination in quantitative magnetic resonance imaging. British Journal of Radiology 60: 1142–1143

Pusey E, Kortman K E, Flannigan B D, Tsuruda J, Bradley W G 1987 MR of craniopharyngiomas: tumor delineation and characterization. American Journal of Roentgenology 149: 383–388

Quint L E, Glazer G M, Chenevert T L et al 1988 In vivo and in vitro MR imaging of renal tumors: histopathologic correlation and pulse sequence optimization. Radiology 169: 359–362

Rafto S E, Gefter W B 1988 MRI of the upper aerodigestive tract and neck. Radiologic Clinics of North America 26: 547–571

Reiser M, Erlemann R, Peters P E 1988 MRI of the musculoskeletal system: value of intravenous Gd-DTPA. Diagnostic Imaging International (suppl) November: 46–49

Santoni R, Bucciolini M, Cionini L, Ciraolo L, Renzi R 1987 Modifications of relaxation times induced by radiation therapy in cervical carcinoma: preliminary results. Clinical Radiology 38: 569–573

Sartoris D J, Resnick D 1987 MR imaging of the musculoskeletal system: current and future status. American Journal of Roentgenology 149: 457–467

Schad L, Lott S, Schmitt F, Sturm V, Lorenz W J 1987 Correction of spatial distortion in MR imaging: a prerequisite for accurate stereotaxy. Journal of Computer Assisted Tomography 11: 499–505

Scotti G, C-Y Yu, Dillon W P et al 1988 MR Imaging of cavernous sinus involvement by pituitary adenomas. American Journal of Roentgenology 151: 799–806

Segebarth C M, Balériaux D F, Arnold D L, Luyten P R, den Hollander J A 1987 MR image-guided P-31 MR spectroscopy in the evaluation of brain tumor treatment. Radiology 165: 215–219

Semmler W, Gademann G, Bachert-Baumann P, Zabel H-J, Lorenz W J, van Kaick G 1988 Monitoring human tumor response to therapy by means of P-31 MR spectroscopy. Radiology 166: 533–539

Smith M A 1985 The technology of magnetic resonance imaging. Clinical Radiology 36: 553–559

Som P M, Braun I F, Shapiro M D, Reede D L, Curtin H D, Zimmerman R A 1987 Tumors of the parapharyngeal space and upper neck: MR imaging characteristics. Radiology 164: 823–829

Som P M, Shapiro M D, Biller H F, Sasaki C, Lawson W 1988a Sinonasal tumors and inflammatory tissues: differentiation with MR imaging. Radiology 167: 803–808

Som P M, Sacher M, Stollman A L, Biller H F, Lawson W 1988b Common tumors of the parapharyngeal space: refined imaging diagnosis. Radiology 169: 81–85

Stack J P, Antoun N M, Jenkins J P R, Metcalfe R, Isherwood I 1988a Gadolinium-DTPA as a contrast agent in magnetic resonance imaging of the brain. Neuroradiology 30: 145–154

Stack J P, Ramsden R T, Antoun N M, Lye R H, Isherwood I, Jenkins J P R 1988b magnetic resonance imaging of acoustic neuromas: the role of gadolinium-DTPA. British Journal of Radiology 61: 800–805

Stark D D, Bradley W G (eds) 1988 Magnetic resonance imaging. C V Mosby, St Louis

Stark D D, Wittenberg J, Butch R J, Ferrucci J T 1987 Hepatic metastases: randomized, controlled comparison of detection with MR imaging and CT. Radiology 165: 399–406

Stark D D, Weissleder R, Elizondo G et al 1988 Superparamagnetic iron oxide: clinical application as a contrast agent for MR imaging of the liver. Radiology 168: 297–301

Sundaram M, McGuire M H, Schajowicz F 1987 Soft-tissue masses: histologic basis for decreased signal (short T_2) on T_2-weighted MR images. American Journal of Roentgenology 148: 1247–1250

Sze G 1988 Gadolinium-DTPA in spinal disease. Radiologic Clinics of North America 26: 1009–1024

Teresi L M, Lufkin R B, Vinuela F et al 1987 MR imaging of the nasopharynx and floor of the middle cranial fossa. Part II Malignant tumors. Radiology 164: 817–821

Thomsen C, Sorensen P G, Karle H, Christoffersen P, Henriksen O 1987 Prolonged bone marrow T_1-relaxation in acute leukaemia. In vivo tissue characterization by magnetic resonance imaging. Magnetic Resonance Imaging 5: 251–257

Toonkel L M, Soila K, Gilbert D, Sheldon J 1988 MRI assisted treatment planning for radiation therapy of the head and neck. Magnetic Resonance Imaging 6: 315–319

Tscholakoff D, Hricak H, Thoeni R, Winkler M L, Margulis A R 1987 MR imaging in the diagnosis of pancreatic disease. American Journal of Roentgenology 148: 703–709

Tsuruda J S, Kortman K E, Bradley W G, Wheeler D C, Dalsem W V, Bradley T P 1987 Radiation effects on cerebral white matter: MR evaluation. American Journal of Roentgenology 149: 165–171

Vanel D, Di Paola R, Contesso G 1987 Magnetic resonance imaging in musculoskeletal primary malignant tumour. In: Kressel H Y (ed) Magnetic resonance annual. Raven Press, New York, pp 237–261

Vogl T, Brüning R, Grevers G, Mees K, Bauer M, Lissner J 1988 MR imaging of the oropharynx and tongue: comparison of plain and Gd-DTPA studies. Journal of Computer Assisted Tomography 12: 427–433

Vogler III J B, Murphy W A 1988 Bone marrow imaging. Radiology 168: 679–693

Weinreb J C, Brateman L, Maravilla K R 1984 Magnetic resonance imaging of hepatic lymphoma. Americal Journal of Roentgenology 143: 1211–1214

Weissleder R, Hahn P F, Stark D D et al 1988 Superparamagnetic iron oxide: enhanced detection of focal splenic tumours with MR imaging. Radiology 169: 399–403

Wittenberg J, Stark D D, Forman B H et al 1988 Differentiation of hepatic metastases from hepatic hemangiomas by using MR imaging. American Journal of Roentgenology 151: 79–84

Yuh W T C, Kathol M H, Sein M A, Ehara S, Chiu L 1987 Hemangiomas of skeletal muscle: MR findings in five patients. American Journal of Roentgenology 149: 765–768

Zimmerman R A, Bilaniuk L T 1988a Ocular MR imaging. Radiology 168: 875–876

Zimmerman R A, Bilaniuk L T 1988b Imaging of tumors of the spinal canal and cord. Radiologic Clinics of North America 26: 965–1007

3. Childhood malignancy

I. W. Turnbull   R. K. Levick

I. W. Turnbull   R. K. Levick

PART 1
THE CENTRAL NERVOUS SYSTEM
I. W. Turnbull

INTRODUCTION

In this chapter primary neoplasms arising within the cranium will be discussed first and the relatively rare primary intraspinal neoplasms will be discussed separately. Most large series have shown that approximately 95% of all central nervous system tumours occurring in children are intracranial in location with only 5% being found in relation to the spinal cord or its coverings.

Paediatric brain tumours constitute between 15 and 20% of all primary brain tumours and represent almost 15% of all paediatric tumours, being the second most common malignancy of childhood (Farwell et al 1977, Naidich & Zimmerman 1984, Tomita & McLone 1985). Posterior fossa neoplasms are more frequent than supratentorial tumours when all paediatric ages are grouped together, but the reverse is true in the first three years of life when approximately 60% of brain tumours will be supratentorial. Posterior fossa lesions predominate from 4 to 11 years of age and both locations are equally frequent throughout the rest of the paediatric period (Farwell et al 1977, Jooma et al 1984).

General principles of imaging brain tumours

As most centres nowadays adopt a multidisciplinary approach to the treatment of paediatric brain tumours, imaging techniques are called upon to provide information for surgeons, radiotherapists and medical oncologists, all of whom may view the disease process from different aspects and may request specialized information pertaining to their particular speciality and interest in the case. In general, however, the following principles can be applied to any imaging modality which may be employed in management.

Detection

Confirming the presence of disease is the primary function of imaging and techniques such as computed tomography (CT) and magnetic resonance imaging (MRI) are extremely sensitive at detecting pathology with an almost negligible false negative rate.

Location

Surgeons in particular will require three-dimensional information as to the location of the tumour and its relationship to known anatomical landmarks such as the tentorium. It will also be helpful to define the anatomy of the tumour in respect of adjacent blood vessels and cerebrospinal fluid (CSF) pathways including the ventricular system.

Tissue characterization

Determining whether the tumour is solid or cystic and whether it contains necrotic areas is obviously of surgical import and, in certain tumours, may have prognostic significance. The presence of calcification in the lesion or recent haemorrhage into the tumour will often have clinical and histological significance. An ideal imaging technique would be required to characterize the tissues comprising the neoplasm with a high degree of specificity. The vascularity of the tumour and the extent to which the blood–brain barrier has been breached might provide valuable information to the surgeon or to the medical oncologist who is considering systemic chemotherapy. Precise definition of the boundary or contour of the tumour and its clear differentiation from adjacent normal brain is essential in defining the true extent of the disease process and it is obviously important to be able to distinguish peritumoural oedema from tumour infiltration. This is particularly important when radiotherapy is considered as the primary treatment, the aim of which is to eradicate all malignant cells within the target volume whilst sparing, as far as possible, the surrounding normal brain.

Extent of disease

Features should be sought which determine the relative malignancy of the neoplasm and its possible rate of growth. The operability of a tumour, the best initial treatment option and the likely prognosis can be obtained for certain tumour groups and these will be discussed under the individual tumour headings.

Imaging complications of the primary tumour

Hydrocephalus is a common accompaniment of many paediatric brain tumours and is readily detected, as is the occasional haemorrhage into a neoplasm. Herniation of brain under the falx, through the tentorial hiatus or into foramen magnum is usually well appreciated. Intracranial or intraspinal subarachnoid seeding of tumour must be sought when the natural history of the lesion suggests that this is a likely consequence and the value of routine screening for clinically silent intraspinal seeding in particular is discussed later.

Restaging of patients during/after treatment

Response to treatment will be monitored and imaging will be required to determine whether a surgical removal has been complete. Tumour shrinkage, resolution of peritumoural oedema and

control of hydrocephalus are further considerations. Later in the follow-up period, detection of tumour recurrence or reactivation will be of paramount importance and distinguishing this from postoperative gliosis, radiation or drug effects poses serious difficulties. The radiological management of early and late complications of treatment, particularly radiation and drug effects on the CNS, require special mention and the problems of immunosuppression and opportunist infection will be considered.

AVAILABLE IMAGING TECHNIQUES

Although skull radiographs may be expected to show some abnormality in between 60 and 90% of children with brain tumours, largely depending on the age at presentation, they are not obtained routinely, but may be required following CT scanning for findings that suggest extradural extension, bone erosion or calcification. There may be specific instances in which sinus development or vault contour may influence the surgical approach. Although skull radiographs may therefore be employed as a screening or first line investigation, they offer very little assistance in solving the radiological problems of management mentioned above (Fig. 3.1).

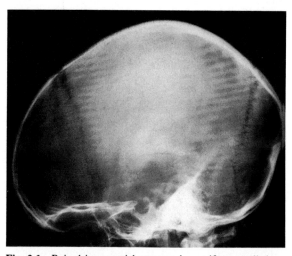

Fig. 3.1 Raised intracranial pressure is manifest as splitting of the sutures. Florid pathological calcification is seen throughout the posterior fossa and there is some localized expansion of the floor of the posterior fossa in this child with medulloblastoma.

Transcranial ultrasound scanning uses the anterior fontanelle as a 'window' for imaging the brain and, as such, is only applicable to the very small baby, although it is possible to employ burr holes or craniectomy defects as a means of postsurgical monitoring (Winkler & Helmke 1985), especially of ventricular size (Fig. 3.2). This subject will be discussed further when the special radiological problems associated with tumours in the first two years of life are discussed.

Arteriography is not used routinely for evaluation of posterior fossa lesions unless features on the CT scan raise the possibility of aneurysm, vascular malformation or a very vascular tumour. Within the supratentorial compartment, however, arteriography still has a rôle in (i) defining the vascular anatomy in relation to the surgical approach, (ii) assessing the safety of surgical approach to the peritumoural bridging veins and venous sinuses,

(iii) defining the vascular pedicle of a particularly hypervascular tumour, and (iv) excluding aneurysm of angioma when appropriate (Naidich & Zimmerman 1984).

Computed tomography (CT) is currently the single most useful method of neuroradiological assessment and all children with a suspected brain tumour should have both non-contrast and contrast-enhanced CT in the transaxial plane with supplementary postcontrast direct coronal and sagittal images depending on the location of the tumour and the ability of the child to cooperate with the posturing needed to generate these pictures. The standard slice thickness employed for most scans is 8–10 mm, but for babies and very small children 4–6 mm slices should be obtained in order to minimize partial volume effect and offer maximal information about tissue characterization of small lesions. Children are naturally restless and sick infants all the more so, therefore some form of sedation is usually necessary. The choice of drug will vary according to local preferences, but it should be capable of being administered orally. As many children have to travel to a specialized centre for their examination, the dose may need to be repeated nearer to the time of the study and, consequently, a relatively mild-acting drug is preferable. Furthermore, it should be realized that a warm, well fed and well hydrated infant will tolerate any type of examination much more readily than a cold hungry one, no matter how much sedation is given. As already mentioned, the initial CT study will include a postcontrast scan and this will be necessary at follow-up examinations unless limited information is required, e.g. the current state of the ventricles. Parental consent is required except in emergency situations.

The basis for the use of intravenous contrast agents is to produce a change of density in the tissues under review, such that the recognition of abnormalities is facilitated. It may also provide information about the nature of the tumour tissue, its vascularity and the relationship of the mass to adjacent vessels, for example, the displacement of the internal carotid arteries by an intrasellar or suprasellar tumour (Burman & Rosenbaum 1982). A number of factors affect the concentration of contrast medium within the tissues after

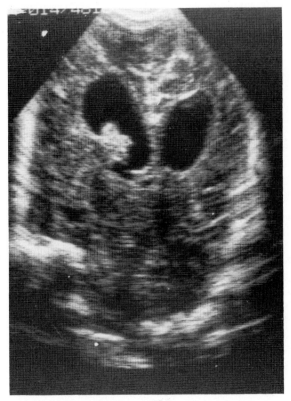

Fig. 3.2 Transcranial ultrasound examination demonstrates an ependymal mass within the right lateral ventricle. Both ventricles are dilated.

intravenous injection and this in turn influences the local attenuation values measured at CT: (i) plasma concentration, (ii) permeability of the capillaries and (iii) rates of diffusion of contrast medium among the fluid compartments of the tissues. Plasma concentration is determined by: (i) dose, (ii) rate of injection, (iii) rate of renal excretion and (iv) equilibration with the extravascular fluid compartment. After intravenous injection, contrast medium disappears from the intravascular space to the extravascular space with a half-time of less than one minute, so that the great majority of the administered dose is removed from the vascular compartment within a few minutes of the injection. The situation within the brain is rather different, where the presence of an intact blood–brain barrier prevents the extravasation of contrast medium to extravascular sites, with certain well known exceptions such as the pituitary stalk and pineal gland where the blood–brain barrier is normally deficient. The use of intravenous contrast for optimal imaging of an intracranial abnormality depends upon altering (usually increasing) the density of pathological tissue relative to normal adjacent brain. As mentioned above, the intravascular concentration, i.e. the vascularity of the tumour, will have some effect on the local attenuation levels within the tissue but this is relatively minor and the greatest portion of abnormal enhancement of the tumour results from passage of the contrast medium into the extravascular space of the lesion through a deficiency in the blood–brain barrier (Fig. 3.3a and b). On occasions, this process may occur slowly and it may be necessary to undertake delayed scans of the suspicious area 30 to 60 minutes after the injection to allow for accumulation of contrast material within the neoplasm. With modern scanners it is possible to assess the vascularity of a tumour, but this requires a modification of the technique whereby a series of rapid scans are made at a predetermined level during the injection of contrast medium. By this means the first pass of contrast through the tumour may be studied, not only allowing estimation of tumour vascularity, but sometimes permitting visualization of the ves-

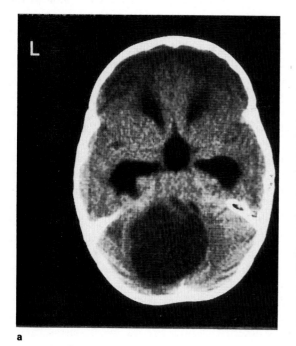
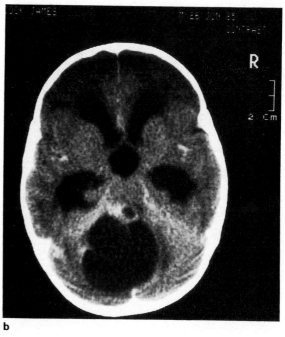

a

b

Fig. 3.3 (a) Non-contrast CT shows large cystic mass in posterior fossa obstructing the fourth ventricle with resultant hydrocephalus. (b) Same patient a few minutes after intravenous contrast showing variable enhancement of the cyst wall and an intramural nodule.

sels themselves as they enter or leave a hypervascular mass. Radiotherapy, cytotoxic drugs, and especially steroids may all influence the permeability of the blood–brain barrier which, in turn, will influence the capacity of the tumour to enhance. The particular relevance of this will be discussed in the section of the chapter dealing with the radiological management of the complications of treatment, including opportunist infections where steroids in particular may suppress the enhancement of an infective lesion such as an abscess, so delaying its recognition and treatment.

Magnetic resonance imaging (MRI) is not widely enough available, certainly not in the UK, for it to be regarded as a routine investigation. Problems of patient cooperation may be encountered as the examination takes longer than CT and the child is more enclosed. However, unlike CT, no hazard is associated with MRI and, unlike sonography, its application in children is not limited by the closure of the fontanelles. Many tumours are located in the posterior fossa where MRI will readily allow their identification, owing to the absence of bony artefacts which are commonly met with in CT scanning (Radkowski et al 1988). It is possible to distinguish intrinsic from extrinsic tumours and to recognize subtle changes in brain stem glioma with MRI (Levene et al 1982, Johnson et al 1983, Lee et al 1985). In a recent major review, Peterman et al (1984) studied 25 children and adolescents with a suspected or proven diagnosis of intracranial tumour and compared their findings with CT. MR scans showed more extensive abnormality than did third generation CT scans in 8 out of 10 cases and mass effects were better demonstrated with MRI in 14 of the 16 cases in whom they were seen. Furthermore, MRI showed cysts or necrosis in the tumours of four patients of which two had no internal structure demonstrated on CT. Some difficulties were encountered, however. For example, CT demonstrated calcification far better than MRI and the tumour–oedema interface was better shown on CT, particularly when there was marked pathological contrast enhancement within the tumour. Thus, although MRI shows more extensive abnormality than does CT, the results of an MR scan are somewhat non-specific and a differential diagnosis of a tumour is primarily dependent on the site of the lesion and the age and gender of the patient. Further disadvantages of MRI include its cost and slow scanning time, although the development of volume and multislice scanning has significantly cut the total examination time and this should become much less of a problem in the future. The technique has also been applied in the follow-up of patients who have been treated and the role of MRI in attempting to distinguish radiation necrosis from tumour recurrence has been studied (Dooms et al 1986).

IMAGING IN RELATION TO SPECIFIC CLINICAL PROBLEMS

Tumours in the first 24 months of life

Brain tumours in infants under the age of 2 years represent about 10% of cerebral neoplasms seen in children (Tadmor et al 1980, Tomita & McLone 1985). The relative elasticity of the infant's skull and the capacity of the immature nervous system for functional adaptations allow tumours to reach a remarkable size prior to diagnosis. As the developing brain is particularly vulnerable to the effects of raised intracranial pressure, it is imperative to make the diagnosis early if profound retardation is to be avoided after successful surgical treatment. These tumours differ in anatomical distribution and morphological features from those presenting in later childhood and this has led some observers to regard many of them as congenital, particularly those detected in the first year of life (Jooma et al 1984, Radkowski et al 1988). In the first year of life, two-thirds of neoplasms will be supratentorial and of these, approximately half will be located within the cerebral hemisphere, lateral ventricle or thalamus and most of the remainder will be in the suprasellar region including the optic chiasm and third ventricle. During the second year of life, the incidence of posterior fossa and supratentorial tumours is about equal. The frequency and type of tumour encountered in children under 2 years is quite different from the pattern seen throughout the paediatric age group generally. Brain stem tumours, craniopharyngiomas and pineal region tumours are rare and cerebellar astrocytomas much less frequent. Medulloblastomas have a similar frequency to that seen in the preadolescent age group, but are often more aggressive in their behaviour. The great majority (80%) of posterior fossa tumours are histologically malignant and in over 90% of cases they will be associated with hydrocephalus, a frequency which is significantly higher than in older children. Despite this, papilloedema is seen in less than 30% of cases, presumably because the elevated intracranial pressure is compensated for by suture diastasis, whereas in older children this is not possible and papilloedema is found in about 70% of cases (Tomita 1983).

Supratentorial astrocytomas are a common tumour in this age group and approximately half are hemispheric and almost invariably very large; most of the remainder occur in the suprasellar–third ventricular region as gliomas of the optic chiasm or hypothalamus. The optic glioma is a very important tumour of the younger age group and up to 30% of cases include symptoms first appearing in children under 2 years of age, although in a significant number these symptoms are missed (Jooma et al 1984, Davis et al 1984).

Although overall an uncommon tumour, choroid plexus papilloma is a relatively frequent finding in this age group, with 20% of all such tumours occurring in the first year of life, particularly in the trigone of the lateral ventricles and often associated with excess production of CSF leading to hydrocephalus and entrapment of the temporal horn (Hawkins 1980). The third and fourth ventricles are rare sites for this tumour (Van Swieten et al 1987).

Ependymomas constitute about 10% of all intracranial gliomas in children and have a peak incidence from 1 to 5 years, accounting for up to 20% of tumours seen in the first 24 months of life. Over 90% of these are infratentorial in this age group (Swartz et al 1982, Zee et al 1983, Rawlings et al 1988).

Finally, Hart & Earle (1973) first described primitive neuroectodermal tumour (PNET) as a highly malignant, highly cellular tumour composed of over 90% non-differentiated cells with variable foci of differentiation along glial or neuronal lines. They are most often found in the deep white matter of a cerebral hemisphere, may seed within the CSF pathways or metastasize to lungs, liver, bone marrow or lymph nodes (Rorke 1983, Hinshaw et al 1983).

Radiology

Macrocrania due to hydrocephalus, tumour bulk or a combination of both is a most important physical sign of an infant with a brain tumour, the skull circumference being greater than the 98th percentile in 65–70% of patients. The raised intracranial pressure which is the basis for this observation results in suture diastasis which occurs readily in the young infant, such that skull radiographs can provide positive evidence of brain tumour in 85–90% of children under the age of 1 year (Fig. 3.1). Even during the second year of life, the skull radiograph has proved useful, by demonstrating either spread sutures, local erosion of bone or local expansion of a compartment such as the posterior fossa (Fig. 3.1) For this reason skull radiographs may be of some value in screening symptomatic children for brain tumours, but only in this age group when such neoplasms are relatively rare in any case.

As 70% or so of all tumours in children under 2 years are found in the ventricles or along the midline, transcranial ultrasound has played an increasing rôle in basic screening of all infants suspected of a neurological abnormality (Chuang & Harwood-Nash 1986). The open fontanelles or sutures may be used as a window on the brain. As mentioned in the previous statistical review, many of the tumours and huge and a very large proportion are associated with hydrocephalus. Ultrasound readily detects hydrocephalus and recent advances in technology now permit a most accurate display of tumour site, size and anatomical relationships. The majority of masses appear to be echodense, but areas of cystic degeneration and calcification are well demonstrated (Han et al 1984, Chuang & Harwood-Nash 1986). Unfortunately, attempts at tissue characterization have not, so far, come anywhere near matching those of CT and information is lacking about tumour vascularity, breaches in the blood–brain barrier and tumour–oedema interface. It is not always possible to detect haemorrhage within a tumour, especially if the latter is by its own nature an echodense lesion, and haematoma has been mistaken for tumour on occasion (Chuang & Harwood-Nash 1986). Thus, although ultrasound is not very specific for brain tumour, it does show the presence of a mass and indicates the need for additional investigation by CT and possibly angiography. Ultrasound also has great versatility as an intraoperative technique for localizing tumours and any cystic components within these tumours, and is now widely accepted in this rôle (Knake et al 1982, Gooding et al 1983, Knake et al 1984). Ultrasound-guided biopsy of deep-seated masses has also proved reliable (Tsutsumi et al 1982). It has the advantage over stereotactic CT that the whole tumour can be clearly localized after craniotomy and that cysts may be aspirated from any part of the surgical field (Shlosnik et al 1983). Whatever the rôle of skull radiographs and ultrasound, all children should be submitted to CT for a fuller evaluation of their suspected tumour.

CT of supratentorial neoplasia

The major tumour groups comprise (i) hemispheric tumours, usually astrocytomas, occasionally PNET; (ii) lateral ventricular tumours, usually choroid plexus papillomas; and (iii) suprasellar–third ventricular masses, usually optic or hypothalamic gliomas. Ependymomas are rarely encountered as a supratentorial mass in this age group.

Hemisphere astrocytoma

On CT these tumours present as large masses, the majority (55%) having a large cyst with a peripherally situated mural nodule (Fig. 3.4). 90–280 ml of fluid may be found in the cyst (Naidich & Zimmerman 1984). A solid tumour is found in 45% of cases. The most frequent sites, in decreasing order of frequency, are the temporal lobe, where cystic tumours are twice as common as solid masses; the frontal lobe where cystic and solid lesions are found with equal frequency; and the parietal lobe where solid tumours are twice as common. Unfortunately, there is considerable variation in the CT appearances which may, at times, resemble the adult glioma or glioblastoma.

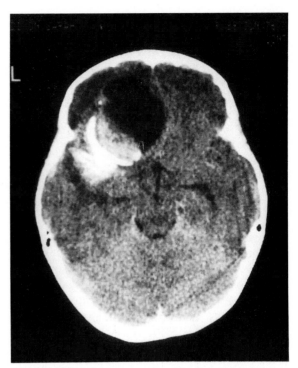

Fig. 3.4 Hemisphere astrocytoma. Note large cyst, peripherally situated mural nodule and local invasion of adjacent temporal lobe.

The pattern of contrast enhancement is also unhelpful as a guide to the relative malignancy of the tumour and bears no relation to neovascularity as shown by angiography. It is therefore not possible on CT grounds alone to differentiate benign from malignant tumours or to offer any reliable prognostic guidance.

Angiography has a rôle because there is a fairly strong correlation between the extent of neovascularity of the mass and grade of malignancy and it is the author's view that catheter arteriography should be undertaken in most, if not all, cases as a prelude to surgery. Angiography also defines the relationship of the lesion to the vessels, thereby assisting the safe surgical resection of the peritumoural bridging veins and venous sinuses.

PNET

This tumour constitutes the major differential diagnosis of a large hemisphere mass and usually occupies the deep white matter where it presents a varied CT appearance. It is almost always very sharply marginated (Fig. 3.5a and b), but despite this, tumour will frequently be found well beyond the boundary suggested by CT, and this examination is therefore a very poor determinant of infiltration into the surrounding brain. On the non-contrasted scan, the tumour is hypodense in 55%, isodense in 22%, of mixed isodensity/hyperdensity in 22% and virtually never purely hyperdense. Calcification, often gross, is seen in 50–70% (as compared with astrocytoma where this is exceedingly rare) and cyst-like necrotic areas are found within the tumour in 30–60% of cases (Altman et al 1985). Intratumoural haemorrhage is relatively common (10%) and may be a presenting feature (Zimmerman & Bilaniuk 1980). Peritumoural oedema, often extensive, is the rule (90%), a feature which is also usually lacking in astrocytomas. Contrast enhancement may be homogeneous, patchy or ring-like, the pattern having no clinical significance.

Angiography has a dual purpose. Firstly, as these tumours have a propensity for growing along the falx or tentorium and often frankly invade the meninges (Priest et al 1981), arteriography may show a meningeal blood supply derived from the external carotid artery. Direct invasion of a venous sinus with tumour occlusion may also be demonstrated. These are not features of the other large hemisphere mass, the astrocytoma, and therefore arteriography is useful in distinguishing between the two. Furthermore, external carotid embolization prior to surgery has been found to reduce the vascularity of the mass sufficient to aid its removal (Hinshaw et al 1983).

Seeding into the CSF pathways has been reported in up to 50% of cases. The value of screening myelography is debatable. These tumours have a bad prognosis and, if radiation

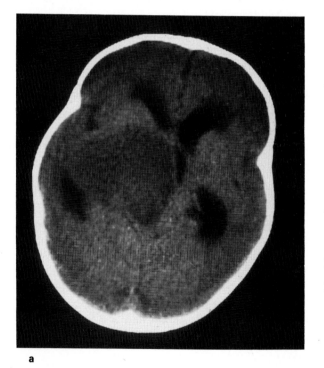
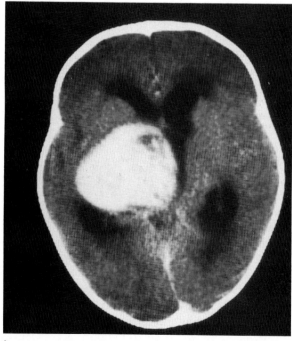

a   b

Fig. 3.5 (a) PNET. Non-contrast scan shows well defined, slightly hypodense mass within the deep white matter of the left hemisphere associated with hydrocephalus due to obstruction of the third ventricle. (b) Postcontrast CT demonstrates intense enhancement of the tumour which appears well marginated. Despite this, tumour is frequently found well beyond the boundaries suggested on CT. A small area of peripheral tumour necrosis is seen (top right).

therapy is contemplated, some argue that it should be applied to the whole neuraxis empirically.

Ependymoma

Supratentorial ependymomas are rare tumours, occurring more commonly in boys, and are typically malignant (86%). They are usually seen on CT as a single large tumour of the cerebral white matter, most frequently in the frontal lobe and sometimes within the parietal lobe. Very occasionally they may be intraventricular. Calcification is seen in 50% of cases and the tumours are cystic in around 70% of cases. Intratumoural haemorrhage has also been recorded. The CT features are not diagnostic and considerable difficulty may arise in distinguishing this tumour from a PNET. The only distinguishing feature appears to be the presence of peritumoural oedema which is observed in 90% of cases of PNET and is a rare finding with ependymoma. Both these tumour groups are uncommon and a cerebral hemisphere mass in this age group is much more likely to be an astrocytoma, the features of which have already been discussed.

Choroid plexus papilloma

This rare tumour is seen as a coarsely lobulated, round, mixed or high density intraventricular mass showing marked contrast enhancement. It is usually located in the trigone of a lateral ventricle, rarely in the third or fourth ventricles. Associated hydrocephalus is common, either due to excess CSF production or to obstruction of the foramen of Monroe by tumour bulk. The CT diagnosis is largely based on the site of the tumour as the appearances are non-specific. The diagnosis has also been made on ultrasound, but distinguishing a choroid plexus haematoma from a papilloma can be difficult (Chuang & Harwood-Nash 1986).

Arteriography will confirm the intraventricular origin by demonstrating a typical blood supply via the choroidal arteries. This has some surgical significance because papillomas are known to be highly vascular and, in order to minimize life-threatening blood loss, neurosurgeons stress the importance of securing the major arterial supply at the outset (Hawkins 1980, Jooma et al 1984). For this reason it may be necessary to consider vertebral angiography if carotid studies have not opacified the whole tumour.

Histologically, some of these neoplasms are benign and surgery may offer the chance of a cure, whilst a somewhat larger proportion are malignant with a correspondingly poor prognosis. Experience to date does not suggest that any neuroradiological investigation on reliably distinguish between these two groups.

Optic and hypothalamic gliomas

Up to 30% of optic gliomas will be associated with symptoms first appearing in children under 2 years and 80% of these tumours will occur in the first decade of life. They represent benign hamartomatous tumours of childhood (juvenile pilocytic astrocytoma) which may involve any part of the visual pathways and are associated with neurofibromatosis in 25–50% of cases (Stern et al 1980). They are characterized by slow growth and present with an insidious visual loss in one or both eyes with or without proptosis. Over 50% of these lesions are mainly or entirely intracranial with little or no involvement of the intraorbital optic nerves. Extension of the tumour into the hypothalamic and third ventricular area is common and this is the usual finding at the time of neuroradiological assessment when distinction from a hypothalamic glioma is one of the diagnostic problems encountered. Such extensive lesions may be associated with a survival of many years, although patients with tumours confined to the chiasm and optic nerves generally have a better prognosis (Fletcher et al 1986). This contrasts with optic and chiasmatic gliomas encountered in adults which are almost invariably highly malignant tumours which readily spread to the adjacent neuraxis and are associated with a very poor prognosis. When diabetes insipidus, a short stature, delayed puberty, the diencephalic syndrome or hydrocephalus are the presenting symptoms, a hypothalamic glioma is more likely. Such tumours may spread to involve the chiasm and visual pathways and, when large, may be indistinguishable from large posterior optic gliomas. Although they are usually low grade astrocytomas, they are more likely than optic chiasm gliomas to exhibit aggressive behaviour.

Radiologically, the examination of choice is CT, although plain radiographs will assist in determining whether one or both optic canals are expanded or eroded, which they will do better than CT in most cases. This is an important observation to make, as the majority of optic gliomas will expand the canal whereas this is uncommon even with huge hypothalamic tumours (Fig. 3.6).

With optic chiasm glioma, contrast-enhanced CT frequently shows the characteristic appearance of an enhancing mass lesion enlarging the chiasm and extending into the optic nerves on one or both sides, often with dilatation and elevation of the third ventricles. Recently Patronas et al (1987) have evaluated the contributions of CT and MRI in imaging these tumours and concluded that all tumours were identified with both techniques, but in the majority of cases the posterior extension of the tumour and its relationship to adjacent brain were shown better by MRI.

Hypothalamic gliomas are associated with more subtle enhancement although this can usually be detected in up to two-thirds of tumours, and obliteration of the third ventricle with resultant hydrocephalus is the rule rather than the exception.

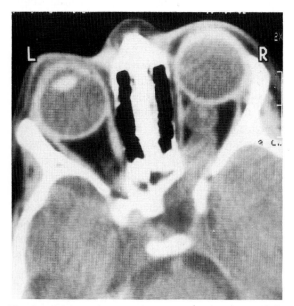

Fig. 3.6 Right optic nerve glioma. Suprasellar tumour with contiguous globular expansion of the optic nerve and characteristic expansion of the optic canal.

Calcification is very rare in either tumour except after radiotherapy (Savoiardo et al 1981), a feature which distinguishes these lesions from craniopharyngiomas, especially in older children.

When the intraorbital optic nerves are involved, CT will show a fusiform enlargement of a part of the optic nerve, the tumour being concentrically situated around the axis of the nerve. It is generally homogeneous in density and usually enhances. Calcification is very rare. The density of the tumour on the non-contrast scan is of no clinical help in determining prognosis and is probably a measure of the partial volume effect, small tumours appearing less dense because of the incorporation of low density intraorbital fat within the CT slice. Thus, the rarer, purely intraorbital optic nerve gliomas are relatively easy to diagnose and the main problems arise with large chiasmatic/suprasellar masses. Even here, it will be possible in the majority of patients to distinguish between optic chiasm and hypothalamic gliomas if one relies on the plain film and CT differences discussed above, along with the clinical history and presentation. In a few cases the distinction is impossible and neither angiography nor MRI (so far) will solve the problem (Lourie et al 1986). In fact, angiography usually underestimates the tumour extent as these lesions are generally hypovascular (Davis et al 1984).

Various fundamental questions may be asked of CT in relation to chiasmal gliomas:

1. Can the potential for tumour growth be predicted from the initial CT appearance?

2. Are there any correlations between CT features and the presence or absence of neurofibromatosis?

3. Is it possible to establish a correlation between CT changes and the level of visual function at diagnosis and with any subsequent change?

4 How useful is CT in monitoring the beneficial or adverse effects of radiation therapy and surgery?

These matters were addressed by Fletcher et al (1986) who found three distinct patterns of disease which were diagnostic of optic chiasm glioma: (i) tubular thickening of the optic nerve and chiasm; (ii) a suprasellar tumour with contiguous optic nerve expansion (Fig. 3.6); and (iii) a suprasellar tumour with optic tract involvement. In contrast, globular suprasellar tumours without optic nerve or tract involvement required a histological examination for diagnosis. Biopsy could therefore be reserved for this group of tumours and the diagnosis of chiasmal gliomas safely assumed on the CT appearances alone if these fell into one of the three patterns already mentioned. Tumour growth was documented by serial CT in only 3 out of a total of 22 patients – all were of the globular type. Chiasmal gliomas with optic nerve or tract involvement tended to remain the same year after year. The presence and degree of pathological contrast enhancement had no prognostic value. Tubular optic nerve and chiasmal thickening was only found in patients with neurofibromatosis, and chiasmal gliomas with contiguous intraorbital optic nerve expansion were observed predominantly in patients with neurofibromatosis. On the other hand, globular chiasmal gliomas without optic nerve or tract involvement were very seldom associated with neurofibromatosis. The CT appearances showed no correlation with visual function either at diagnosis or on follow-up. Failing visual function did not reflect chiasmal tumour growth and stable vision did not exclude it.

Five out of 16 patients receiving radiation therapy showed post-treatment tumour shrinkage and in all there was a corresponding reduction of pathological contrast enhancement. Three patients showed significant tumour enlargement after radiotherapy whilst the remaining eight lesions remained unaltered. Unfortunately, there was very little correlation between alterations in tumour size and visual improvement or deterioration and CT was unable to predict those tumours which would shrink following radiotherapy. Postradiation effects mainly consisted of progressive calcification within the surrounding brain, particularly in the region of the lentform nuclei, and cerebral infarction outside the primary beam.

In conclusion, CT has modified and refined the role of neurosurgery in the management of chiasmal gliomas. It facilitates both detection of hydrocephalus and monitoring of shunt function. The specificity of CT in establishing the diagnosis of most types of chiasmal glioma obviates the need for craniotomy. Its lack of specificity in the case of a globular suprasellar mass constitutes a clear indication for surgical exploration and biopsy.

CT posterior fossa neoplasia

Ependymoma

Ependymoma is a neoplasm composed of and usually derived from differentiated ependymal cells. It therefore tends to arise in close relationship to the ventricles. Ependymal cell rests may, however, be found far from the ventricular linings, particularly (i) where the ventricles are sharply angled, (ii) posterior to the occipital horns, (iii) adjacent to the foramina of Luschka, and (iv) along the tela choroidea. Tumour origin from such rests may explain intraparenchymal and cerebello-pontine angle ependymomas (Naidich & Zimmerman 1984). These tumours constitute approximately 8% of all intracranial gliomas in children, affecting boys more than girls and having a peak age incidence from 1 to 5 years (and again in adults at around 35 years). Posterior fossa ependymomas constitute 70% of those seen in childhood but this figure rises to over 90% in children under 2 years of age. Almost 50% of cases of posterior fossa ependymoma are malignant, and in a third there is tumour dissemination throughout the subarachnoid space, usually of the intraspinal region. In 80% of cases, posterior fossa ependymoma grows within the fourth ventricle. About 15% extend into the cerebello-pontine angle cistern and involve the lateral recess of the fourth ventricle. Development within a cerebellar hemisphere is relatively uncommon (8%). Intraventricular ependymoma may also grow downwards through the foramen of Magendie to the vallecula and into the brain stem or cerebellum or through the foramen magnum into the cervical spinal canal.

The CT findings are usually those of a midline mass, poorly defined and situated within an expanded fourth ventricle. A characteristic feature of ependymoma is the production of hydrocephalus at an early stage of tumour growth, with the result that these tumours are generally smaller than most others at the time of presentation. The non-contrast study may show a tumour of virtually any density. Calcification, often dense, is seen in 50% of cases and small intratumoural lucencies, presumably representing areas of necrosis, are also seen in half the cases. Acute haemorrhage into the tumour may be detected in between 10 and 15%

of patients (Swartz et al 1982, Zee et al 1983). Varying degrees of enhancement will usually be seen in the solid portion of the tumour in about 85% of cases. Posterior fossa ependymoma thus has a very variable CT appearance, the single most common and useful characteristic being the presence of prominant calcification within a moderately enhancing fourth ventricular mass. In the first 2 years of life, the principal differential diagnosis is from a medulloblastoma and just possibly from ependymal seeding of the fourth ventricle by a supratentorial tumour. In older children an astrocytoma would also have to be considered.

Initial CT studies may document dissemination of ependymoma to the basal cisterns and lateral ventricles and, in older children, a case can be made out for examining the spinal subarachnoid space at myelography. Whether this should also be undertaken in the younger age group under discussion remains a contentious issue. Stanley et al (1985) have shown that ependymoma is the second most common tumour to seed throughout the intraspinal subarachnoid space and maintain that all children with posterior fossa ependymomas, irrespective of age, should have routine postoperative myelography even though they have no spinal symptoms. In very young infants this will often necessitate the use of general anaesthesia, which therefore adds a further invasive aspect to the investigation.

Common tumours in the older child

Medulloblastoma

Medulloblastoma is a highly malignant tumour composed of primitive embryonal cells capable of differentiating into glial or neuronal elements (Camins et al 1980). The tumour originates from primitive glial cells most frequently found in the germinative zone of the posterior medullary velum. These cells migrate from the roof of the fourth ventricle to form the external granular layer of the cerebellar hemispheres, and medulloblastomas may therefore develop anywhere along the path of migration. They constitute 15–20% of all intracranial neoplasms in childhood and, along with cerebellar astrocytomas, are the commonest

posterior fossa tumour in children. They affect boys twice as often as girls. Anatomically, medulloblastomas are usually found within the cerebellar vermis (93%), being confined to the vermis in 30%, extending from the vermis into the cerebellar hemisphere in 31% and invading the brain stem by direct extension across the fourth ventricle in 32%. In 7% of cases, the tumour is confined to the cerebellar hemispheres (Naidich & Zimmerman 1984). Spontaneous haemorrhage may be seen in around 5% of cases at presentation, and can also occur spontaneously after radiotherapy or following preoperative ventricular drainage (Park et al 1983).

Medulloblastomas are usually classified into four histological types: (i) classical (80%); (ii) desmoplastic (15%); (iii) pleomorphic (4%); and (iv) melanotic (1%). Classical medulloblastomas occur with almost equal frequency among the different age groups, whereas the age distribution of desmoplastic medulloblastomas is skewed towards younger children with 52% occurring in children under 5 years and 95% in children under 10 years. Tumour dissemination is frequent and often widespread. Subarachnoid seeding and direct arachnoid invasion are commonly observed preoperatively or at postmortem (McComb et al 1981, Tomita & McLone 1983) when they are often found involving the skull base and within the sylvian fissures where a thick layer of tumour cells may form along the inferior and lateral surfaces of the cerebrum, brain stem and cerebellum.

Spinal cord and cauda equina metastases are reported in 10–45% of patients and are cervical in location in 10%, thoracic in 30%, lumbo-sacral in 22% and involve multiple sites in 38% (Deutsch & Reigel 1980, Allen & Epstein 1982, Park et al 1983). The majority are intradural/extramedullary lesions but true intramedullary metastases have been described. They are usually clinically silent, even when large. Systemic metastases are found in about 10–15% of patients and may occur prior to surgical intervention although it is noteworthy that the incidence rises to almost 20% when preoperative ventricular shunts are performed without a millipore filter (Park et al 1983). The most frequent site of distal metastasis is the skeleton (86%) followed by the peritoneum (via shunt) (43%), lymph nodes (30%), lung (7%) and liver.

Radiological management

A detailed appreciation of the pathology and natural history of medulloblastomas as outlined above is required to obtain the best use of neuroradiology in diagnosing the tumour, documenting any complications at presentation, seeking prognostic features and monitoring treatment, as well as studying the biology of the disease.

Tumour diagnosis

Presumably owing to their high degree of cellularity, medulloblastomas tend to appear uniformly hyperdense on non-contrast CT (70%) and less often isodense (20%) or of mixed density (10%) (Fig. 3.7a). They are very rarely hypodense. Characteristically, they will present as a large, round to oval, discreetly marginated, non-calcified, midline mass situated in the inferior vermis behind the fourth ventricle. As the tumour enlarges, it invaginates the fourth ventricle dis-placing it anteriorly and finally obstructing it. The mass may be circumscribed by a lucent halo of CSF compromising invaginated fourth ventricle anteriorly and compressed cisterna magna posteriorly.

Contrast enhancement is the rule (95%) and is typically homogeneous (Fig. 3.7b), being due in part to breakdown of the blood–brain barrier and in part to the hypervascularity of the tumour. The pattern of enhancement may be modified if the patient is given steroids prior to the examination and this has been the usual explanation for the rare instances when the neoplasm has failed to enhance or has done so only very faintly. The mass may, of course, arise within a cerebellar hemisphere or extend from the midline into it and lateral growth into an adjacent cerebello-pontine angle cistern may occur. Brain stem compression or frank invasion can be discerned in just under a third of cases. Calcification is infrequent (under 10%) and cystic or necrotic areas are uncommon. Differential diagnosis is mainly from ependymoma, especially in the very young infant. The principal

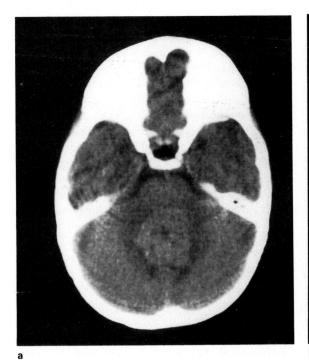
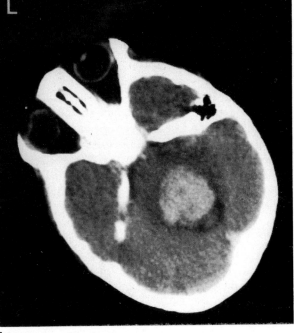

a   b

Fig. 3.7 (a) Medulloblastoma. Non-contrast CT with uniformly hyperdense, midline posterior fossa mass. (b) Same patient after intravenous contrast showing typical homogeneous enhancement.

features distinguishing an ependymoma are the presence of dense calcification in 50%, a greater frequency of mixed or low density tumours before contrast and the relatively small size of the tumour compared with medulloblastomas which are nearly always very large at presentation.

In the author's view, angiography has little merit nowadays in the assessment of posterior fossa tumours but a few workers still employ this technique in an attempt to distinguish ependymoma from medulloblastoma in difficult cases. Medulloblastomas may display a subtle blush, but never show frank neovascularity or early-draining veins. A vermian mass effect displaces the choroidal loops of the posterior inferior cerebellar artery downward and forward, and generally speaking, both choroidal points are displaced to the contralateral side. This is in contrast to the intraventricular ependymoma which will usually spread the choroidal points apart in the frontal projection and displace them posteriorly in the lateral projection. It seems highly unlikely that the surgical management of the patient will be affected by subtle angiographic distinctions and the examination is now less often employed.

Complications

Hydrocephalus is almost invariable at the time of presentation. Spontaneous haemorrhage within the tumour is poorly documented but probably occurs as an acute event in 4–5% of cases and may, therefore, be a presenting feature. One should also take into account the fact that per-operative shunts or other ventricular drainage devices have been implicated in the development of haemorrhage in posterior fossa tumours (Epstein & Murali 1978, Vaquero et al 1981).

Prognosis

Two distinct but related prognostic factors have been clearly identified: age of the child and tumour dissemination at diagnosis. Children under 2 years of age have the worst prognosis and children under 5 years generally do badly compared with those in the older age groups (Berry et al 1981, Allen & Epstein 1982, Park et al 1983, Kaputy et al 1987). Younger children also have a greater likelihood of having dissemination of disease at diagnosis. Two possible explanations for the association of age and disease dissemination are late diagnosis and tumour biology. There is no evidence that the duration of symptoms prior to diagnosis is any longer in the younger age groups. Since it is unlikely that an operation in a young child is any more likely to disseminate tumour than in an older child, the tumour probably seeds throughout the neuraxis prior to surgery, reflecting a higher degree of malignancy of the neoplasm in the younger patient.

CT is ideal for demonstrating early intracranial subarachnoid seeding. This is usually manifest as intense leptomeningeal enhancement around the base of the brain and into the sylvian fissures with obliteration of the quadrigeminal cistern. Occasionally, nodular masses may be seen within the cisterns or larger masses within the lateral ventricles (North et al 1985). The occurrence of these metastases has been attributed to poor encapsulation of the primary tumour, local invasion of the fourth ventricle and/or extension into the subarachnoid space, the primitive nature of the tumour cells themselves, and the viability of the tumour cells in CSF. It is interesting to note that North et al (1985) noted a strong positive correlation between the appearance on the initial CT and myelography. Five of their cases with intracranial subarachnoid seeding also had myelography, and in all 5 cases they demonstrated metastases in the spinal subarachnoid space. They further emphasized the low incidence of positive CSF cytology (1 positive out of 7 cases) and this poor correlation between abnormal myelography and normal CSF cytology was also commented upon by Deutsch & Reigel (1980) in their study of 16 patients with medulloblastoma, 7 of whom had abnormal myelograms, but in 5 of whom the CSF findings were normal. These two studies suggest that CSF cytology may be a poor indicator of disseminated subarachnoid seeding and the latter authors in particular strongly recommended myelography on all children with medulloblastoma, irrespective of the CSF cytology findings. In a further study, Stanley et al (1985) found myelographic evidence of subarachnoid metastatic seeding in 12 out of 16 children with medulloblastoma and commented upon the associated poor prognosis in this group. At myelography, a variety of patterns of intraspinal spread are seen. In the lumbo-sacral region, nodularity and irregularity of the distal sac is common, as is nodular thickening of the nerve roots with obliteration of the root sleeves. The high incidence of involvement of the lumbo-sacral region is probably an effect of gravity on the CSF-borne metastases. Diffuse thickening with adhesions of the nerve roots and irregular obliteration of the subarachnoid space may resemble chemical or postinfective arachnoiditis.

In the cervical and thoracic regions a variety of appearances are seen reflecting involvement of the cord and surrounding membranes. Nodularity or cloaking of the cord with plaques of tumour is common, a finding often observed at post mortem. A degree of caution is required in interpreting widening of the cord which is nearly always the result of compression from extensive extramedullary plaques and not from intramedullary metastases, which are rare. However, metastatic disease may invade the cord parenchyma from the surface, a feature which it is not possible to assess accurately in radiological studies. From a technical viewpoint, several aspects need emphasizing. As the metastatic tumour seedlings have a predilection for the dorsal surface of the cord, supine myelography is essential. The detail provided by careful myelography is entirely sufficient, so CT of the spine following myelography is rarely required, but might be helpful in some cases where there is apparent widening of the cord. Early reports on the rôle of MRI in screening the spine for asymptomatic disease were disappointing, mainly because most studies were performed using a body coil with a slice thickness in the 0.8 cm to 1.5 cm range (Paushter et al 1985). The recent introduction of surface coil technology has allowed a 4 mm slice thickness owing to improvement in the signal-to-noise ratio, and more encouraging results have been found (Barloon et al 1987).

The International Society of Paediatric Oncology (Bloom 1979) and the Children's Cancer Study Group (Evans et al 1979) have amassed evidence identifying the importance of such prognostic factors as tumour size, extent of tumour infiltration and degree of surgical resection. Modern CT scanners can readily measure tumour size and volume, particularly after contrast enhancement. According to the earlier work of Chang et al (1969), tumours of 3 cm or greater in diameter were associated with the worst prognosis, findings confirmed by Kopelson et al (1983), although many observers have challenged this assertion and as most neurosurgeons agree that the primary tumour should be resected completely whenever this is practical, the preoperative tumour size and volume have assumed less importance. Prognosis is related to the completeness or otherwise of tumour excision and this, in its turn, is dependent on the site and extent of infiltration present. Part of a cerebellar hemisphere and vermis can frequently be sacrificed to obtain a complete clearance, but this is not the case with brain stem involvement or extension into the peduncles. CT parameters of infiltration in childhood posterior fossa tumours have been elegantly studied by Kingsley & Harwood-Nash (1984) who used high resolution scanner and compared their findings with detailed operative reports to evaluate morphological features indicative of infiltration. Their study suggested that the line of demarcation between the tumour and normal tissue, and hence the degree of infiltration, is problematical. Only where there was a sharp demarcation between densely-enhancing tumour tissue and the surrounding oedema or normal brain was a plane of cleavage usually found, and even then this was not consistent. Where there was a gradual decrease in the degree of enhancement towards the tumour edge, or where the whole tumour did not enhance to a great degree, a relatively infrequent CT finding, infiltration was usually present. Brain stem infiltration was frequently impossible to assess, even when the fourth ventricle could be seen. The position and appearance of the fourth ventricle on CT was compared with the operative findings. They attempted to determine whether the ventricle was displaced by or filled with tumour, and they were successful in their interpretation in 60% of cases. In four instances apparent displacement of the ventricle was, in reality, a ventricle filled with tumour and where the fourth ventricle was not visualized, there was an approximately equal chance of it being displaced and compressed by, or filled with, tumour. There was no relationship between the extent or appearance of peritumoural oedema and the presence or absence of infiltration. CT has, therefore, proved rather disappointing in its ability to record the presence and degree of infiltration, particularly of vital structures such as the brain stem.

MRI has clear advantages over CT in the posterior fossa and is especially valuable in demonstrating midline and deep-seated lesions. It shows more extensive abnormality than does CT and provides much greater detail about the internal structures of tumours particularly in relation to cystic or necrotic areas (Peterman et al 1984). Potentially, it should display a greater accuracy in determining the extent of infiltration, although a possible disadvantage is the relative inability of MRI to identify the tumour–oedema interface (Johnson et al 1983).

At least one paper has highlighted the discrepancy between CT and MR imaging in a case of medulloblastoma which was diagnosed on CT as a brain stem glioma, but where MRI demonstrated the lesion to be extrinsic to the brain stem and posterior fossa exploration disclosed a medulloblastoma filling the fourth ventricle (Heafner et al 1985).

Post treatment management

In assessing the extent of surgical resection, the timing of the postoperative CT study is crucial and contrast enhancement is essential. During the first 5 days following surgery, no enhancement is seen if all the tumour has been removed. Postoperative enhancement along the line of surgical resection first appears at 6 to 8 days, is maximal at 11 to 18 days and then fades, sometimes over several months. The mechanism for this is ill understood but the phenomenon appears to be a 'physiological' reaction following resection of virtually any brain tumour and is not significantly affected by steroids. It only occurs along the margins of 'raw' exposed brain and is not found at any time following a complete lobectomy. Pathological enhancement before 5 days therefore equals residual tumour, and this represents the optimum time for scanning the patient for this purpose. After 6 to 8 days, pathological enhancement has to be interpreted with great caution. In the early postoperative period, CT may be employed to monitor the efficacy of a shunting procedure or to seek complications related to it such as infection.

Ventriculitis is relatively easy to diagnose, either by ultrasound (in infants) where the key feature is increased echodensity of the ventricular walls, or by contrast-enhanced CT where there is pathological enhancement of the ventricular ependyma. On the other hand, infection at the operative site may pose something of a problem since the hallmark of an abscess is the presence of ring-like enhancement within an area of oedema, and differentiation from residual tumour in the first few days, and resection-line enhancement thereafter, is problematical especially as one can reasonably expect oedema to be present in any case. A further difficulty is encountered if the patient is on steroids, as this may greatly reduce the potential contrast enhancement within an abscess capsule.

On later follow-up CT, it may be difficult to distinguish residual calcified tumour from dystrophic calcification within the tumour bed as a result of radiation treatment with or without adjuvant chemotherapy (Kingsley & Kendall 1981, Davis et al 1986). Radiotherapy may also induce haemorrhage within residual tumour (*vide infra*).

Cerebellar astrocytoma

As the name implies, this tumour is composed of astrocytes displaying varying degrees of maturity and is often subcategorized into ascending grades of malignancy from 1 to 4. Fortunately, most are grade 1, and a few grade 2. They may be further classified as juvenile type, which form the great majority of those seen in children (25 year survival rate, 94%), or diffuse/adult type which may occasionally be seen in this age group and have a much poorer prognosis (25 year survival rate, 38%) (Gjerris & Klinken 1978). Overall, they constitute 10% of paediatric brain tumours and affect both sexes with equal frequency. They may arise in any part of the cerebellum but classical teaching has the majority of juvenile type occurring in the midline, possibly extending into one or both hemispheres (80%), whereas in adults they usually arise de novo within the hemisphere. Most midline and combined midline/hemisphere tumours bulge into the fourth ventricle and 10% are found predominantly within the ventricle (Szenasy & Slowik 1983).

Cerebellar astrocytomas may be solid or cystic,

the incidence being approximately equal for midline lesions, while lateral tumours are cystic in over 80%. The cyst wall may consist of non-neoplastic compressed glial cerebellar tissue, in which case the tumour itself lies along the cyst wall as a mural nodule, while in other cases necrosis within solid tumour creates a true neoplastic cavity, often multilocular, and lined entirely by tumour. This distinction can be observed on CT by the presence or absence of enhancement of the wall. It appears that contrast enhancement of the wall only occurs when it is composed of tumour elements. Interesting though this observation is, Gjerris & Klinken (1978) found no correlation with patient survival.

On CT, cerebellar astrocytomas are usually large and their solid or cystic propensity readily determined. The CT number (Hounsfield Units) of the cysts is generally well above that of CSF because of the high protein content within them. On non-

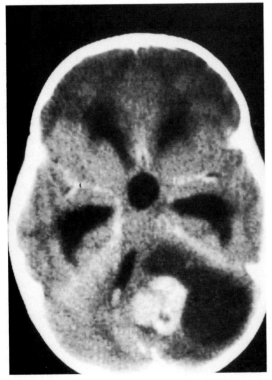

Fig. 3.8 Cerebellar juvenile astrocytoma. Postcontrast CT demonstrates large cyst with enhancement of intramural tumour mass. Note the absence of enhancement of the cyst wall which is composed of compressed cerebellar tissue.

contrast CT, the mural nodule is virtually always solitary, tends to be isodense with cerebellum and, after intravenous contrast, shows a well defined intense homogeneous tumour blush. One would not expect there to be any enhancement of the wall of the cyst as it is composed of compressed cerebellar tissue (Fig. 3.8), but when a cyst forms as a result of necrosis within a previously solid astrocytoma, the cyst is usually multilocular and its walls, being composed of necrotic tumour tissue, will enhance with contrast (Turnbull & Hughes, unpublished observation). In this situation there will, of course, be no evidence of a mural nodule.

Solid astrocytomas are usually round, lobulated and moderately well defined. They are of variable density relative to brain and show a wide pattern of pathological enhancement including ring-like, dense, homogeneous or hardly any at all. Calcification is not a feature of either solid or cystic astrocytomas. The CT diagnosis of a classical cystic cerebellar astrocytoma therefore poses very few diagnostic problems in the majority of instances. With solid tumours, however, the differentiation from medulloblastoma (in all age groups) and ependymoma (particularly in young infants) can be extremely difficult.

Brain stem glioma

This term is used to encompass a group of glial tumours intrinsic to the medulla, pons or midbrain and they constitute 10–20% of all intracranial childhood tumours. About 70% of brain stem gliomas are anaplastic astrocytomas or glioblastoma multiforme. A few represent a subgroup of atypical benign glioma (Hoffman et al 1980). Girls and boys are affected equally with a peak incidence between 4 and 13 years. Whilst specific subgroups may achieve a 5 year survival of 55%, the great majority of patients show a steady deterioration to death with a median survival of 4–15 months (Epstein 1985, Albright et al 1986, Epstein & McCleary 1986, Stroink et al 1986, Jenkin et al 1987). Thus, despite being a relatively common neoplasm, the management remains controversial because of the differing biological behaviour of these tumours. This has prompted several workers to seek a CT classification of these lesions based on their location, whether they are focal or diffuse, solid or cystic and whether they have any specific contrast enhancing features. Epstein (1985) proposed a staging system based mainly on tumour location describing tumours as (i) intrinsic, (ii) exophytic or (iii) disseminated. Neoplasms of less than 2 cm were regarded as focal and those greater than 2 cm as diffuse. Exophytic tumours were considered in relation to the cerebello-pontine angle anterolaterally, the brachium pontis posterolaterally and the fourth ventricle behind. Disseminated tumour was diagnosed by routine spinal fluid cytology supplemented by myelography in specific cases. Epstein showed that all diffuse neoplasms were malignant and had an extremely poor prognosis. The great majority of anterolateral and posterolateral exophytic tumours were also malignant and shared a similarly poor outcome. A relatively unique group of exophytic brain stem tumours grew posteriorly into the fourth ventricle, tending to occur in very young children and to cause symptoms as a result of hydrocephalus. These neoplasms were commonly found to be low grade astrocytomas which were subependymal in origin and grew posteriorly rather than anteriorly into the brain stem. He concluded that surgery should only be considered as potentially beneficial for focal astrocytomas of grade 1 or 2, and experienced considerable difficulty in distinguishing peritumoural oedema from malignant infiltration based on CT criteria. The best results appeared to be related to tumours found at the cervico-medullary junction. Substantially similar results were reported by Albright et al (1986), who were also unable to show any relationship between prognosis and the enhancement of the tumour.

Possibly the best CT classification of brain stem tumours as it relates to prognosis has been reported by Stroink et al (1986) who categorized these tumours into the following groups based on CT criteria:

1. Group 1 represented tumours which were isodense or slightly hypodense on the plain scan, and all extended posteriorly from the brain stem into the fourth ventricle which they filled. Tumours in this group all enhanced brightly. This cohort had the best outcome with 10 out of 11 patients alive after a mean follow-up period of 4.5 years.

2. Group 2(a) were diffuse tumours intrinsic to the brain stem which were hypodense and did not enhance. All these tumours were of high grade malignancy and the prognosis for these patients was dismal, none in the group surviving beyond 20 months from the time of diagnosis. Group 2(b) patients had a diffuse tumour intrinsic to the brain stem with hyperdense, exophytic, contrast-enhancing components extending into the cerebello-pontine angle anterolaterally. A similarly hopeless outcome was recorded in this population with a mean survival time of 12 months.

3. Group 3 contained tumours which were intrinsic to the brain stem, focal and cystic with a contrast-enhancing capsule. Despite cyst aspiration and radiotherapy, virtually all the patients in this group were dead within 12 months.

4. In group 4 there was a solid focal isodense tumour intrinsic to the brain stem which showed marked contrast enhancement with usually clear margins. This group had the second best outcome, 7 out of 9 patients being alive with a mean follow-up period of 2.3 years.

From these various study groups we can conclude that CT is vital in classifying brain stem tumours into those in which a reasonable outcome might be predicted and which probably warrant surgical intervention, and those in which the prognosis is so dismal that surgery is not indicated, even for biopsy, and alternative treatment with radiotherapy and chemotherapy is the management of choice. If surgery is being contemplated based on the CT criteria discussed above, then it may be worth remembering that as many as 25% of brain stem tumours disseminate throughout the spinal axis some time between diagnosis and death. This not only has implications for treatment but may provide a basis for routine myelography in this small group of patients.

Finally, most workers agree that it is important when offering radiotherapy to include the entire tumour volume within the radiation field. The boundaries of those fields should, ideally, be based on MRI, since the extent of paediatric brain stem gliomas on MRI exceeds that visible on CT scan in up to 50% of cases (Packer et al 1985). These workers found that MRI demonstrated more extensive disease in 50% of the cases, especially in the cervico-medullary region where tumours carry the best prognosis. MRI also seems to be better than CT in following the response of brain stem gliomas to therapy and in confirming relapses.

Craniopharyngioma

This is an epithelial neoplasm believed to originate from nests of squamous epithelial cells in the pars tuberalis or Rathke's pouch. Structurally, they are closely affiliated to the epidermoid cysts found in other sites and have been described under a bewildering collection of names. They constitute about 4% of all intracranial tumours and account for 17% of supratentorial neoplasms found in children.

CT reveals a lobulated mass lesion within the suprasellar cistern with prominent tumoural calcification seen in 80% of childhood cases (compared with 30% in adults), being ring-like in two-thirds and nodular in the remainder (Fig. 3.9a). The presence of calcification is not related to the size of the tumour nor to whether it is solid or cystic (Cabezudo et al 1981). At least 60% of craniopharyngiomas presenting in childhood con-

tain cystic areas (Fig. 3.9b) (compared with 15% in adults), but the incidence rises to almost 100% with giant tumours (Al-Mefty et al 1985) and with recurrent disease (Cabezudo et al 1981). Pathological contrast enhancement is readily detected in 50–75% of lesions presenting in children and may be seen within the tumour wall or consist of ill defined blush throughout the whole tumour mass. Recurrent tumours, however, virtually always display some enhancement.

The accuracy of CT in diagnosing a suprasellar mass as a craniopharyngioma depends on whether the tumour is cystic, contains calcification, and displays contrast enhancement. It approaches 100% when all the features are present, which they are in 70% of cases. When any two of these criteria are present (25%), the accuracy falls to 85%. On the rare occasions when only one of them is evident, accuracy falls to 50% with difficulty in distinguishing other lesions such as hypothalamic or chiasmal gliomas, dermoids or interventricular meningiomas. A further diagnostic difficulty arises in respect of the 20% of craniopharyngiomas which have an intrasellar origin. Fortunately the majority of these occur in

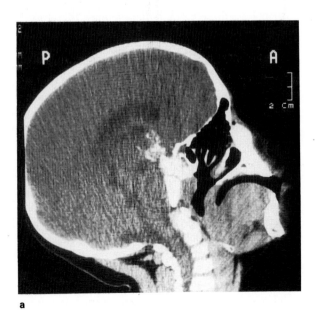

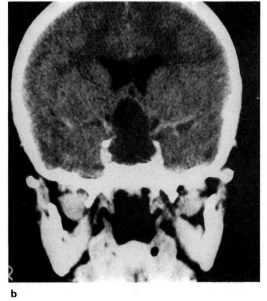

a   b

Fig. 3.9 (a) Direct sagittal CT reveals suprasellar mass with prominent tumoural calcification which is observed in 80% of childhood craniopharyngiomas. (b) Direct, coronal CT demonstrates a large intrasellar and suprasellar cystic mass. Cysts are found in at least 60% of craniopharyngiomas.

adults where, unless the tumour is calcified, it may be indistinguishable from a pituitary adenoma.

Cerebral angiography is a valuable aid in planning surgical treatment, probably in most cases, but certainly when tumours are large. At carotid angiography there is usually lateral displacement of one or both internal carotid arteries (ICA) and evidence of zones of narrowing of the intracranial segment of the ICAs or anterior cerebral arteries (ACA) should be sought, as this usually implies encirclement and compression of these arteries by tumour. A further important observation is the relationship of the A1 segment of the ACA to the mass. Most often this will be elevated and stretched, but if it is *not* elevated this suggests a prefixed optic chiasm with retrochiasmatic growth of the tumour which will require a combined unilateral subfrontal and pterional surgical approach rather than one of the more standard techniques. Vertebral angiography is also helpful in identifying the posterior extent of the tumour. Angiographic techniques are perhaps most pertinent in young children who will require a general anaesthetic, thus adding an element of invasiveness. For older children, much of this information can be provided by digital intravenous angiography (DIVA) provided the child can cooperate with the study.

Since calcification and cyst formation are hallmarks of craniopharyngioma, CT is more specific than MRI in the diagnosis of these tumours, but MRI offers a more accurate assessment of tumour extent (Freeman et al 1987).

DISTINGUISHING RECURRENT DISEASE FROM RADIATION OR CHEMOTHERAPEUTIC INJURY

Introduction

Radiotherapy may be given to a tumour as a primary or postoperative option. Prophylactic irradiation of a wider area such as the spine is given to control CSF seeding which has occurred from the original tumour site.

Chemotherapeutic agents may also be used, alone or in conjunction with radiotherapy. Sterilization of the primary tumour is the aim of radiotherapy, but the effects inevitably extend to the surrounding normal tissues. The sequelae of any radiation therapy depend on the magnitude of the damage and the capacity of the brain to repair it. The brain removes necrotic debris slowly and residual necrotic material often results in surrounding oedema which may be severe and can even exceed the amount of oedema which surrounded the original tumour (Deck 1980, Mikhael 1980). Although partial recovery takes place between fractionated radiation doses, the neuronal component of the brain has practically no repair function and persistence or progression of residual damage may continue after the course of treatment is complete. The extent of radiation damage, its clinical significance and any progression depend on the total dose, the number of fractions, the size of the fractions and the duration of radiation therapy. It is important to recognize the nature of postradiation changes, since the surgical removal of a mass resulting from radiation necrosis may significantly improve, and can even reverse, the neurological deterioration of the patient. On the other hand, re-irradiation of brain already damaged by radiation therapy is highly undesirable and can be disastrous (Danoff et al 1982, Hohweiler et al 1986). Clinical deterioration during or after CNS radiation may therefore be due to recurrent disease, or to an adverse effect of the radiation on nervous tissue or vessels within the beam, or to an alteration in the blood–brain barrier, thus influencing the effects of drug therapy. Improved survival times have increased awareness of these complications and distinguishing recurrent tumour from radiation injury to the brain has become a major radiological problem. In examining the rôle of radiology in addressing this problem, it is necessary to review briefly the known pathological effects of radiation treatment on the brain and to determine which of these effects can be imaged. In their excellent review of the subject, Leibel & Sheline (1987) grouped reactions to radiation according to the time of their appearance: (i) acute reactions (that is, those occurring during a course of treatment); (ii) early delayed reactions which appear from a few weeks to 2–3 months after treatment; and (iii) late delayed reactions which typically appear from several months to many years later.

Acute reactions

With conventional fractionation, acute reactions are seldom of any clinical consequence. When they do occur, they are usually manifest by evidence of raised intracranial pressure or by an exacerbation of the signs and symptoms relating to the lesion being treated. Evidence suggests that the underlying pathology is oedema associated with a perivascular lymphocytic exudation similar to that observed in experimental animals, and there is usually a dramatic response to steroids. No specific CT changes have been described at this stage (Kingsley & Kendall 1981) and there is consequently no need to scan these patients.

Early delayed reactions

These tend to appear from a few weeks to a few months after treatment and are usually transient, disappearing without specific therapy. There is often a characteristic clinical syndrome of somnolence, lethargy, anorexia and irritability. Children are prone to this reaction with an incidence approaching 80% (Freeman et al 1973, Danoff et al 1982, Chin & Maruyama 1984, Tomita & McLone 1986). Many of these children also received aggressive systemic chemotherapy, sometimes with additional intrathecal methotrexate, so that radiotherapy alone may not always be the cause of this symptom complex.

Reversible CT changes have been reported in very few children and usually consist of diffuse areas of low attenuation within the periventricular white matter, serial scans three and six months later showing a gradual return to normal, coinciding with clinical resolution (Kingsley & Kendall 1981). The importance of recognizing the early delayed syndrome lies in the fact that it is generally transient and the appearance of new symptoms at this time does not necessarily indicate failure of treatment, nor the need for a change in therapy (Leibel & Sheline 1987).

Late delayed reactions

Reactions in this category are generally irreversible and frequently progressive. Clinical findings depend on the area and volume of brain irradiated

and range from mild impairment of function to death (Marks et al 1981, Bloom 1982, Jenkin et al 1987). Classical permanent radiation effects include (i) atrophy, (ii) radionecrosis, (iii) vascular effects, (iv) calcification, (v) necrotizing leukoencephalopathy, (vi) tumour induction, and (vii) others such as progressive multifocal leukoencephalopathy and opportunist infections.

Atrophy

CT appearances consistent with cerebral atrophy will be seen in up to two-thirds of children following radiotherapy, depending on the volume of brain irradiated, the total radiation dose received and whether concurrent chemotherapy was given, especially methotrexate (Lund & Hamborg-Pederson 1984, Davis et al 1986). The changes seen range from mild to severe (Fig. 3.10). Although the term 'atrophy' is used widely in literature, there is very little support from pathological studies to justify the term as it is generally

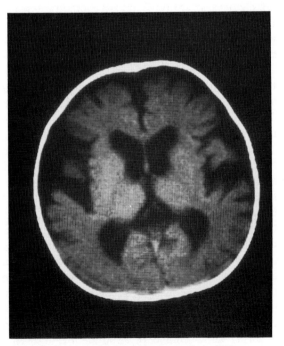

Fig. 3.10 Gross cerebral atrophy is seen in a child following whole brain irradiation. Note the shrinkage of cerebral tissue, the enlarged subarachnoid spaces and cortical sulci and the passive dilatation of the ventricles.

conceived. Wang et al (1983), in a retrospective correlation of CT and autopsy findings in 50 patients who had undergone whole brain irradiation, found radiological evidence of atrophy in 18 patients (36%), but only 2 of these cases showed gross atrophy on post mortem examination, and even in these cases the cortex was histologically normal. No histological abnormality consistent with tissue loss or damage (e.g. neuronal drop-out, neurofibrillary tangles) was seen in any of these 18 cases, and they suggested that the observed CT changes may not be structurally fixed, as in Alzheimer's disease or senile atrophy, but might represent a dynamic or reversible alteration in the brain. Reversible ventricular and subarachnoid space enlargement on CT is well known following steroid therapy and is known to occur in alcoholics and those with anorexia nervosa or Cushing's syndrome. The precise cause of these changes is not known, but variations in the water content of the brain or increased protein catabolism have been suggested as mechanisms underlying the observed CT changes. It is also important to remember that there is a poor correlation between CT changes of 'atrophy' and psychometric testing. De Reuck et al (1979), as well as others, have suggested that the appearances may be due to communicating hydrocephalus from a high convexity block. In the relatively rare instances when this diagnosis needs to be confirmed, the author has developed a technique for studying CSF dynamics with CT following the introduction of intrathecal contrast, usually via lumbar puncture (Turnbull 1986). Water soluble contrast medium is introduced into the lumbar subarachnoid space and gravity-directed towards the head. The passage of contrast through the basal cisterns and intracranial subarachnoid spaces is monitored by CT and it is then a simple matter to determine whether there is any obstruction in the flow of contrast medium (and hence CSF) to the site of absorption at the arachnoid villae. Atrophy can thus be distinguished from communicating hydrocephalus. Furthermore, extracerebral fluid collections can be confidently compartmentalized as either subarachnoid or subdural by observing whether the injected contrast medium enters the collections or not (Fig. 3.11). If it does, then communicating hydrocephalus is diagnosed and

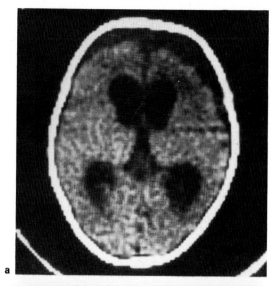

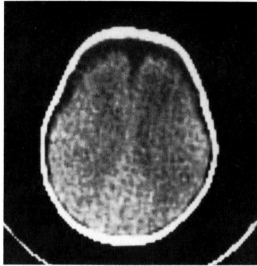

Fig. 3.11 (a) Non-contrast CT shows enlarged ventricles and bilateral extracerebral fluid collections. Communicating hydrocephalus or bilateral subdural collections? (b) Same patient after lumbar intrathecal injection of contrast medium. Contrast has entered the ventricles rendering them isodense with brain but has not entered extracerebral fluid collections which must, therefore, be subdural in location.

appropriate CSF diversion considered, whereas bilateral subdural collections will be approached differently.

Radionecrosis

Radionecrosis of the brain is a result of delayed

radiation effect and is characterized by an insidious onset of clinical features which may suggest tumour recurrence. It can commence as early as six months after completion of radiotherapy, but may develop up to 15 or more years later (Martins et al 1977, Deck 1980, Hohweiler et al 1986). Various hypotheses have been advanced to explain the pathology of delayed radiation necrosis of the brain, but the most widely accepted is that radiation affects the small and medium-sized arteries causing endarteritis obliterans and leading to ischaemia and necrosis. This hypothesis is supported by animal experiments and by observation in humans (Fike et al 1982, 1984). As the white matter has a poorer blood supply than the grey matter, this theory would explain the greater susceptibility of the white matter to radiation damage.

CT scanning is the most widely used imaging technique for detecting radionecrosis and, as it is non-invasive, it can be repeated as required in the follow-up of patients receiving radiotherapy to the head. In those centres having a stereotaxic system linked to the CT scanner, needle biopsy of the lesion under CT guidance can result in a tissue diagnosis. The varied appearance of radiation necrosis on CT depends, amongst other things, on the dose given (Mikhael 1979).

In patients receiving 5000 to 5500 rads (50–55 Gy) total dose using standard fractionation, radiation necrosis is usually shown on CT as diffuse low density lesions in the white matter, having no mass effect and showing no contrast enhancement. They usually appear after a latent period of 18 to 28 months after radiotherapy. In patients who receive 6000 to 7000 rads (60–70 Gy) total dose, or more, radionecrosis is usually observed as:

1. a localized mass with pathological contrast enhancement which is of varied appearence, sometimes peripheral, sometimes central. The enhancement is invariably present even when the original lesion, before treatment, did not show enhancement. This particular pattern of necrosis usually occurs after a latent period of about 9 to 19 months (Littman et al 1977, Wang et al 1983);

2. diffuse low density lesions affecting the white matter, without mass effect and with patchy contrast enhancement in about half the cases (Littman et al 1977, Wang et al 1983).

The differential diagnosis of these appearances creates major radiological problems. Diffuse low density areas without mass effect may be due to infarction, either as a result of intracranial vascular occlusions or as a consequence of various types of arteritis. Necrotizing leukoencephalopathy, progressive multifocal leukoencephalopathy and white matter oedema associated with tumour recurrence can present similar appearances, albeit usually with mass effect. Contrast enhancing mass lesions may be indistinguishable from tumour recurrence unless they are found remote from the original tumour site, but within the radiation field. The role of angiography in differentiating radionecrosis and tumour recurrence can be summarized as follows:

1. Virtually all radionecrotic masses of the brain are avascular.

2. A significant number of recurrent tumours are avascular.

3. Masses which show pathological new vessels within them are nearly always tumour recurrence.

Thus, angiography may be helpful, but only when a pathological circulation has been demonstrated. The lack of specificity of CT in discriminating reliably between these two major pathological entities has been confirmed in the laboratory by Fike et al (1984) who carried out a CT analysis of the canine brain following irradiation. The same workers have studied the accumulation and washout of iodinated contrast medium in canine brain tumours and irradiated normal brain using serial CT. Their preliminary results suggest that rapid sequence serial CT scanning during intravenous contrast infusion may allow a distinction between tumour and tissue necrosis to be made based on the differing effect of these two pathologies on the blood–brain barrier (Fike & Cann 1984). If human research can confirm these differences, then a potential may exist in the future for determining with greater accuracy than at present the nature of an enhancing mass in a treated patient.

Unfortunately, recent research with MR imaging has concluded that recurrent or residual brain tumour cannot be distinguished from radiation brain damage, despite the fact that MRI can detect and display radiation lesions with greater sensitivity than CT (Dooms et al 1986, Di Chiro et al 1988). Following animal experiments by Ito et al (1986), subsequent work on humans by Doyle et al (1987) and Di Chiro et al (1988) has suggested a potential solution to the difficulty in distinguishing tumour recurrence from radiation necrosis and/or intra-arterial chemotherapeutic effects on the brain. By studying glucose metabolism with positron emission tomography (PET), these workers demonstrated a focal reduction of glucose metabolism in the area of radionecrosis which contrasted with the hypermetabolism associated with residual/recurrent tumour. Di Chiro et al (1988) also found that cerebral necrosis following intra-arterial chemotherapy was likewise characterized by a marked reduction in glucose metabolism. They were able to verify their results with neuropathological studies. The availability of PET is limited to those centres with a nearby cyclotron, but nevertheless this research offers exciting possibilities in the future.

Brain necrosis should be easier to prevent than treat. Hohweiler et al (1986) have argued that if CT or MRI could adequately delineate the true extent of the original tumour and could show it to be truly focal, then radiotherapy could be collimated to this area and there would be no need to irradiate the whole brain. In Hohweiler's submission, many malignant brain tumours are focal diseases with tumour cells infiltrating variable distances from their contrast-enhancing margins demonstrated on CT scans. The precise distance of neoplastic cell migration probably varies from tumour to tumour, and to date neither CT nor MRI provides a completely reliable measure of neoplastic cell infiltration. Nevertheless, Hohweiler suggests that the majority of functional tumour cells reside locally. From this it may be suggested that when, following a tissue diagnosis, the natural behaviour of a tumour suggests that any recurrence is likely to be local and that subarachnoid dissemination is exceedingly unlikely, these patients should be referred for MRI as it is more sensitive than CT in delineating the full extent of the tumour and radiation might then be confined to this volume. Decisions of this sort depend on the views of the people treating the individual child, however, and not all workers will agree with the basic premise underlying Hohweiler's arguments.

Haemorrhage may occur within necrotic tissue at any time after radiotherapy. Recent blood clot is readily demonstrated by CT, but unless the underlying necrosis was documented previously, the true state of affairs may not be apparent. Not surprisingly, infection has also been reported in necrotic tissue but this is frequently not recognized in its early stages. The diagnostic difficulties are compounded by a low index of suspicion for infection clinically, and a CT picture which can be extremely variable. A thin, ring-enhancing capsule with extensive oedema (the usual appearance of an intracerebral abscess) is rarely observed. More often, the enhancement is patchy and diffuse with poorly defined borders and the degree of enhancement and the extent of the surrounding oedema may be profoundly modified by the use of steroids so that CT signs of infection may be masked.

Vascular

The vascular consequences of radiation therapy may present from three months to many years after treatment. As the endothelium is the most radiosensitive layer of a vessel, the capillaries, which are proportionately more largely composed of endothelial tissue, are affected more than medium or large vessels. Young children are particularly vulnerable to radiation vasculopathy which is usually manifest as stenoses or occlusions of intracranial arteries. This may result in a rich collateral network of vessels, either in the basal ganglia territory or at the base of the brain when a 'moya-moya' pattern may be simulated. Stenosis, occlusions and collateral vessels are readily appreciated angiographically and the wide availability of DIVA can allow this to be conducted with less disturbance to be child.

Postradiation calcification

It is perhaps surprising that calcification of the brain is such an uncommon entity when the relative high frequency of calcification in tumours is considered. Calcification of the basal ganglia after radiation therapy has been well recognized for many years, and in young children, particularly those under 3 years of age, the frequency of calcification on CT in non-tumourous tissue can be as high as 28% (Davis et al 1986). In this group, the most frequently identified site is subcortical at the grey–white junction and the calcification can be progressive over several years. Correlation with available pathology suggests that this subcortical calcification is either the result of radiation-induced vasculopathy with perivascular calcification (mineralizing microangiopathy) or the result of demyelenation and tissue necrosis followed by dystrophic calcification. Although mineralizing microangiopathy and dystrophic calcification are thought to be specific to the combination of methotrexate and radiation therapy, Davis et al (1986) recorded several cases which occurred with radiation alone. Mineralizing microangiopathy may affect other areas of grey matter within the CNS such as the putamen of the lentiform nucleus or, less frequently, the cerebellar folial grey matter. Although it produces permanent destructive

changes in specific regions of the brain, its effect on cerebral function may be minimal. Certainly, the clinical significance of mineralizing microangiopathy is less apparent than the sequelae of leukoencephalopathy (Deck 1980). Calcification within tumours may become more marked after radiotherapy and occasionally calcification within areas of primary or metastatic tumour may appear for the first time after radiation treatment (Pearson et al 1983) (Fig. 3.12).

Necrotizing leukoencephalopathy

Leukoencephalopathy is characterized histologically by demyelination, beginning with axonal swelling and fragmentation and progressing to coagulative necrosis and gliosis. Initially, the lesion presents as multifocal coalescing areas of coagulation and necrosis in the white matter with sparing of the grey matter of the cortex and basal ganglia. Clinically, this is a rare but serious debilitating condition and it is thought to occur when radiotherapy is employed in combination

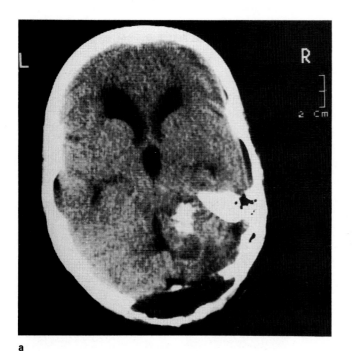
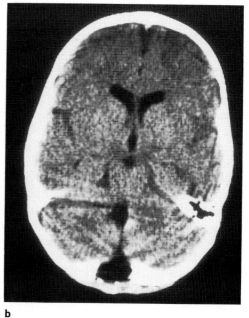

a   **b**

Fig. 3.12 (a) There was no evidence of calcification at presentation, CT 17 months after treatment showing tumour recurrence associated with dense calcification. (b) 14 months after surgery and radiotherapy for medulloblastoma, two small foci of calcification are seen immediately to the right of the 4th ventricle. This proved to be dystrophic calcification.

with systemic and intrathecal methotrexate. Children under 10 years are especially at risk, presumably because immature tissues are particularly susceptible. Radiologically, it is seen as diffuse areas of low attenuation within the deep matter which are devoid of mass effect and do not show pathological contrast enhancement. The distinction from cerebral necrosis following low dose radiation is not possible on radiological grounds alone. Following higher doses of radiation, contrast enhancement is usually present either in a localized mass or within the diffuse low density lesion.

Induction of second primary tumour

With high or repeated doses of radiation, various types of tumour may develop some years later. The incidence is very low, however, less that 2% at 20 years, and this begs the question of whether the second primary brain tumour was radiation-induced or occurred spontaneously (Haselow et al 1978, Danoff et al 1982). There are no known distinguishing features on CT or MRI which would answer this question in an individual child.

Other complications of cancer treatment

Progressive multifocal leukoencephalopathy (PML) was first recognized as a distinct neuropathological entity by Astrom et al in 1958 and was thought to be a disease contracted by patients suffering from leukaemia and the lymphoproliferative disorders, but it is now known that any immunocompromised patient may be at risk (Bernick & Gregorios 1984, Brooks & Walker 1984). The condition is caused by polyoma viruses and a positive diagnosis can only be reliably made by direct examination of brain tissue. PML is an apparently lethal disease: although prolonged clinical courses have been reported, survival for more than one year after diagnosis is unusual (Brooks & Walker 1984).

CT demonstrates a low density lesion confined to the white matter, generally without mass effect or contrast enhancement (Schlitt et al 1986) although seepage of contrast into the lesions can sometimes be demonstrated when delayed scans are obtained 60 minutes after a double dose of in-

travenous contrast (Carroll et al 1977, Krupp et al 1985) (Fig. 3.13). Schlitt et al (1986) have argued the use of CT as a means of localizing areas most likely to be abnormal, which can be safely biopsied. They presented three patients diagnosed in this way, two of whom had longterm survival after discontinuation of their immunosuppressive therapy. Whilst the safety of biopsy is generally agreed, there is concern in the literature about the possible contamination of operating instruments with slow viruses which are difficult to eradicate by ordinary sterilization processes.

It is very important to appreciate the various ways in which radiation, chemotherapy and especially a depressed immunological response in a child can greatly modify the radiological appearances of common, as well as less frequent, conditions. For example, opportunist infections of the brain may present as a non-enhancing mass or only show enhancement if delayed scans are obtained after a double dose (Kelly & Brant-Zawadzki 1983, Whelan et al 1983, Post et al 1985). They do not evolve as typical abscesses with a clearly defined capsule and liquefied centre. In the absence of enhancement, the lesions may be misdiagnosed as radiation necrosis, for example, and their infective aetiology not appreciated (Sze

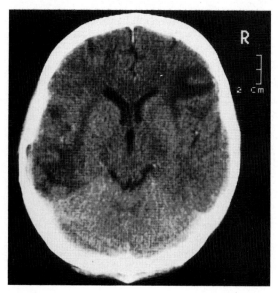

Fig. 3.13 PML. CT reveals bilateral low density areas without mass effect or contrast enhancement confined to the white matter.

et al 1987). Both radiation and chemotherapy may affect the blood–brain barrier and allow contrast to enter areas of the brain previously appearing on CT as non-enhancing, and a poorly or non-enhancing tumour may show increasing enhancement after treatment which is the result of an altered permeability of the blood–brain barrier due to treatment and not because the tumour has changed its biological behaviour or degree of malignancy. Recent research on the CNS manifestations of opportunist infections in AIDS patients has added to our knowledge of the neuropathology and CT/MRI appearances of infections occurring in the immunocompromised host (Levy et al 1986, Post et al 1988).

Finally, a number of clinical problems may disclose themselves after radiation treatment of children, especially the very young, which are not well-served by radiology, either in its ability to predict their occurrence or in imaging the abnormalities responsible for them. Behaviour disorders, mental retardation and endocrine deficiencies, especially impaired growth hormone secretion, are all commonly encountered and radiology has little to offer in their management.

INTRASPINAL TUMOURS

Reference has already been made to the role of myelography in detecting tumours which may have seeded from primary neoplasms in the brain. This section is concerned with the relatively rare primary intraspinal tumours in children which comprise at most 5% of childhood CNS neoplasms (Farwell et al 1977). Although ultrasound has firmly established itself as a diagnostic tool for imaging the spinal contents of neonates and young children (Naidich & Zimmerman 1984, Gusnard et al 1986), this has largely been in relation to congenital anomalies of one sort or another and it would not normally be regarded as a primary imaging method for evaluating tumours. It has been employed per-operatively for localizing intramedullary neoplasms with excellent results (Raghavendra et al 1984, Montalvo & Quencer 1986).

The neoplasms may be situated within the spinal cord (intramedullary), within the dura but outside the cord (intradural/extramedullary), or in the extradural space. On rare occasions, they may occupy two or three of these compartments (Harwood-Nash and Fitz 1980).

Plain films are important in demonstrating signs of an expanding lesion within the canal and will be abnormal in 55–75% of cases (Farwell & Dohrmann 1977, DeSousa et al 1979). Early radiological signs may, however, be subtle and by the time they are established, primary intraspinal tumours are often quite large. The three main radiological features are: (i) changes in the pedicles with erosion or flattening (Fig. 3.14); (ii) scoliosis; and (iii) deformity of the paraspinal shadows (the latter being seen mainly in association with sarcomas and neuroblastomas and other metastatic lesions which are not our concern here). If a lesion can be localized in this way, it allows the radiologist the option of deciding whether a myelogram is better performed from above or below. Myelography remains the most widely employed investigative technique for imaging these tumours, the purpose of which is to show the upper and lower extent of the neoplasm and to demonstrate its relationship to the cord in those instances when the tumour is extramedullary. Even though a 'block' is present at myelography with apparent obstruction of contrast medium at the site of the tumour, it is usually possible to coax modern water soluble contrast media around the tumour and so determine its whole extent. For this reason the author prefers to perform the examination from below as this is technically easier, requires simpler equipment and is possibly safer. Having identified a mass in this way, transaxial CT slices through the lesion may then be used to localise it with respect to the cord and its dural covering.

The use of CT in this way has its advocates, the Toronto group having pioneered its use with excellent results (Pettersson & Harwood-Nash 1982). They advocate CT myelography (CTM) as the primary investigation and have tended to abandon conventional myelography. It is important to recognize the difference between conventional myelography followed by CT, and primary CTM. The former requires a larger volume of contrast medium of increased concentration which will be gravity-directed to allow complete visualization of the spinal subarachnoid space, with CT being

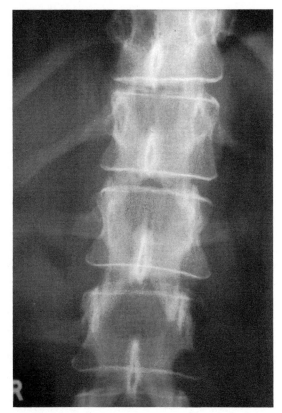

Fig. 3.14 AP radiograph of the thoraco-lumbar spine in a child with an ependymoma showing an increased interpedicular diameter in association with erosion and flattening of the pedicles. These changes are long standing and imply an expanding lesion with the spinal canal.

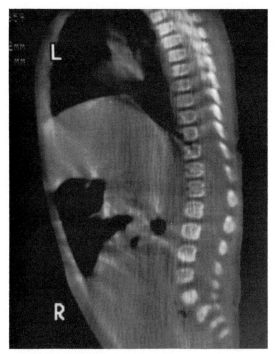

Fig. 3.15 Direct sagittal CTM of the lower thoracic, lumbar and sacral spines. Isotonic intrathecal contrast medium is identified in the thoracic region but there is no subarachnoid contrast from the thoraco-lumbar junction downwards owing to the presence of a large soft tissue mass which is filling and expanding the spinal canal. Diagnosis ependymoma.

reserved for any area of abnormality disclosed by this method, most images being made in the transaxial plane. The technique involves more manipulation of the child which will adversely affect patient cooperation and thus appropriate sedation or general anaesthesia assumes critical importance. With primary CTM, much smaller volumes of isotonic contrast medium are introduced at lumbar puncture and the contrast is allowed to diffuse throughout the subarachnoid space. Thereafter, direct coronal and sagittal CT of the whole spine is attempted with selected transaxial views being employed as above to localize the lesion as intramedullary, intradural or extradural (Fig. 3.15). There is potentially less handling of the child and sedation is said to be less critical. In practice, however, one sees intraspinal tumours relatively infrequently and in most cases

the myelogram provides sufficient information about the location and probable nature of the neoplasm for treatment decisions to be made. CT can thus be reserved for those few cases where there is diagnostic difficulty. There is no doubt that MRI depicts the spinal cord with remarkable clarity of detail and it is likely to supplement myelography as the investigation of choice in the future (Barloon et al 1987). The reader is referred to Chapter 2 on this specialized technique.

Primary neoplasms of neural origin

Astrocytoma, ependymoma and neurofibroma account for the great majority of primary intraspinal tumours.

Astrocytoma

Although this is an uncommon tumour, it is the

most frequent glioma of the cord in children and constitutes around 8% of intraspinal mass lesions (Harwood-Nash & Fitz 1976). They are most often located in the cervical region and may extend over several vertebral segments, occasionally involving almost the entire cord. They are slow-growing tumours and the cord is often extensively involved before symptoms are sufficiently manifest for a thorough neuroradiological assessment to be undertaken.

Both myelography and CTM will reveal a large intramedullary tumour, the margins of which are often irregular and there may be areas of adherence of tumour to the dura. The mass can be cystic or solid although in practice it is often difficult to distinguish these variants, even with CT. MRI is more accurate in this respect. Handel et al (1978) have shown that a portion of these tumours may enhance following intravenous contrast medium. Unfortunately, pathological contrast enhancement of the spinal cord and roots is not specific to tumours and may be seen in children who have had previous irradiation of the neuraxis where it is thought that this probably represents a subclinical myelitis induced by the radiation (Pettersson et al 1981).

Ependymoma

This tumour comprises around 6% of all intraspinal mass lesions (Harwood-Nash & Fitz 1976) and arises from ependymal cells in the spinal cord or filum terminale, the lumbar region being most commonly involved. The tumour is depicted at myelography or CTM either as a gradual widening of the cord or filum terminale, or as a more focal and eccentric nodular expansion. As with the astrocytoma, the ependymoma may be solid or cystic and it can be impossible, even with myelography and CTM, to distinguish an intramedullary ependymoma from an astrocytoma or a teratodermoid, or even from syringohydromyelia.

Neurofibroma

This is a histologically benign tumour of neural origin composed of cells derived from the nerve sheath. It may appear as a solitary lesion or as multiple tumour nodules in Von Recklinghausen's disease and can be intradural, extradural or both.

REFERENCES

Albright A L, Guthkelch A N, Packer R J, Price R A, Rourke L B 1986 Prognostic factors in paediatric brain stem gliomas. Journal of Neurosurgery 65: 751–755

Allen J C, Epstein F 1982 Medulloblastoma and other primary malignant neuroectodermal tumors of the CNS. Journal of Neurosurgery 57: 466–451

Al-Mefty O, Hassounah M, Weaver P, Sakati N, Jinkins J R, Fox J L 1985 Microsurgery for giant craniopharyngioma in children. Neurosurgery 17: 585–595

Altman N, Fitz C R, Chuang S, Harwood-Nash D, Cotter C, Armstrong D 1985 Radiological characteristics of primitive neuroectodermal tumours in children. American Journal of Neuroradiology 6: 15–18

Astrom K E, Mancall E L, Richardson E P Jr 1958 Progressive multifocal leukoencephalopathy. Brain 81: 93–111

Barloon T J, Yuh W T C, Yang C J C, Schultz D H 1987 Spinal subarachnoid tumor seeding from intracranial metastasis: MR findings. Journal of Computer Assisted Tomography 11: 242–244

Bernick C, Gregorios J B 1984 Progressive multifocal leukoencephalopathy in a patient with acquired immune deficiency syndrome. Archives of Neurology 41: 780–782

Berry M P, Jenkin R D T, Keen C W, Nair B D, Simpson W J 1981 Radiation treatment for medulloblastoma. A 21-year review. Journal of Neurosurgery 55: 43–51

Bloom H J G 1979 Prospects for increasing survival in children with medulloblastoma; present and future studies. In: Paoletti P, Walker M D, Butti G et al (eds) Multidisciplinary aspects of brain tumor therapy. Elsevier North-Holland, New York, pp 245–260

Bloom H J G 1982 Intracranial tumors: response and resistance to therapeutic endeavors, 1970–1980. International Journal of Radiation Oncology and Biological Physics 8: 1083–1113

Brooks B R, Walker D L 1984 Progressive multifocal leukoencephalopathy. In: Johnson K P (ed) Neurologic clinics (neurovirology) 2: 299–313

Burman S, Rosenbaum A E 1982 Rationale and techniques for intravenous enhancement in computed tomography. Radiological Clinics of North America 20: 15–22

Cabezudo J M Vaquero J, Garcia-de-Sola R, Lenda G, Nombela L, Bravo G 1981 Craniopharyngioma. Surgical Neurology 15: 422–427

Camins M B, Cravioto H M, Epstein F et al 1980 Medulloblastoma: an ultrastructural study – evidence of astrocytic and neuronal differentiation. Neurosurgery 6: 398–411

Carroll B A, Lane B, Norman D, Enzmann D 1977 Diagnosis of progressive multifocal leukoencephalopathy by computed tomography. Radiology 122: 127–141

Chang C H, Housepian E M, Herbert C 1969 An operative

staging system and a megavoltage radiotherapeutic technique for cerebellar medulloblastomas. Radiology 93: 1351–1359

Chin H W, Maruyama Y 1984 Age at treatment and long-term performance results in medulloblastoma. Cancer 53: 1952–1958

Chuang S, Harwood-Nash D 1986 Tumors and cysts. Neuroradiology 28: 463–475

Danoff B F, Cowchock F S, Marquette C, Mulgrew L, Kramer S 1982 Assessment of the long-term effect of primary radiation therapy for brain tumors in children. Cancer 49: 1580–1586

Davis P C, Hoffman J C Jr, Weidenheim K M 1984 Large hypothalamic and optic chiasm gliomas in infants: Difficulties in distinction. American Journal of Neuroradiology 5: 579–585

Davis P C, Hoffman J C Jr, Pearl J S, Braun I F 1986 CT evaluation of effects of cranial radiation therapy in children. American Journal of Neuroradiology 7: 639–644

Deck M D F 1980 Imaging techniques in the diagnosis of radiation damage to the central nervous system. In: Gilbert H A, Kagan A R (eds) Radiation damage to the nervous system. A delayed therapeutic hazard. Raven Press, New York, pp 107–127

De Reuck J, De Coster W, Vander E, Eecken H 1979 Communicating hydrocephalus in treated leukaemia patients. European Neurology 18: 8–14

DeSousa A L, Kalsbeck J E, Mealey J Jr, Campbell R L, Hockey A 1979 Intraspinal tumors in children. A review of 81 cases. Journal of Neurosurgery 51: 437–445

Deutsch M, Reigel D H 1980 The value of myelography in the management of childhood medulloblastoma. Cancer 45: 2194–2197

Di Chiro G, Oldfield E, Wright D C et al 1988 Cerebral necrosis after radiotherapy and/or intraarterial chemotherapy for brain tumors: PET and neuropathologic studies. American Journal of Radiology 150: 189–197

Dooms G C, Hecht S, Brant-Zawadzki M, Berthiaume Y, Norman D, Newton T H 1986 Brain radiation lesions: MR imaging. Radiology 158: 149–155

Doyle W K, Budinger T F, Valk P E, Levin V A, Gutin P H 1987 Differentiation of cerebral radiation necrosis from tumor recurrence by (18F) FDG and 82Rb positron emission tomography. Journal of Computer Assisted Tomography 11: 563–570

Epstein F 1985 A staging system for brain stem gliomas. Cancer 56: 1804–1806

Epstein F, McCleary E L 1986 Intrinsic brain stem tumours of childhood: surgical indications. Journal of Neurosurgery 64: 11–15

Epstein F, Murali R 1978 Pediatric posterior fossa tumors: hazards of the 'preoperative' shunt. Neurosurgery 3: 348–350

Evans A E, Anderson J, Chang C et al 1979 Adjuvant chemotherapy for medulloblastoma and ependymoma. In: Paoletti P, Walker M D, Butti G et al (eds) Multidisciplinary aspects of brain tumor therapy. Elsevier North-Holland, New York, pp 219–222

Farwell J R, Dohrmann G J 1977 Intraspinal neoplasms in children. Paraplegia 15: 262–273

Farwell J R, Dohrmann G J, Flannery J T 1977 Central nervous system tumors in children. Cancer 40: 3123–3132

Fike J R, Cann C E 1984 Contrast medium accumulation and washout in canine brain tumors and irradiated normal brain: A CT study of kinetics. Radiology 151: 115–120

Fike J R, Cann C E, Davis R L, Phillips T L 1982 Radiation effects in the canine brain evaluated by quantitative computed tomography. Radiology 144/3: 603–608

Fike J R, Cann C E, Davis R L et al 1984 Computed tomography analysis of the canine brain: effects of hemibrain X irradiation. Radiation Research 99/2: 294–310

Fletcher W A, Imes R K, Hoyt W F 1986 Chiasmal gliomas: appearance and long-term changes demonstrated by computerized tomography. Journal of Neurosurgery 65: 154–159

Freeman J E, Johnston P G B, Voke J M 1973 Somnolence after prophylactic cranial irradiation in children with acute lymphoblastic leukaemia. British Medical Journal 4: 523–525

Freeman M P, Kessler R M, Allen J H, Price A C 1987 Craniopharyngioma: CT and MR imaging in nine cases. Journal of Computer Assisted Tomography 11: 810–814

Gjerris F, Klinken L 1978 Long-term prognosis in children with benign cerebellar astrocytoma. Journal of Neurosurgery 49: 179–184

Gooding G A W, Edwards M S B, Rabkin A E, Powers S K 1983 Intraoperative real-time ultrasound in the localization of intracranial neoplasms. Radiology 146: 459–462

Gusnard D A, Naidich T P, Yousefzadeh D K, Haughton V M 1986 Ultrasonic anatomy of the normal neonatal and infant spine: correlation with cryomicrotome sections and CT. Neuroradiology 28: 493–511

Han B K, Babcock D S, Oestreich A E 1984 Sonography of brain tumours in infants. American Journal of Neuroradiology 5: 253–258

Handel S, Grossman R, Sarwar M 1978 Computed tomography in the diagnosis of spinal cord astrocytoma. Journal of Computer Assisted Tomography 2: 226–228

Hart M N, Earle K M 1973 Primitive neuroectodermal tumours of the brain in children. Cancer 32: 890–897

Harwood-Nash D C, Fitz C R 1976 Neuroradiology in infants and children. C V Mosey, St Louis

Harwood-Nash D C, Fitz C R 1980 Computed tomography and the pediatric spine: computed tomographic metrizamide myelography in children. In: Post M J D (ed) Radiographic evaluation of the spine. Masson, New York, pp 4–33

Haselow R E, Nesbit M, Dehner L P, Khan F M, McHugh R, Levitt S H 1978 Second neoplasms following megavoltage radiation in a pediatric population. Cancer 42: 1185–1191

Hawkins J C 1980 Treatment of choroid plexus papillomas in children: A brief analysis of twenty years' experience. Neurosurgery 6: 380–384

Heafner M D, Schut L, Packer R J, Bruce D A, Bilaniuk L T, Sutton L N 1985 Discrepancy between computed tomography and magnetic resonance imaging in a case of medulloblastoma. Neurosurgery 17: 487–489

Hinshaw D B Jr, Ashwal S, Thompson J R, Hasso A N 1983 Neuroradiology of primitive neuroectodermal tumors. Neuroradiology 25: 87–92

Hoffman H J, Becker L, Craven M A 1980 A clinically and pathologically distinct group of benign brain stem gliomas. Neurosurgery 7: 243–248

Hohweiler M L, Lo T C M, Silverman M L, Freidberg S R 1986 Brain necrosis after radiotherapy for primary intracerebral tumour. Neurosurgery 18: 67–74

Ito M, Patronas N J, Di Chiro G, Mansi L, Kennedy C

1986 Effect of moderate level X-radiation to brain on cerebral glucose utilization. Journal of Computer Assisted Tomography 10(4): 584–588

Jenkin R D T, Boesel C, Ertel I et al 1987 Brain stem tumors in childhood: a prospective randomized trial of irradiation with and without adjuvant CCNU, VCR and prednisone. A report of the children's cancer study group. Journal of Neurosurgery 66: 227–233

Johnson M A, Pennock J M, Bydder G M et al 1983 Clinical NMR imaging of the brain in children. American Journal of Radiology 141: 1005–1018

Jooma R, Hayward R D, Grant D N 1984 Intracranial neoplasms during the first year of life: Analysis of one hundred consecutive cases. Neurosurgery 14: 31–41

Kaputy A J, McCullough D C, Manz H J, Patterson K, Hammock M K 1987 A review of the factors influencing the prognosis of medulloblastoma. The importance of cell differentiation. Journal of Neurosurgery 66: 80–87

Kelly W M, Brant-Zawadzki M 1983 Acquired immunodeficiency syndrome: neuroradiologic findings. Radiology 149: 485–491

Kingsley D P E, Harwood-Nash D C 1984 Parameters of infiltration in posterior fossa tumours of childhood using a high resolution CT scanner. Neuroradiology 26: 347–350

Kingsley D P E, Kendall B E 1981 Review article – CT of the adverse effect of therapeutic radiation of the central nervous system. American Journal of Neuroradiology 2: 453–460

Knake J E, Chandler W F, McGillicuddy J E, Silver T M, Gabrielsen T O 1982 Intraoperative sonography for brain tumour localization and ventricular shunt placement. American Journal of Radiology 139: 733–738

Knake J E, Chandler W F, Gabrielsen T O, Latack J T, Gebarski S S 1984 Intraoperative sonographic delineation of low grade brain neoplasms defined poorly by computed tomography. Radiology 151: 735–739

Kopelson G, Linggood R M, Kleinman G M 1983 Medulloblastoma. The identification of prognostic subgroups and implications for multimodality management. Cancer 51: 312–319

Krupp L B Lipton R B, Swerdlow M L et al 1985 Progressive multifocal leukoencephalopathy: clinical and radiographic features. Annals of Neurology 17: 344–349

Lee B C P, Zimmerman R D, Manning J J, Deck M D F 1985 MR imaging of syringomyelia and hydromyelia. American Journal of Neuroradiology 6: 221–228

Leibel S A, Sheline G E 1987 Review article. Radiation therapy for neoplasms of the brain. Journal of Neurosurgery 66: 1–22

Levene M I, Whitelaw A, Dubowitz V, Bydder G M, Steiner R E, Randell C P, Young I R 1982 Nuclear magnetic imaging of the brain in children. British Medical Journal 285: 774–776

Littman P, James H, Zimmerman R A, Slater R 1977 Radionecrosis of the brain presenting as a mass lesion. Journal of Neurology, Neurosurgery and Psychiatry 40: 827–829

Lund E, Hamborg-Pederson B 1984 Computed tomography of the brain following prophylactic treatment with irradiation therapy and intraspinal methotrexate in children with acute lymphoblastic leukaemia. Neuroradiology 26: 351–358

McComb J G, Davis R L, Isaacs H Jr 1981 Extraneural metastatic medulloblastoma during childhood. Neurosurgery 9: 548–551

Marks J E, Baglan R J, Prassad S C et al 1981 Cerebral radionecrosis: incidence and risk in relation to dose, time, fractionation and volume. International Journal of Radiation Oncology and Biological Physics 7: 243–252

Martins A N, Johnston J S, Henry J M, Stoffel T J, de Chiro G 1977 Delayed radiation necrosis of the brain. Journal of Neurosurgery 37: 336–345

Mikhael M A 1979 Radiation necrosis of the brain; correlation between patterns on computed tomography and dose of radiation. Journal of Computer Assisted Tomography 3: 241–249

Mikhael M A 1980 Dosimetric considerations in the diagnosis of radiation necrosis of the brain. In: Gilbert H A, Kagan A R (eds) Radiation damage to the nervous system. A delayed therapeutic hazard. Raven Press, New York, pp 59–91

Montalvo B M, Quencer R M 1986 Intraoperative sonography in spinal surgery: current state of the art. Neuroradiology 28: 551–590

Naidich T P, Zimmerman R A 1984 Primary brain tumors in children. Seminars in Roentgenology 19: 100–114

North C, Segall H D, Stanley P, Zee C-S, Ahmadi J, McComb J G 1985 Early CT detection of intracranial seeding from medulloblastoma. American Journal of Neuroradiology 6: 11–13

Packer R J, Zimmerman R A, Luerssen T G et al 1985 Brain stem gliomas of childhood: magnetic resonance imaging. Neurology 35: 397–401

Park T S, Hoffman H J, Hendrick E B, Humphreys R P, Becker L E 1983 Medulloblastoma: clinical presentation and management. Experience at the Hospital for Sick Children, Toronto, 1950–1980. Journal of Neurosurgery 58: 543–552

Patronas N J, Dwyer A J, Papathanasiou M, Schiebler M L, Schellinger D 1987 Contributions of magnetic resonance imaging in the evaluation of optic gliomas. Surgical Neurology 28: 367–371

Paushter D M, Modic M T, Masaryk T J 1985 Magnetic resonance imaging of the spine: applications and limitations. Radiological Clinics of North America 23: 551–562

Pearson A D J, Campbell A N, McAllister V L and Pearson G L 1983 Intracranial calcification in survivors of childhood medulloblastoma. Archives of Diseases of Children 58: 133–136

Pederson H, Clausen N 1981 The development of cerebral CT changes during treatment of acute lymphocytic leukaemia in childhood. Neuroradiology 22: 79–84

Peterman S B, Steiner R E, Bydder G M 1984 Magnetic resonance imaging of intracranial tumours in children and adolescents. American Journal of Neuroradiology 4: 703–709

Pettersson H, Harwood-Nash D C F 1982 CT and myelography of the spine and cord. Techniques, anatomy and pathology in children. Springer-Verlag, Berlin

Pettersson H, Harwood-Nash D C F, Fitz C R, Chuang S, Armstrong E 1981 Computed tomographic intravenous myelography of the irradiated spinal cord in children. American Journal of Neororadiology 2: 581–584

Post M J D, Kursunoglu S J, Hensley G T et al 1985 Cranial CT in acquired immunodeficiency syndrome: spectrum of diseases and optimal contrast enhancement technique. American Journal of Radiology 145: 929–940

Priest J, Dehner L P, Sung J, Nesbit M E 1981 Primitive neuroectodermal tumors (embryonal gliomas) of childhood. A clinicopathologic study of 12 cases. In: Humphrey G B et al (eds) Pediatric oncology, vol 1. Nijhoff, The Hague, pp. 247–264

Radkowski M A, Naidich T P, Tomita T, Byrd S E, McLone D G 1988 Neonatal brain tumors: CT and MR findings. Journal of Computer Assisted Tomography 12: 10–20.

Raghavendra B N, Epstein S J, McCleary L 1984 Intramedullary spinal cord tumours in children: localisation by intraoperative sonography. American Journal of Neuroradiology 5: 395–397

Rawlings C E, Giangaspero F, Burger P C, Bullard D E 1988 Ependymomas: A clinicopathologic study. Surgical Neurology 29: 271–81

Savoiardo M, Harwood-Nash D, Tadmor R et al 1981 Gliomas of the intracranial anterior optic pathways in children. Radiology 138: 601–610

Schlitt M, Morawetz R B, Bonnin J et al 1986 Progressive multifocal leukoencephalopathy: three patients diagnosed by brain biopsy, with prolonged survival in two. Neurosurgery 18: 407–414

Shlosnik A, Tomita T, Raimondi A I, Hahn Y S, McLone D G 1983 Intraoperative neurosurgical ultrasound. Localisation of brain tumours in infants and children. Radiology 148: 525–527

Stanley P, Senac M O Jr, Segall H D 1985 Intraspinal seeding from intracranial tumours in children. American Journal of Radiology 144: 157–161

Stern J, Jakobiecfa A, Housepain E M 1980 The architecture of optic nerve gliomas with and without neurofibromatosis. Archives of Ophthalmology 98: 505

Stroink A R, Hoffman H J, Hendrick E B, Humphreys R P 1986 Diagnosis and management of paediatric brain-stem gliomas. Journal of Neurosurgery 65: 745–750

Swartz J D, Zimmerman R A, Bilaniuk L T 1982 Computed tomography of intracranial ependymomas. Radiology 143: 97–101

Sze G, Brant-Zawadzki M N, Norman D, Newton T H 1987 The neuroradiology of AIDS. Seminars in Roentgenology 22: 42–53

Szenasy J, Slowik F 1983 Prognosis of benign cerebellar astrocytomas in children. Child Brain 10: 39–47

Tadmor R, Harwood-Nash D C, Savoiardo M et al 1980 Brain tumors in the first two years of life: CT diagnosis. American Journal of Neuroradiology 1: 411–417

Tomita T 1983 Statistical analysis of symptoms and signs in cerebellar astrocytoma and medulloblastoma. In: Charles C T, Amador L (eds) Brain tumors in the young. C C Thomas, Springfield IL, pp. 514–525

Tomita T, McLone D G 1983 Spontaneous seeding of medulloblastoma: results of cerebrospinal fluid cytology and arachnoid biopsy from the cisterna magna. Neurosurgery 12: 265–267

Tomita T, McLone D G 1985 Brain tumours during the first 24 months of life. Neurosurgery 17: 913–919

Tomita T, McLone D G 1986 Medulloblastoma in childhood: results of radical resection and low-dose neuraxis radiation therapy. Journal of Neurosurgery 64: 238–242

Tsutsumi Y, Andoh Y, Inoue N 1982 Ultrasound-guided biopsy for deep-seated brain tumours. Journal of Neurosurgery 57: 164–167

Turnbull I W 1986 Computed tomography and dynamic cerebrospinal fluid studies in the evaluation of extracerebral fluid collections in infants with hydrocephalus. Acta Radiologica, Supplementum 369: 683–685

Van Swieten J C, Thomeer R T W M, Vielvoye G J, Bots G T A M 1987 Choroid plexus papilloma in the posterior fossa. Surgical Neurology 28: 129–134

Vaquero J, Cabezudo J M, de Sola R G et al 1981 Intratumoral hemorrhage in posterior fossa tumors after ventricular drainage. Report of two cases. Journal of Neurosurgery 54: 406–408

Wang A, Skias D D, Rumbaugh C L, Schoene W C, Zamani A 1983 Central nervous system changes after radiation therapy and/or chemotherapy: correlation of CT and autopsy findings. American Journal of Neuroradiology 4: 466–471

Whelan M A, Kricheff I I, Handler M et al 1983 Acquired immunodeficiency syndrome: cerebral computed tomographic manifestations. Radiology 149: 477–484

Winkler P, Helmke K 1985 Ultrasonic diagnosis and follow-up of malignant brain tumours in childhood. A report of 4 cases and a review of the literature. Paediatric Radiology 15: 215–219

Zee C S, Segall H D, Ahmadi J, Becker T S, McComb J G, Miller J H 1983 Computed tomography of posterior fossa ependymomas in childhood. Surgical Neurology 20: 221–226

Zimmerman R A, Bilaniuk L T 1980 CT of primary and secondary craniocerebral neuroblastoma. American Journal of Neuroradiology 1: 431–434

FURTHER READING

Abrams D 1986 Idiopathic thrombocytopenic purpura update. AIDS file, San Francisco General Hospital 162: 3

Al-Mefty O, Al-Rodhan N R F, Phillips R L, El-Senossi M, Fox J L 1987 Factors affecting survival of children with malignant gliomas. Neurosurgery 20: 416–420

Alvord E C Jr, Lofton S 1988 Gliomas of the optic nerve or chiasm. Outcome by patients' age, tumor site, and treatment. Journal of Neurosurgery 68: 85–98

Barnes P D, Lester P D, Yamanashi W S, Prince J R 1986 Magnetic resonance imaging in infants and children with spinal dysraphism. American Journal of Neuroradiology 7: 465–472

Bentson J, Reza M, Winter J, Wilson G 1978 Steroids and apparent cerebral atrophy on computer tomography scans. Journal of Computer Assisted Tomography 2: 16–23

Bilaniuk L T, Zimmerman R A, Littman T S, Gallo E, Rorke L B, Bruce D A, Schut L 1980 Computed tomography of brain stem gliomas in children. Radiology 134: 89–95

Bleyer W A, Griffin G W 1980 White matter necrosis, mineralising microangiopathy, and intellectual abilities in survivors of childhood leukaemia: associations with central nervous system irradiation and Methotrexate therapy. In: Gilbert H A, Kagan A R (eds) Radiation damage to the nervous system. A delayed therapeutic hazard. Raven Press, New York, pp 155–174

Boyd M C, Steinbok P 1987 Choroid plexus tumors: problems in diagnosis and management. Journal of Neurosurgery 66: 800–805

Brandt-Zawadzki M, Anderson M, De Armond S J, Conley F K, Jahnke R W 1980 Radiation induced large intracranial vessel occlusive vasculopathy. American Journal of Radiology 134: 51–55

Brown E W, Riccardi V M, Mawad M, Handel S, Goldman A, Bryan R N 1987 MR imaging of optic pathways in patients with neurofibromatosis. American Journal of Neuroradiology 8: 1031–1036

Burger P C, Dubois P J, Shold S C Jr et al 1983 Computerised tomographic and pathological studies of the untreated, quiescent, and recurrent glioblastoma multiforme. Journal of Neurosurgery 58: 159–169

Caputy A J, McCullough D C, Manz H J, Patterson K, Hammock M K 1987 A review of the factors influencing the prognosis of medulloblastoma. The importance of cell differentiation. Journal of Neurosurgery 66: 80–87

Coffey R J, Lunsford L D 1985 Stereotactic surgery for mass lesions of the mid brain and pons. Neurosurgery 17: 12–18

Davis P C, Hoffman J C Jr, Ball T I et al 1988 Spinal abnormalities in pediatric patients: MR imaging findings compared with clinical, myelographic and surgical findings. Radiology 166: 679–685

Dhellemmes P, Demaille M C, Lejeune J P, Baranzelli M C, Combelles G, Torrealba G 1986 Cerebellar medulloblastoma: results of multidisciplinary treatment. Report of 120 cases. Surgical Neurology 25: 290–294

Edwards M S, Wilson C B 1980 Treatment of radiation necrosis. In: Gilbert H A, Kagan A R (eds) Radiation damage to the nervous system. A delayed therapeutic hazard. Raven Press, New York, pp 129–143

Edwards M S B, Hudgins R J, Wilson C B, Levin V A, Wara W M 1988 Pineal region tumors in children. Journal of Neurosurgery 68: 689–697

Ellenberg L, McComb J G, Siegel S E, Stowe S 1987 Factors affecting intellectual outcome in pediatric brain tumor patients. Neurosurgery 21: 638–644

Epstein F, Wisoff J 1987 Intra-axial tumors of the cervicomedullary junction. Journal of Neurosurgery 67: 483–487

Fortuna A, Nolletti A, Nardi P, Caruso R 1981 Spinal neurinomas and meningiomas in children. ACTA Neurochir (Wien) 55: 329–341

Futrell N N, Osborn A G, Cheson B D 1981 Pineal region tumors: computed tomographic-pathologic spectrum. American Journal of Neuroradiology 2: 415–420

Gilbert H A, Kagan A R 1980 Radiation damage to the nervous system. A delayed therapeutic hazard, Raven Press, New York

Goldberg M B, Sheline G E, Malamud J 1963 Malignant intracranial neoplasms following radiation therapy for acromegaly. Radiology 80: 465–470

Grant E G, White E M, Schellinger D, Rosenbach D 1987 Low-level echogenicity in intraventricular hemorrhage versus ventriculitis. Radiology 165: 471–474

Gregorios J B, Green B, Page L, Thomsen S, Monforte H 1986 Spinal cord tumors presenting with neural tube defects. Neurosurgery 19: 962–966

Hall W A, Yunis E J, Albright A L 1986 Anaplastic ganglioglioma in an infant: Case report and review of the literature. Neurosurgery 19: 1016–1020

Han J S, Benson J E, Kaufman B et al 1985 Demonstration of diastematomyelia and associated abnormalities with MR imaging. American Journal of Neuroradiology 6: 215–219

Handel S F, Miller M H, Danziger J 1979 Brain and spinal cord. In: Libshitz H I (ed) Diagnostic roentgenology of radiotherapy change. Williams & Wilkins, Baltimore, pp 167–184

Harwood-Nash D C F, Riley B J 1970 Calcification of basal ganglia following radiation therapy. American Journal of Radiology 108: 392–395

Hochberg S H, Pruitt A 1980 Assumptions in the radiotherapy of glioblastoma. Neurology (NY) 30: 907–911

Hoffman H J, Neill J, Crone K R, Hendrick E B, Humphreys R P 1987 Hydrosyringomyelia and its management in childhood. Neurosurgery 21: 347–351

Honig P J, Charney E B 1982 Children with brain tumor headaches. Distinguishing features. American Journal of Diseases of Children 136: 121–124

Hosoda K, Tamaki N, Masumura M, Matsumoto S 1987 Magnetic resonance images of brain-stem encephalitis. Case report. Journal of Neurosurgery 66: 283–285

Kaiser M C, Pettersson H, Harwood-Nash D C, Fitz C R, Armstrong E 1981 Direct coronal CT of the spine in infants and children. American Journal of Neuroradiology 2: 465–466

Kangarloo H, Gold R H, Diament M J, Boechat M I, Barrett C 1984 High-resolution spinal sonography in infants. American Journal of Radiology 142: 1243–1247

Katayama Y, Tsubokawa T, Yoshida K 1986 Cystic meningiomas in infancy. Surgical Neurology 25: 43–48

Kendall B, Reider-Grosswasser I, Valentine A 1983 Diagnosis of masses presenting within the ventricles on computed tomography. Neuroradiology 25: 11–22

Kingsley D P E, Kendall B E 1978 Cranial computed tomography in leukaemia. Neuroradiology 16: 543–546

Kramer S, Lee K F 1974 Complications of radiation therapy: central nervous system. Seminars in Roentgenology 9: 75–83

Lee B C P, Kneelend J B, Walker R W, Posner J B, Cahill P T, Deck M D F 1985 MR imaging of brain stem tumours. American Journal of Neuroradiology 6: 159–163

Lee B C P, Lipper E, Nass R, Ehrlich M E, de Ciccio-Bloom E, Auld P A M 1986 MRI of the central nervous system in neonates and young children. American Journal of Neuroradiology 7: 605–616

Lemire R J, Loeser J D, Leech R W et al 1975 Normal and abnormal development of the human nervous system. Harper and Rowe, Hagerstown, Md. pp 84–94

Levy R M, Rosenbloom S, Perrett L V 1986 Neuroradiology findings in AIDS: a review of 200 cases. American Journal of Neuroradiology 7: 833–839

Littman P, Jarrett P, Bilaniuk L T et al 1980 Pediatric brain stem gliomas. Cancer 45: 2787–2792

Liu J C, De Armond S J, Edwards M S B 1985 An unusual spinal meningioma in a child: case report. Neurosurgery 17: 313–316

Lockman L A, Mastri A, Priest J R, Nesbit M 1980 Dural venous sinus thrombosis in acute lymphoblastic leukaemia. Paediatrics 66: 943–950

Lourie G L, Osborne D R, Kirks D R 1986 Involvement of posterior visual pathways by optic nerve gliomas. Pediatric Radiology 16: 271–274

McAllister M D, O'Leary D H 1987 CT myelography of subarachnoid leukemic infiltration of the lumbar thecal sac and lumbar nerve roots. American Journal of Neuroradiology 8: 568–569

McDonnell P, Miller N R 1983 Chiasmatic and hypothalamic extension of optic nerve glioma. Archives of Ophthalmology 101: 1412–1415

McLone D G, Raimondi A J, Naidich T P 1982 Craniopharyngiomas. Child's Brain 9: 188–200

Marin G, Carollo C, Perilongo G et al 1983 Cerebral changes shown by computed tomography in children with acute lymphatic leukemia after therapy. Radiologia Medica (Torino) 69 (7–8): 554–558

Martin W H, Kail W S, Morris J L, Constable W C 1980 Fibrosarcoma after high energy radiation therapy for pituitary adenoma. American Journal of Neuroradiology 1: 469–472

Massad M, Haddad F, Slim M et al 1985 Spinal cord compression in neuroblastoma. Surgical Neurology 23: 567–572

Mechanick J I, Hochberg F H, LaRocque A 1986 Hypothalamic dysfunction following whole-brain irradiation. Journal of Neurosurgery 65: 490–494

Mikhael M A 1978 Radiation necrosis of the brain; correlation between computed tomography, pathology and dose distribution. Journal of Computer Assisted Tomography 2: 71–80

Miller J H, Weinblatt M E, Smith J C, Fishman L S, Segall H D, Ortega J A 1983 Combined computed tomographic and radionuclide imaging in the long-term follow-up of children with primary intra-axial intracranial neoplasms. Radiology 146: 681–686

Murovic J A, Nagashima T, Hoshino T, Edwards M S B, Davis R L 1986 Pediatric central nervous system tumors: A cell kinetic study with bromodeoxyuridine. Neurosurgery 19: 900–904

Nobuhiko A, Masuzawa H 1986 Subdural hematomas in abused children: report of six cases from Japan. Neurosurgery 18: 475–477

Numaguchi Y, Hoffman J C, Sones P J 1975 Basal ganglia calcification; a late radiation effect. American Journal of Radiology 123: 27–30

Oi S, Raimondi A J 1981 Hydrocephalus associated with intraspinal neoplasms in childhood. American Journal of Diseases of Children 135: 1122–1124

Olsen W L, Winkler M L, Ross D A 1987 Carcinomatous encephalitis: CT and MR findings. American Journal of Neuroradiology 8: 553–554

Peylan Ramu N, Poplak D G, Blei C L, Herdt J R, Vermess M, Di Chiro G 1979 Computer assisted tomography in methotrexate encephalopathy. Journal of Computer Assisted Tomography 1: 216–221

Post M J D, Tate L G, Quencer R M, Hensley G T, Berger J R, Sheremata W A, Maul G 1988 CT, MR, and pathology in HIV encephalitis and meningitis. American Journal of Neuroradiology 9: 469–476

Price D B, Hotson G C, Loh J P 1988 Pontine calcification following radiotherapy: CT demonstration. Journal of Computer Assisted Tomography 12: 45–46

Price R A, Birdwell D A 1978 The central nervous system in childhood leukaemia III mineralising microangiopathy and dystrophic calcification. Cancer 42: 717–728

Pusey E, Kortman K E, Flannigan B D, Tsuruda J, Bradley W G 1987 MR of craniopharyngiomas: tumour delineation and characterisation. American Journal of Neuroradiology 8: 439–444

Ramsey R G, Zacharias C E 1985 MR imaging of the spine after radiation therapy: easily recognisable effects. American Journal of Neuroradiology 6: 247–251

Rorke L B 1983 The cerebellar medulloblastoma and its relationship to primitive neuroectodermal tumors. Journal of Neuropathology and Experimental Neurology 42: 1–15

Rubenstein L J, Herman M M, Long T F, Wilburn J R 1975 Disseminated necrotising leukoencephalopathy; a complication of treated central nervous system leukaemia and lymphoma. Cancer 35: 291–305

Sandhu A, Kendall B 1987 Computed tomography in management of medulloblastomas. Neuroradiology 29: 444–452

Savoiardo M, Harwood-Nash D, Tadmor R et al 1982 Glioma of the intracranial anterior optic pathways in children. Radiology 138: 601

Schott L H, Naidich T P, Gan J 1983 Common paediatric brain tumours. Typical computed tomographic appearances. The Journal of Computed Tomography 7: 3–15

Scotti G, Scialfa G, Colombo N, Landoni L 1987 Magnetic resonance diagnosis of intramedullary tumors of the spinal cord. Neuroradiology 29: 130–135

Segall H D, Zee C S, Naidich T P, Ahmadi J, Becker T S 1982 Computed tomography in neoplasms of the posterior fossa in children. Radiologic Clinics of North America 20: 237–253

Shuman R M, Alvord E C Jr, Leach R W 1975 The biology of childhood ependymomas. Archives of Neurology 32: 731–739

Stroink A R, Hoffman H J, Hendrick E B, Humphreys R P, Davidson G 1987 Transependymal benign dorsally exophytic brain stem gliomas in childhood: diagnosis and treatment recommendations. Neurosurgery 20: 439–444

Sundaresan N, Galicich J H, Deck M D F, Tomita T 1981 Radiation necrosis after treatment of solitary intracranial metastases. Neurosurgery 8/3: 329–333

Tomita T, McLone D G, Naidich T P 1986 Mural tumors with cysts in the cerebral hemispheres of children. Neurosurgery 19: 998–1005

Vandenberg S R, May E E, Rubinstein L J et al 1987 Desmoplastic supratentorial neuroepithelial tumors of infancy with divergent differentiation potential ("desmoplastic infantile gangliogliomas"). Report on 11 cases of a distinctive embryonal tumor with favorable prognosis. Journal of Neurosurgery 66: 58–71

Wang A N, Carson B S 1987 Upward herniation of the posterior fossa cyst in the shunted child. Surgical Neurology 28: 215–220

West C G H 1987 Optic nerve gliomas in children: a reappraisal. British Journal of Neurosurgery 1: 99–104

Williams A L, Haughton V M, Pojunas K W, Daniels D L, Kilgore D P 1987 Differentiation of intranedullary neoplasms and cysts by MR. American Journal of Neuroradiology 8: 527–532

Woo E, Lam K, Yu Y L, Lee P W H, Huang C Y 1987 Cerebral radionecrosis: is surgery necessary? Journal of Neurology, Neurosurgery and Psychiatry 50: 1407–1414

Wright T L, Bresnan M J 1976 Radiation induced cerebrovascular disease in children. Neurology (NY) 26: 540–543

PART 2
THE LYMPHORETICULAR SYSTEM; PRIMARY TUMOURS OF THE ABDOMEN, PELVIS AND RETROPERITONEUM; MISCELLANEOUS SOLID TUMOURS
R. K. Levick

The recent decline in mortality from childhood malignancy is due mainly to improved methods of treatment. However, earlier and more accurate diagnosis is also a contributory factor. Imaging techniques have been extended from conventional X-rays to include isotopes, ultrasound, X-ray computed tomography (CT) and, most recently, magnetic resonance imaging (MRI) and monoclonal antibody techniques. Guided biopsy techniques, using ultrasound and CT, are now widely available for primary diagnosis and follow-up.

LEUKAEMIA

Leukaemia in its various forms accounts for about one third of all childhood malignancy, acute lymphocytic leukaemia (ALL) being by far the commonest type. Staging is not normally required at the time of initial diagnosis as the condition is usually widespread. For example, the identification of areas of bone destruction by radiographic or isotope methods has no prognostic value. Imaging techniques are used mainly in an attempt to identify areas of disease which may remain after treatment in sanctuary sites.

Bone and bone marrow

Sites of leukaemic tissue in the bone marrow following treatment may be identified by isotope scanning with technetium-99m sulphur colloid which is taken up by the reticulo-endothelial cells outside affected areas. However, 'cold-spots' may represent either tumour tissue or areas of fibrosis.

Bone lesions occurring during or after treatment include osteoporosis, ischaemic necrosis and osteomyelitis. Plain radiographs are usually helpful but an isotope scan using e.g. technetium-99m methyldiphosphonate (MDP) is preferred for detecting bone necrosis.

Genitourinary tract

Widespread involvement is common and the rôle of the testes as sanctuary sites has been recognized for some years (Hustu & Aur 1978). Ultrasound is normally employed for testicular imaging, with enlarged testes containing hypoechoic areas indicating leukaemic infiltration. However, these areas may require biopsy for confirmation of tumour involvement. Ovarian involvement has been described and manifests as an adnexal mass on ultrasound or as diffuse ovarian enlargement on CT scans. Neither technique is tissue characteristic. Ultrasound scanning of the kidneys may show enlargement, with or without areas of increased echogenicity. When associated with hepatosplenomegaly, this usually represents leukaemic involvement, and a localized leukaemoid tumour may be present. Renal colic, due to blood clot or to uric acid calculi, should be investigated with ultrasound (Fig. 3.16).

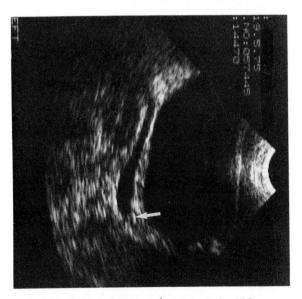

Fig. 3.16 Child aged 10 years on treatment for ALL. Longitudinal scan through the bladder showing a dilated ureter obstructed by a uric acid calculus (arrow).

Gastrointestinal tract

Infiltration of the mucosa or submucosa may be present but symptoms are rare unless due to complications such as intussusception. Double contrast barium studies may show mucosal infiltration. Hydrostatic reduction of intussusception is usually preferred to surgery. Typhlitis is a necrotizing enteritis affecting the colon, probably induced by chemotherapy and secondary infection of the compromised mucosa. Contrast studies are rarely needed but can show ulceration, pseudopolyps and thumb-printing (Wagner et al 1970). Low osmolality contrast should be used.

Central nervous system (CNS)

Symptoms occurring at diagnosis or in early treatment are likely to be due to intracranial bleeding in the presence of low platelet levels; CT evaluation is employed. Rarely initial presentation is due to a mass effect from a leukaemoid tumour. Sanctuary sites are often leptomeningeal and are difficult to define but magnetic resonance imaging may be of help in the future. Ventricular dilatation may follow treatment, and the development of periventricular areas of contrast enhancement on CT suggests a leukoencephalopathy. (*Vide supra*)

Thorax

On a frontal chest radiograph, upper mediastinal widening due to thymic enlargement is very suggestive of T-cell disease. A lateral radiograph will often show the anterior mass. Enlarged hilar and mediastinal glands are also shown by chest radiography (Fig. 3.17). CT scanning is usually reserved for complications such as superior mediastinal syndrome, when enlarged lymph nodes can be identified. In this situation angiography will only show vascular compression and gallium-67 isotope scans do not differentiate infection from tumour.

Opportunistic infections are common. Radiographic patterns are very rarely diagnostic although pneumocystis is suggested by a fine stippling and mycoplasma by patchy consolidation. Central venous line position is noted on the chest radiograph and possible blockage investigated by a screened injection of contrast with appropriate aseptic technique.

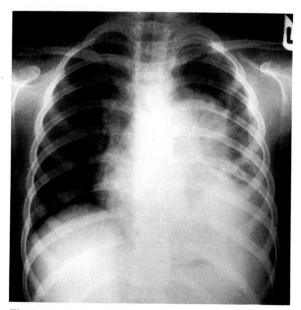

Fig. 3.17 A girl aged 12 years with T-cell leukaemia. This frontal chest radiograph demonstrates bulk mediastinal lymphadenopathy, probably with thymic involvement. There is a left pleural effusion.

LYMPHOMA

The lymphomas comprise Hodgkin's disease (HD) and non-Hodgkin's lymphoma (NHL) and are the third most common form of childhood malignancy. NHL arises mainly from extranodal sites particularly in the abdomen, around the appendix, caecum and terminal ileum. Spread occurs locally, and to the CNS, bone marrow and kidneys. The mediastinum is the next most common primary site. There is considerable overlap between NHL and acute lymphocytic leukaemia (Murphy 1978).

Staging

Once a diagnosis of lymphoma is made, imaging is directed to identifying the number of involved areas. Several staging systems are used, the Ann Arbor system being almost universal for HD occurring in childhood:

Stage 1. Involvement of a single lymph node region or of a single extralymphatic organ or site.

Stage 2. Involvement of two or more lymph node regions on the same side of the diaphragm, or localized involvement of an extralymphatic organ or site and of one or more lymph node regions on the same side of the diaphragm.

Stage 3. Involvement of lymph node regions on both sides of the diaphragm which may also be accompanied by localized involvement of an extralymphatic organ or site or involvement of the spleen or both.

Stage 4. Diffuse or disseminated involvement of one or more extralymphatic organs or tissues with or without associated lymph node involvement.

Staging laparotomy is rarely performed in children. Chest radiographs, CT of the thorax and abdomen, ultrasound and a gallium-67 isotope scan are used to define involved sites and provide a base line so that response to treatment can be monitored. Other investigations may be required as clinically indicated.

In children there is no agreed staging system for NHL. The St Jude scheme is commonly used:

Stage 1. A single tumour (extranodal) or single anatomical area (nodal) with the exclusion of the mediastinum or abdomen.

Stage 2. A single tumour (extranodal) with regional node involvement. Two or more nodal areas on the same side of the diaphragm. Two single (extranodal) tumours with or without node involvement, on the same side of the diaphragm. A primary gastrointestinal tract tumour with or without involvement of associated mesenteric nodes.

Stage 3. Two single tumours (extranodal) on opposite sides of the diaphragm. Two or more nodal areas above or below the diaphragm. All primary intrathoracic tumours. All extensive primary intra-abdominal disease. All paraspinal or epidural tumours.

Abdomen

Plain radiographs may show mass effect displacement of bowel and evidence of splenomegaly. Ultrasound is valuable in demonstrating nodal masses or individual nodes more than 2 cm in diameter. The typical involved node shows a hypoechoic pattern, as can areas of bowel involvement. Displacement of the aorta and inferior vena cava can be identified. CT scanning is, how-ever, the method of choice for initial assessment, its most notable failure being an inability to recognize involved but non-enlarged nodes and diffuse splenic involvement. The bowel should be opacified with oral contrast. Involvement of the terminal ileum, caecum and appendix are seen as encircling areas of adjacent masses of soft tissue density. Intravenous contrast enables displacement or encasement of vessels to be identified, the latter by the loss of vessel outline. In the upper abdomen it may be difficult to differentiate tumour adjacent to an organ from invasion, but preservation of fat planes usually excludes invasion. Liver involvement is most commonly diffuse and associated with enlargement. Only if there are focal lesions will areas of decreased attenuation be visible. Similar problems are found in splenic imaging despite its importance in staging, and ultrasound is no more accurate. Nodal involvement at the splenic hilum suggests splenic involvement. Isotope imaging with gallium-67 will identify disseminated areas of involvement but not non-enlarged nodes. It is normally used as a whole body scanning technique; during treatment involved nodes may fail to take up isotope (Sty et al 1983). The liver and spleen may be imaged with technetium-99m sulphur colloid but accuracy is no greater than CT or ultrasound, and is usually reserved for patients with doubtful results from these methods. In summary, baseline ultrasound is routine, and CT is used in initial staging but less often to monitor progress. The rôle of lymphangiography is disputed. Involved nodes of normal size, especially those in the iliac and para-aortic groups, are usually demonstrated when ultrasound and CT are ineffective. Accuracy is lower in the upper abdomen, and the contrast may interfere with subsequent gallium-67 scanning (Hays 1975). There are technical problems in children and this examination is rarely attempted in those under 4 years of age.

Thorax

Tumour is most commonly found in the anterior mediastinum when the superior vena cava and airway may be compressed; hilar involvement is commoner in HD. Pleural, pericardial and lung parenchymal involvement may occur. Plain chest radiographs, PA and lateral are required and form a baseline; conventional tomography has been replaced by CT. Certainly in HD a CT scan is required for proper evaluation of the mediastinum and hila, including vascular and tracheal displacement and narrowing. CT scanning should normally extend into the upper abdomen. Blood-borne spread to the lungs produces a variety of reticulo-nodular patterns including pseudomiliary tuberculosis (Fig. 3.18). These are seen on chest radiographs as well as on CT. Gallium-67 isotope scans will show these pulmonary infiltrations as well as involved hilar and mediastinal nodes.

Head and neck

Approximately 10% of patients with NHL present with a primary tumour involving the head and neck. Lymphoma in the nasopharynx, paranasal sinuses and orbits together with bone involvement is best demonstrated by CT scan or MRI, and gallium-67 isotope scanning may be of value. Cervical nodes may be continuous with those in the mediastinum.

Genitourinary tract

Renal involvement is most common in Burkitt's

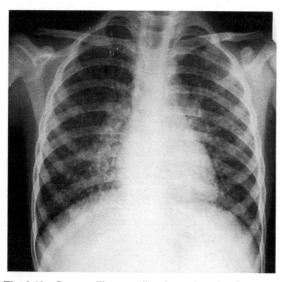

Fig. 3.18 Coarse miliary mottling due to lung involvement in a 10-year-old asian boy with HD. At presentation the history of cough, night sweats and a contact history led to a period of antituberculous therapy.

lymphoma. On ultrasound scans the kidneys are enlarged and may show hypoechogenicity or focal areas of increased echoes due to tumour or to haemorrhage. Dilatation of the collecting systems may be seen due to extrinsic ureteric obstruction by tumour. Gonadal involvement is almost always secondary and produces hypoechoic areas.

Bone

Lesions are assessed on plain radiographs; they may be destructive or sclerotic and periosteal reaction is occasionally marked. Isotope bone scans will provide a full skeletal survey.

Central nervous system

Involvement is seen as leptomeningeal disease in NHL. Dural lesions may cause cord compression and are shown by myelography (with water soluble low-osmolar contrast) followed by a CT scan if necessary. CT will also display focal infiltration in the brain or spinal cord, appearing as contrast-enhancing areas (Brant–Zawadzki & Enzmann 1978). As in leukaemia, MRI may prove to be of a greater value.

GENITOURINARY TUMOURS

Abdominal masses in children most frequently arise from the kidney, adrenal gland or the sympathetic chain ganglia. Plain radiographs of the chest and abdomen are obtained to identify any calcification associated with the mass, metastases in lung or bone, paravertebral masses and evidence of enlargement of the liver or spleen. An ultrasound scan is usually performed next and may identify a non-malignant mass such as a hydronephrosis or a duplication cyst. In the case of a solid tumour an assessment of the extent of disease should be undertaken and if the tumour is inoperable a guided biopsy for diagnosis can be performed. CT scanning may be required as an additional staging procedure. Intravenous urography (IVU) and arteriography are used much less since the advent of ultrasound and CT. Specific forms of isotope scan, such as [123]I-*meta*-iodobenzyl guanidine (MIBG) in neuroectodermal tumours, are used to define the primary tumour site and extent. At the same time estimations of tumour secretions, such as catecholamines from neuroblastoma, may identify the tumour type and therefore the likely site.

Wilms' tumour

This is the most common solid childhood abdominal tumour and is usually seen in the under 5-year-olds with a peak incidence at 3.5 years. There is an association with hemihypertrophy, Beckwith–Weidermann syndrome and non-familial aniridia. The tumour probably arises from the metanephric mesoderm. The staging system used is:

Stage 1. Tumour limited to the kidney and removed completely at surgery.
Stage 2. Local spread but excision complete, local flank spillage. This includes renal vein thrombus.
Stage 3. Residual tumour in the abdomen in subcategories (a)–(e):
  (a) lymph nodes in the hilum or para-aortic chain
  (b) diffuse peritoneal spread including operative spill
  (c) peritoneal tumour implants
  (d) tumour beyond areas of excision, gross or on histology
  (e) tumour spread into adjacent vital structures
Stage 4. Blood-borne deposits in liver, brain, lung and bone.
Stage 5. Initial evidence of bilateral tumour.

Plain radiographs may show a mass in the renal area; calcification is seen in only about 5%. The pattern of bowel displacement may indicate a large mass which crosses the midline. A plain chest radiograph is mandatory and may show a solitary or multiple rounded metastases. On ultrasound Wilms' tumour masses are of mixed reflectivity and may show ill-defined cystic areas due to tumour necrosis and haemorrhage (Levick 1970). Part of the affected kidney is often normal but ureteric compression by tumour produces dilatation of otherwise unaffected calyces. Invasion of the renal vein and inferior vena cava may also be seen. The contralateral kidney must be assessed as approximately 5% of Wilms' tumours are bilateral.

A normal ultrasound scan virtually excludes tumour but minute areas of potential tumour cannot be detected. An intravenous urogram is rarely indicated. If an absent or ectopic contralateral kidney is suspected on ultrasound, an isotope scan with an appropriate agent is usually performed. If an IVU is carried out, it is traditional to inject contrast into a leg vein and screen the inferior vena cava whilst compressing the opposite femoral vein in order to show caval narrowing or occlusion by tumour. Arteriography is normally reserved for the assessment of the renal vessels when bilateral disease is present and partial nephrectomy considered, or for recurrence in the remaining kidney. CT provides the best preoperative information about tumour in retroperitoneal nodes and in the liver. Contrast enhancement may make the demarcation between tumour and normal kidney clearer. Staging involves the identification of local spread up to stage 3, the finding of blood-borne metastases in lung, liver, brain and bone in stage 4, and of bilateral renal involvement in stage 5. A combination of plain chest and abdominal radiographs, upper abdominal ultrasound and a CT scan of the thorax and abdomen will usually provide this information. Bone metastases are rare in Wilms' tumour in the absence of prior lung involvement (Levick & Steiner 1983), and their early appearance suggests a

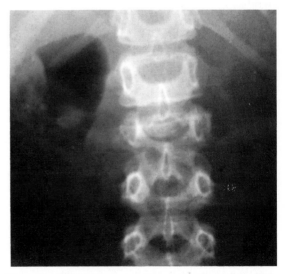

Fig. 3.19 Partial destruction of a vertebral body in a child with a renal mass. Histology showed a clear-cell sarcoma.

non-Wilms' type of tumour (Fig. 3.19). When multiple bone lesions are suspected an isotope bone scan should be performed. Staging may be predicted on imaging findings but operative findings are an essential part of the process, particularly in identifying intra-abdominal spread.

Following surgery or when preoperative tumour shrinkage is carried out, ultrasound is usually performed to monitor progress. However, bowel loops may fill the renal bed making ultrasound technically unsatisfactory and CT scanning may be necessary. Regular ultrasound of the remaining kidney should be carried out for at least five years to detect the appearance of a contralateral tumour. Hypertrophy is usually found, sometimes in the form of pseudotumours which may be distinguished from true tumour by isotope scanning using technetium-99m glucoheptonate.

NEUROBLASTOMA

Neuroblastoma arise in the adrenal glands or in sympathetic chain ganglia. They are the commonest solid malignant tumours in infancy and the first decade of life. Histologically, tumours can be differentiated into neuroblastoma, ganglioneuroblastoma and ganglioneuroma. Some neuroblastoma may regress and apparently differentiate to benign lesions.

Staging is as follows (Evans et al 1971 (modified)):

Stage 1. Tumour confined to structure of origin.
Stage 2. Extension in continuity not crossing the midline. Lymph nodes on the same side may be involved.
Stage 3. Extension in continuity which crosses the midline.
Stage 4. Spread to bone, other organs, soft tissues or distant lymph nodes.
Stage 4a. Stage 1 or 2 plus remote disease in liver, skin or bone marrow but with no radiographic evidence of bone destruction.

Because patients in stage 2 without local lymph node involvement have a better prognosis, Stage 2a may be used to denote no nodal tumour and Stage 2b to denote involved nodes.

Recent advances have made imaging in primary staging and follow-up less complex and more accurate than previously. Plain radiographs of the abdomen and thorax are usually obtained, often prior to diagnosis, and are complemented, ideally, by a thoraco-abdominal CT scan. An isotope scan using ^{123}I MIBG may reveal occult metastases as well as better definition of bone involvement (Bomanji et al 1988). Ultrasound scans will demonstrate most of the lesions found on CT and are used to measure tumour regression in response to chemotherapy in preference to repeat CT scans.

Where surgery is contemplated following chemotherapy preoperative staging should be performed. [123]I MIBG will provide whole body screening enabling a tailored CT scan to be performed which provides better anatomical detail of residual tumour.

The rôles of magnetic resonance imaging (Siegel et al 1986) and monoclonal antibody techniques (Matthay 1985) are still being assessed. For example, bone marrow involvement may be demonstrated by MR and relapse identified. Monoclonal techniques show promise in detecting unsuspected secondary deposits.

On the plain radiographs the tumour may be identified as a thoracic or abdominal mass with calcification visible in nearly two-thirds of cases. On the CT and ultrasound scans it is important to identify the involvement of adjacent structures, involvement of regional lymph nodes, encasement of vessels, the presence of liver metastases and extension of abdominal disease into the thorax. Identification of tumour crossing the midline is an important finding for accurate staging and if this occurs through the root of the mesentery, the pancreas and common bile duct may be involved. Contrast-enhanced CT scans may be required to identify involvement of the liver, kidney or vessel encasement and tumour thrombus. CT is superior to ultrasound in assessing extension of tumour into the thorax.

Invasion of the kidney may mimic a primary renal tumour. However, the tumour pattern is different and raised catecholamine levels will indicate an extrarenal origin; isotope scanning with ^{131}I MIBG (Ackery et al 1984) or ^{123}I MIBG (Bomanji et al 1988) will confirm the neuroectodermal origin. CNS involvement is rarely primary, and secondary lesions are predominantly dural with local extension and may cause sutural separation.

Phaeochromocytoma may also be identified by MIBG scanning with greater accuracy than CT or ultrasound. Recent recognition of amine precursor uptake and decarboxylation (APUD) pathways has explained the relationship between various endocrine-secreting tumours; thus a thoracic ganglioneuroma may secrete a vasoactive intestinal peptide (Swift et al 1975). In a patient with neuroblastoma receiving treatment, a rising level of 4-hydroxy-3-methoxymandelic acid indicates increased tumour activity and the need for further imaging of the primary and metastatic tumour sites.

TESTICULAR AND OVARIAN TUMOURS

These may spread to adjacent structures, regional lymph nodes, the lungs and mediastinum, bones and, less commonly, to the brain. Initial tumour identification is often possible with ultrasound but pelvic, abdominal and thoracic CT are used to determine spread; brain CT is reserved for patients with clinical evidence of involvement. Isotope scanning is used to detect bone metastases.

RHABDOMYOSARCOMA

These arise in connective tissues and are differentiated histologically into the embryonal and alveolar types. They account for up to 8% of childhood malignancies (Sutow 1981). Embryonal rhabdomyosarcoma is usually found in infants, affecting the head and neck and genitourinary tract. Sarcoma botryoides is an embryonal variant. The alveolar type is often found in peripheral sites in older children and has a less favourable prognosis. The simplest staging system is the Saint Jude:

Stage 1. Localized tumour with complete resection.
Stage 2. Regional tumour with adjacent spread, local or regional lymph nodes involved. Stage 2a indicates that the tumour is fully resected, if not 2b.
Stage 3. Generalized tumour spread. Stage 3a with normal bone marrow, 3b with marrow involvement.

It will be seen that staging depends largely on operative results and bone marrow examination. Preoperative staging can be undertaken to provide useful information. Plain radiographs may show a mass lesion with adjacent bone involvement. Contrast bladder studies can demonstrate the extent of intravesical tumour. CT with or without IV contrast and ultrasound can be used to image the primary tumour and its intrapelvic or intra-abdominal extent. CT is the investigation of choice to detect lung metastases, which are common, and CNS tumour, usually due to meningeal spread. Assessment of any site after removal of the primary tumour is difficult, particularly the distinction between residual tumour and postoperative changes.

OSTEOGENIC SARCOMA

Osteosarcoma is the commonest primary malignant bone tumour with most patients presenting between 10 and 25 years of age. It is most commonly seen in the lower femoral or upper tibial metaphysis. The pelvis and upper humerus are the next most commonly involved sites. Periosteal new bone patterns such as Codman's triangle and spiculation at right angles to the shaft axis are highly suggestive of osteosarcoma in the presence of bone destruction and some irregular new bone formation. However, the distinction between sarcoma and infection can be difficult and a biopsy may be needed to establish malignancy as well as to identify tumour type. Modern imaging techniques are concerned mainly with better definition of the bony and soft tissue limits of the primary tumour and more accurate assessment of metastatic involvement of other structures, notably the lungs. Plain radiographs will undoubtedly be obtained in the initial diagnosis, including the primary lesion and the lungs. Treatment protocols then demand CT scans of the entire bone containing the tumour and of the lungs. Scans of the bony lesion reveal the extent of soft tissue spread and spread within the bone marrow whilst thoracic scans show metastases too small to be seen on plain radiographs. Contrast enhancement may define the soft tissue tumour boundary better. Ultrasound can be used to define soft tissue extensions, especially in the pelvis. MRI with its superior tissue contrast may well replace CT when it is more readily available. Isotope scans are not mandatory in all protocols. Technetium-99m methyl-diphosphonate images show, in the blood pool phase, the hyperaemic response to the tumour; later whole body images demonstrate the sites of metastases, which may require confirmation by radiographs or CT (Hudson et al 1983). During treatment routine chest radiographs are obtained and CT repeated at prescribed intervals, especially before surgery.

Ewing sarcoma of bone and reticulum cell sarcoma (non-Hodgkin's lymphoma) are quantified and followed up in a manner similar to that described for osteogenic sarcoma. Isotope scans using technetium-99m sulphur colloid may give a good indication of areas of marrow involvement.

HEPATIC TUMOURS

Hepatoblastoma and hepatocellular carcinoma account for about 5% of paediatric tumours. The former occur mainly in children under 3 years of age; the latter occur later in childhood and may follow liver damage from conditions such as tyrosinaemia and glycogen storage disease. Plain radiographs in hepatoblastoma may show fine calcification; larger areas of calcification suggest a haemangioma, but can be seen in thrombosed tumour vessels. Vascular malformations are sometimes difficult to distinguish from malignancy and tumour markers such as alpha-fetoprotein are used both in diagnosis and in follow-up. This marker is initially positive in about two-thirds of cases. Most tumours arise in the right lobe. Ultrasound scans show liver enlargement, the tumour being poorly defined and of increased echogenicity compared with surrounding tissue; there may be hypoechoic areas representing necrosis. Spread to the other lobe of the liver, porta hepatis and regional nodes should be sought. Tumour thrombus in the hepatic veins and inferior vena cava may be seen. Doppler ultrasound is used to confirm abnormal flow in these vessels. Scans with technetium-99m sulphur colloid may show a tumour 'blush' in blood pool phase; more commonly the tumour appears as a void. CT scans will provide information similar to ultrasound and contrast enhancement will help to distinguish an isodense tumour on unenhanced scans from nor-

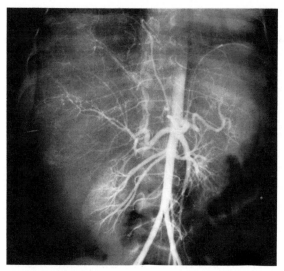

Fig. 3.20 Aortogram in a 2-year-old with massive liver enlargement due to hepatoblastoma. There is an abnormal circulation involving the right lobe of the liver. The right kidney is displaced but not involved.

mal liver. Angiography is used occasionally to define tumour limits and blood supply prior to surgery (Fig. 3.20).

The lungs should be assessed for metastases with plain radiographs and CT. Bone and CNS involvement is uncommon and may only require assessment if clinically indicated. Serial ultrasound scans are used to assess tumour involution, often accompanied by cystic necrosis. Repeat isotope scans may be difficult to evaluate as tumour size may initially increase and become more or less vascular. Fatty degeneration may occur with chemotherapy and can be assessed by ultrasound (Foster et al 1980).

HISTIOCYTOSIS

The recognition of a common pattern of Langerhans cell proliferation has linked together the various forms of histiocytosis X on a firm histological basis. The group comprises eosinophil granuloma, Hand–Schuller–Christian syndrome and Letterer–Siwe disease. Malignant histiocytosis is a lymphohistiocytosis and not a Langerhans cell disorder.

Bone lesions

These may be single or multiple and soft tissue extension is fairly common. Plain radiographs are usually employed to detect and follow up lesions, which appear initially as clearly defined areas of bone destruction with non-reactive margins. In skull lesions there may be a central area of dense bone (Fig. 3.21). In the ribs and long bones expansion and considerable periosteal reaction may occur, mimicking infection. Bowing and pathological fracture occur. Vertebral body lesions may lead to collapse and vertebra plana. Healing is evidenced by blurring of the margins and filling in of the defect, sometimes preceded by spotty calcification. Isotope scanning will also reveal affected areas and may be used to avoid skeletal surveys in older children; however, in infants lesions adjacent to growth plates are difficult to identify. Soft tissue extensions can be assessed by ultrasound or by CT.

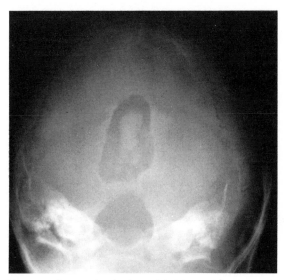

Fig. 3.21 Destruction in the occipital bone with preserved central bone island. Histologically proven Langerhans histiocytosis.

Pulmonary lesions

Interstitial involvement produces a reticulonodular pattern. Plain radiographs usually suffice for recognition and follow-up. Gallium-67 isotope scans will also demonstrate the infiltration and can be used for diagnosis and follow-up.

Abdomen

Hepatosplenomegaly is common in multisystem disease. On ultrasound the liver shows a diffuse increase in echogenicity whereas the spleen is often hypoechoic. Bile duct dilatation may be seen due to areas of nodular infiltration (Lichtenstein 1953).

Central nervous system

The well-known association with diabetes insipidus is due to an extension of bone disease into the pituitary fossa, usually demonstrable by CT. Alternatively there may be a suprasellar mass which enhances on CT. Multiple CNS lesions are rare.

Malignant histiocytosis

This is a lymphohistiocytic reticulosis associated with multiple areas of bone destruction, lung infiltration and hepatosplenomegaly. Leptomeningeal infiltration may occur. Imaging appearances suggest severe and widespread histiocytosis X-like changes.

REFERENCES

Ackery D, Tippet P, Condon B, Sutton H, Wyeth P 1984 New approach to the localisation of phaeochromocytoma: Imaging with [131]I-*meta*-iodobenzyl guanidine. British Medical Journal 288: 1587–1591

Bomanji J, Conry B G, Britton K E, Reznek R H 1988 Imaging neural crest tumours with [123]I-*meta*-iodobenzyl guanidine and X-ray computed tomography: A comparative study. Clinical Radiology 39: 502–506

Brant-Zawadzki M, Enzmann D R 1978 Computed tomographic brain scanning in patients with lymphoma. Radiology 129: 67–71

Evans A E, D'Angio G J, Randolph J 1971 A proposed staging for children with neuroblastoma. Cancer 31: 374–378

Foster K J, Dewbury K C, Griffiths A H, Wright R 1980 The accuracy of ultrasound in the detection of fatty infiltration of the liver. British Journal of Radiology 53: 440–442

Hays D M 1975 Staging of Hodgkin's disease in children reviewed. Cancer 35: 973–978

Hudson T M, Schiebler M, Springfield D S, Hawkins I F, Enneking W F, Spanier S S 1983 Radiologic imaging of osteosarcoma. Skeletal Radiology 10: 137–146

Hustu H O, Aur R J A 1978 Extramedullary leukaemia. Clinical Haematology 7: 313–337

Levick R K 1970 Radiology and ultrasound in Wilms' tumour diagnosis. Annales de Radiologie 13: 3–4, 209

Levick R K, Steiner G M 1983 Skeletal survey in Wilms' tumour assessment. Annales de Radiologie 26: 2–3, 235–236

Lichtenstein L 1953 Histiocytosis X. Archives of Pathology 56: 84–102

Matthay K K 1985 Monoclonal antibodies in the diagnosis and treatment of childhood diseases. Advances in Paediatrics 32: 101–137

Murphy S B 1978 Current concepts in cancer. Childhood non-Hodgkin's lymphoma. New England Journal of Medicine 299: 1446–1448

Siegel M J, Nadel S N, Glazer H S, Sagel S S 1986 Mediastinal lesions in children: comparison of CT and MR. Radiology 160: 241–244

Sty J R, Starshak R J, Miller J H 1983 Pediatric nuclear medicine (Current Practice in Nuclear Medicine series). MTP Press, Norwalk, Connecticut, pp 121–135 (lymphoma) and pp 167–199 (Wilms' tumour)

Sutow W W 1981 Childhood rhabdomyosarcoma. In: Malignant solid tumours in children. Raven Press, New York, pp 129–147

Swift P G F, Bloom S R, Harris F 1975 Watery diarrhoea and ganglioneuroma with secretion of a VIP. Archives of Disease in Childhood 50: 896–899

Wagner M L, Rosenberg H S, Fernbach D J, Singleton E B 1970 Typhlitis: A complication of leukaemia in childhood. American Journal of Roentgenology 109: 341–350

4. The lung

E. Sawicka   P. Gishen

INTRODUCTION

Cancer of the lung is the most common form of cancer in British men, and indeed the incidence of lung cancer amongst males in some parts of the UK is the highest in the world (Miller 1980). During 1984 it was the cause of 36 000 deaths per year in England and Wales (Office of Population Censuses and Surveys 1985). The risk of developing lung cancer is directly related to smoking habits, and for the heavy smoker is thirty times that for a non-smoker (Doll & Hill 1964). At present breast and bowel cancers are still more common amongst women in this country, but with the recent increase in smoking by women a rapid rise in the incidence of lung tumours is ocurring in this group. There is an increased risk of developing lung cancer with occupational exposure to some chemicals, minerals and radioactive aerosols. In particular, a smoker with heavy asbestos exposure has a 100 fold increase in the risk of developing lung cancer compared to a non-smoker, who has no increased risk even if exposed to asbestos. The effect of exposure to these two substances has an additive, if not a multiple effect (Selikoff et al 1968).

Survival following a diagnosis of lung cancer is poor (vide infra), but varies considerably with cell type so that an understanding of the pathology of these tumours is necessary to evaluate the most appropriate steps in the investigation and treatment.

PATHOLOGY OF TUMOURS OF THE CHEST

Tumours in the chest may arise from the bronchi, trachea, pleura and lymphoid tissue and can be benign or malignant. Only the latter will be considered here.

Classifications of epithelial tumours of the lung have been suggested by a number of groups, including the World Health Organization (WHO 1981), Veterans' Administration Lung Cancer Chemotherapy Study (Matthews 1976), Working Party for Therapy of Lung Cancer (Matthews 1976), and the Armed Forces Institute of Pathology (AFIP) (Carter & Eggleston 1980). There are differences between these classifications, but all recognize four major types: (i) squamous cell (epidermoid); (ii) adenocarcinoma; (iii) large cell, the three non-small cell cancers; and (iv) small cell tumours. In the WHO and AFIP classification a mixed adenocarcinoma and squamous cell type is included. An acceptable classification of the major subtypes of malignant tumours of the lung based on the Edinburgh system (Lamb 1984) is shown in Table 4.1. The accuracy with which this may be applied varies with the sampling, biopsy size or cytological techniques used (Payne et al 1981), and recognition of these is important as the prognosis and response to treatment of the subtypes vary considerably. The major differences between the classifications is in the division of subgroups of different cell types; in most cases this includes an assessment of differentiation.

Squamous cell carcinoma

This is the most common type of bronchogenic carcinoma, occurring in about 50% of patients (Mountain 1976). These tumours usually arise in the mucosa of a large bronchus, and bronchial obstruction may occur at an early stage with secondary infection and abscess formation.

Table 4.1 Edinburgh classification of epithelial tumours of the lung (Lamb 1984)

Squamous carcinoma
    well differentiated
    moderately differentiated
    poorly differentiated
    undifferentiated

Small cell carcinoma
    oat cell
    intermediate (polygonal)
    combined (oat cell with squamous and/or adenocarcinoma)

Adenocarcinoma
    well differentiated
    moderately differentiated
    poorly differentiated
    bronchoalveolar

Large cell carcinoma
    large cell undifferentiated

Mixed tumours
    adeno-squamous
    other

Carcinoid
    classical carcinoid
    atypical (malginant) carcinoid

Bronchial gland carcinoma
    adenoid cystic
    muco-epidermoid
    other

Miscellaneous epithelial tumours
    giant cells
    clear cell
    carcinosarcoma
    spindle cell variant of squamous carcinoma

Undiagnosable

Squamous cell carcinoma is related to smoking and the occurrence of the tumour may be preceded by squamous metaplasia and the finding of dysplastic cells in the sputum (Doll et al 1957, Heard & Payling-Wright 1976). Squamous cell tumours of multicentric origin are frequently seen (Shimosato 1980), and this may account for the high incidence of second primary tumours of the lung in those patients who have survived with a curative resection.

The characteristic microscopic features are masses of tumour cells with keratinization and pearl formation often traversed by strands of fibrous stroma. The less well differentiated tumours have less keratin formation and/or intercellular bridges (prickles), while poorly differentiated varieties may consist of large spindle-shaped cells.

The larger tumours of this type may cavitate, causing complications including haemorrhage. Distant metastases are less common in squamous cell carcinoma than in other types, and the well differentiated varieties are commonly localized to the thorax at autopsy (Heard & Payling-Wright 1976).

Small cell carcinoma

In contrast to the squamous cell variety, small cell tumours are highly malignant with doubling times of 30 days (Geddes 1979), and often present with symptoms due to distant metastases. They usually arise in the large airways, and are smoking-related. Early regional gland involvement, usually of the hilar glands, is characteristic. They account for 15–30% of cases of bronchogenic carcinoma (Weiss 1981).

The cells are poorly differentiated in character and as they contain neurosecretory granules are thought to be derived from cells associated with amine precursor uptake and decarboxylation (APUD) and peptide production. This accounts for the endocrine activity which may be found with these tumours. There is good histological and other evidence that these cells derive from the bronchial endoderm, like all other bronchogenic carcinomas (Yesner & Carter 1982).

The tumours may be subdivided into oat cell (lymphocyte-like), intermediate (polygonal) or combined types. The oat cell tumours consist of small oval or oat-shaped cells with little cytoplasm. Mitoses are common and there is little host response with inflammatory cells, unlike squamous cell types. The intermediate cell tumours also contain larger cells with slightly more cytoplasm and more prominent nuclei. The cells may show ribboning or rosette formation. Combined small cell tumours include features of either squamous cell or adenocarcinoma, and are rare in untreated diagnostic material (Aisner & Matthews 1985).

Adenocarcinoma

Adenocarcinomas account for approximately 25% of bronchogenic carcinomas. They are commoner among smokers than non-smokers, but the relationship with smoking is not as clear as with squamous or small cell tumours and they are equally common in males and females (Shimosato 1980). They usually occur in the periphery of the lung and may arise in scar tissue (Ochs et at 1982) (Fig. 4.1), though as scar tissue is a feature of this type of tumour, Shimosato (1980) have suggested that fibrotic foci form after the development of cancer. Cagle et al (1985) believe that the development of the scar is secondary to the tumour.

Adenocarcinomas of the lung may be divided into four groups: acinar, papillary, bronchoalveolar

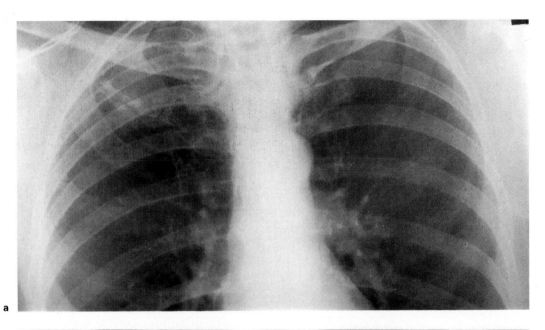

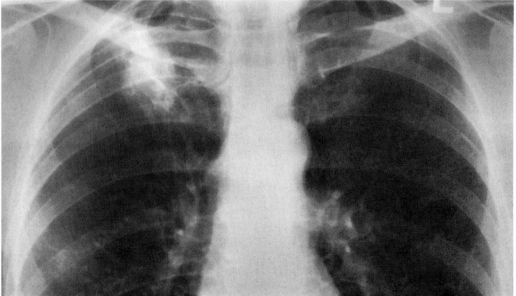

Fig. 4.1 (a) Frontal chest radiograph showing a scar at the right apex. In radiograph (b) a carcinoma has developed and there is right paratracheal lymphadenopathy.

(bronchioloalveolar or alveolar cell) and solid carcinoma with mucus secretion, and these may be further subdivided into well, moderately or poorly differentiated types. The characteristic microscopic features are the formation of acinar, tubular and papillary patterns with mucus secretion. The papillary type is the usual peripheral adenocarcinoma. Convergence of bronchi and vessels toward the tumour is common and may cause pleural distortion. A pleural effusion is more common in this type of non-small cell cancer than others. It may be difficult to distinguish adenocarcinoma of the lung with pleural involvement from mesothelioma, or primary bronchogenic adenocarcinoma from a solitary pulmonary metastasis. Distant metastases to the lung, liver, bone, adrenal and central nervous system are common (Fig. 4.2).

Bronchoalveolar carcinoma arises from terminal bronchoalveolar regions, and accounts for 1–9% of bronchogenic cancers (Knudson et al 1965, St J Thomas et al 1985). It may consist of mucin secreting, non-ciliated bronchiolar cells, Clara cells and type II pneumocytes, which spread along surfaces of alveoli and bronchi without forming a distinct border (Fig. 4.3). Occasionally this gives rise to gross appearances of pneumonic consolid-

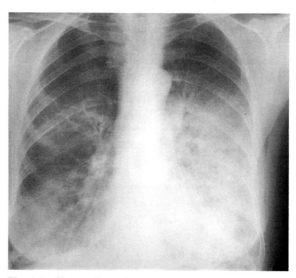

Fig. 4.3 Chest radiograph showing diffuse consolidation in both lungs. The patient was producing copious amounts of white mucoid material. Bronchoalveolar cell carcinoma was diagnosed by transbronchial biopsy.

ation. Classical bronchorrhoea is an uncommon but often quoted presentation of this tumour (Edwards 1984, St J Thomas et al 1985). Once these tumours have invaded the pleural surfaces and metastasized to the regional lymph nodes, their behaviour is indistinguishable from that of other adenocarcinomas, but several authors suggest that widespread metastases occur in only about 15% of cases (Bell & Knudtson 1961, St J Thomas et al 1985). There is some evidence that this tumour is also associated with localized scars (Ochs et al 1982, Edwards 1984) and there is a reported association with diffuse interstitial lung disease, particularly scleroderma (Twersky et al 1976). A study of 205 patients with cryptogenic fibrosing alveolitis showed a ten-fold increase in the risk of developing lung cancer relative to males who smoke, but the distribution of histological types was similar to that in patients without fibrosis. There was no excess of cases of bronchoalveolar or adenocarcinoma (Turner-Warwick et al 1980) (Fig. 4.4).

Large cell carcinoma

This group accounts for up to 9% of bronchogenic carcinomas (Carr 1980). It is a group that is

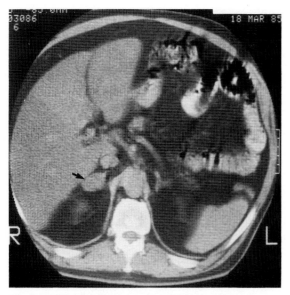

Fig. 4.2 CT scan taken through the adrenal glands showing a tumour mass in the right adrenal gland (arrow) due to a secondary deposit from a primary adenocarcinoma of the lung. The left adrenal is normal.

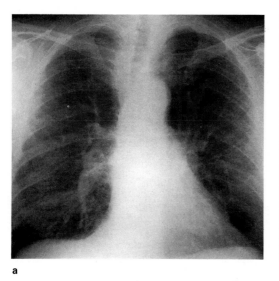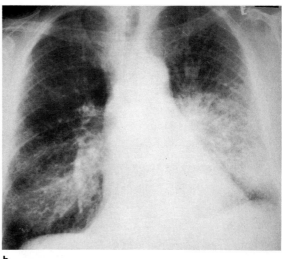

a   b

Fig. 4.4   (a) A chest radiograph of a patient with interstitial fibrosis. In radiograph (b) malignant change has developed with diffuse shadowing at both bases and elevation of the left dome of the diaphragm.

defined by exclusion, in that it is an undifferentiated carcinoma with no light microscopic features of squamous cell, small cell or adenocarcinoma. The cells grow diffusely or in solid nests, cytoplasm is abundant and nucleoli often prominent. The tumours are usually large at presentation and arise from subsegmental or distal bronchi. Giant cell and clear cell tumours are variants of this group in some classifications, but are classified separately in the Edinburgh classification (Lamb 1984). The incidence of metastases and survival is similar to that of adenocarcinoma (Yesner & Carter 1982), although the giant cell variant has a particularly poor prognosis (Shin et al 1986).

Adenosquamous carcinoma

This group forms only 1–2% of bronchogenic tumours diagnosed by light microscopy. There is distinct evidence of glandular and squamous differentiation, and they are usually more peripheral than squamous cell tumours. The survival of patients with this type of tumour is uncertain as there is no adequate data.

Carcinoid tumours

Carcinoid tumours account for less than 1% of bronchogenic tumours. They generally occur at an earlier age than other forms of carcinoma. The tumour develops in one of the larger bronchi, and appears to be a smooth red mass at bronchoscopy, though the majority of the tumour lies outside the bronchus and may best be visualized by CT. Infection and collapse distal to the obstruction are common.

The microscopic appearances are of masses of small uniform polygonal cells, which contain neurosecretory granules and are derived from the APUD cell system. Thus they are related to the small cell tumour in origin. The tumour is slow growing, compresses rather than invades local structures and rarely metastasizes.

Bronchial gland carcinoma

Adenoid cystic, incorporating the previously labelled cylindromas, and mucoepidermoid carcinomas are included in this group of tumours of low grade malignancy. The former usually arises at the carina or in the trachea (Fig. 4.5). It consists of small pleomorphic cells forming tubules. Mucoepidermoid tumours arise from the mucus glands in the bronchi.

Other rare primary tumours of the lung include sarcomas and lymphomas.

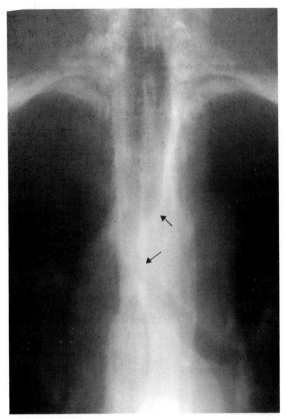

Fig. 4.5 Linear tomogram showing a tumour of the trachea extending onto and narrowing the orifice of the left main bronchus as well as the trachea (shown by arrows).

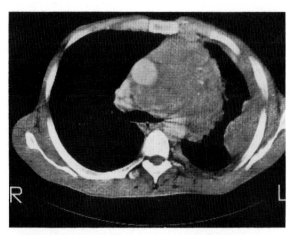

Fig. 4.6 CT scan at the level of the carina showing extensive mediastinal and pleural involvement by mesothelioma with reduction in the size of the left hemithorax.

Malignant mesotheliomas

Primary malignant tumours of the pleura have been found in individuals 20 years after industrial or environmental exposure to asbestos, particularly of crocidolite variety (Parkes 1982). They arise in the parietal pleura and grow to form a mass of white tissue encasing and compressing the lung. Spread within the thorax and to local nodes is common, but distant metastases are less frequent (Fig. 4.6).

Microscopically the appearance of the tumour is varied, either epithelium-like, forming tubules or sheets, or sarcoma-like.

SCREENING FOR LUNG CANCER

At the time of presentation with symptoms, patients with lung cancer usually have advanced disease, so that the overall 5-year relative survival rate is approximately 7.5%. (Office of Population Censuses and Surveys 1988). The prognosis is improved in patients with localized disease, particularly those in whom the tumour is amenable to curative resection. Thus the aim of screening would be to detect new cases at this early stage.

Any screening technique should be repeatable, without inconvenience or risk to the patient, and have a high yield. Currently these criteria are only met by radiography and sputum cytology and as the overall prevalence of lung cancer in the population is low, screening is confined to a high risk group only, smokers over the age of 45 years.

The earliest studies to assess the value of screening were carried out 2–3 decades ago, and used either regular chest radiography (Nash et al 1968, Brett 1968, 1969) or radiography with sputum examination (Lilienfield et al 1966). The studies of Nash et al (1968) and Brett (1968, 1969) suggested that there may be some benefit, with a few long surviving cases among those detected by routine radiographic screening, though annual mortality was unaltered despite earlier treatment. This benefit was not confirmed by Weiss et al (1981) during a 10-year prospective study, nor by Lilienfield et al (1966) who were unable to show an improvement in survival.

Recent improvement in diagnostic and surgical techniques may alter these results. The advent of fibreoptic bronchoscopy has enabled localization of tumours detected by sputum cytology alone. The study undertaken by the Johns Hopkins Hospital, the Mayo Clinic and the Sloan–Kettering Cancer Centre is currently attempting to assess the value of modern screening methods and whether with appropriate treatment earlier detection would lead to a reduction in mortality (Berlin et al 1984). There are minor differences in the designs of the studies in the three centres, but essentially they compare screening with regular chest radiographs (4 or 12-monthly) and sputum examination (4-monthly) to regular annual follow-up by questionnaire alone or with a radiograph. 31 360 high risk male smokers aged over 45 years have been screened and 223 cases of lung cancer detected, approximately one case per hundred. 77% of tumours found in patients screened by both techniques were detected by radiology alone, and 23% by cytology alone. Lung cancers detected solely by radiographic examination were either adeno- or large cell undifferentiated in more than 50% of cases, and most were peripheral.

The study has shown that both radiographic and cytological methods of screening were highly specific ($\geq$90%) while the sensitivity could not be assessed as it was not possible to determine how many cases of lung cancer were missed. There was an improvement in 5-year survival after treatment in these patients, particularly in the radiographically negative, cytology positive group; however, the apparently optimistic outcome of this data must be viewed with caution, as it is weighted towards detection of slow growing tumours with a better prognosis which may have remained dormant through the remainder of the subject's life. There is no clear evidence from this phase of the study that overall mortality from lung cancer is significantly affected (Anonymous 1984, Berlin et al 1984).

Further information will be gained from the incidence study of this multicentre trial. This phase of the study is not yet complete, but preliminary reports have been published (Melamed et al 1981, Taylor et al 1981, Tockman et al 1985). These show that cases of lung cancer were detected at an early stage in the screened group. 60% of cases were detected by the screening technique, but a further 30% were detected by other methods, including symptoms and non-study chest radiograph, and these tended to be later stage cases. Despite screening, approximately 50% of the tumours were already advanced, thus no impact was made on overall mortality from lung cancer in the screened population. These results may of course be more favourable when data from the completed study is available, but at present the rôle of screening in improving survival is dubious.

There is no programme for using CT scanning as a screening test for carcinoma of the lung. This would provide a more sensitive method than chest radiographs for determining the presence of an asymptomatic pulmonary nodule. However, the cost, limited availability, low specificity and high radiation exposure of this examination make it unlikely that it will gain in popularity for screening.

RADIOLOGICAL INVESTIGATION OF BRONCHOGENIC CARCINOMA

The first investigation usually performed is the chest radiograph, which remains the cornerstone of the investigation of lung pathology. The importance of obtaining previous radiographs if they are available cannot be stressed sufficiently, as they may alter the entire investigation of any lung mass. A tumour may be centrally sited (56%), usually endobronchial, or peripheral (40%) (Theros 1977). Rarely the tumour is found in the trachea, a site particularly associated with bronchial gland carcinomas.

Different cell types of tumour are associated with radiographic appearances which reflect pathological characteristics (Byrd et al 1969). 66% of squamous cell tumours present as a hilar or perihilar mass associated with distal infection, collapse and consolidation. They may cavitate and on very rare occasions a pneumothorax may occur as a result of this (Wright 1976). Small cell tumours usually appear as a central mass due to early local gland involvement, particularly of the hilar glands. Distal infection, collapse or consolidation due to obstruction are less common than in squamous cell tumours.

Peripheral lesions occur in only 25% of radiographs and cavitation is rare. 75% of adenocarcinoma are peripheral lesions, usually in the upper lobe. These tumours tend to be smaller in size than squamous cell or large cell types. Hilar or mediastinal enlargement and secondary changes due to obstruction of the airway are also uncommon (Lehan et al 1967). The radiographic appearances of bronchoalveolar carcinoma may be localized, as a single nodule, or diffuse with multiple nodules of varying size, which can coalesce to give the appearance of pneumonic consolidation (Marzano et al 1984) (Fig. 4.3). Large cell carcinoma is characterized by a peripheral site on the chest radiograph; the lesions tend to be large, usually greater than 4 cm in diameter, but rarely cavitate. In approximately 50% of cases mediastinal node involvement is present.

Malignant peripheral lesions are usually rounded masses. The edge of the lesion is often indistinct and tomography may be needed to provide more detail. A malignant lesion usually has an ill-defined spiky edge which is also seen on CT. This represents a combination of tumour infiltration, oedema and fibrosis extending from the main body of the mass into the surrounding tissue. Growth in the tumour is often uneven so that the mass may become lobulated. 28% of 1267 neoplasms seen by Theros (1977) were lobulated. Occasionally a tumour can develop a notch which is referred to as umbilication. Some primary lung tumours, particularly slow growing, well-differentiated carcinoma, have a sharply defined edge (Theros 1977), while some granulomas of the lung, particularly tuberculosis, have irregular spiculated edges. Thus although the edge of the mass is an important radiological sign, it is not specific in distinguishing benign from maligant lesions. Digital postprocessing of conventional postero-anterior chest radiographs in patients with subtle changes due to lung cancer has been used to enhance the edge of the tumour but has not improved diagnostic accuracy (Oestmann et al 1988). If the mass contains calcification visible on plain radiography it is likely to be a benign lesion, either a granuloma or hamartoma, but CT has shown that up to 13% of carcinoma of the lung contain some calcification (Siegelman et al 1986b). These are North American findings and the situation could be different in Europe and other continents. Before the advent of CT, calcification of a tumour was considered to be a rare finding, occurring in only 1% of radiographs (Theros 1977).

A peripheral asymptomatic bronchogenic carcinoma may present as a pulmonary nodule. The problem is in distinguishing a carcinoma from a benign lesion, particularly in the USA where there is a greater incidence of benign nodules in the lung field than in the UK (Edwards & Kelsey Fry 1982). It would be ideal if benign nodules could be differentiated from malignant ones by using a non-invasive method like CT, but there is a lack of standardization in performance of CT scanners and even between scanners of the same type and model. Nodules which have dense diffuse calcification are commonly benign, and large spiculated soft tissue density nodules are almost always malignant. CT is more sensitive than conventional tomography in assessing the density of pulmonary nodules (Siegelman et al 1980). Benign hamartoma may contain fat and about 50% have some calcification in them, so can be diagnosed on CT (Siegelman et al 1986a). Partial volume averaging affects the CT number (Hounsfield units), and in order to be as accurate as possible, 2 mm thick slices need to be taken through the lesion (Fig. 4.7). In practice 8–10 mm thick contiguous slices are taken through the lung and this is sufficient to identify the mass. Additional 2 mm thick contiguous slices are then made through the mass to assess the density and edge of

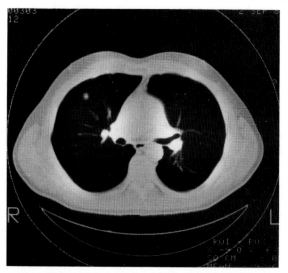

Fig. 4.7 Thin section CT scan showing calcification within the right anterior lung lesion.

the lesion. If these thin sections show dense calcification and a clear edge then the lesion is likely to be benign and needs no further investigation, bearing in mind that benign hamartomas may grow. Siegelman et al (1986b) advise resection for rapidly growing masses or those exceeding 2.5 cm in diameter and regular review of smaller lesions. If a mass is considered to be 'not obviously benign' further investigation must be performed, although some physicians and surgeons believe that this should take the form of thoracotomy and excision.

Malignant mesothelioma may be detected on plain radiography, but CT has greatly enhanced the diagnosis (Kreel 1981). Mesothelioma is usually one-sided but is occasionally bilateral. The tumour takes on a plaque-like lobular appearance and encases the lung, invading the mediastinum, diaphragm, and often the pericardium as well. Tumour invasion of the fissures may be found, but some of the thickening is due to fibrous tissue and fluid. The tumour may infiltrate along the bronchi producing narrowing. Pleural effusions vary in size, but are commonly large, persistent and haemorrhagic. Nodes are not apparent because of the total infiltration of the mediastinum. The lower chest is more involved than the upper chest, and the encased lung produces a constricted hemithorax. Rib destruction and expansion represent spread into the thoracic wall. Irregular calcification may be seen within or on the edge of the tumour.

Although there is a strong link to asbestos exposure, only a third of patients with mesothelioma are shown to have calcified or fibrous plaques on the opposite side (Mintzer & Cugell 1982).

Abdominal extension of tumour is common; about 50% of patients have retroperitoneal spread, and tumour in the liver, kidneys and adrenal glands. Involvement of the contralateral lung also occurs. The main differential diagnosis is adenocarcinoma, but thymoma and lymphoma can mimic mesothelioma if the disease is more localized.

THE ROLE OF LUNG BIOPSY

Percutaneous fine needle lung biopsy is the method of choice for obtaining cytological confir-

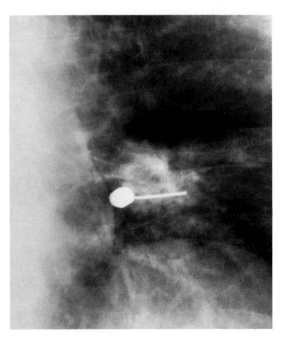
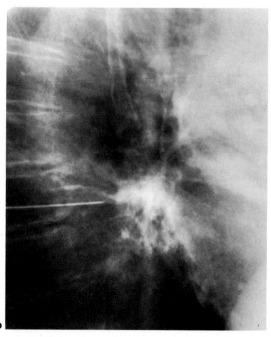

a   b

Fig. 4.8 Lung biopsy with the needle position shown on both anteroposterior (a) and lateral (b) views. A 20 gauge, 15 cm long, short bevelled needle has been used and is seen approaching the tumour.

mation of peripheral lung cancer (Fig. 4.8) The biopsy procedure is achieved using frontal and/or lateral screening and when necessary making use of CT (Khouri et al 1985) and ultrasound (Centi & Hawkins 1984) for the localization. Many reported series have claimed an accuracy for diagnosis varying from 74–99% (Sinner 1979). The incidence of false positive diagnosis is extremely low, being approximately 1%. It is difficult to establish a definite diagnosis of a benign lesion as there is always the possibility that the lesion was inadequately sampled during the biopsy, resulting in a false negative result which occurred in 14% of biopsies in one series (Veale et al 1988). Most authors use two or three passes to obtain specimens. The yield for the correct diagnosis, either true positive or true negative for malignancy is dependent on the number of passes made (Nahman et al 1985) and it is because of this that some operators will make more biopsy passes. However, the necessity for this is dependent on the processing of specimens, which varies from immediate to a delay of a few days. If the policy of immediate cytology is adhered to, multiple passes can be avoided and rebiopsy is possible. Our policy is to take two good specimens and to send these to the cytology laboratory where they are stained and analysed, usually within the hour. If the biopsy proves to be negative then a second and rarely a third biopsy can be undertaken at the time of admission.

A number of other factors play an important rôle in the accuracy of diagnosis. Most series fail to mention the size of the lesion being biopsied though it is significantly easier to biopsy large peripheral pulmonary tumours than small centrally placed nodules of under 1 cm in size. Various authors have advocated different types of needle to improve the collection of specimens varying from a fine Chiba needle (Chin & Yee 1978) to the Rotex screw which has become more popular (Sinner 1982, Nahman et al 1985). A recent report by Nahman et al (1985) using a Rotex needle yielded a true positive rate of 98% with two false negative diagnoses. The use of cutting needles for histology is less widely used because of the greater associated morbidity and mortality (Herman & Hessel 1977).

After the biopsy is taken a chest radiograph is obtained to look for the presence of a pneumothorax. The optimal time for the radiograph to be taken is within the first four hours of the biopsy. 89% of pneumothoraces are diagnosable immediately (Perlmutt et al 1986). The patient may leave the hospital 3–4 hours after the biopsy (Sinner 1982) but the more conservative approach, favoured by the authors, is to admit the patient overnight. A further chest radiograph is taken prior to discharge the following morning to check for the presence of a pneumothorax, as 2% of patients will develop a pneumothorax four hours or more after the procedure. It also has the advantage of allowing further management decisions to be made regarding the patient during that admission. The injection of autologous partly clotted blood through an introducing needle as it is withdrawn after biopsy has not lowered the incidence of pneumothorax (Bourgouin et al 1988). Other complications are haemoptysis and intrapulmonary haemorrhage. Both of these are usually self-limiting and very rarely produce further respiratory symptoms, but it is advisable to warn the patient of these risks before carrying out the procedure. An extremely rare complication is implantation of tumour which has been reported as occuring as seldom as 1 in 5300 biopsies (Sinner 1979). The incidence of death is said to rise sharply when cutting needles are used (Herman & Hessel 1977).

The contraindications to lung biopsy are all relative. Severe chronic airflow obstruction will usually preclude the patient from undergoing biopsy as severe respiratory failure may ensue if a pneumothorax results. The doctor undertaking the biopsy should be circumspect and assess the risks in relation to the future management of the individual patient. It is more dangerous to carry out a biopsy on a lung if the patient has undergone a previous contralateral pneumonectomy. Bleeding diathesis and pulmonary hypertension are two contraindications as in both of these conditions haemorrhage may be severe, and if this occurs respiratory distress and even cardiac side-effects may develop. If a central lesion is being biopsied and bleeding is anticipated, the biopsy can be undertaken using general anaesthesia with a double lumen endotracheal tube in place to allow immediate suction and clearing of blood from the bronchi, and protection of the contralateral lung. In almost all instances bleeding will stop spontaneously; if not pulmonary or bronchial artery embolization or surgery may be used to deal with this very rare complication. It is said to be contraindicated to knowingly biopsy echinococcus of the lung, but viable, non-infected cysts have been biopsied and aspirated unintentionally without deleterious effects (McCorkell 1984).

STAGING OF BRONCHOGENIC CARCINOMA

Staging of tumours is important to assess extent of disease and thus operability in those with limited disease. It is important that this be carried out accurately and standardized if reliable comparisons between trials of treatment and assessment of prognosis are to be made. The widely used TNM classification (Tables 4.2 and 4.3) has been applied to staging of lung cancer (Mountain 1986), and has proved useful in all cell types except small cell

Table 4.2 TNM staging of lung cancer

Symbol	
T	Primary tumour size and location
N	Regional lymph node involvement
M	Distant metastases outside mediastinum or hemithorax
T0	No evidence of tumour
Tx	Tumour proven by presence of malignant cells only
Tis	Carcinoma in situ
T1	Tumour of less than 3 cm diameter, surrounded by lung tissue or visceral pleura, and localized to a lobar bronchus
T2	Tumour within a lobar bronchus, greater than 3 cm diameter, or invading visceral pleura or with associated collapse or infection, extending to the hilum but at least 2 cm distal to the carina
T3	Tumour of any size extending to the chest wall, diaphragm, mediastinal pleura or pericardium, without involvement of the heart, great vessels, trachea, oesophagus or vertebral bodies or within 2 cm of the carina
T4	Any size tumour involving the heart, great vessels, trachea, oesophagus, vertebral body or the presence of malignant effusion
N0	No regional node involvement
N1	Peribronchial and/or ipsilateral hilar node involvement
N2	Ipsilateral mediastinal or subcarinal node involvement
N3	Contralateral hilar, mediastinal and any scalene or supraclavicular nodes
M0	No distant metastases
M1	Distant metastases in the contralateral lung or outside the thorax

Table 4.3 Tumour stages

Occult carcinoma	TX N0 M0
Stage 0	Tis N0 M0
Stage I	T1 N0 M0
	T2 N0 M0
Stage II	T1 N1 M0
	T2 N1 M0
Stage IIIA	T3 N0 M0
	T3 N1 M0
	T1 N2 M0
	T2 N2 M0
	T3 N2 M0
Stage IIIB	Any T, N3 M0
	T4, Any N M0
Stage IV	Any T, Any N, M1

tumours, where a simpler staging technique is generally used (see pp. 122, 123). Although physical examination, blood tests and invasive investigations are used for staging, radiological investigations are the most important.

Radiological staging of bronchogenic carcinoma

There are a number of indications on the chest radiograph of tumour spread and inoperability, bearing in mind that the criteria for the latter may vary between different centres. Tumour spread to the opposite lung is seen as single or multiple opacities in the lung fields and each lung opacity must be carefully assessed. Multiple opacities which vary in size and are distributed throughout the lung fields are almost certainly due to secondary deposits (Fig. 4.9). However, if there is a primary malignancy in one lung and a second nodule is present either in the same or the other lung this may represent different pathology.

Spread into the mediastinum or hilum of the lung can be diagnosed by widening or thickening of the paratracheal strip. Deviation of the trachea and bronchi from the tumour mass or extrinsic compression of the trachea or bronchus may occur if nodes are particularly large. Hilar lymphadenopathy may be difficult to distinguish from pulmonary vessels and it is in this area that tomography, either conventional antero-posterior, lateral or oblique, or CT may be used for differentiation (Goldstraw 1986). It is usually simpler

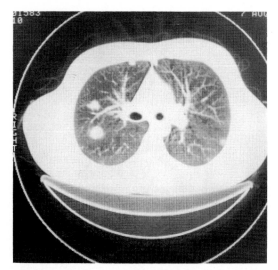

Fig. 4.9 CT scan at a level 2 cm below the carina showing multiple rounded densities varying in size in both lung fields due to intrapulmonary spread from primary carcinoma of the lung. The deposit in the left lung adjacent to the anterior pleural reflection would be difficult to detect using any other method of examination.

and most effective to use CT and bolus intravenous contrast enhancement scans to differentiate the blood vessels from hilar nodes and to reserve plain tomography for the rare occasions when the radiographs and CT have been unhelpful. On the radiographs the vessels have parallel walls whereas the presence of nodes produces lobulation and a lumpy appearance of the hilum. The hilar point is a radiographic landmark formed where the lateral blood vessels from the upper lobe cross the basal artery. An obtuse angle is seen on the chest radiograph and this angle may be filled in by abnormal lymph nodes. Subcarinal spread of tumour produces widening of the carina and spreading of the major bronchi. This appearance can be mistaken for left atrial enlargement, but there will not be any associated left atrial appendage prominence on the left heart border and no evidence of redistribution of blood from the lower lobes to the upper lobes, a sign associated with mitral valve disease or left heart failure.

Another indication of inoperability is elevation of the dome of the diaphragm on the same side as the tumour (Fig. 4.4). This suggests involvement of the phrenic nerve and screening of the diaphragm during respiration, coughing and sniff-

ing will show paradoxical movement if this is so. If the diaphragm is seen to move normally there may be a benign cause but hepatomegaly due to secondary deposits should be excluded. When tumour is present in the periphery of the lung, invasion of the pleura and destruction of the underlying rib can be seen. In the apex of the lung a peripheral tumour can destroy ribs and invade the vertebrae and the brachial plexus producing a Pancoast tumour, the clinical signs of which are Horner's syndrome and pain with sensori-motor deficit in the hand and forearm.

The development of pleural fluid associated with a lung mass invariably indicates pleural metastases. This diagnosis may be difficult to establish. Aspiration will yield either straw-coloured or bloody fluid and multiple biopsies may have to be made to establish the presence of secondary deposits if fluid analysis is unrewarding. If the amount of fluid in the pleural space is small, it may be localized more accurately, to facilitate diagnostic tapping, by performing an ultrasound scan (Lipscomb & Flower 1980). If this proves unhelpful CT scanning can be used to assess the position and mobility of the fluid, the patient being scanned in different positions if necessary. Another advantage gained from CT is the differentiation between fluid and solid tumour in the pleural space. Secondary deposits may be localized or fairly diffusely sited in the pleura, but can usually be differentiated from mesothelioma which

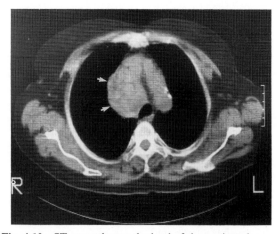

Fig. 4.10 CT scan taken at the level of the aortic arch, showing metastatic tumour in the azygos nodes (arrowed) from adenocarcinoma of the lung.

characteristically spreads throughout the pleural space and encases the entire lung. Thoracoscopy of the pleural space will reveal the deposits which can be biopsied under direct vision and the effusion can be drained and treated on the same occasion by instillation of corynebacterium parvum, tetracycline, talc or bleomycin (Weissberg et al 1980). Mediastinal spread of tumour may produce occlusion of the superior vena cava, particularly when the azygos vein is invaded (Fig. 4.10). This is suspected clinically when the patient

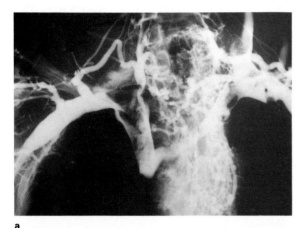

a

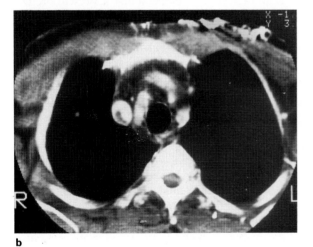

b

Fig. 4.11 Bilateral upper limb venogram (a) and CT scan (b) showing occlusion of the superior vena cava with intraluminal filling defects due to either thrombus or tumour. Multiple collateral vessels are visualized on the chest wall. The diffuse nature of these collaterals can be appreciated on the CT scan with vessels seen anteriorly, laterally and posteriorly on the left.

complains of swelling of the face or arms and collateral vessels are noted on the chest wall. The diagnosis cannot be proved by radiographs alone and the use of intravenous contrast, digital angiography or CT (Moncado et al 1984) is necessary (Fig. 4.11).

The development or presence of interstitial lines on the chest radiograph, either peripherally or centrally situated, and in the absence of left heart failure, dust exposure or a drug reaction, usually suggests the development of lymphangitis carcinomatosa, a grave prognostic sign.

When an endobronchial tumour produces obstruction of a bronchus, the major radiological sign on the chest radiograph is loss of volume of a segment or a lobe of the lung. Unless obstruction is present, the radiograph may be completely normal. If there is volume loss the lung may move towards the side of abnormality. The hilar point is a sensitive indicator and moves towards the area of volume loss, as does the trachea, the heart and the diaphragm. This volume loss can be associated with opaque non-aerated lung which may be seen adjacent to the trachea in upper lobe collapse, obliterating the right or left heart border in right middle lobe or lingular collapse, and obliterating the clarity of part of the diaphragm in lower lobe collapse. If volume loss is a new sign on the chest radiograph of a patient, even if the examination was done for a routine reason, then bronchoscopy is an essential investigation in spite of the possibility of other causes of pulmonary collapse and subjection of the patient to an unnecessary procedure.

The rôle of fibreoptic bronchoscopy

The development of fibreoptic bronchoscopy has greatly simplified the investigation of symptoms, signs or radiographic abnormalities suggestive of malignant disease. It is a safe procedure with a mortality of 0.04% or less (Simpson et al 1986). It is usually carried out via the transnasal route after appropriate premedication with sedative and anticholinergic drugs and application of local anaesthetic to the nasal passage and larynx. The upper airway may be examined simultaneously, the presence of vocal cord paresis, usually the left, implying that a tumour is inoperable. Very few patients are considered unfit to undergo this examination, though care is taken when examining patients with greatly reduced spirometry or hypoxaemia, particularly in the presence of ischaemic heart disease.

All the major airways may be examined to the subsegmental level, so that 70% of radiographically identified tumours are visualized by this method. Bronchoscopy remains the investigation of choice in determining the presence or extent of endobronchial abnormality, and even CT has failed to supercede this (Colice et al 1985). Suspicious areas may be biopsied with forceps passed through the instrument, and cytological specimens are obtained by aspirating saline washed over the area and brushing the surface of the lesion. The diagnostic yield from biopsy increases with the experience of the operator (Gellert 1982a) and the number of biopsies taken (Gellert 1982b). The likelihood of achieving a positive result is increased further if both histological and cytological specimens are taken and a diagnosis should be possible in more than 90% of cases (Matsuda et al 1986).

The location of the tumour is important in assessing operability, though many surgeons believe that submucosal tumour infiltration may be assessed accurately only by testing the compliance of the airway with the rigid bronchoscope. Widening of a subcarina and loss of variation in the calibre with respiration suggest infiltration. Compression of the airways may be due to extrabronchial tumour or lymphadenopathy while widening of the main carina implies invasion of the subcarinal glands and inoperability. Tumour occurring within 0.5 cm of the main carina or invading the trachea, apart from minor extension along the right lateral wall, would generally be considered unresectable.

Extrabronchial tumour may be biopsied in patients with normal blood coagulation via the transbronchial route, using fluoroscopy to check that the forceps are in the correct position. The method will produce a diagnosis in about 60% of cases (Mitchell et al 1981). The technique has a higher mortality and morbidity than endobronchial biopsy, the major complications being haemorrhage and pneumothorax (Simpson et al 1986). As the diagnostic yield from percutaneous needle biopsy is higher (more than 80%), many physicians reserve transbronchial biopsy for the diagnosis of diffuse rather than localized lung disease (Winning et al 1986).

Mediastinal lymph nodes may also be sampled using transbronchial needle aspiration and fluoroscopic screening (Wang & Terry 1983, Wang et al 1983). Subcarinal nodes may be sampled without screening (Shure & Fedullo 1984). Although this method has few reported complications it is not yet widely used for staging of bronchogenic carcinoma and has not superceded mediastinotomy or mediastinoscopy in the UK.

ASSESSMENT OF TUMOUR OPERABILITY

In the past, assessment for surgery involved clinical assessment, simple radiographic techniques and rigid bronchoscopy. A decision regarding resectability was often made at exploratory thoracotomy. Thus during the 1950s only 67% of patients undergoing exploration for primary lung cancer of all cell types had a resection, of which 60% were considered to be 'curative' (Galofre et al 1964, Goldman 1965). Resection and survival rates suggest that many of the patients subjected to thoracotomy had more advanced disease which could not be detected by the methods of staging in use at that time.

If an indication of inoperability is present on the chest radiograph, further costly and often distressing investigations may be deemed unnecessary as treatment is palliative. On the other hand, if the chest radiograph shows a peripheral mass or collapse of part of the lung and no obvious tumour spread then further investigations including fibreoptic bronchoscopy are undertaken. The indications on the radiograph of operability are very unreliable and insensitive compared to tomography.

Plain tomography has a limited rôle in diagnosing hilar or mediastinal spread of tumour, and CT has virtually superceded this investigation (Goldstraw 1986). CT scanning using contiguous slices enables tumours to be staged more accurately, resulting in better selection of cases for surgery. Hilar or mediastinal masses not visible on conventional chest radiography are better detected using CT, the use of high dose, bolus injections of intravenous contrast improving accuracy (Rea et al 1981, Haponik & Wang 1985). This produces enhancement of the blood vessels, will highlight non-vascular structures such as tumour and will also differentiate pathology such as dissection of blood vessels which may mimic tumour on both radiographs and CT. However, the accuracy and specificity of CT scanning is still being researched. Nodes of over 2 cm in diameter are more likely to contain tumour than those under 1 cm in diameter. This rule of thumb is not completely reliable. Libshitz & McKenna (1984) examined 86 patients with nodes under 1 cm in diameter and showed that 21 contained metastatic tumour. Where possible thin needle sampling for cytological analysis should be carried out, but biopsy of central masses even using a fine needle carries some risk (Wiesbrod et al 1984). Underwood et al (1979) noted that in a series of 18 patients with carcinoma of the lung, CT scans gave a 30% false negative result compared with mediastinoscopy and thoracotomy, though they were more accurate than chest radiographs. Goldstraw et al (1983), comparing CT scanning, mediastinoscopy and mediastinotomy to surgical exploration, also found a high false positive rate (11 out of 23 positive scans), but there were no false negative results.

The sensitivity and specificity of CT scanning were 57 and 85% respectively compared to 67 and 100% for mediastinotomy, but CT scanning was superior in detecting direct mediastinal invasion, particularly with lower lobe tumours. Rea et al (1981), in a similar study with similar results, concluded that patients with a negative scan should proceed to surgery, while those with evidence of possible mediastinal metastases should undergo further histological investigation. The CT scan was helpful in deciding which was the most appropriate approach. Later studies using faster, higher resolution scanners have found a considerable improvement in results, with specificity of 94–100% and sensitivity of 88–89% (Faling et al 1981, Graves et al 1985). CT and mediastinoscopy were compared after all accessible nodes were removed or sampled at thoracotomy. Nodes seen on CT with a long axis greater than 10 mm should be regarded as enlarged. Nodes of this size produce a sensitivity for detecting mediastinal node metastases equal to mediastinoscopy (79%), but the specificity with CT was only 65% compared to 100% on mediastinoscopy. When

abnormal nodes are present, normal sized nodes at a different site may be invaded by tumour. CT may provide additional information about possible involvement of nodes not accessible to mediastinoscopy (Staples et al 1988). This progress may continue but in the meantime the conclusions of Rea et al (1981) summarize the accepted views.

Unsuspected spread of tumour to the ipsilateral or contralateral lung may be shown on CT scans by the presence of rounded nodules which may vary in size and even demonstrate cavitation (Muhm et al 1977). Tumour nodules adjacent to the pericardium or lying anterior or posterior to the heart may be missed even on high quality chest radiographs. When basal pleural fluid is present the patient should be scanned both supine and prone in case the fluid is obscuring pulmonary masses. CT scanning has proved insensitive, inaccurate and non-specific in assessing chest wall invasion by bronchogenic tumour (Pennes et al 1985) and, unless entirely unequivocal and gross, should not be relied upon. Bronchial compression and invasion is usually more easily appreciated on CT scans. The extrabronchial spread of endobronchial, centrally situated tumour can be assessed by CT scanning. Rarely the pericardium may be seen to be involved by tumour.

More distal spread should also be excluded if the patient is to undergo thoracotomy and lung resection. Scans should be obtained through the liver and both adrenal glands (Fig. 4.2), and through the brain in the case of small cell and adenocarcinoma even in asymptomatic patients (Jacobs et al 1977).

It is hoped that with further development of magnetic resonance imaging (MRI), tissue characterization and differentiation between benign and malignant lesions may be possible (Webb et al 1984). Malignant tumour and inflammatory tissue have a T_1 value longer than that of normal tissue. Well-differentiated adenocarcinoma, however, has a short T_1 value, possibly due to the presence of fibrous tissue, as does necrotic tumour. In vitro investigations suggest that T_2-weighted images may be able to discriminate between viable and necrotic tumour and inflammatory tissue (Shioya et al 1988). The accuracy of MRI and CT in staging bronchogenic carcinoma for curative resection was compared in 37 patients by Levitt et al (1985) and found to be equal. CT was successful in assessing 35 and MRI 36 cases, but the antomical detail was greater with CT. Musset et al (1986) showed similar results. Small lung nodules may be undetected by MRI due to respiratory motion and partial volume averaging. Some patients, for example those with cardiac pacemakers, will prove unsuitable for MRI scans. At this stage it appears that CT is still the examination of choice for staging patients with bronchogenic carcinoma and hilar and mediastinal masses, whilst MRI has the ability to show the blood vessels without intravenous contrast and may be able to distinguish other pathological processes (Shioya et al 1988).

RADIO-ISOTOPE SCANNING

Radio-isotope scanning for tumour spread is most commonly carried out when looking for tumour in bone. ^{99m}Technetium methyldiphosphonate (MDP) injected intravenously is a sensitive method of detecting spread of tumour. Localized radiographs of any abnormality may be required as increased isotope activity is seen in conditions other than secondary deposits, where bone turnover is increased or inflammation is present (see Chapter 1).

Patients may have tumour diagnosed after presenting with unusual symptoms. The presence of hypertrophic pulmonary osteoarthropathy can best be shown by radiographs of the painful limbs. Symmetrical well-organized new bone formation is seen. Radio-isotope scanning will show increased activity in the affected bones. The most common cause for the finding is a carcinoma of the lung and this may be associated with any histological type, though it is most often seen in squamous cell tumours.

The detection of hepatic metastases is a complex problem. It is far too simplistic to compare ultrasound, radio-isotope, CT and MRI scanning; each modality must be compared using state of the art equipment. There are multiple methods which can be employed using most of these techniques. Radio-isotope scanning can be achieved using different radiopharmaceuticals i.e. ^{99m} technetium sulphur colloid, ^{99m} technetium HIDA or ^{67}gallium as well as tomographic imaging (Ashare 1980). CT may be carried out by giving a large bolus dose of

intravenous contrast and then performing dynamic immediate scans as well as delayed scans after 4–6 hours. CT arteriography may also be used and ethiodized oil emulsion (EOE 13) as a contrast agent to improve the detection of secondary deposits (Bernadino et al 1986). MRI has also been used and compared with CT in an attempt to define the best method of detecting secondary deposits (Heiken et al 1985, Reinig et al 1987, Stark et al 1987).

When comparisons between each modality have been made, all methods, i.e. radio-isotope, ultrasound, CT and MRI have not been used. Different statistical analysis may also influence the results (Smith et al 1982, Alderson et al 1983).

A practical approach would be to employ two or three imaging modalities. In our institution ultrasound scanning is the first choice and, if negative, dynamic immediate pre- and post-intravenous bolus contrast CT is used. Very rarely radio-isotope scanning would also be employed. If MRI were more freely available it would be an alternative choice to CT.

TREATMENT

The long term survival with untreated bronchogenic carcinoma is poor, and the only opportunity for cure in all histological types is by resection or radical radiotherapy. It is estimated that 20–30% of patients presenting with these tumours should be considered for surgery (Shields 1982, Spiro 1984, Martini 1985), though Le Roux (1968) found that only about 12% of referred patients were fit and had localized disease amenable to curative surgery. Small cell carcinoma is associated with widespread metastases at presentation, and thus although there are reports of long term survival after resection (Shields et al 1982, Sorensen et al 1986), in practice this is rarely feasible.

Improvements in diagnostic and staging techniques have been aimed at reducing the need for thoracotomy in inoperable cases, where it does not improve prognosis and carries considerable morbidity and mortality. The involvement of mediastinal nodes with tumour has long been recognized to reduce the prognosis greatly (Haponik & Wang 1985). Surgical mortality is increased in this group, and the 5-year survival after resection is only 5–7% compared to 40% in patients without mediastinal disease (Sarin and Nohl-Oser 1969, Paulson & Reisch 1976).

Widespread metastases having been excluded, information regarding the site and spread of the tumour assessed by PA and lateral chest radiograph and CT scan, as well as bronchoscopic information, enables the surgeon to decide on the operative approach.

Tumours which are not visualized by radiography and are diagnosed by cytology alone tend to be squamous cell in type, and the source of cells is sought using fibreoptic bronchoscopy. These rare tumours have a good prognosis with resection, with no recurrence of the original tumour during follow-up of 27 patients for up to 20 years in a series reported by Martini & Melamed (1980). However, 45% of these patients may develop a second carcinoma, usually of the airway. As this may be amenable to surgery, indefinite follow-up with regular screening is necessary (Martini & Melamed 1980, Mathison et al 1984).

Small peripheral lesions on the chest radiograph are likely to be tumours with a probability that increases with age (40% at 40 years, 60% at 60 years) and this reflects the increasing incidence of carcinoma of the bronchus with age (Berlin et al 1984). In these cases a previous film for comparison may be helpful in the initial diagnosis. These tumours should be treated by surgical resection in all cases of non-small cell type where age, lung function and general condition permit. Lobectomy or pneumonectomy is the treatment of choice, and the operation selected depends on the site of the tumour and the presence of local node involvement. Wherever possible lobectomy is preferable as it spares lung tissue and has a lower operative mortality (Shields 1982). A segmentectomy or wedge resection further spares lung tissue, but at present there are no controlled trials to determine whether this is the preferred procedure in peripheral tumours. The operative mortality of patients over the age of 70 years is 7%, approximately twice that below the age of 70 years (Thompson-Evans 1973, Ginsberg et al 1983), and this should be considered when deciding upon treatment. Similarly, a forced expiratory volume in one second (FEV1) less than 2 litres or 50% predicted and a reduction in forced vital capacity (FVC) of 50% are critical values for satisfactory survival after surgery (Spiro 1984). In such cases regional ventilation/perfusion lung scanning (Ali et al 1980, Williams et al 1984) or regional assessment of lung function (Pierce et al 1986) may be helpful in the preoperative assessment. The former technique appears to be more accurate in determining volume loss associated with pneumonectomy than with lobectomy.

A survey of 115 non-small cell stage I cases treated surgically, including mediastinal lymph node dissection, and re-staged at operation, showed a 74% survival free of disease at three years; the rate was better in patients with smaller T1 tumours than in those T2 tumours (Martini & Beattie 1977, Melamed et al 1981). At the moment there is no evidence that adjuvant therapy prolongs survival, and clearly careful follow-up with regular chest radiographs and perhaps even CT scanning is justified to detect relapse. CT is particularly useful in follow-up of patients with a pneumonectomy, as recurrence within the pleural space or mediastinum is more readily detected than by plain radiographs, and the scan may be helpful in defining radiation ports for therapy (Glazer et al 1984).

Stage II disease will generally require pneumonectomy, and the prognosis for these patients is not as good as for those with stage I disease (Shields et al 1980). Some patients with stage III disease present with major airway obstruction. The advent of laser therapy via the bronchoscope has enabled these patients to be treated to alleviate symptoms, and subsequent surgical treatment, even with bronchoplastic procedures, has been successful (Fujimura et al 1985, George et al 1986). This advance in treatment has been of particular importance in the management of bronchial gland carcinomas which are of low grade malignancy, locally invasive and potentially curable but may present with extreme breathlessness due to their central location in the trachea.

Many surgeons no longer regard peripheral extension of the tumour to involve the chest wall as a contraindication to surgery, particularly in the absence of nodal metastases, and these may be treated by excision of the involved part of the chest wall, and if necessary repair with synthetic material (Le Roux 1984, Martini 1985), though survival is better if the tumour is confined to the parietal pleura (McCaughan et al 1986). In contrast, chest wall invasion at the apex with radiological evidence of bone destruction is rarely considered suitable for a surgical approach, though some workers suggest that a combined approach of preoperative radiotherapy and surgery produces the best results (Hilaris et al 1971, Shields 1982).

In the long term, survival after resection in non-small cell carcinoma is related to tumour stage preoperatively (Paulson & Reisch 1976, Shields et al 1980) and a favourable prognosis is associated with age less than 60 years (Shields et al 1972, Higgins et al 1975). By contrast, weight loss, chest pain, tumour size and cell type, particularly large cell anaplastic, have the most significant adverse effects (Clee et al 1984).

The rôle of surgery in the treatment of peripheral small cell tumours is still debated. An early controlled trial comparing surgery to radical radiotherapy (Miller et al 1969, Fox & Scadding 1973) and a more recent multicentre, retrospective survey of cases staged with mediastinoscopy, peritoneoscopy, bone marrow and liver biopsy comparing treatment with surgery, chemotherapy and radiotherapy to chemotherapy and radiotherapy alone (Osterlind et al 1985) have failed to demonstrate additional benefit from surgery.

In contrast to these studies are the results of surgery on isolated pulmonary nodules which showed no difference in 5- or 10-year survival of small cell tumours which had been resected compared to other cell types, the overall 10-year survival being 20% (Higgins et al 1975). Similar favourable results have been demonstrated by Shore & Paneth (1980), Li et al (1981) and Sorensen et al (1986), the former demonstrating prolonged survival of 11 out of 40 patients treated for small cell lung cancer with curative surgery even with hilar and mediastinal node involvement, and a 5-year survival of 27%.

It is reasonable to conclude from these studies that prolonged survival may be achieved in patients with peripheral stage I small cell tumours, but patient selection must include CT scanning and mediastinoscopy as a minimum. Shields (1982) suggests that staging should also include 55° oblique tomograms of the hilum, and surgery should be limited to patients without lymph node involvement or distant metastases.

Radiotherapy

As already discussed, surgery holds the best prospect of cure for patients with lung cancer, especially non-small cell, and radiotherapy is used largely to treat patients with inoperable non-small cell tumours or those who are medically unfit for surgery, a group with a poor prognosis. Treatment may be aimed at achieving survival (radical radiotherapy) or alleviating symptoms which may arise from the primary site or from distant metastases (palliative radiotherapy). The response to radiotherapy may be followed up by clinical symptoms and signs and by chest radiography. Radiation is damaging to normal tissue, particularly the lung, causing pneumonitis and later fibrosis (Fig. 4.12), and to the spinal cord, causing myelitis if normal tissue tolerance is exceeded. Therapeutic fields must therefore be planned to avoid unnecessary irradiation (see Chapter 18). Histological type is an important prognostic factor because it determines the natural history of the disease and the susceptibility of the tumour to radiation. The best results from radical radiotherapy are obtained in patients with squamous cell carcinoma, with poorer survival in

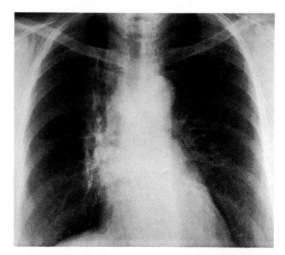

Fig. 4.12 Frontal chest radiograph demonstrating fibrosis with a sharp lateral border corresponding to the radiotherapy field.

adeno- and large cell tumours (Coy & Kennelly 1980). Patients treated in this way die largely from local disease in squamous cell carcinoma, while 57% of patients with adeno-, 55% of patients with large cell, and 70% of patients with small cell carcinoma die with disseminated disease (Cox et al 1979). Aristizabal and Caldwell (1976) were able to show that patients with moderately or well-differentiated tumours have a better chance of survival, with a 3-year survival of 16% compared to 3% in those with poorly differentiated tumours. These and other studies have also shown that the presence of supraclavicular nodes, local bone erosion and the presence of superior vena caval obstruction (except in small cell lung cancer) are associated with a worse prognosis.

Short course, low dose radiotherapy has long been recognized to be of value in symptom relief in lung cancer. Specific symptoms respond better than generalized symptoms such as weight loss or paraneoplastic syndromes (Gregor 1984).

Haemoptysis and cough are readily controlled by radiotherapy with up to 80% symptom relief. Breathlessness also improves temporarily in about half the cases, though re-expansion of an aetelectatic area is only achieved in about one quarter of cases (Slawson & Scott 1979). Patients most likely to benefit have greater ventilation/perfusion mismatching than would be expected from the radiographic appearances alone. Re-expansion of a completely collapsed lung or lobe can be achieved in about 30% of cases treated by radiotherapy or Nd-YAG laser, but symptomatic and functional improvement occurs in 60–85% of patients where symptoms are due to partial obstruction of a major bronchus or trachea by tumour. Haemoptysis may also be stopped or reduced by this technique in approximately 60% of cases irrespective of cell type (Arabian & Spagnolo 1984, Gelb & Epstein 1984, Hetzel et al 1985) compared to 80% of cases of non-small cell lung cancer treated by radiotherapy (Gregor 1984). Laser therapy remains a second line of treatment as it does not achieve better results than radiotherapy and is an invasive method of treatment requiring general anaesthesia and rigid bronchoscopy. When mediastinal lymph node enlargement cases dysphagia, radiotherapy may be helpful in control of symptoms, but if there is evidence of involvement of the oesophageal mucosa, worsening of symptoms or a

fistula may result. Radiotherapy should be avoided in the latter situation.

One of the complications of lung cancer which requires early treatment is superior vena caval obstruction. It may be the presenting feature, particularly of right-sided squamous cell carcinoma and small cell tumour. In non-small cell tumours radiotherapy remains the treatment of choice, but in small cell cancer chemotherapy is as effective (Spiro et al 1983). In most cases it is advisable to attempt to make a histological diagnosis before commencing treatment, as the management varies with cause, and in younger patients in particular this may rarely be due to other mediastinal tumours such as lymphomas which are amenable to curative treatment. Despite venous congestion, causing a slight increase in bleeding, fibreoptic bronchoscopy and biopsy is usually easily and safely performed. Other ways of obtaining a histological diagnosis such as percutaneous lung biopsy, mediastinotomy or thoracotomy are not readily undertaken under these circumstances, and in such cases biopsy material is obtained after treatment. Bone marrow aspiration may be diagnostic, particularly in small cell tumours. In some cases it may be necessary to perform CT scanning, venography or radionuclide angiography to determine the extent of the tumour and the radiation field. If the obstruction is not complicated by extensive thrombosis oedema will be cleared, though symptomatic relief is generally achieved before there is objective evidence.

Distant metastases are common in the later stages of bronchogenic carcinoma, particularly the non-squamous types. Those most likely to cause symptoms are bone and cerebral metastases. Pain due to bone metastases usually responds very well to radiotherapy, with about 50% of patients obtaining complete relief of pain (Tong et al 1982). Involvement of the vertebrae may lead to collapse and spinal cord compression. This should be rapidly investigated and treated with radiotherapy, as there is no additional benefit from surgical intervention (Gilbert et al 1978) and response and recovery is best in those patients with minimal signs. Decompressive laminectomy may be required in patients where the nature of the lesion is uncertain, after previous radiotherapy, or if there is marked progression of the signs during treatment.

Cerebral metastases are particularly common in the non-squamous varieties of lung cancer. When a diagnosis of carcinoma has been previously established and the patient presents with neurological signs, a radio-isotope scan may be sufficient to confirm the presence of metastases, but CT which shows better anatomical detail remains the preferable investigation. Generally multiple cerebral metastases are found, and though symptomatic improvement may be achieved with corticosteroids, such cases have a poor prognosis (Borgelt et al 1980), and should be selected for radiotherapy with care.

Following radiotherapy to the lung some degree of fibrosis is universal (Hellman et al 1964, Slawson & Scott 1979) and in 10–15% of cases will produce symptoms of cough and breathlessness. These symptoms are usually transient and develop 8–12 weeks after treatment. Clinical signs are rarely present, but the chest radiograph is abnormal with either a ground glass appearance or indistinct pulmonary markings, with sharp margins corresponding to the radiotherapy field and not to any anatomical landmarks (Fig. 4.12). When severe symptoms occur they may be controlled with steroids. Over six months after treatment these changes can progress to fibrosis which is irreversible. Streaky shadowing and loss of lung volume are present on the chest radiograph and may even lead to skeletal deformity. In cases where fibrosis is not visible on the radiograph it may be clearly seen on the CT scan.

These changes must be distinguished from tumour recurrence, lymphangitis or infection as a cause of breathlessness. The presence of sharp borders reflecting the field of radiotherapy on the chest radiograph are very helpful distinguishing features, but in cases where doubt remains as to the aetiology, fibreoptic bronchoscopy with transbronchial biopsy is most likely to yield the answer.

Oesophagitis is a common symptom during radiotherapy, and occurs in all patients whose oesophagus is inside the treatment field. It usually responds to symptomatic treatment, but may be more troublesome in cases treated with higher doses or concomitant drug therapy. Rarely it may lead months later to the development of a stricture requiring balloon dilatation, and in these cases radiographic and endoscopic techniques will help to exclude the presence of malignant tissue as the cause. Oesophageal obstruction is more commonly due to recurrent disease.

Drug therapy for non-small cell lung cancer

A large proportion of patients with non-small cell carcinoma present with widespread disease, and for the young patient, particularly, there is an anxiety to provide some form of treatment. A number of drugs are currently being evaluated, and at the moment ifosfamide, etoposide, cisplatin, mitomycin C and vindesine appear to be the most useful (Bakowski & Crouch 1983, Joss et al 1984, Souhami 1985, Sorensen et al 1987). These drugs are toxic and when given in large doses cause marrow suppression, leading to neutropaenia and possible life-threatening infection, most commonly gram negative septicaemia. At present the complete response rate with single agents is negligible, though the overall response rate is up to 26% (Bakowski & Crouch 1983, Souhami 1984). Combination therapy with ifosfamide, mitomycin C and cis-platin is more encouraging with a complete response rate in 20% and overall response rate of 60% (Giron et al 1987). Attempts are being made to improve on this figure by giving higher induction doses, and using autologous bone marrow transplantation for rescue. These methods of treatment have a high morbidity and mortality, and in view of the limited response should only be given to carefully selected patients in regional centres where careful assessment and staging of response to treatment may be carried out.

Chemotherapy of small cell lung cancer

Small cell cancer of the lung is associated with the shortest survival of all types, the median being 1.5 months if untreated (Slevin et al 1983). Most patients already have metastases at presentation, the common sites being liver, abdominal lymph nodes, adrenals, bone, brain, pancreas and kidneys. Detailed TNM staging is therefore of little value and has little bearing on prognosis, so a simpler limited/extensive disease staging system is generally used (Arnold & Williams 1979, Smyth

1984). Limited disease is confined to one hemithorax but includes ipsilateral mediastinal and supraclavicular nodes. Extensive disease includes all that not included in the above definition. Using this staging system it has been shown that patients with limited disease have a better prognosis and a greater chance of long term survival or cure (Livingston et al 1978, Cooksey et al 1979), though performance status, age, weight loss and clinical or biochemical evidence of liver, bone or central nervous system metastases are also important (Hansen et al 1985, Poplin et al 1987).

The widespread dissemination of this tumour at presentation makes any local treatment inadequate (Fox & Scadding 1973, Slevin et al 1983) and improved survival has only been achieved since the development of systemic therapy. Fortunately, because of the rapid replication of these tumour cells they are sensitive to the cidal action of drugs and radiotherapy (Arnold & Williams 1979). Single agents have been used and will improve survival, but rarely produce the complete response necessary for prolonging survival. Present regimes of combination therapy will produce an objective response in 80% of patients, with a complete response in 15–50%, the latter being more common in patients with limited disease (Smyth 1984). Median survival is increased to eight months or more in patients with extensive disease, and 8–20% of patients with limited disease survive two years or more without recurrence (Hansen et al 1985, Richards & Scarantino 1985). Higher dose combination regimes produce slightly better response rates with more disease-free long term survivors, but this is associated with fatal toxicity in a proportion of cases, the most serious being bone marrow suppression (Mehta & Vogl 1982, Brower et al 1983). Among the agents widely used are cyclophosphamide, adriamycin, vincristine, etoposide, ifosfamide and platinum compounds. A complete response is defined on clinical, radiological and bronchoscopic grounds as clearing of tumour for a minimum of four weeks. If used, CT scanning of the chest may reduce the number of apparent complete responders. In general, chemotherapy is given in a number of courses three to four weeks apart, and if a response is going to occur, there is usually radiographic evidence by the third course of treatment. The risk of relapse is reduced in patients remaining disease free for two years.

Palliative treatment of lung cancer

In the terminal stages of lung cancer when other forms of treatment have failed symptom relief remains the only form of treatment which the clinician may have to offer the patient. Breathlessness and pain are the most common symptoms encountered. Methods of relief of the former have already been discussed, and whilst analgesics of all forms are widely used for the latter, local anaesthesia may be used with excellent results in some patients who would otherwise require high doses of opiates with unwanted side-effects. The most useful of these techniques are the paravertebral and epidural blocks for chest wall and bone pain, and brachial plexus block for Pancoast tumours.

PROGNOSIS OF BRONCHOGENIC CARCINOMA AND MESOTHELIMOA

The prognosis of lung cancer is dependent on a number of factors including histological type, size, spread of the tumour, patient's age and performance status, assessed on the Karnofsky (Karnofsky & Burchenal 1949) or ECOG/Zubrod (Zubrod et al 1960) scale, weight loss and treatment. The relative importance of these for the prognosis depends on the stage, so that in easily resectable tumours the outcome will be dependent largely on the histology, while in the later stages with distant metastases histological type is less important than the performance status (Stanley 1985).

The prognosis of squamous cell carcinoma is better than that of any other cell type, with a 5-year survival of about 40% of all patients with stage 1 disease, and 10% in stage 3 disease. The most important factor affecting prognosis is surgical intervention, which may increase 5-year survival to approaching 60% in stage 1 disease (Carr 1980). Overall the 5-year survival of this type of tumour is 25% (Spiro & Goldstraw 1984).

Adenocarcinoma has a more favourable natural history than large cell tumours, although not as good as that of the squamous cell type. The 5-year survival of patients with adeno- and large cell carcinoma is similar, of the order of 15%, but patients with T1 adenocarcinoma have a better prognosis (38% 5-year survival) than those with large cell tumours (17% 5-year survival) (Mountain 1976). Survival curves of different types of tumours separated for stage of disease have shown that widespread metastases have a more deleterious effect on survival in adenocarcinoma than on any other cell type, and the size of the primary tumour is a poor prognostic sign in large cell tumours. Although slow-growing, broncho-alveolar carcinoma has a poor prognosis, with a mean survival of four months due to the late presentation and lack of response to radio- or chemotherapy (St J Thomas et al 1985).

Small cell carcinoma has a very poor prognosis, and most patients present with disseminated disease; their survival and response to treatment with either chemotherapy or chemotherapy and radio-therapy is considerably worse than those with limited disease. Only 2% of patients with extensive disease survive more than two years, compared with 13% with limited disease (Spiro 1985). In the rare cases where the disease is resectable, figures of 60% 5-year survival have been quoted (Mountain et al 1976, Shields et al 1982). Overall median survival time has increased from 1.5 to 10.85 months with chemotherapy (Slevin et al 1983, Aisner 1987).

The prognosis of mesothelioma is poor, with a median survival of one year from the onset of symptoms. Radical pleuropneumonectomy in cases with disease confined to the parietal pleura of one hemithorax has only been shown to be effective in one study (de Laria et al 1978). Other forms of therapy have not made any impact on survival though radiotherapy may have a place in relief of chest pain.

REFERENCES

Aisner J 1987 Identification of new drugs in small cell lung cancer: phase II agents first? Cancer Treatment Reports 71: 1131–1133

Aisner S C, Matthews M J 1985 The pathology of lung cancer. In: Aisner J (ed) Lung cancer. Churchill Livingstone, New York, pp 1–23

Alderson P O, Adams D F, McNeil B J et al 1983 Computed tomography, ultrasound and scintography of the liver in patients with colon or breast carcinoma: a prospective comparison. Radiology 149: 225–230

Ali M K, Mountain C F, Ewer M S, Johnston D, Haynie T P 1980 Predicting loss of pulmonary function after pulmonary resection for bronchogenic carcinoma. Chest 77: 337–342

Anonymous 1984 Early lung cancer detection: summary and conclusions. American Review of Respiratory Disease 130: 565–570

Arabian A, Spagnolo S V 1984 Laser therapy in patients with primary lung cancer. Chest 86: 519–523

Aristizabal S A, Caldwell W L 1976 Radical irradiation with the split course technique in carcinoma of the lung. Cancer 37: 2630–2635

Arnold A M, Williams C J 1979 Small cell lung cancer: a curable disease? British Journal of Diseases of the Chest 73: 327–348

Ashare A B 1980 Radiocolloid liver scintography. Radiologic Clinics of North America 18: 315–320

Bakowski M T, Crouch J C 1983 Chemotherapy of non-small cell lung cancer: a reappraisal and look to the future. Cancer Treatment Reviews 10: 159–172

Bell J W, Knudtson K P 1961 Observations on the natural history of bronchiolo-alveolar cell carcinoma: experience with 21 cases. American Review of Respiratory Diseases 83: 660–667

Berlin N I, Buncher C R, Fontana R S, Frost J K,

Melamed M R 1984 The National Cancer Institute Cooperative Early Lung Cancer Detection Program: results of the initial screen (prevalence). American Review of Respiratory Diseases 130: 545–549

Bernadino M E, Erwin B C, Steinberg H V, Baumgartner H V, Torres W E, Gadgaudas-McLees R C 1986 Delayed hepatic CT scanning: increased confidence and improved detection of hepatic metastases. Radiology 159: 71–74

Borgelt B, Gelber R, Kramer S et al 1980 The palliation of brain metastases: final results of the first two studies by the Radiation Therapy Oncology Group. International Journal of Radiation Oncology, Biology and Physics 6: 1–10

Bourgouin P M, Shepard J A O, McLoud T C, Spizarny D L, Dedrick C G 1988 Transthoracic needle aspiration biopsy: evaluation of the blood patch technique. Radiology 166: 93–95

Brett G Z 1968 The value of lung cancer detection by six-monthly chest radiographs. Thorax 23: 414–420

Brett G Z 1969 Earlier diagnosis and survival in lung cancer. British Medical Journal 4: 260–262

Brower M, Ihde D C, Johnston-Early A et al 1983 Treatment of extensive stage small cell bronchogenic carcinoma. American Journal of Medicine 75: 993–1000

Byrd R B, Carr D T, Miller W E, Payne W S, Woolner L B 1969 Radiographic abnormalities of the lung as related to histological cell type. Thorax 24: 573–576

Cagle P T, Cohle S D, Greenberg S D 1985 Natural history of pulmonary scar carcinomas: clinical and pathologic implications. Cancer 56: 2031–2035

Carr D T 1980 Diagnosis and staging. In: Hansen H H, Rorth M (eds) Lung cancer 1980. (II World Conference on Lung Cancer, Copenhagen). Excerpta Medica, Amsterdam, pp 49–70

Carter D, Eggleston J C 1980 Tumours of the lower

respiratory tract. In: Atlas of tumour pathology, second series. Fascicle 17. Armed Forces Institute of Pathology, Washington DC, pp 59–161

Centi D, Hawkins H B 1984 Aspiration biopsy of peripheral pulmonary masses using real time sonographic guidance. American Journal of Roentgenology 142: 1115–1116

Chin W S, Yee I S T 1978 Percutaneous aspiration biopsy of malignant lesions using a Chiba needle: an initial experience. Clinical Radiology 29: 617–619

Clee M D, Hockings N F, Johnston R N 1984 Bronchial carcinoma: factors influencing post-operative survival. British Journal of Diseases of the Chest 78: 225–235

Colice G L, Chappell G J, Frenchman S M, Solomon D A 1985 Comparison of computerized tomography with fibreoptic bronchoscopy in identifying endobronchial abnormalities in patients with known or suspected lung cancer. American Review of Respiratory Diseases 131, 397–400

Cooksey J A, Bitran J D, Desser R K et al 1979 Small cell carcinoma of the lung: the prognostic significance of stage on survival. European Journal of Cancer 15: 859–865

Cox J, Yesner R, Mietlowski W, Petrovich Z 1979 Influence of cell type on failure pattern after irradiation for locally advanced carcinoma of lung. Cancer 44: 94–98

Coy P, Kennelly G M 1980 The role of curative radiotherapy in the treatment of lung cancer. Cancer 45: 698–701

de Laria G A, Jensik R, Faber L P, Kittle C F 1978 Surgical management of malignant mesothelioma. Annals of Thoracic Sugery 26: 375–382

Doll R, Hill A B 1964 Mortality in relation to smoking: ten years' observations of British doctors. British Medical Journal 1: 1399–1410

Doll R, Hill A B, Kreyberg L 1957 The significance of cell type in relation to the aetiology of lung cancer. British Journal of Cancer 11: 43–48

Edwards C W 1984 Alveolar carcinoma: a review. Thorax 39: 166–174

Edwards S E, Kelsey Fry I 1982 Prevalance of lung nodules on computed tomography of patients without known malignant disease. British Journal of Radiology 55: 715–716

Faling L J, Pugatch R D, Jung-Legg Y et al 1981 Computed tomographic scanning of the mediastinum in the staging of bronchogenic carcinoma. American Review of Respiratory Diseases 124: 690–695

Fox W, Scadding J G 1973 Medical Research Council comparative trial of surgery and radiotherapy for primary small celled or oat-celled carcinoma of bronchus. Lancet 2: 63–65

Fujimara S, Kondo T, Imai T et al 1985 Prognostic evaluation of tracheobronchial reconstruction for bronchogenic carcinoma. Journal of Thoracic and Cardiovascular Surgery 90: 161–166

Galofre M, Payne W S, Woolner L B, Claggett O T, Gage R P 1964 Pathologic classification and surgical treatment of bronchogenic carcinoma. Surgery, Gynaecology and Obstetrics 119: 51–61

Geddes D M 1979 The natural history of lung cancer: a review based on rates of tumour growth. British Journal of Diseases of the Chest 73: 1–17

Gelb A F, Epstein J D 1984 Lasers in treatment of lung cancer. Chest 86: 662–666

Gellert A R, Rudd R M, Sinha G, Geddes D M 1982a Fibreoptic bronchoscopy: effect of experience of operator on diagnostic yield of bronchial biopsy in bronchial carcinoma. British Journal of Diseases of the Chest 76: 397–399

Gellert A R, Rudd R M, Sinha G, Geddes D M 1982b Fibreoptic bronchoscopy: effect of multiple bronchial biopsies on diagnostic yield in bronchial carcinoma. Thorax 87: 684–687

George P J M, Garrett C P O, Goldstraw P, Hetzel M R, Ramsay A D 1986 Resuscitative laser photoresection of a tracheal tumour before elective surgery. Thorax 41: 812–813

Gilbert R W, Kim J H, Posner J B 1978 Epidural spinal cord compression from metastatic tumour: diagnosis and treatment. Annals of Neurology 3: 40–51

Ginsberg R J, Hill L D, Eagan R T et al 1983 Modern 30-day operative mortality for surgical resections in lung cancer. Journal of Thoracic and Cardiovascular Surgery 86: 654–658

Giron C C, Ordonez A, Jalon J I, Baron M G 1987 Combination chemotherapy with ifosfamide, mitomycin and cisplatin in advanced non-small cell lung cancer. Cancer Treatment Reports 71: 851–853

Glazer H S, Aronberg D J, Sagel S S, Emami B 1984 Utility of CT in detecting post-pneumonectomy carcinoma recurrence. American Journal of Roentgenology 142: 487–494

Goldman K P 1965 Histology of lung cancer in relation to prognosis. Thorax 20: 298–302

Goldstraw P G 1986 CT scanning in the pre-operative assessment of non-small cell lung cancer. In: Hansen H H (ed) Lung cancer: basic and clinical aspects. Martinus Nijhoff, Boston, pp 183–199

Goldstraw P G, Kurzer M, Edwards D 1983 Pre-operative staging of lung cancer: accuracy of computed tomography versus mediastinoscopy. Thorax 38: 10–15

Graves W G, Martinez M J, Carter P L, Barry M J, Clark J S 1985 The value of computed tomography in staging bronchogenic carcinoma: a changing rôle for mediastinoscopy. Annals of Thoracic Surgery 40: 57–60

Gregor A 1984 Radiotherapy for inoperable non-small cell carcinoma of the bronchus. In: Smyth J F (ed) The management of lung cancer. Edward Arnold, London, pp 91–131

Hansen H H, Rorth M, Aisner J 1985 Management of small cell lung cancer. In: Aisner J (ed) Lung cancer. Churchill Livingstone, New York, pp 269–285

Haponik E F, Wang K 1985 New methods for the diagnosis and staging of mediastinal disease. In: Aisner J (ed) Lung cancer. Churchill Livingstone, New York, pp 67–100

Harper P G, Houang M, Spiro S G, Geddes D M, Hodson M, Souhami R L 1981 Computerized tomography in the pre-treatment assessment of small cell carcinoma of the bronchus. Cancer 47: 1775–1780

Heard B E, Payling-Wright G 1976 The lungs. In: Symmers W D (ed) Systemic Pathology. vol 1. Churchill Livingstone, Edinburgh, pp 392–414

Heiken J P, Lee J K T, Glazer H S, Ling D 1985 Hepatic metastases studied with MR and CT. Radiology 156: 423–427

Hellman S, Kligerman M, Von Essen C F, Scibetta M D 1964 Sequelae of radical radiotherapy of carcinoma of the lung. Radiology 82: 1055–1061

Herman P G, Hessel S J 1977 The diagnostic accuracy and complications of closed lung biopsies. Radiology 125: 11–14

Hetzel M R, Nixon C, Edmonstone W M et al 1985 Laser therapy in 100 tracheobronchial tumours. Thorax 40: 341–345

Higgins G A, Sheilds T W, Keehn R J 1975 The solitary pulmonary nodule: ten year follow-up of Veterans Administration Armed Forces Cooperative Study. Archives of Surgery 110: 570–575

Hilaris B S, Luomanen R K, Beattie E J 1971 Integrated irradiation and surgery in the treatment of apical lung cancer. Cancer 27: 1369–1373

Jacobs L, Kinkel W R, Vincent R C 1977 Silent brain metastases from lung carcinoma determined by computerized tomography. Archives of Neurology 34: 690–693

Joss R A, Cavalli F, Goldmirsch A, Mermillod B, Brunner K W 1984 New agents in non-small cell lung cancer. Cancer Treatment Reviews 11: 205–236

Karnofsky D A, Burchenal J H 1949 The clinical evaluation of chemotherapeutic agents in cancer. In: MacLeod C M (ed) Evaluation of chemotherapeutic agents. (Symposium, Microbiology Section, New York Academy of Medicine, New York 1949). Columbia University Press, New York, pp 191–205

Khouri N F, Stitik F P, Erozan Y S et al 1985 Transthoracic needle aspiration of benign and malignant lung lesions. American Journal of Roentgenology 144: 281–288

Knudtson R J, Hatch H B, Mitchell W T, Ochsner A 1965 Unusual carcinoma of the lung II. Bronchiolar carcinoma of the lung. Diseases of the Chest 48: 628–633

Kreel L 1981 Computed tomography in mesothelioma. Seminars in Oncology 8: 302–312

Lamb D 1984 The pathology and classification of lung cancer. In: Smyth J F (ed) The management of lung cancer. Edward Arnold, London, pp 19–35

Lehan T J, Carr D T, Miller W E, Payne W S, Woolner L B 1967 Roentgenographic appearance of bronchogenic adenocarcinoma. American Review of Respiratory Diseases 96: 245–248

Le Roux B T 1968 Bronchial carcinoma. Thorax 23: 136–143

Le Roux B T 1984 The surgical management of bronchial carcinoma. In: Smyth J F (ed) The management of lung cancer. Edward Arnold, London, pp 53–90

Levitt R G, Glazer H S, Roper C L, Lee J K T, Murphy W A 1985 Magnetic resonance imaging of mediastinal and hilar masses: comparison with CT. American Journal of Roentgenology 145: 9–14

Li W, Hammar S P, Jolly P C, Hill L D, Anderson R P 1981 Unpredictable course of small cell undifferentiated lung carcinoma. Journal of Thoracic and Cardiovascular Surgery 81(1): 34–43

Libshitz H I, McKenna R J 1984 Mediastinal lymph node size in lung cancer. American Journal of Roentgenology 143: 715–718

Lilienfield A, Archer P G, Burnett C H et al 1966 An evaluation of radiographic and cytologic screening for the early detection of lung cancer: a cooperative pilot study of the American Cancer Society and the Veterans Administration. Cancer Research 26: 2083–2121

Lipscomb D J, Flower C D R 1980 Ultrasound in the diagnosis and management of pleural disease. British Journal of Diseases of the Chest 74: 353–361

Livingston R B, Moore T N, Heibrun L, Bottomley R, Lehaned R T 1978 Small cell carcinoma of the lung: combined chemotherapy and radiation. Annals of Internal Medicine 98: 194–199

McCaughan B C, Martini N, Bains M S, McCormack P M 1986 Chest wall invasion in carcinoma of the lung. Journal of Thoracic and Cardiovascular Surgery 89: 836–841

McCorkell S J 1984 Unintended percutaneous aspiration of pulmonary echinococchal cysts. American Journal of Radiology 143: 123–126

Martini N 1985 Pre-operative staging and surgery for non-small cell lung cancer. In: Aisner J (ed) Lung cancer. Churchill Livingstone, New York, pp 101–130

Martini N, Beattie E J 1977 Results of treatment in stage 1 lung cancer. Journal of Thoracic and Cardiovascular Surgery 74: 499–505

Martini N, Melamed M R 1980 Occult carcinomas of the lung. Annals of Thoracic Surgery 30: 215–223

Marzano M J, Deschler T, Mintzer R A 1984 Alveolar cell carcinoma. Chest 86: 123–128

Mathison D J, Jensik R J, Faber L P, Kittle C F 1984 Survival following resection for second and third primary lung cancers. Journal of Thoracic and Cardiovascular Surgery 88: 502–510

Matthews M J 1976 Problems in morphology and behaviour of bronchopulmonary malignant disease. In: Israel I, Chahinian A P (eds) Lung cancer — natural history, prognosis and therapy. Academic Press, New York, pp 23–63

Matsuda M, Horai T, Nakamura S et al 1986 Bronchial brushing and biopsy: comparison of diagnostic accuracy and cell typing reliability in lung cancer. Thorax 41: 475–478

Mehta C, Vogl S E 1982 High dose cyclophosphamide in the induction chemotherapy of small cell lung cancer: minor improvement in rate of remission and survival. Proceedings of the American Association for Cancer Research 23: 155

Melamed M R, Flehinger B J, Zaman M B, Heelan R T, Hallerman E T, Martini N 1981 Detection of true pathologic stage 1 lung cancer in a screening program and the effect on survival. Cancer 47: 1182–1187

Miller A B 1980 Epidemiology and etiology of lung cancer. In: Hansen H H, Rorth M (eds) Lung cancer 1980. (II World Conference on Lung Cancer, Copenhagen). Excerpta Medica, Amsterdam, pp 9–26

Miller A B, Fox W, Tall R 1969 Five year follow-up of the Medical Research Council comparative trial of surgery and radiotherapy for primary treatment of small celled or oat-celled carcinoma. Lancet 2: 501–505

Mintzer R A, Cugell D W 1982 The association of asbestos-induced pleural disease and rounded atelectasis. Chest 81: 457–460

Mitchell D M, Emerson C J, Collins J V, Stableforth D E 1981 Transbronchial lung biopsy with fibreoptic bronchoscope: analysis of results in 433 patients. British Journal of Diseases of the Chest 75: 258–262

Moncado R, Cardella R, Demos T C et al 1984 Evaluation of superior vena cava obstruction by axial CT and CT phlebography. American Journal of Roentgenology 143: 731–736

Mountain C F 1976 The relationship of prognosis to morphology and the anatomic extent of disease: studies on a new clinical staging system. In: Israel L, Chahinian A P (eds) Lung cancer — natural history, prognosis and therapy. Academic Press, New York, pp 107–140

Mountain C F 1986 A new international staging system for lung cancer. Chest 89 (suppl): 2255–2335

Muhm J R, Brown L R, Crowe J K 1977 Detection of

pulmonary nodules by computed tomography. American Journal of Roentgenology 128: 267–279

Musset D, Grenier P, Carette M F et al 1986 Primary lung cancer staging: prospective comparative study of MR imaging with CT. Radiology 160: 607–611

Nahman B J, van Aman M E, McLemore W E, O'Toole R V 1985 Use of the Rotex needle in percutaneous biopsy of pulmonary malignancy. American Journal of Roentgenology 145: 97–99

Nash F A, Morgan J M, Tomkins J G 1968 South London lung cancer study. British Medical Journal 2: 715–721

Ochs R H, Katz A S, Edmonds L H, Miller C L, Epstein D M 1982 Prognosis of pulmonary scar carcinoma. Journal of Thoracic and Cardiovascular Surgery 84: 359–366

Oestmann I W, Kushner D C, Bourgouin P M, Llewellyn H J, Mockbee B W, Greene R 1988 Subtle lung cancers: impact of edge enhancement and grey scale reversal on detection with digitized chest radiographs. Radiology 167: 657–658

Office of Population Censuses and Surveys Monitor M.B1. 88/1 1988

Office of Population Censuses and Surveys 1985 Mortality statistics: cause, 1984. HMSO, London, p 10

Osterlind K, Hansen M, Hansen H H, Dombernowsky P, Rorth M 1985 Treatment policy of surgery in small cell carcinoma of the lung: retrospective analysis of 874 consecutive patients. Thorax 40: 272–277

Parkes W R 1982 Silicates and lung disease. In: Parkes W R (ed) Occupational lung disorders. Butterworth, London, pp 275–293

Paulson D L, Reisch J S 1976 Long-term survival after resection for bronchogenic carcinoma. Annals of Surgery 184: 324–332

Payne C R, Hadfield J W, Stove P G H, Barker V, Heard B E, Stark J W 1981 Diagnostic accuracy of cytology and biopsy in primary bronchial carcinoma. Journal of Clinical Pathology 34: 773–778

Pennes D R, Glazer G M, Wimbish K J, Gross B H, Long R W, Orringer M B 1985 Chest wall invasion by lung cancer: limitations of CT evaluation. American Journal of Roentgenology 144: 507–511

Perlmutt L M, Braun S D, Newman G E, Oke E J, Dunnick N R 1986 Timing of chest film follow-up after transthoracic needle aspiration. American Journal of Roentgenology 146: 1049–1050

Pierce R J, Pretto J J, Rochford P D, McDonald C F, Hanan J A, Barter C E 1986 Lobar occlusion in the pre-operative assessment of patients with lung cancer. British Journal of Diseases of the Chest 80: 27–36

Poplin E, Thompson B, Whitacre M, Aisner J 1987 Small cell carcinoma of the lung. Influence of age on treatment outcome. Cancer Treatment Reports 71: 291–296

Rea H H, Sherland J E, House A J S 1981 Accuracy of computed tomographic scanning in assessment of the mediastinum in bronchial carcinoma. Journal of Thoracic and Cardiovascular Surgery 81: 825–829

Reinig J W, Dwyer A J, Miller D L et al 1987 Liver metastases detection: comparative sensitivities of MR imaging and CT scanning. Radiology 162: 43–47

Richards F Scarantino C W 1985 Results of clinical trials and basis for future therapeutics. In: Scarantino C W (ed) Lung cancer. Springer Verlag, Berlin, pp 97–125

St J Thomas J, Tullett W M, Stack B H R 1985

Bronchioloalveolar cell carcinoma: a 21 year retrospective study of cases at the Western Infirmary, Glasgow. British Journal of Diseases of the Chest 79: 132–140

Sarin C L, Nohl-Oser H C 1969 Mediastinoscopy: a clinical evaluation of 400 consecutive cases. Thorax 24: 585–588

Selikoff I J, Hammond E C, Churg J 1968 Asbestos exposure, smoking and neoplasia. Journal of the American Medical Association 204: 106–112

Shields T W 1982 Surgical therapy for carcinoma of the lung. In: Matthay R A (ed) Recent advances in lung cancer. Clinics in Chest Medicine 3: 369–387

Shields T W, Higgins G A, Keehn R J 1972 Factors influencing survival after resection for bronchial carcinoma. Journal of Thoracic and Cardiovascular Surgery 64: 391–399

Shields T W, Humphrey E W, Matthews M, Eastridge C E, Keehn R J 1980 Pathological stage grouping of patients with resected carcinoma of the lung. Journal of Thoracic and Cardiovascular Surgery 80: 400–405

Shields T W, Higgins G A, Matthews M J, Kahn R J 1982 Surgical resection in the management of small cell carcinoma of the lung. Journal of Thoracic and Cardiovascular Surgery 84: 481–488

Shimosato Y 1980 Pathology of lung cancer. In: Hansen H H, Rorth M (eds) Lung cancer 1980. (II World Conference on Lung Cancer, Copenhagen). Excerpta Medica, Amsterdam, pp 27–48

Shin M S, Jackson L K, Shelton R W, Greene R E 1986 Giant cell carcinoma of the lung. Chest 89: 366–369

Shioya S, Haida M, Ono Y, Fukizaki M, Yamabayashi H 1988 Lung cancer: differentiation of tumour necrosis and atelectasis by means of T1 and T2 values measured in vitro. Radiology 167: 105–109

Shore D S F, Paneth M 1980 Survival after resection of small cell carcinoma of the bronchus. Thorax 35(11): 819–822

Shure D, Fedullo P F 1984 The role of transcarinal needle aspiration in the staging of bronchogenic carcinoma. Chest 86: 693–696

Siegelman S S, Zerhouni E A, Leo F P, Khouri N F, Stitik F P 1980 CT of the solitary pulmonary nodule. American Journal of Roentgenology 135: 1–13

Siegelman S S, Khouri N F, Scott W W et al 1986a Pulmonary hamartoma: CT findings. Radiology 160: 313–317

Siegelman S S, Khouri N F, Leo F P, Fishman E K, Braverman R M, Zerhouni E A 1986b Solitary pulmonary nodules: CT assessment. Radiology 160: 307–312

Simpson F G, Arnold A G, Purvis A, Belfield P W, Muers M F, Cooke N J 1986 Postal survey of the bronchoscopic practice of physicians in the United Kingdom. Thorax 41: 311–317

Sinner W N 1979 Pulmonary neoplasms diagnosed with transthoracic needle biopsy. Cancer 43: 1533–1540

Sinner W N 1982 Fine needle biopsy of hamartoma of the lung. American Journal of Roentgenology 138: 65–69

Slawson R G, Scott R M 1979 Radiation therapy for bronchogenic carcinoma. Radiology 132: 175–176

Slevin M L, Harvey V J, Ponder B A J et al 1983 Small cell lung carcinoma: survival after combination chemotherapy, radiotherapy or symptomatic treatment. British Journal of Diseases of the Chest 77: 381–389

Smith T J, Kemeny M M, Sugarbaker P H et al 1982 A prospective study of hepatic imaging in the detection of metastatic disease. Annals of Surgery 195: 486–491

Smyth J F 1984 The management of small cell anaplastic lung cancer. In: Smyth J F (ed) The management of lung cancer. Edward Arnold, London, pp 115–131

Sorensen H R, Claus L, Alstrup P 1986 Survival in small cell lung carcinoma after surgery. Thorax 41: 479–482

Sorensen J B, Osterlind K, Hansen H H 1987 Vinca alkaloids in the treatment of non-small cell lung cancer. Cancer Treatment Reviews 14: 29–51

Souhami R L 1984 The management of advanced non-small cell lung carcinoma of the bronchus. In: Smyth J F (ed) The management of lung cancer. Edward Arnold, London, pp 132–149

Souhami R L 1985 Chemotherapy in non-small cell bronchial carcinoma. Thorax 40: 641–646

Spiro S G 1984 The diagnosis and staging of lung cancer. In: Smyth J F (ed) The management of lung cancer. Edward Arnold, London, pp 36–51

Spiro S G 1985 Chemotherapy of small cell lung cancer. Clinics in Oncology 4: 105–120

Spiro S G, Goldstraw P 1984 The staging of lung cancer. Thorax 39: 401–407

Spiro S G, Shah S, Harper P G, Tobias J S, Geddes D M, Souhami R L 1983 Treatment of obstruction of the superior vena cava by combination chemotherapy with and without irradiation in small-cell carcinoma of the bronchus. Thorax 38: 501–505

Stanley K E 1985 Prognostic factors in lung cancer. In: Aisner J (ed) Lung cancer. Churchill Livingstone, New York, pp 41–65

Staples C A, Muller N L, Miller R R, Evans K G, Nelems B 1988 Mediastinal nodes in bronchogenic carcinoma: comparison between CT and mediastinoscopy. Radiology 167: 367–372

Stark D D, Wittenberg J, Butch R J, Ferrucci J T 1987 Hepatic metastases: a randomized, controlled comparison of detection with MR and CT. Radiology 165: 399–406

Taylor W F, Fontana, R S, Unlenhopp M A, Davis C S 1981 Some results of screening for early lung cancer. Cancer 47: 1114–1120

Theros E G 1977 Varying manifestations of peripheral pulmonary neoplasms: a radiologic–pathologic correlative study. American Journal of Roentgenology 128: 893–914

Thompson-Evans E W 1973 Resection for bronchial carcinoma in the elderly. Thorax 28: 86–88

Tockman M S, Frost J K, Stitik F P, Levin M L, Ball W C, Marsh B R 1985 Screening and detection of lung cancer. In: Aisner J (ed) Lung cancer. Churchill Livingstone, New York, pp 25–40

Tong D, Gillick L, Hendrickson F R 1982 The palliation of symptomatic osseous metastases: final result of the study by the radiation oncology group. Cancer 50: 893–899

Turner-Warwick M, Lebowitz M, Burrows B, Johnson A 1980 Cryptogenic fibrosing alveolitis and lung cancer. Thorax 35: 496–499

Twersky J, Twersky N, Lehr C 1976 Scleroderma and carcinoma of the lung. Clinical Radiology 27: 203–209

Underwood G H, Hooper R G, Axelbaum S P, Goodwin D W 1979 Computed tomographic scanning of the thorax in staging of bronchogenic carcinoma. New England Journal of Medicine 300: 777–778

Veale D, Gilmartin J J, Sumerling M D, Wadehra V, Gibson G J 1988 Prospective evaluation of fine needle aspiration in the diagnosis of lung cancer. Thorax 43: 540–544

Wang K P, Terry P B 1983 Transbronchial needle aspiration in the diagnosis and staging of bronchogenic carcinoma. American Review of Respiratory Disease 127: 344–347

Wang K P, Brower R, Haponik E F, Siegelman S 1983 Flexible transbronchial needle aspiration for staging of bronchogenic carcinoma. Chest 84: 571–576

Webb W R, Gamsu G, Stark D D, Moon K L, Moore E H 1984 The evaluation of magnetic resonance sequences in imaging mediastinal tumours. American Journal of Roentgenology 143: 723–727

Weisbrod G L, Lyons D J, Tao L C, Chamberlain D W 1984 Percutaneous fine needle aspiration biopsy of mediastinal lesions. American Journal of Roentgenology 143: 525–529

Weiss W 1981 Small cell carcinoma of the lung: epidemiology and etiology. In: Greco F A, Oldham R K, Bunn P A (eds) Small cell lung cancer. Grune & Stratton, New York, pp 1–34

Weiss W, Boucot K R, Cooper D A 1981 The Philadelphia Pulmonary Neoplasm Research Project: survival factors in bronchogenic carcinoma. Journal of the American Medical Association 216: 2119–2123

Weissberg D, Kaufman M, Zurkowski Z 1980 Pleuroscopy in patients with pleural effusion and pleural masses. Annals of Thoracic Surgery 29: 205–208

Williams A J, Cayton R M, Harding L K, Mostafa A B, Matthews H R 1984 Quantitative lung scintigrams and lung function in the selection of patients for pneumonectomy. British Journal of Diseases of the Chest 78: 105–110

Winning A J, McIvor J, Seed W A, Husain O A N, Metaxes N 1986 Interpretation of negative results in fine needle aspiration of discrete pulmonary lesions. Thorax 41: 875–879

World Health Organization 1981 Histological typing of lung tumours. In: International histological classification of tumours, 2nd edn. World Health Organization, Geneva, pp 19–32

Wright F W 1976 Spontaneous pneumothorax and pulmonary malignant disease — a syndrome sometimes associated with cavitating tumours. Clinical Radiology 27: 221–222

Yesner R, Carter D 1982 Pathology of carcinoma of the lung. In: Matthay R A (ed) Recent advances in lung cancer. Clinics in Chest Medicine 3: 257–289

Zubrod C G, Schneiderman M, Frei E et al 1960 Appraisal of methods for the study of chemotherapy of cancer in man: comparative therapeutic trial of nitrogen mustard and triethylene thiophosphoramide. Journal of Chronic Disease 11: 7–33

5. The breast

I. H. Gravelle

INTRODUCTION

Radiological examination has played an important rôle over the years in the management and assessment of patients with breast cancer. Conventional radiography of the breast and skeleton have been the traditional physical methods of detection of dissemination of the disease. These are still retained but newer, sophisticated imaging modalities have now become available which have increased the radiologist's rôle in the management of breast cancer and have improved the accuracy of staging (Gravelle 1982).

In addition to the advances in the demonstration of dissemination there is now a general acceptance of the value of imaging of the primary lesion. In this situation mammography is still the method of choice, but with more recent refinements. Other modalities are also available but have not supplanted the original radiographic method. Some have complementary uses, however.

STAGING

The imaging methods available for staging of breast cancer include plain radiography of the lungs, mediastinum and skeleton together with radiographic tomography of these structures. Additional techniques, now widely used, are scintigraphy, ultrasound and CT. Magnetic resonance imaging (MRI) is under assessment but is not yet readily available.

The value of the available modalities varies in different clinical situations. There is no point in duplicating or even triplicating investigations in order to confirm and reconfirm an abnormality shown by simple plain radiography. Further inves-

tigation of an equivocal finding or characterization of a particular soft tissue mass is acceptable. The investigative enthusiasm of both clinician and radiologist should be curbed and channelled to suit the needs of the individual patient. The selection of a particular imaging modality in a clinical situation will depend on that situation and on the availability of apparatus and expertise. In general, two situations will arise; the detection of spread to soft tissues and skeletal dissemination.

In breast carcinoma, Cutler et al (1969) reported that in women with one site of metastasis 58% had skeletal disease, 26% had pulmonary or pleural involvement and 16% had secondary spread to lymph nodes other than the ipsilateral axillary group. Even though the lungs are the second commonest site for metastatic involvement, local invasion may rarely cause intrathoracic spread before distant metastases occur.

Soft tissue metastases

The soft tissues most frequently involved in metastatic disease are the lungs, pleura, thoracic wall, mediastinum, liver and brain. Lymph nodes are commonly affected and extranodal abdominal and pelvic masses occur.

The thorax

In the assessment of thoracic involvement by metastases, ultrasound is of no value in the detection of pulmonary or mediastinal spread and of little practical value in pleural involvement, apart from occasional guidance for diagnostic aspiration in small effusions difficult to detect clinically. Scintigraphy is also of very limited use, but may possibly be of use in the differentiation of abscess, granuloma or embolism.

The most important technique in detecting metastases is still the plain chest radiograph. A high kV technique is preferred and an appropriate lateral view should be obtained. In the presence of obvious pulmonary or mediastinal metastases the chest radiograph can be accepted as the definitive procedure and used to assess response to therapy. If there is any doubt as to the presence of metastases then conventional whole lung and mediastinal tomography can be undertaken and will elucidate a proportion of problems. However, CT is the investigation of choice in this situation. It is more sensitive than chest radiography and conventional tomography in the detection of metastases, and is particularly useful in the demonstration of peripheral deposits and those situated in the costophrenic recesses, retrohilar and retrosternal areas (Fig. 5.1). Metastases as small as 3 mm in diameter may be shown but their differentiation from granulomata will not be possible.

CT is the ideal method of demonstrating the presence and extent of thoracic wall involvement and pleural spread. Mediastinal deposits are more readily shown than by conventional radiographic methods. In the problem of differentiation of the nature of pulmonary and mediastinal masses, CT-guided percutaneous, transthoracic needle biopsy or transbronchial biopsy may be necessary to acquire histological characterization. Chiles and Ravin (1985) state that mediastinal lymph nodes under 1 cm in diameter may be considered as normal, those over 1.5 cm in diameter as abnormal and that nodes between 1 cm and 1.5 cm should be regarded with suspicion. Even though CT is superior to chest radiography in the demonstration of mediastinal masses, it has no particular advantage in hilar assessment. Meyer and Munzenrider (1981) consider CT useful in the detection of internal mammary node involvement during local recurrence of tumour. Internal mammary radiocolloid lymphoscintigraphy, as advocated by Ege (1978) for the evaluation of parasternal lymph nodes has not established a rôle in investigation or management.

The occurrence of a pleural effusion, in an individual with a past history, no matter how long, of breast cancer, is an important finding. About 50% of all breast cancer patients will develop an effusion. It may rarely occur at presentation but is more usually the first sign of recurrence of disease. It may indicate local chest wall involvement or pleural metastases. CT examination is the method of choice in the assessment of local thoracic wall infiltration. In effusion, thoracentesis (with cytological analysis) and pleural biopsy will allow a diagnosis of malignancy to be made in 90% of cases (Salyer et al 1975). It is not often that ultrasound-guided needle aspiration will be required.

The decision as to which imaging modality to use for the assessment of dissemination should be made with the full knowledge of clinical or other evidence of metastatic spread elsewhere. If metastases are present at other sites then conventional radiography would seem to be the method of choice, as the demonstration of additional metastatic disease (by conventional or computed tomography) would be unlikely to alter a chemotherapeutic regime.

With no evidence of metastases at other sites, CT may be indicated to exclude the presence of pulmonary or mediastinal lesions, or to elucidate the nature of a lesion of doubtful significance. It is useful when a solitary pulmonary nodule appears

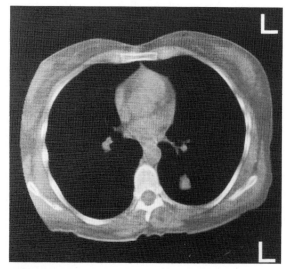

Fig. 5.1 Thoracic CT scan showing a left retrohilar metastasis.

on a follow-up chest radiograph as it may demonstrate the presence of additional lesions. However, final tissue characterization using biopsy techniques may be required. Another important point should be considered, which is that pulmonary nodules do not necessarily demonstrate the presence of viable malignant cells following appropriate chemotherapy, so the failure of disappearance of pulmonary nodules in such a situation is not necessarily significant. Subsequent enlargement, however, is of paramount significance.

The place of magnetic resonance imaging in the assessment of thoracic disease is under investigation. It is probably complementary to CT. They both give similar information but one may prove more informative than the other in selected cases. The advantages of CT include a shorter scanning time and the consequent availability for use with ill patients, the lack of effect on pacemakers, the detection of calcification and the use for guided needle biopsy. MRI has several disadvantages — its limited availability at the present time, relatively long scan times which make it unsuitable for ill patients, the impossibility of examining patients with pacemakers and its failure to demonstrate calcifications consistently. However, there are advantages to the use of MRI. No contrast medium is required and normal hilar structures are readily identified and differentiated from masses: this latter may prove to be its biggest asset.

The ability of MRI to demonstrate and differentiate pulmonary and mediastinal lesions is not significantly different from that of CT. The hope that a characteristic change in the MRI appearance of tumour tissue would occur with successful treatment, and so be recognizable, has as yet not been borne out.

Abdomen and pelvis

Scintigraphy, ultrasound and CT are three modalities used in the assessment of the abdomen and pelvis. Liver and spleen scintigraphy has a sensitivity of the order of 86% in the detection of metastases but a relatively low specificity of around 79% (McClees and Gedgaudas-McClees 1984). In addition, the examination is limited to the assessment of the liver and spleen.

With the introduction of real-time ultrasound the examination of the abdomen and pelvis has been simplified and enhanced, with increased accuracy in the detection of metastatic disease. The ultrasonic appearances of hepatic and splenic metastases are variable. Lesions may be hyperechoic, hypoechoic or show mixed echogenicity. In addition, necrotic lesions may be fluid-filled and transonic, with or without echoes in the necrotic area.

Focal lesions of 1 cm diameter and over may be demonstrated but metastases may be recognized on the basis of distorted anatomy and/or the presence of a diffuse, abnormal sonographic pattern. Differentiation from benign hepatic lesions such as adenoma, nodular hyperplasia, haemangioma, cirrhosis and even cysts may be difficult at times. Specificity and sensitivity of around 90% may now be achieved. When taken in conjunction with the clinical picture, the demonstration of multiple, solid, hepatic lesions is usually adequate to indicate the presence of metastatic infiltration. If the clinical picture is at variance with the sonographic findings, or if there is doubt as to the nature of the lesions, then percutaneous, fine needle biopsy is indicated and is very conveniently carried out under ultrasound guidance. When splenic metastases are shown then there are invariably hepatic metastases as well, but the reverse situation is not true. Consequently, if a splenic lesion is shown in the absence of hepatic abnormality, a diagnosis of metastasis should be questioned. Sonography can also show abdominal lymph node involvement and the presence of abdominal and pelvic extranodal masses. Renal lesions are readily shown but adrenal deposits can be difficult to detect. Usually, there is little difficulty in the identification of the presence of ascites.

CT can detect hepatic and splenic metastases under 1 cm in size and with modern equipment is more sensitive than scintigraphy and sonography. In the author's experience its specificity is similar to that of ultrasound. The technique of dynamic scanning during bolus enhancement has improved the sensitivity of this technique (Zeman et al 1985). Needle biopsy may still be necessary to obtain histology. CT is a more accurate technique than sonography for the demonstration of retroperitonal structures including the adrenal glands and lymph nodes, but preparation of the patient is required and scanning time, especially if contrast enhancement is utilized, is relatively long.

Hepatic metastases are unlikely to be present in early stage disease, the incidence of detectable metastases in such a situation being about 1% and the question therefore arises as to whether abdominal scanning should be carried out at presentation. As ultrasound examination of the liver, the spleen and the rest of the upper abdomen is easily and quickly carried out, without upset or discomfort to the patient, it is recommended in all cases, including clinically confined cancers with a normal clinical examination. If spread to the axillary or supraclavicular nodes is clinically evident, or if there is hepatosplenomegaly or a mass in the abdomen or pelvis, then sonography is the primary investigation of choice and can be complemented by ultrasound-guided biopsy when necessary. CT examinations can be confined to those cases where there are equivocal findings on ultrasound or where sonography does not confirm clinical opinion. In addition, CT of the upper abdomen may conveniently be carried out as an extension of a thoracic examination.

Sonography or CT may be used to assess response of metastases to therapy. At least a 25% reduction in lesion volume should occur before considering the changes to be significant, as it is difficult to measure the same parameters on consecutive scans. A further difficulty in the assessment of response is that sometimes some lesions can be shown to decrease in size while others become larger in the same patient. Other factors such as the clinical state of the patient and the appearance of metastases elsewhere must be taken into consideration when assessing overall response.

Hepatic angiography has little or no place in the management of metastases from carcinoma of the breast. Together with CT it may assist in the differentiation of haemangioma from metastases. At present, MRI has little to add to sonography or CT in the detection and assessment of abdominal metastatic disease.

Brain

At present, the optimum procedure for the demonstration of cerebral metastases is CT. It has replaced angiographic and encephalographic techniques and for the most part scintigraphy (Grossman et al 1987). It is more accurate and comfortable for the patient and less hazardous, even with the use of intravenous contrast. It should be used only when cerebral metastases are suspected clinically. Most brain metastases from breast carcinoma are solid and isodense but some are hypodense and others hyperdense. Occasional 'cystic', necrotic deposits occur. Lesions are frequently multiple and characteristically have surrounding oedema. Contrast enhancement is necessary to show deposits poorly defined on unenhanced scans. Metastases may show enhancement, ring enhancement or may be delineated as a result of the enhancement of surrounding brain tissue. Dearnley et al (1981) consider that CT may give prognostic information, as in their experience metastases over 5 cm in diameter respond poorly to whole brain irradiation.

MRI has already been shown to be a sensitive, new technique in the assessment of intracranial disease (Bydder 1984) and no doubt will become the method of choice with future development and increased availability. It is also likely to become the most important method of assessment of lesions in the central spinal axis.

Lymph nodes

It may be easy or difficult to judge clinically whether axillary lymph nodes are involved by metastases from breast carcinoma. The same applies for physical methods of assessment.

The axillary nodes may be well seen on properly positioned lateral oblique mammograms (Fig. 5.2). Nodes over 1 cm in diameter are considered to be possibly involved by metastases but node enlargement may be due to hyperplasia. Nodes under 1 cm in diameter are not necessarily free of metastases. Enlarged nodes may be shown mammographically to be composed mainly of fatty tissue but this does not exclude the presence of metastases. When the axillary nodes are shown to contain fine microcalcifications similar to those found in mammary carcinoma then metastatic spread is likely, but this finding is rare. Ultrasound examination is also non-specific and scintigraphic methods have been disappointing be-

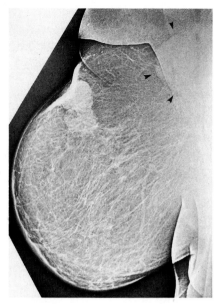

Fig. 5.2 Lateral-oblique negative mode xeromammogram showing a carcinoma and enlarged axillary lymph nodes (black arrow heads).

cause of the large number of lymph nodes and their extensive drainage areas.

Internal mammary lymph node scintigraphy as propounded by Ege (1978) has not found favour as a method of assessment of internal mammary node involvement.

CT is the method of choice for assessment of distant lymph node involvement in the mediastinal or retroperitoneal areas. MRI has been shown to be superior to it in the hilar regions.

Skeletal metastases

Plain radiography and scintigraphy are the modalities usually employed to detect skeletal metastases.

Edelstyn et al (1967) have shown that from 50–70% of the cancellous portion of a bone may be destroyed before the lesion becomes radiographically visible. Radiographic tomography and computed tomography may show lesions which are not visible on plain films. The bones most commonly involved are the pelvis, spine, ribs and upper ends of the femora. The skull is less commonly involved and metastases distal to the elbows and knees are rare.

Consequently, a skeletal survey should include frontal views of the pelvis and upper femora, the chest, thoracic and lumbosacral spine and lateral views of the spine and skull. These may be supplemented by additional views of any symptomatic area in individual cases.

Metastatic lesions may be osteolytic, osteoblastic or may show a mixture of these changes. The commonest finding is an osteolytic lesion, occurring in about 80% of cases. Approximately 10% are osteoblastic and the further 10% are of the mixed variety. A solitary deposit is a rare finding. The lesions are usually circumscribed but generalized diffuse loss, or increase, of bone density can occur.

Pathological fractures are more common in the osteolytic type and callus may readily form. Periosteal reaction is usually an indication of the presence of fracture. Osteoblastic lesions are more readily seen in skeletal radiographs than osteolytic ones. Mixed lesions may be seen as a presenting feature or may occur as an indication that some sites are healing while others are progressing. Furthermore, serial skeletal surveys can show a response to treatment by an increase in density in previous osteolytic lesions or in areas which were originally unsuspected as sites of metastatic involvement. Escape from therapeutic control is not uncommonly demonstrated where previous evidence of repair reverts to bone lysis.

Nowadays the most important application of scintigraphy in breast carcinoma is the assessment of skeletal metastases. Technetium-labelled phosphate compounds are usually used. Normally there is a symmetrical uptake; metastases are usually multiple and asymmetrical in distribution in the appendicular skeleton and uneven in the axial skeleton. The vertebral pedicles are usually prominently affected. Many benign conditions, however, give rise to abnormal scintigrams, with conditions such as Paget's disease, fibrodysplasia, osteomyelitis, spondylarthrosis and vertebral collapse due to osteoporosis giving 'positive' scans.

Skeletal scintigraphy is more sensitive in the demonstration of metastases than conventional radiography. The initial skeletal assessment should be by scintigraphy supplemented by conventional radiography of the abnormal areas to exclude benign disease as the cause of scintigraphic abnormality (Roberts et al 1976). This will not always be necessary as uneven changes with multiple pedicular involvement in the presence of breast malignancy will provide adequate evidence of metastasis. In the presence of a solitary scintigraphic abnormality, radiographic, conventional tomography or CT of the abnormal area are indicated. The use of skeletal CT should be restricted to such problem cases.

Occasionally, radiography may show metastases when scintigraphy is normal. This arises either when there is marked bone destruction or when there is appreciable healing following therapy. Combined radiography and scintigraphy is therefore also of use in the assessment of therapeutic response.

A potential disadvantage of MRI in skeletal investigation is the lack of MR signal from calcifications and cortical bone (Paushter et al 1985). Even so, metastases involving the vertebral column are well demonstrated and their relationship to the cord and theca shown without the use of contrast medium. Another advantage from the point of view of assessment of response to radiotherapy is that MRI can detect the effects of radiation on the vertebrae and can potentially distiguish between radiation changes and recurrent tumour.

ASSESSMENT OF THE PRIMARY LESION

The methods of imaging breast carcinoma include mammography, thermography, diaphanography, ultrasound, CT and MRI.

Mammography

Mammography has been assessed over many years and is a well tried and accurate method of detecting breast cancer. Stewart et al (1969) reported a mammographic accuracy of 93% and an 88% accuracy for clinical examination. They point out that when both modalities are employed then 97% of the cancers are found. This is an important point and in our practice mammography and clinical examination are regarded as complementary methods of examination. A good radiographic technique is essential and full clinical information is necessary for rational interpretation of the images.

Mammography has developed considerably since its introduction in the early 1950s (Leborgne and Dominguez 1951, Leborgne 1953). There are two major techniques in use; xeromammography and film/screen mammography with grid. Both these methods allow penetration of dense breasts and xeromammography also provides enhancement of the edges of breast structures and lesions with highlighting of microcalcifications.

Proper positioning of the patient and adequate compression of the breast allow excellent mammograms to be obtained with a 'mean breast dose' of the order of 3–8 mGy per exposure for a film screen technique using a molybdenum anode and grid. Negative mode xeromammography with tungsten anode and 2.5 mm aluminium filtration gives a 'mean breast dose' of the order of 1.5–2.0 mGy. This level of radiation dosage gives an extremely low risk of development of breast cancer, of the order of one excess cancer per 2 million women examined (Feig 1984). If the death rate for breast cancer is taken to be 50% then the risk would be one excess death per 4 million women examined. According to Pochin (1978) this risk level is similar to the risk of travelling 100 miles by air or 15 miles by car. The incidence of naturally occurring breast cancer according to Seidman (1980) is 800 cases per million women per year at the age of 40 years and 2500 cases per million women per year at 65 years, so that the risk of breast cancer induction as a result of a properly executed mammographic examination is minimal. Arguments for the use of other modalities in breast cancer screening on the basis of radiation carcinogenesis are unacceptable.

Thermography

This method involves the detection and recording of the infrared radiation emitted by the breasts. The apparatus records the naturally emitted radiation and consequently the technique is harmless. This is its most important feature and only advantage. The increased vascularity, increased heat emission from the nipple and circumscribed areas seen in breasts affected by cancer may be found in benign disease and even in clinically and mammographically normal breasts. The method is non-specific and a diagnosis of breast cancer cannot be made with certainty (Evans & Gravelle 1973). Clark et al (1978), however, maintained that it is useful as an indicator of those women likely to develop breast cancer. They believe that a positive thermogram, even with normal clinical and mammographic examinations, indicates a high risk of future development of breast cancer. Approximately 20% of women screened show an abnormal thermogram but only a small percentage of these develop cancer subsequently. It is unlikely to be a significant risk indicator.

Diaphanography

There has been a resurgence of interest in transillumination of the breast. Halliday and Blamey (1981) reported a sensitivity of 75% for the detection of breast cancer. Bartrum & Crow (1984) point out that the method has a poor sensitivity for cancers under 1 cm and there is difficulty in demonstrating lesions located more than 2 cm beneath the skin surface. It is unable to show microcalcifications. Tucker (1986) maintains that the method is too slow for a screening procedure; at present it should be used only as an adjunct to clinical examination.

Ultrasound

Practically all reports on the use of ultrasound in breast examination stress that it can readily differentiate between cystic and solid lesions. Jellins et al (1977) reported a sensitivity of 95% for the detection of cysts. In clinical practice this ability is not important: if the lesion is palpable then needle aspiration will not only prove the nature of the lesion but will treat the cyst as well. Impalpable smooth rounded lesions on mammography are most likely to be small cysts or fibroadenomata. The ultrasonic demonstration that the lesion is a cyst is of little consequence. In addition it is not logistically possible to biopsy every solid lesion detected by ultrasound. If there are features of malignancy, then of course biopsy is indicated. However, so called 'fibrocystic disease' may show ultrasonic features of malignancy (Fig. 5.3). These signs include a well defined, highly echogenic, anterior margin to the lesion, which is often irregular. The lesion is usually hypoechoic but increased echogenicity occurs with increased

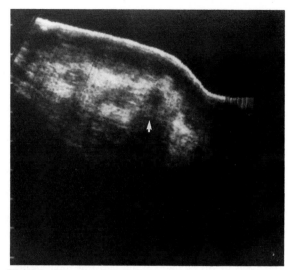

Fig. 5.3 Ultrasound of the breast. Nodular breast due to 'fibrocystic disease'. The arrowed lesion shows the features of malignancy.

sonar intensity. Attenuation of the ultrasonic beam usually gives a posterior shadow. Skin thickening and disruption of architecture may be shown and sometimes an increased 'reactive' perifocal echogenicity.

Well defined, smooth, circumscribed cancers may simulate benign lesions with distal enhancement and a homogeneous echo pattern (Fig. 5.4).

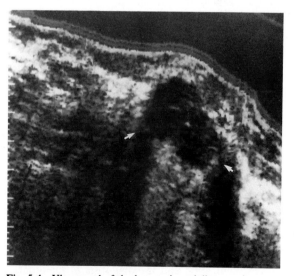

Fig. 5.4 Ultrasound of the breast. A medullary carcinoma (arrow) showing posterior enhancement and lateral shadowing — benign features.

Sickles et al (1983) have compared mammography with ultrasound in symptomatic and clinically well women. Of the 64 histologically confirmed cancers 97% were detected by mammography, sonar detecting only 58%. Of the tumours smaller than 1 cm only 8% were detected by sonar. Many reports state that ultrasound of the breast is of value in the examination of the radiologically dense breast. Most of these have been series utilizing suboptimal mammographic technique i.e. without grid facilities or without xeromammography. They do not give a true assessment of the relative values of ultrasound and mammography.

The disadvantages of sonar are that it does not show fine microcalcifications, lesions less than 1 cm are very difficult to demonstrate whatever the type of breast, and some cancers have benign ultrasonic features. In addition, multiple scans or a videotape of each breast have to be examined.

Sonography could be useful as a complementary method to mammography when there is a lesion with equivocal mammographic appearances. In such a situation it could be used for guided needle aspiration biopsy. Alternatively the needle could be employed to introduce a convenient dye for localization at open biopsy.

Computed tomography

Breast cancers can be shown by CT (Fig. 5.5) either using body scanners or dedicated breast scanners. Sensitivities of 94% have been reported by Chang et al (1977) but false positive results occur due to inflammatory disease and fibroadenoma. The technique does not show fine microcalcifications, is time consuming, involves radiation to other parts of the thorax, requires intravenous contrast and has a relatively high cost. It has a possible use in the detection of a primary tumour in a clinically and mammographically normal breast when axillary node metastases are present.

Magnetic resonance imaging

MRI has little to offer at present. It cannot detect microcalcification and the diagnosis of malignancy is made on the basis of morphological change and the configuration of the lesion. This can be done

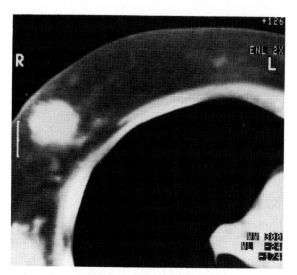

Fig. 5.5 CT of right breast showing a carcinoma with skin thickening. Enlarged axillary nodes are present.

more easily, more clearly, at less expense and quite safely by means of mammography.

MAMMOGRAPHY

Well performed mammography is the method of choice in the physical examination of the breast. Both xeromammography and film screen, grid mammography are acceptable. Magnification mammography has been advocated by Sickles (1980). Devotees state that more numerous calcifications are seen on magnification, but this does not necessarily make the diagnosis any easier or more certain. Similarly, the margins of small mass lesions are said to be more clearly shown but again this may not contribute to the diagnosis and the use of a simple magnifying glass gives the same information. More importantly, the technique quadruples the radiation dose.

Mammography is indicated in the following situations:

1. In the presence of a palpable lesion whether this is clinically malignant, benign or of uncertain nature. Mammography may confirm or refute the clinical diagnosis and may show unsuspected carcinomas.

2. In the investigation of breast pain especially if this is a persistent, non-periodic or unusual type of pain.

3. The diagnosis of the underlying cause of nipple discharge, particularly if the discharge is from one duct. Ductography can be additionally useful in this situation.

4. The pretreatment assessment and follow-up of patients undergoing radiotherapy or chemotherapy. It gives a more accurate measurement of response of the primary tumour than does clinical assessment (Fig. 5.6). However, following radiotherapy to the breast the mammographic changes can be confusing. There is inevitable hypervascularity and skin thickening with increased prominence of trabeculae so that it is not possible to be certain whether these features are those of further malignant change or due to radiotherapy. Skin thickening due to radiotherapy may take up to one year to regress, and any increase after this period is an indication of progression, infection, or (less likely) fat necrosis. In our experience,

microcalcifications may disappear or occur for the first time following radiotherapy and are not necessarily an indication of failure of treatment or recurrence of tumour. Re-examination will be necessary in such a situation – after three months initially and, if there is no change, then six months later. If there is still no change then annual mammography should be carried out thereafter. Coarse calcification occurs in areas of fat necrosis following radiotherapy (Fig. 5.7). The form of the tumour mass may change following radical or even palliative radiotherapy but the persistence of a mass does not necessarily indicate continuing malignancy. Serial examination gives an assessment of the response of the breast lesion to palliative radiotherapy. The mammograms provide an excellent record for future review.

5. In the management of the locally invasive or non-invasive carcinoma treated by 'lumpectomy' or excision of an area of microcalcification. In such cases it is advisable to carry out mammography two months after the operation to obtain a baseline mammogram for future reference. This will show any postoperative distortion liable to remain.

6. Management of the contralateral breast following mastectomy or other therapy. There is an increased incidence of carcinoma in the contralateral breast, which may be by cross-lymphatic spread or the development of a second primary. Cross-lymphatic spread may be shown on craniocaudal mammograms by skin thickening over the medial aspect of the contralateral breast, and this may be the first indication of tumour spread. Stewart et al (1969) reported a series of contralateral tumours in 384 patients over a period of five years: 39 were detected, a 10% incidence, and 11 of these 39 cancers were unsuspected clinically.

7. When a suspicious mammographic lesion is impalpable radiological localization of the lesion is necessary.

8. Demonstration of an impalpable primary breast malignancy presenting with metastases (Fig. 5.8).

9. Mammography has been shown to be an accurate method of population screening for breast cancer (Lundgren & Jakobssan 1976). Mammography often shows specific characteristic features which enable a diagnosis of benign or malignant

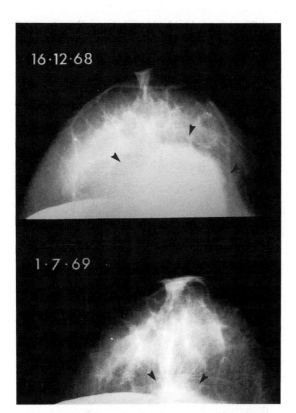

Fig. 5.6 Mammogram showing the response of carcinoma to chemotherapy. The tumour has changed from a large nodular lesion (upper) to a small spiculated lesion (lower).

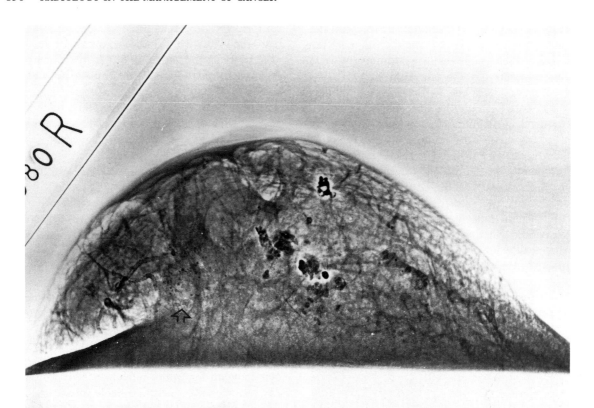

Fig. 5.7 Positive mode xeromammogram following radiotherapy. Calcifications are shown as black areas. There is coarse calcification due to fat necrosis and fine tumour calcifications (arrow).

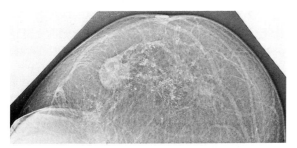

Fig. 5.8 Negative mode xeromammogram showing an impalpable carcinoma. There is a mass and microcalcifications (white dots). The patient presented with low back pain due to metastatic disease.

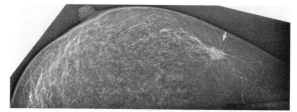

Fig. 5.9 Negative mode xerogram showing a spiculated carcinoma clinically throught to be a fibroadenoma.

disease to be made, and can lead to earlier diagnosis of breast cancer.

Unrecognized cancers

These are either palpable tumours, misdiagnosed clinically as benign, or are impalpable. Four groups may be considered:

1. A palpable lesion is present which is clinically benign, or of uncertain significance. Mammography is of value in three ways:

a. It may show conclusively that the lesion is malignant. Figure 5.9 is a xerogram of a 40-year-old women with a palpable, mobile lesion which was clinically thought to be fibroadenoma. It is clearly a carcinoma. The lesion in Figure 5.10 was thought clinically to be a lipoma, but is in fact a carcinoma with a surrounding area of distorted fat – a radiological psuedolipoma.

b. It may confirm the benign nature of the palpable lesion but identify a malignant lesion in the same or contralateral breast. The 39-year-old patient whose mammogram is shown in Figure 5.11 complained of lumps in the breast which were clinically consistent with fibroadenosis. No mammographic abnormality is demonstrable on the right side but a posterior tumour is seen on the left, which is infiltrating the pectoral muscles.

c. Mammography may show that the lesion is a carcinoma and there may be an impalpable,

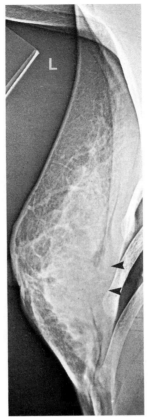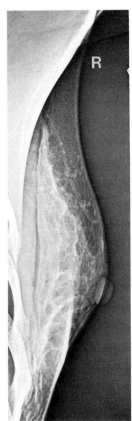

Fig. 5.11 Negative mode xeromammograms. These breasts show a DY pattern. There is a posterior infiltrating carcinoma on the left side (arrowed).

simultaneous cancer in the contralateral breast or multiple lesions in the same breast. Figure 5.12 is of a patient who had a lumpectomy for carcinoma without prior mammography. The mammogram taken six

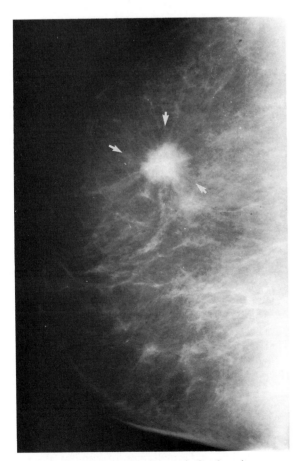

Fig. 5.10 Mammogram showing a spiculated carcinoma with surrounding 'pseudolipoma' (arrowed).

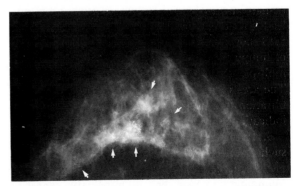

Fig. 5.12 Film screen mammogram. There are multiple impalpable malignant lesions (arrowed).

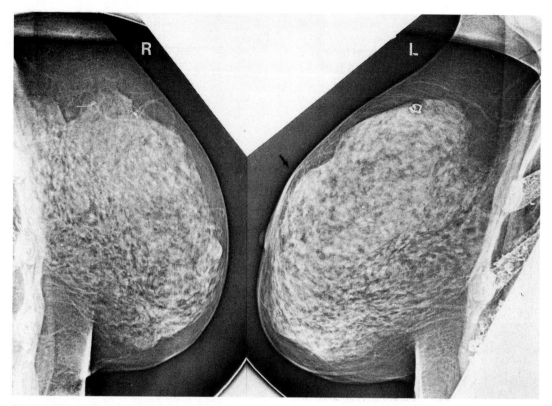

Fig. 5.13 Breasts showing prominent ducts (P2 grade). Impalpable carcinoma of left breast. Localized skin thickening (arrowed) and increased parenchymal density.

weeks later demonstrated several foci of malignant disease which must have been present at the time of excision of the clinically diagnosed breast mass.

2. Multiple palpable lesions are present, often bilaterally. Unsuspected malignancies may occur in such lumpy breasts in the absence of a dominant mass. Mammography can distinguish between benign and malignant lesions in such cases and lead to earlier diagnosis of malignancy. Figure 5.13 shows the xerograms of a woman complaining of lumpy breasts. There are prominent ducts and multiple small rounded lesions in both breasts. The area of skin thickening and subcutaneous infiltration above the left nipple were the only indications of malignancy.

3. In this group the patient has vague symptoms such as breast discomfort or pain, eczema or nipple discharge, and there is no palpable lesion. Mammography may show an impalpable cancer in three types of cases:

a. Intraduct carcinoma may be shown due to the presence of highly characteristic microcalcification occurring in a defined area of the breast. Figure 5.14 is the xerogram of a woman presenting with breast discomfort, showing the presence of a wedge-shaped area of microcalcification which is characteristic of intraduct carcinoma.

b. The tumour is impalpable because it is small and the breast large. 5 mm tumours can readily be shown, especially in fatty breasts where radiographic contrast is enhanced. The mammogram in Figure 5.15 is of a patient presenting with localized breast pain. The small spiculated carcinoma was not palpable.

c. Mammography may show a combination of breast distortion and microcalcification (Fig. 5.16).

Impalpability and small size of tumour do not necessarily indicate 'early' breast cancer. Wide-

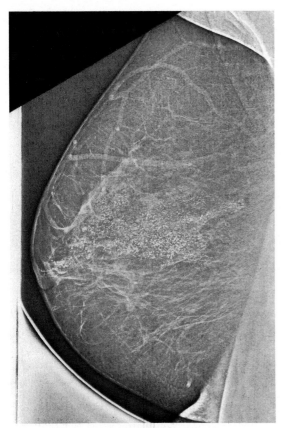

Fig. 5.14 Extensive microcalcification indicating intraduct carcinoma. No clinical abnormality.

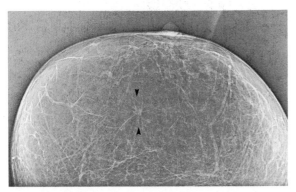

Fig. 5.15 Small spiculated carcinoma in a large fatty breast. N1 type of breast.

spread metastases may be present with occult breast cancer.

Mammography is a very sensitive method of demonstrating skin thickening and may do so when it is not clinically evident (Figs 5.13 and 5.16). We have measured skin oedema in a series of patients with non-inflammatory breast cancer. The mean skin oedema was obtained by taking the mean of five measurements from separate areas on the mammogram – the superior, inferior, medial and lateral areas and the areola – and subtracting the corresponding measurements from the normal breast (Fig. 5.17) (Shukla et al 1984). Oedema of over 0.25 mm was considered appreciable and its prevalence was found to be 70% for cancers less than 1 cm and 100% for cancers over 3 cm in diameter. This measure of oedema correlated significantly with tumour size and node status. With tumours less than 2 cm in diameter skin oedema indicated a poor prognosis, but with tumours greater than 5 cm and without oedema the prognosis was relatively good. Patients who developed recurrence had significantly greater oedema originally. The degree of oedema was a more accurate predictor of recurrence than lymph node status, tumour size or tumour stage. The degree of oedema and tumour size are measurements available preoperatively, and they may be combined to provide a means of assessing prognosis before deciding which treatment is appropriate in an individual case. Treatment failure occurred often in patients with skin oedema greater than 2 mm and invariably if oedema was greater than 4 mm.

4. This final group is composed of clinically well women. These tumours can only be discovered by screening programmes and present a problem in management. A localization procedure is necessary to guide the surgeon to the appropriate area and to ascertain that the pathologist is presented with the tissue containing the radiological abnormality. There are several techniques of localization (Feig 1983): it is of little consequence which method is employed as long as it is reliable. We favour the 'double dye' technique described and discussed by Preece et al (1977). The localization can be carried out at least 24 h prior to biopsy but is conveniently done 3–4 h before.

The patient is brought to the X-ray Department and previous mammograms are inspected by the radiologist. The position of the abnormality within the breast is estimated. A mixture of 1 ml of

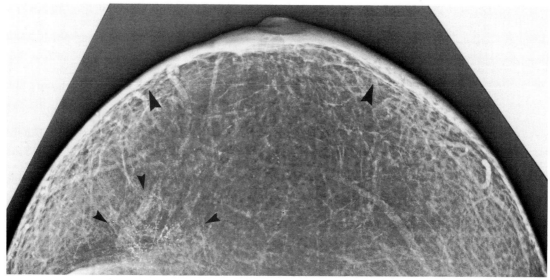

Fig. 5.16 Paget's disease of the nipple. No clinical evidence of skin thickening or malignancy. Both features are arrowed.

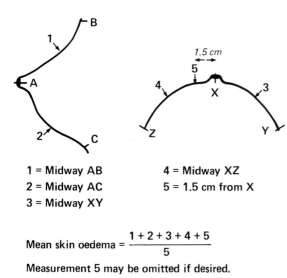

1 = Midway AB
2 = Midway AC
3 = Midway XY
4 = Midway XZ
5 = 1.5 cm from X

$$\text{Mean skin oedema} = \frac{1 + 2 + 3 + 4 + 5}{5}$$

Measurement 5 may be omitted if desired.

Fig. 5.17 Method of measurement of skin thickening.

sodium diatrizoate solution with 2 drops of Patent Blue Violet dye is prepared and drawn into a 2 ml syringe. The patient is placed on the X-ray table in the appropriate lateral-oblique position. The syringe with the mixture is attached to a needle which is then inserted by the radiologist to the estimated position of the radiological abnormality. 0.5 ml of the mixture is then injected and

craniocaudal and lateral-oblique views taken. The distance of the radio-opaque contrast from the radiological abnormality can then be measured (Fig. 5.18). This is the same distance as the visible blue dye is from the abnormal area. The images with their recorded measurements are sent with the patient. The surgeon displays the dye at operation and removes the appropriate tissue. The next vital step is to X-ray the specimen (Fig. 5.19) to ensure that the radiological abnormality has been

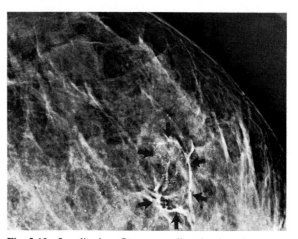

Fig. 5.18 Localization. Contrast medium has been injected into the area containing the microcalcifications (arrowed).

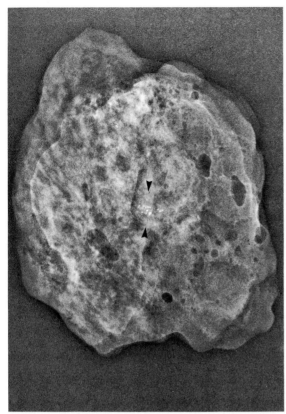

Fig. 5.19 X-ray of breast biopsy confirming the presence of microcalcifications (arrowed).

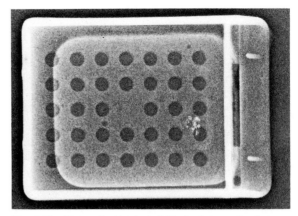

Fig. 5.20 X-ray of a histological block of tissue showing microcalcifications.

5.21): nowadays this is a medically and legally unacceptable procedure. Abandonment of frozen section analysis is due to the high incidence of sclerosing adenosis as a cause for these minimal radiological lesions and the difficulty in distinguishing this pathological entity from carcinoma on frozen section. In addition, distinguishing between carcinoma-in-situ and early invasive changes is more readily achieved on paraffin section and this decides whether conservative surgical methods or mastectomy will be employed.

removed. The specimen may then be further divided to isolate the abnormal area.

The specimen should not be examined by frozen section. Either immediate or delayed paraffin section examination is essential and the patient should be advised accordingly. If immediate paraffin section examination is available then the patient may be advised that if the biopsy is positive the surgeon may proceed to more definitive surgery. If immediate paraffin section is not available then further surgery should be postponed until the result of paraffin section is available. Frozen section is not an acceptable technique in this particular situation. Even the interpretation of paraffin sections may be difficult or uncertain in this type of case.

Radiography of the pathologist's tissue blocks (Fig. 5.20) can indicate the area of interest. What should not be done is surgical removal of the breast before localized biopsy and histological examination of the radiological abnormality (Fig.

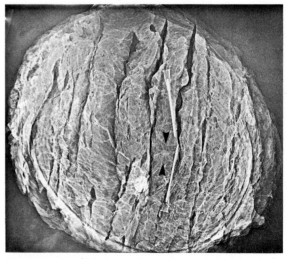

Fig. 5.21 X-ray of mastectomy specimen: the impalpable cancer is arrowed. See also Figure 5.15. Mastectomy without prior localization and histological examination is unacceptable.

Ductography and cystography

These can be useful additional techniques in suitable circumstances.

Following preliminary mammography and inspection of the films ductography is carried out if no definite diagnosis can be made. The nipple is cleaned and the affected duct dilated by means of a probe. This is replaced by a 20 gauge cannula fitted to a 2 or 5 ml syringe containing bubble free water-soluble contrast medium. 25% sodium diatrizoate solution is used for mammography but is diluted with 1 in 3 parts water if xeroradiography is being used. The contrast is injected until the patient experiences a feeling of fullness (this is usually 0.5–3.0 ml). The cannula is withdrawn and the duct sealed with adhesive tape. Craniocaudal and lateral-oblique views are then taken. The only complication in practice is penetration of the duct wall with tissue injection. This is accompanied by pain and the examination should be terminated and repeated after 1–2 weeks. Contraindications include breast and nipple infection and possible iodine sensitivity.

When the only presenting feature is nipple discharge, ductography should be considered. This is especially true when the discharge is from one duct orifice. If more than one duct is discharging the underlying process is likely to be benign, usually duct ectasia or fibroadenosis. If, however, one of these ducts shows a different colour of discharge then that particular duct should be injected. The colour of the discharge may give an indication of the underlying cause, e.g. a milky discharge is usually postlactational or due to duct ectasia but this condition can also give a clear serous discharge or bloodstaining. A black, brownish or green discharge is commonly due to fibroadenosis with cysts but may be due to altered blood. A bloody discharge is most commonly due to papilloma but may indicate duct ectasia, granuloma or carcinoma. An important point to remember is that malignancy may be present with any kind of discharge and may quite frequently be the cause of a profuse watery discharge from one duct. The fluid should be cytologically examined for red blood cells, leukocytes, benign and malignant cells.

Figure 5.22 shows the xerograms of a 51-year-

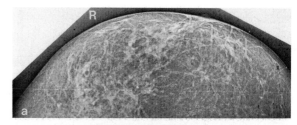
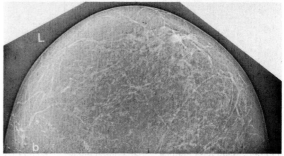
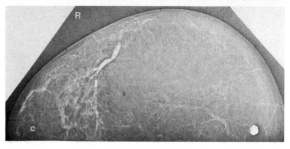

Fig. 5.22 The xerograms (a) and (b) show unilateral ductal enlargement. (c) The ductogram shows extensive proximal intraduct carcinoma.

old woman presenting with copious clear discharge from one duct in the right breast. The left breast is normal but there are dilated ducts in the right breast which were clinically palpable and considered to represent duct ectasia. However, duct ectasia is a bilateral condition. Ductography shows multiple filling defects within the ducts, irregularities of the ducts and periductal opacities. The appearances are those of intraductal carcinoma.

Aspiration of a cyst is an excellent method of confirming the diagnosis and treating the patient. Mammography should be carried out as well especially if the cyst refills (Fig. 5.23) as this may indicate the presence of a neoplasm close to the cyst. If a bloodstained aspirate is obtained pneumocystography should be considered. In this situation, and in repeat filling of a cyst following

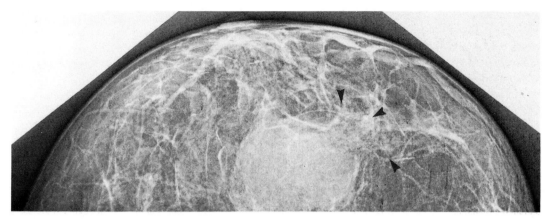

Fig. 5.23 A cyst with adjacent carcinoma arrowed.

aspiration, cytological examination of the aspirate is indicated as well as cystography. The possible causes of a bloodstained aspirate are intracystic papilloma or carcinoma. Haematoma is also a possibility in the presence of trauma, anticoagulant overdosage or blood dyscrasia. The procedure is easily carried out: the skin is cleaned and the needle inserted, the cyst is completely aspirated and an equal volume of air introduced. The breast is then radiographed. The aspirated fluid is sent for bacteriological and cytological examination. Figure 5.24 illustrates the pneumocystogram of a patient with a solitary palpable cystic lesion – posterior lesion. The aspirate was bloodstained. Pneumocystography showed a dominant cystic lesion posteriorly with a broad-based solid lesion with an extra cystic extension. The small anterior intracystic papilliferous lesion showed microcalcifications and was connected to the dominant lesion.

The technique is relatively free of complications. Infection occurs infrequently, usually due to examination of an infected cyst rather than the introduction of infection. Haematoma is rare. Contraindications are the presence of skin infection, blood dyscrasia or anticoagulant therapy.

Screening

There can be no doubt that the detection of mammary cancer is more accurate by means of

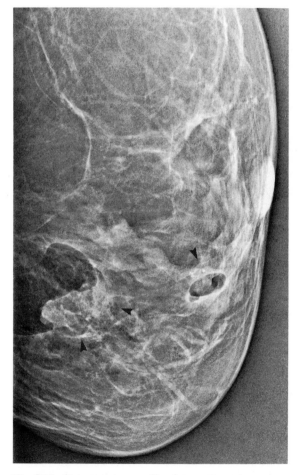

Fig. 5.24 Pneumocystogram. Two intracystic carcinomas (arrowed). Only the posterior cyst was insufflated.

mammography than by clinical examination. However, a palpable lesion which is clinically suspicious of malignancy, even though mammographically benign or not even demonstrated, should be biopsied. Many suspicious lesions are shown on mammography which are not clinically detectable and a percentage of these are 'early' breast carcinomas. It is this situation that has led to the insistence that generalized mammographic screening for breast cancer should be carried out.

The available facts do not point unequivocally towards the necessity for mass mammographic screening. The results of many breast screening programmes have been reported in the literature but very few of these have been adequate, controlled and randomized. In the presentation of results few have acknowledged the misleading effects of lead-time bias and length bias. In addition, women attending a screening programme are those most likely to attend their own general practitioner in the event of any abnormality presenting. A further consideration is that the demonstration of malignancy on microscopy does not necessarily indicate a malignant biological outcome. Skrabanek (1985) has forcefully stated his opposition to breast cancer screening by mammography.

There are two randomized controlled studies of the effect of mammographic screening on breast cancer mortality: one is by Tabar et al (1985) in Sweden and the other by Shapiro et al (1982) in America. In this latter trial the results at 14 years are available. After 10 years the mortality due to breast cancer in the screened group was about 30% less than the mortality in the non-screened group. Arithmetic gains due to screening were maintained at the fourteenth year but there was a decline in relative gains. With the longer follow-up periods, cumulative survival rates in the group screened by mammography alone decreased more rapidly than survival rates in the other subgroups. The exact extent of benefit in the mammographically screened group is difficult to calculate accurately but may be of the order of two years prolongation of life. The Swedish trial reported by Tabar confirms the early results of the American trial.

The Shapiro study, or 'HIP' (Hospital Insurance Plan) as it is popularly known, has been analysed independently by Aron and Prorok (1986). They point out that the overall mortality in the study group (i.e. the screened group) was 6.7% as compared with 6.8% in the control group (i.e. the unscreened group). From Shapiro's assessment it would appear that the mortality was 704 per 10 000 women per 10 years in the screened group and 710 per 10 000 women per 10 years in the non-screened group so that the 30% reduction in mortality in the 'HIP' survey is the difference between 5 deaths per 1000 women per year in the screened group and 7 deaths per 1000 women per year in the non-screened group (Skrabanek 1987).

The recommendations of the Forrest report on breast cancer screening (1986) are largely based on the 'HIP' study and the Swedish study. The results of both of these studies are similar and the main conclusions have been stated above. The Swedish survey employed a modern and more sophisticated mammographic technique but achieved no significant improvement in reduction in mortality rate in the screened population. Neither study showed a statistically significant reduction in mortality in screened women under the age of 50 years. This is the reason for the Forrest recommendation that mammographic screening should be restricted to women over 50 years of age and 50–64 year age group was recommended for screening. Swedish results showed reduced compliance over the age of 64 years: screening in the over 64s would be carried out on request. The general feeling, however, amongst radiologists committed to breast cancer screening by mammography is that screening should also be offered to the 40–49 year age group even though there is no statistical proof of its value in this group.

The frequency of screening by mammography is another controversial and unresolved matter. On the basis that there was in the Swedish study 'a substantial benefit in women aged 50 and over with a screening interval of nearly three years' the Forrest committee recommended that the screening interval should be three years. Many screeners will insist that this interval is too long, but no statistical proof is available to the contrary. However, sound, significant statistical proof is difficult to find for many aspects of breast cancer screening.

The report also recommended that single lateral-oblique view mammography should be the method of choice in screening. This recommendation was also based on Swedish experience as reported by Lundgren and Jakobssan (1976) and Tabar et al (1985). However, Sickles et al (1986) pointed out that by using two-view mammography instead of one-view mammography, eight extra cancers would be detected per 10 000 women, i.e. in the number of women expected to be examined in a single basic screening unit per year in the UK. In addition, fewer women would be recalled for additional views — amounting to 7% in two-view mammography as against 26% in the single-view group. This would lead to reduced psychological trauma to the individual and reduced cost.

Two-view mammography would lead to a higher cancer detection rate and lower recall rate. It would only need to be used for the initial 'prevalent' screen. At interval, single-view screening, previous films would be available for comparison.

Whether a national breast cancer screening programme will lead to a statistically significant reduction in breast cancer mortality remains to be seen. This result cannot be assumed on the basis of the statistical knowledge presently available.

Who should receive mammography? In general any woman who develops a palpable lesion, becomes symptomatic or is to have breast surgery, certainly if over 35 years of age and some would maintain at any age in these situations. The devotees of breast cancer screening maintain that all women over 50 should be screened annually. Some would advise a 'base-line' mammogram at 35 years of age and thereafter regular biennial or triennial screens up to the age of 50 years depending on the mammographic pattern or the presence or absence of high risk factors in the individual. The epidemiological factors usually considered to be associated with high risk of development of breast cancer are nulliparity, low parity, late age at birth of first child, early menarche and a family history of breast cancer in close relatives. Wolfe (1974, 1976) has claimed that the risk of developing breast cancer can be predicted from mammographic patterns. Four main patterns are described as follows:

1. N1 – Normal:low density of parenchyma with large fat content (Fig. 5.15);
2. P1 – Ductal prominence involving less than a quarter of the breast;
3. P2 – Ductal prominence involving more than a quarter of the breast and often with a nodular component (Fig. 5.13);
4. DY – Increased density of the parenchyma with or without nodular areas (Fig. 5.11).

The two high risk groups are the DY and P2 groups. Wolfe found that the highest risk group, the DY group, contained 37 times the number of breast cancers than the N1 group, the lowest risk group. In a series of 5000 mammograms of women over 30, 97% of the cancers were in 57% of this population, that is the DY and P2 groups. The majority of subsequent reports have confirmed his results but the absolute risk to women with DY and P2 patterns has been found to be much smaller than originally described and in some instances no association between breast patterns and risk has been found (Boyd et al 1984). In addition Gravelle et al (1980, 1986) have shown that variables such as age, weight, age at birth of first child and parity are highly related to the proportion of high risk mammographic patterns found in a population. In their prospective study Gravelle and colleagues found that women with DY and P2 grades had approximately four times the risk of developing cancer compared with those with N1 or P1 grades. Their results suggest that Wolfe grades in conjunction with anamnestic variables may indicate groups of potential breast cancer cases.

Whether screening for breast cancer by means of mammography significantly improves prognosis is still uncertain. There are two opposing views: one view is that breast screening is beneficial and a worthwhile procedure, while the opposing view is that the necessity for screening is an indication of the failure of current therapeutic options and that the continued search for the cause of breast cancer is the rational approach to the problem.

REFERENCES

Aron J L, Prorok P C 1986 An analysis of the age mortality effect in a breast cancer screening study. International Journal of Epidemiology 15: 36–43

Bartrum R J, Crow H C 1984 Transillumination light scanning to diagnose breast cancer. American Journal of Roentgenology 142: 409–414

Boyd N F, O'Sullivan B, Fishell E, Simor I, Cooke G 1984 Mammographic patterns and breast cancer risk: methodological standards and contradictory results. Journal of the National Cancer Institute 72: 1253–1259

Bydder G M 1984 Magnetic resonance imaging of the brain. Radiological Clinics of North America 22: 779–793

Chang C H, Sibala J L, Gallagher J H 1977 Computed tomography of the breast: a preliminary report. Radiology 124: 827–829

Chiles C, Ravin C E 1985 Intrathoracic metastasis from an extrathoracic malignancy. Radiological Clinics of North America 23: 427–438

Clark R M, Rideout D F, Chart P L 1978 Thermography of the breast: experiences in diagnosis and follow-up in a cancer treatment centre. Acta Thermographica 3: 155–161

Cutler S J, Asire A J, Taylor S G 1969 Classification of patients with disseminated cancer of the breast. Cancer 24: 861–869

Dearnley D P, Kingsley D P E, Hesband J E, Horwich A, Coombes R C 1981 The rôle of computed tomography of the brain in the investigation of breast cancer patients with suspected intracranial metastases. Clinical Radiology 32: 375–382

Edelstyn G A, Gillespie A J, Grebell F S 1967 The radiological demonstration of osseous metastases. Experimental observations. Clinical Radiology 18: 158–162

Ege G N 1978 Internal mammary lymphoscintigraphy: a rational adjunct to the staging and management of breast cancer. Clinical Radiology 29: 453–456

Evans K T, Gravelle I H 1973 Mammography, thermography and ultrasonography in breast disease. Radiology in clinical diagnosis series, Butterworth, London

Feig S A 1983 Biopsy localization of non-palpable breast lesions. In: Wolfe J N (ed) Xeroradiography of the breast, 2nd edn, Charles C Thomas, Springfield, Illinois, pp 648–671

Feig S A 1984 Hypothetical breast cancer risk from mammography. In: Brunner S, Langfeldt B, Anderson P E (eds) Recent results in cancer research. Early detection of breast cancer, Springer-Verlag, Berlin, pp 1–10

Forrest P 1986 Breast cancer screening. Report to the Health Ministers of England, Wales, Scotland and Northern Ireland, HMSO, London

Gravelle I H 1982 Diagnostic imaging in breast cancer. Clinics in Oncology 1: 795–820

Gravelle I H, Bulstrode J C, Wang D Y, Hayward J L 1980 The relation between radiographic features and determinants of risk of breast cancer. British Journal of Radiology 53: 107–113

Gravelle I H, Bulstrode J C, Bulbrook R D, Wang D Y, Allen D, Hayward J L 1986 A prospective study of mammographic parenchymal patterns and risk of breast cancer. British Journal of Radiology 59: 487–491

Grossman Z D, Chew F S, Ellis D A, Brigham S C 1987 Cerebral metastases. The clinician's guide to diagnostic imaging, 2nd edn, Raven Press, New York, 27: 132–133

Halliday H W, Blamey R W 1981 Breast transillumination using the sinus diaphanograph. British Medical Journal 283: 411–413

Jellins J, Reeve T S, Kossof G 1977 Detection and classification of liquid filled masses in the breast by grey-scale echography. Radiology 125: 205–212

Leborgne R A 1953 The breast in Roentgen diagnosis. Constable, London

Leborgne R A, Dominguez C M 1951 Diagnosis of tumours of the breast by simple roentgenography. American Journal of Roentgenology 65: 1–11

Lundgren B, Jakobssan S 1976 Single view mammography. A simple and effective approach to breast cancer screening. Cancer 28: 1124–29

McClees E C, Gedgaudas-McClees R K 1984 Screening for diffuse and focal liver disease. The case for hepatic scintigraphy. Journal of Clinical Ultrasound 12: 75–81

Meyer J E, Munzenrider J E 1981 Computed tomographic demonstration of internal mammary lymph node metastasis in patients with locally recurrent breast carcinoma. Radiology 139: 661–663

Paushter D M, Modic M T, Masaryk J J 1985 Magnetic resonance of the spine: applications and limitations. Radiological Clinics of North America 23: 551–562

Pochin E E 1978 Why be quantitative about radiation risk estimates? The Lauriston S Taylor lecture series in radiation protection and measurements, National Council on Radiation Protection and Measurements

Preece P E, Gravelle I H, Hughes L E, Baum M, Fortt R W, Leopold J G 1977 The operative management of subclinical breast cancer. Clinical Oncology 3: 165–169

Roberts J G, Bligh A S, Gravelle I H, Leach K G, Baum M, Hughes L E 1976 Evaluation of radiography and isotopic scintigraphy for detecting skeletal metastases in breast cancer. Lancet 1: 237–239

Salyer W R, Eggleston J C, Erozan Y S 1975 Efficacy of pleural needle biopsy and pleural fluid cytopathology in the diagnosis of malignant neoplasm involving the pleura. Chest 67: 536–539

Seidman H 1980 Statistical and epidemiological data on cancer of the breast. American Cancer Society, New York

Shapiro S, Venet W, Strax P, Venet L, Roeser R 1982 Ten to fourteen year effect of screening on breast cancer mortality. Journal of the National Cancer Institute 69: 349–355

Shukla H S, Gravelle I H, Hughes L E, Newcombe R G, Williams S 1984 Mammary skin oedema: a new prognostic indicator for breast cancer. British Medical Journal 288: 1338–1341

Sickles E A 1980 Further experience with microfocal spot magnification radiography in the assessment of clustered breast microcalcifications. Radiology 131: 599–607

Sickles E A, Filly R A, Callen P W 1983 Breast cancer detection with sonography and mammography: comparison using state-of-the-art equipment. American Journal of Roentgenology 140: 843–845

Sickles E A, Weber W N, Galvin H B, Ominsky S H, Sollitto R A 1986 Baseline screening mammography. One vs two views per breast. American Journal of Roentgenology 147: 1149–1153

Skrabanek P 1985 False premises and false promises of breast cancer screening. Lancet 2: 316–319

Skrabanek P 1987 Personal communication

Stewart H J, Gravelle I H, Apsimon H T 1969 Five years' experience with mammography. British Journal of Surgery 56: 341–344

Tabar L, Gad A, Holmberg L H et al 1985 Reduction in mortality from breast cancer after mass screening with mammography. Lancet 1: 829–832

Tucker A K 1986 Personal communication
Wolfe J N 1974 Analysis of 462 breast carcinomas.
  American Journal of Roentgenology 121: 846–849
Wolfe J N 1976 Risk for breast cancer development
  determined by mammographic parenchymal pattern.

Cancer 37: 2486–2492
Zeman R K, Pauser D M, Scheibler M L, Choyke P L,
  Jaffe M H, Clark L R 1985 Hepatic imaging: current
  status. Radiological Clinics of North America 23: 473–487

6. The oesophagus, stomach and small intestine

P. J. Cadman   D. J. Nolan

THE OESOPHAGUS

Benign neoplasms

Benign neoplasms account for less than 10% of all surgically resected oesophageal neoplasms. The majority of these are leiomyomas; other rare neoplasms include papillomas, neurofibromas (Schatzki and Hawes 1942) and haemangiomas.

Leiomyomas

Leiomyomas have a 3:1 male to female ratio and are most often found in the 20–50 year age group. Approximately half the lesions are found in the distal third of the oesophagus, one-third in the middle third, and one-sixth in the upper third (Johnston et al 1953): they usually measure 2–3 cm in diameter when diagnosed. Presenting symptoms include dysphagia and retrosternal chest pain although 50% of lesions are detected incidentally.

Most leiomyomas are detectable on barium studies (Johnston et al 1953) as an intramural lesion projecting into the oesophageal lumen, at right angles to the oesophageal wall. The surface is smooth and, unlike leiomyomas elsewhere in the gastrointestinal tract, the overlying mucosa is nearly always intact and ulceration is uncommon. About 15% are detectable as a mediastinal mass on plain radiographs (Johnston et al 1953).

Endoscopy usually confirms the intramural location of the lesion but superficial biopsy is often unhelpful as the normal squamous oesophageal epithelium is preserved (Johnston et al 1953).

Other benign oesophageal lesions

True oesophageal papillomas are very rare and many of the earlier reports in the literature are disputed (Gowing 1962). Proven benign lesions are usually found on the posterior aspect of the distal oesophagus in elderly males and are frequently asymptomatic (Schatzki and Hawes 1942, Parnell et al 1978).

Non-neoplastic polyps include the long pedicled simple fibrous polyp usually arising from the post-cricoid region and the inflammatory polyps found in the distal oesophagus associated with thickened oesophageal folds (Bleshman et al 1978).

Malignant neoplasms

These tumours account for 2.5% of all malignant disorders in the UK, 90% being squamous cell carcinomas and most of the remaining 10% adenocarcinomas. Other rare malignant neoplasms include adenosquamous carcinoma, the carcinosarcoma and pseudosarcoma group, leiomyosarcomas, melanomas and oat cell carcinomas.

Squamous carcinomas and adenocarcinomas

Squamous carcinoma is usually seen in elderly males with the majority occurring in the fifth to seventh decades (Le Roux 1961) with a male to female ratio of between 3:2 (Le Roux 1961, Miller 1962) and 4:1 (Raven 1948). Numerous predisposing factors have been identified including smoking, alcohol, lye dye induced strictures, asbestos exposure, oesophageal diverticulae, achalasia, tylosis, coeliac disease, and a history of head and neck squamous carcinoma (Goldstein & Zornosa 1978). Dietary factors have been postulated to explain marked variation in the incidence in different geographical locations.

Approximately 50% of squamous carcinomas originate in the middle third of the oesophagus, 30% in the lower third and 20% in the upper third. Neoplasms confined to the upper third are uncommon in male subjects; most neoplasms found in this region are post-cricoid lesions. These neoplasms have an association with the Paterson–Kelly syndrome in certain geographical areas although this association has not been documented worldwide (Jacobson 1962).

The majority of adenocarcinomas arise in the lower third of the oesophagus on a background of columnar metaplasia which is thought to be induced by gastro-oesophageal reflux and to have premalignant potential (Poleyard et al 1977).

The most common presenting symptom is dysphagia; other less constant symptoms include anorexia, weight loss, odynophagia and the consequences of anaemia. Occasionally respiratory symptoms dominate the clinical picture, secondary to recurrent overflow aspiration, or rarely due to a tracheo-oesophageal fistula.

Adenosquamous carcinomas

Adenosquamous carcinomas, which are very rare, are usually found in the distal oesophagus; they are of uncertain histological origin.

Leiomyosarcomas

These neoplasms are very rare and doubt has been cast upon many of the previously reported cases in the literature. Five new cases were described and the literature critically reviewed by Johnston et al (1953). They reported leiomyosarcomas to be more common in males but, unlike leiomyomas, uncommon under the age of 50. They follow a similar anatomical distribution to leiomyomas but no malignant transformation of the benign lesion has been documented. Some of the neoplasms are polypoid, some infiltrating and some show a combination of both features, thus radiologically simulating the commoner squamous carcinoma. Local invasion of adjacent structures may occur but distant metastases are unusual (Tanner & Smithers 1962).

Pseudosarcomas and carcinosarcomas

These rare oesophageal neoplasms contain both carcinomatous and sarcomatous elements. The epidemiology in terms of the sex distribution and age of presentation along with the clinical manifestations are similar to squamous cell carcinoma. They are characteristically large polypoid neoplasms consisting predominantly of malignant-looking spindle cells with a small localized component of carcinomatous material, usually at the margin of the neoplasm or superficially invading into the mass. They have a significantly more favourable prognosis when treated surgically.

There has been some controversy about the histological origin of these neoplasms, but Mitros (1984), having reviewed 53 of the reported cases, concluded that these neoplasms represent carcinomas which have undergone metaplasia giving rise to sarcomatous elements.

Other rare neoplasms of the oesophagus include melanomas, which like the pseudosarcoma neoplasms often have a polypoid macroscopic appearance but do not share the favourable prognosis; rhabdomyosarcomas (Thorpe & Neiman 1950) and oat cell carcinomas.

Lymphoma only occasionally involves the oesophagus. The oesophagus is the least common site of gastrointestinal involvement and where the gastrointestinal tract is the primary site of disease the oesophagus is only involved in 1% of cases. Most of these occur in the distal oesophagus, in continuity with gastric involvement.

Radiology

The primary investigation in suspected oesophageal carcinoma is a barium swallow examination using single and/or double contrast techniques. Radiographs must be obtained in at least two different projections. Frequently more are required, particularly for a single contrast study when only that part of the wall seen in profile can be adequately assessed. A high kilovoltage is used, particularly crucial during a single contrast study, in an attempt to see through the column of contrast and appreciate any intraluminal pathology. Double contrast studies are now widely used to supplement single contrast views of the oesophagus especially for detecting early oesophageal carcinoma (Suzuki et al 1972, Kohler et al 1976, Itai et al 1978). Techniques combining water with barium have been described although most radiologists now prefer combining barium and air. Air-contrast studies depend on the ability of the patient to swallow an adequate volume of air to obtain oesophageal distension. If this is not achieved by getting the patient to drink rapidly, other methods such as holding the nose while drinking or perforations in the drinking straw may be tried. Some workers have found oesophageal catheterization necessary in a proportion of patients, particularly when studying the distal segment. The use of smooth muscle relaxants can be helpful in achieving good oesphageal distension.

Early carcinoma is usually seen as a sessile or plaque-like lesion of abnormal mucosa, confined to one aspect of the oesophageal lumen. Any polypoid intraluminal component tends to be small. The mucosal pattern overlying the lesion is usually abnormal, showing a granular or nodular appearance with or without areas of ulceration. Polypoid lesions may appear smooth but more frequently have a lobulated surface (Fig. 6.1). The oesophageal wall at the affected site is often rigid and lacks distensibility; a sign which may be best appreciated with fluoroscopy. Rigidity of the wall adjacent to the abnormal area implies submucosal infiltration of the neoplasm.

Some workers have reported a marked improvement in the prognosis when oesophageal carcinoma is detected at an early stage (Suzuki et al 1972, Kohler et al 1976, Itai et al 1978, Yamada 1979). Yamada (1979) reported an improvement in the 5-year survival from 21.5% for all oesophageal carcinomas seen in their hospital to 67% for early oesophageal carcinoma (localized to the mucosa and submucosa). However, only 3.6% of the total number of oesophageal carcinomas were detected at an early stage. Zornoza & Lindell (1980) failed to verify this improved prognosis for early oesophageal carcinoma, although the numbers in this study were small. The major difficulty in the early diagnosis of oesophageal carcinoma is not radiological detection but the tendency to present late, as verified by Yamada (1979).

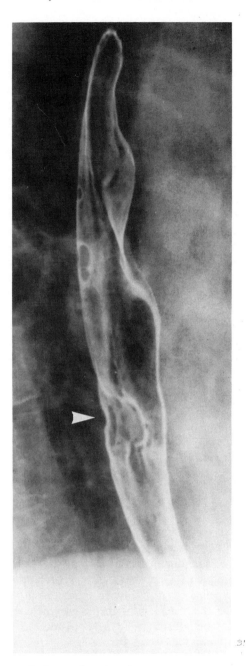

Fig. 6.1 Early oesophageal carcinoma seen as a broad-based sessile lesion with an irregular surface at the junction of the middle and lower thirds of the oesophagus (arrowhead). Histology showed a squamous carcinoma confined to the mucosa and submucosa with no nodal involvement.

In the majority of patients with symptoms referable to an oesophageal carcinoma, the disease process has progressed through the early stage and is easily demonstrated on single or double contrast barium studies. Macroscopically these more advanced carcinomas often show a sessile, fungating tumour, protruding into the oesophageal lumen. Areas of ulceration within the neoplasm may be present and submucosal infiltration of neoplasm around the sessile component may be apparent. The submucosal infiltration is often much more extensive microscopically than the gross appearances would suggest. The radiological patterns produced by the neoplasms reflect the macroscopic changes. When the region of the sessile component is seen in profile it appears as a rolled and undercut edge (Fig. 6.2), typical of a mucosally-based lesion. The surface of the neoplasm usually appears nodular or fungating and ulcer craters may be seen. The process may be confined to the side of the oesophageal wall or may be circumferential, producing an annular stricture with shouldered margins. The zone of transition between such neoplasms is often sharp radiologically, or may be more gradual due to submucosal neoplastic infiltration. Where submucosal infiltration is the dominant abnormality the appearances are those of a relatively smooth stricture of variable length with a gradual transition between normal and diseased oesophagus. The mucosal abnormalities produced by predominantly submucosal neoplasms are often subtle although it is usually possible to appreciate an area of mucosal granularity or nodularity with or without focal ulceration. In other neoplasms most of the tumour mass, apparent radiologically, is ulcerated. The ulcers have characteristically raised rolled edges producing a radiolucent margin around the ulcer crater meniscus when seen in profile and a radiolucent halo around the crater when viewed en face.

A rare variant of the squamous carcinoma is the verrucous carcinoma. Histologically these are low grade, well differentiated neoplasms which macroscopically appear as localized stalked or sessile polyps with a lobulated surface; only seven cases were available in the literature when the subject was reviewed by Sridhar et al (1980). Owing to the histological and macroscopic features, the prognosis of this variety has been thought to be more

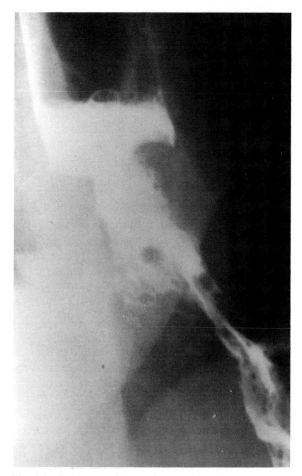

Fig. 6.2 Carcinoma of the lower third of the oesophagus. An annular stricture with mucosal destruction and mucosal shouldering at the proximal aspect of the tumour.

favourable; however, Minielly et al (1967) described five cases of verrucous carcinoma, four of whom died directly as a result of the neoplasm presenting at a late stage.

Adenocarcinomas may be indistinguishable from squamous carcinomas, although any involvement of the gastric fundus makes an adenocarcinoma much more likely. An early lesion in the distal oesophagus may show only slight prominence of the mucosal folds with subsequent progression to a nodular or fungating component and stricture formation. Carlson (1983) stressed the need for careful fluoroscopy to demonstrate loss of peristalsis and rigidity which may be the earliest radiological manifestation.

Adenosquamous carcinomas and leiomyosarcomas appear similar radiologically to squamous carcinomas. Pseudosarcomas, on the other hand, may show a large polypoid component making it possible to suggest the correct diagnosis.

Differential diagnosis

Secondary involvement of the oesophagus, either due to direct invasion from an adjacent primary neoplasm or metastases from a distant site, may simulate many of the appearances of a primary carcinoma. The appearances of metastases involving the oesophagus are discussed later.

Extensive nodular/fungating neoplasms involving a long segment of the oesophagus may resemble varices or severe oesophagitis, particularly oesophagitis secondary to candidiasis. Infiltrating and stenosing neoplasms may be difficult to distinguish from benign oesophageal strictures, particularly in the distal oesophagus when normal or thickened gastric mucosal folds within a hiatus hernia immediately below a stricture may be impossible to differentiate from the nodular component of a neoplasm in the oesophagus. Strictures secondary to an infiltrating neoplasm tend to be more eccentric and asymmetrical and usually show at least a small area of mucosal destruction. Sometimes carcinomatous strictures in the distal oesophagus may assume a 'bird's beak' configuration mimicking achalasia. Features which favour a neoplasm rather than achalasia include a short history, an older patient, high-grade obstruction, an unchanging pattern of obstruction despite forceful drinking, retention of the normal strippling wave, a nodular or polypoid component of the stricture, an associated mass lesion (best appreciated on fluoroscopy by the nature of transmitted pulsations) and an abnormality in the gastric fundus indicating malignant infiltration. The diagnosis of malignancy rather than achalasia may even be missed with endoscopy and biopsy, prompting the suggestion that all older subjects with apparent achalasia should be treated surgically rather than by endoscopy and dilatation (Lawson & Dodds 1976).

Benign ulceration, most commonly found in a columnar-lined oesophagus, may simulate the predominantly ulcerating carcinoma.

Further investigation

In order to understand the need for further investigation and staging of oesophageal carcinomas it is necessary to be familiar with the spread of disease, the treatment and prognosis.

The lack of serosa around the oesophagus and the thin wall explain the early dissemination and poor prognosis of the carcinoma. Contiguous spread into the surrounding mediastinum is common and may involve the trachea and major bronchi, lung parenchyma, pericardium and aorta. Neoplasms in the middle and upper thirds are more frequently inoperable due to involvement of adjacent vital structures than are neoplasms in the lower third (Le Roux 1961, Miller 1962, Moss et al 1980). Lymph node metastases occur early and may involve the perioesophageal, paratracheal, peribronchial, paraoesophageal, posterior mediastinal, coeliac, splenic and deep cervical groups. Approximately 60% of squamous carcinomas show evidence of nodal disease at surgery and the figure is even higher for adenocarcinomas (Le Roux 1961, Miller 1962). Visceral metastases, most frequently involving the liver, lungs and adrenals, are also common and are found in about 70% of cases on postmortem examination (Morson & Dawson 1979), although they are less frequently detected in pretreatment staging studies based on CT and surgical findings where an incidence of 10–17% has been reported (Moss et al 1981a, Schneeblock et al 1983).

The treatment of squamous carcinoma is by surgical resection and/or radiotherapy. The choice remains somewhat controversial as the 5-year survival remains very poor at 4–14% with either treatment (Earlam & Cunha-Melo 1980a, 1980b, Hambraeus et al 1981) although Hambraeus has shown a significant improvement in the 1-year survival from 23 to 50% using a combination of radiotherapy and surgery rather than surgery alone. The major disadvantage of surgery is the very high operative mortality of up to 30% (Earlam & Cunha-Melo 1980a, Giulli & Gignoux 1980, Hambraeus et al 1981).

Adenocarcinomas are normally treated with surgery as these tumours are not very radioresponsive. Some workers have reported a lower operative mortality (Earlam & Cunha-Melo 1980a) although this was not confirmed by Giulli and Gignoux (1980) in a larger retrospective study.

Once oesophageal carcinoma is suspected on barium study, in all but the most moribund patients endoscopy with biopsy and cytological brushings should be performed to confirm the diagnosis and to obtain histology. The accuracy of these techniques is about 96% (Witzel et al 1976). However, if negative, in the presence of suspicious radiological appearances, repeat endoscopy and biopsy is required.

In the cases where definitive treatment is intended, further imaging to assess the spread of the disease is required. This should commence with a chest radiograph to exclude gross mediastinal involvement, metastatic adenopathy and pulmonary metastases. Upper abdominal ultrasound may be performed to assess hepatic involvement and may detect subdiaphragmatic nodal enlargement. Radionuclide imaging is a complementary modality to exclude hepatic metastases and is particularly helpful when the index of suspicion is high, such as patients with abnormal liver function tests but in whom ultrasound appears normal.

CT is the best imaging modality currently available to stage carcinoma of the oesophagus and has completely replaced the other modalities in most centres. Chest radiography and ultrasound may be used to select those patients with advanced disease although even in the presence of distant metastases CT may be of value to demonstrate the volume of mediastinal involvement for palliative radiotherapy planning.

The major advantage of CT is its ability to demonstrate the extent of the mediastinal involvement and thus aid the decision whether or not an attempt at curative surgical resection, palliative surgery or radiotherapy plus or minus the use of bypass Celestin tubes should be employed. Moss et al (1981a) studied the use of CT in staging and used the following criteria to assess extra-oesophageal spread:

1. Loss of fat planes between the oesophagus and contiguous mediastinal structures
2. Enlargement of lymph nodes
3. Contrast leak into paraoesophageal structures
4. Mass extension into trachea or bronchi
5. Presence of hepatic, pulmonary and abdominal metastases.

Moss reported that 87% of patients showed evidence of spread and in those patients treated surgically (one-third of cases), the CT and surgical/pathological staging showed good correlation. Since Moss's work (Moss et al 1981a) further studies have described the use of CT in oesophageal carcinoma, further refining and describing the limitations of these criteria. Knowledge of the normal mediastinal anatomy with particular reference to the normal fat planes is essential (Schneeblock et al 1983). A paucity of mediastinal fat may make the scan interpretation more difficult and Thompson W M et al (1983) encountered 18 such cases out of a total of 76, although in only 6 of these was the scan indeterminate for staging. No fat plane normally separates the oesophagus from the trachea or left main bronchus and hence invasion of the airway can only be predicted by a convex deformity indicating mass extension into the airway. Similarly, in only 40% of normal subjects does a fat plane separate the oesophagus from the descending aorta and aortic arch. Aortic invasion is excluded if a fat plane exists: if no fat plane exists then aortic invasion may be predicted by estimating the angle of contact between the tumour and the aorta. If the angle of contact is greater than 90° of the aortic circumference then invasion is highly probable, but if less than 45° it is unlikely. 45–90° angles of contact are thus indeterminate although Picus et al (1983) only encountered these angles in 6 out of 30 cases. The pericardium is normally separated from the oesophagus by a fat plane. If this fat plane is lost on two consecutive slices at the level of the tumour but preserved on the slices above and below then pericardial invasion exists. Infiltration of the perioesophageal fat without invasion of the surrounding viscera may be suggested by loss of sharpness of the external contour of the tumour, although this criterion was found to be unreliable by Schneeblock et al (1983).

Major problems exist in the detection of perioesophageal nodes. The criteria for enlargement remain imprecise with upper limits of normal size ranging between 5 and 10 mm in different studies. More important, involved perioesophageal nodes are frequently of normal size and are often engulfed by the tumour (Thompson W M et al 1983). Subdiaphragmatic nodes involved by tumour are more accurately predicted with a sensitivity of 70% (Halvorsen et al 1986) but again the inability to detect tumour in normal sized nodes explains the significant number of false negative cases. Thompson W M et al (1983) noted that metastatic nodes in adenocarcinomas are frequently of normal size, partially explaining the less accurate results in the staging of gastro-oesophageal junction tumours.

Despite the limitations of CT in staging oesophageal carcinoma, the overall accuracy of five series reviewed by Thompson W M et al (1983) was 90% for mediastinal invasion and 80% for subdiaphragmatic metastases, although Quint et al (1985a) found only 13 cases out of 39 correctly staged by CT. Halvorsen et al (1986) showed that evidence of mediastinal invasion, liver metastases and abdominal adenopathy as demonstrated on CT predict a shortened survival time regardless of the treatment used, the specific CT criteria for mediastinal invasion being tracheal, aortic and pericardial invasion.

Only limited work using MRI in the staging of oesophageal neoplasms has been reported. Quint showed MRI to be of low accuracy at only 40% although his work has also reported a CT accuracy of only 30% (Quint et al 1985b).

Endoscopic ultrasound (Fig. 6.3) is a new technique which can be used for staging oesophageal carcinoma (Heyder 1987, Murata et al 1987, Shorvon et al 1988). This technique uses high frequency, high resolution, real-time ultrasound images from within the gastrointestinal tract produced by an ultrasound probe incorporated into the tip of a fibreoptic endoscope (Shorvon et al 1987). A rubber balloon attached to the tip and containing deaerated water provides contact between the scanner and the oesophageal wall. The depth of oesophageal invasion is shown by identifying the layers of the oesophageal wall which are involved by the neoplasm. Metastatic involvement of lymph nodes can also be identified. Metastases are usually present in lymph nodes greater than 10 mm in diameter and metastatic lymph nodes

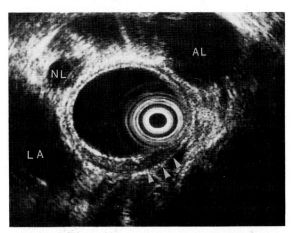

Fig. 6.3 Transoesophageal ultrasound scan of carcinoma. The small oesophageal carcinoma is seen in the oesophageal wall (arrowheads). A normal lymph node (NL) and abnormal lymph node (AL) are seen. The left atrium (LA) can also be identified (Courtesy of Drs P J Shorvon, W R Lees and R A Frost).

are frequently spherical (Murata et al 1987). The incidence of metastases is high in lymph nodes which show a distinct border and heterogeneous internal echoes. It is also possible to determine whether cancer has infiltrated adjacent organs. Murata et al (1987) correctly estimated the extent of invasion in 84% of cases in whom a technically satisfactory ultrasound had been performed prior to surgery.

Secondary neoplasms

Many patients dying from malignant disease have pathological evidence of oesophageal involvement and about 18% in one series had a history of dysphagia (Toreson 1944). In about 70% of cases oesophageal involvement is from a contiguous primary neoplasm such as hypopharyngeal, thyroid, pulmonary or gastric. Radiologically these may be seen as extrinsic compression or actual invasion of the oesophageal wall or lumen which may simulate a primary oesophageal carcinoma. Usually there is, however, an obvious associated mass lesion either clinically or radiologically, and in the case of a gastric primary there will be obvious fundal involvement.

Excluding involvement by contiguous tumours,

secondary involvement of the oesophagus is normally via metastases to contiguous mediastinal lymph nodes and less frequently due to direct metastatic spread to the oesophagus itself. It is often difficult to separate these processes clearly radiologically (Anderson & Harrell 1980). Spread via adjacent node involvement usually affects the middle third of the oesophagus, although examples of breast carcinoma involving the gastroesophageal junction have been described (Toreson 1944). Enlargement of adjacent mediastinal lymph nodes produces radiological evidence of extrinsic compression with a mass protruding into the oesophageal lumen forming obtuse angles with the oesophageal wall. Initially only one wall of the oesophagus may show indentation but as the disease progresses the oesophagus becomes encased and may be displaced. As the neoplasm invades the wall, localized irregularities may develop and it may become impossible to distinguish from a primary carcinoma. Sometimes a desmoplastic reaction to the invading neoplasm, either from adjacent nodes or direct spread, may produce a long smooth stricture which appears radiologically similar to the benign lesion.

Distant metastases are most often from lung or breast cancer although secondary deposits in the oesophagus from renal, bladder, pancreatic and cervical tumours have been described. By the time a breast tumour metastasizes to the oesophagus the primary is usually well known and widely disseminated, whereas oesophageal involvement secondary to a bronchial carcinoma may occur early and dysphagia may be the presenting symptom.

Endoscopy in metastatic disease often confirms the presence of a stricture when the wall is involved rather than simply displaced but even in these circumstances, biopsy is frequently normal as the oesophageal mucosa is preserved.

Gastric lymphoma invading the oesophagus appears radiologically as thickened nodular folds with a non-obstructive narrowing of the distal oesophagus (Carnovale et al 1977). Occasionally the disease extends proximal to the distal third and thickened nodular folds may resemble varices. A single case of multiple, 1–2 cm diameter, lymphomatous intramural nodules throughout the oesophagus has been described where the nodules were radiologically identical to multiple leio-

myomas or polypoid metastatic deposits from melanoma (Carnovale et al 1977).

THE STOMACH

Benign neoplasms

Benign neoplasms of the stomach may be of epithelial or mesenchymal origin. Epithelial neoplasms are usually polypoid in nature and appear radiologically similar to other gastric polyps of non-neoplastic origin. Table 6.1 shows the different types of benign gastric neoplasms and other non-neoplastic polypoid lesions which are considered in the differential diagnosis. Most of the conditions listed are rare; only smooth muscle neoplasms, hyperplastic polyps, adenomatous polyps and pancreatic rests are relatively common.

Epithelial neoplasms

Gastric polyps were detected in 1.6 and 1.7% of cases in two recent large surveys of double contrast examinations (Gordon et al 1980, Montesi et al 1982); some almost certainly represented smooth muscle tumours as endoscopy and biopsy revealed normal gastric mucosa in a number of cases.

In another recent series (Op den Orth & Dekker 1981) gastric adenomas were found in 0.1% of barium studies and Kayima et al (1982) showed

Table 6.1 Benign gastric tumours and non-neoplastic gastric polyps

Benign tumours	Non-neoplastic polyps
Adenomatous polyps	Hyperplastic polyps
Smooth muscle tumours	Eosinophilic granulomatous polyps*
Neurogenic tumours	Aberrant pancreatic rest
Glomus tumours	
Lipomas	
Vascular tumours	
— haemangiomas	
— lymphangiomas	

*Probably inflammatory in aetiology although a neurogenic origin has also been suggested.

that the incidence of gastric adenomas increased with age. Adenomatous polyps account for 20% of all gastric polyps (Ming & Goldman 1965, Tomasulo 1971), nearly all the remainder being non-neoplastic hyperplastic polyps. Adenomatous polyps are composed of intestinal-like epithelium and are usually found on a background of intestinal metaplasia. Predisposing factors include atrophic gastritis, pernicious anaemia, familial polyposis and Gardner's syndrome. Hamartomatous polyps may coexist with adenomas in Gardner's syndrome and familial polyposis.

Gastric adenomas are most common in the antrum and are usually broad-based, single, sessile lesions which form an acute angle rather than a right or obtuse angle with the gastric wall, helping to differentiate them from smooth muscle tumours. Some adenomas are pedunculated and a stalk may be apparent. Most are between 1–2 cm in size when detected (Op de Orth & Dekker 1981, Kayima et al 1982) although some are larger. The surface of the lesion is usually smooth or may show minor irregularities. Villous adenomas are large sessile adenomatous polyps with an irregular surface. Radiologically, adenomatous polyps may be seen as a subtle ring shadow on a double contrast study or as a filling defect on the single contrast part of a biphasic study, often well demonstrated on compression.

The major significance of the adenomatous polyp is its premalignant potential and association with carcinoma of the stomach. The incidence of malignant change is controversial. In a series of 80 cases with long term follow-up, there was an incidence of malignant change in 11% (Ming & Goldman 1965). Adenomatous polyps less than 2 cm in diameter rarely show malignant change (Berg 1958, Monaco et al 1962, Ming and Goldman 1965, Tomasulo 1971). It is generally agreed that only a small minority of gastric carcinomas develop from a previously benign adenomatous polyp.

The major differential diagnosis of an adenomatous polyp is the more common non-neoplastic hyperplastic polyp. These are usually less than 1.5 cm in diameter, pedunculated and more frequently multiple (30% of cases) (Appleman 1984). Biopsy is, however, often necessary to exclude an adenomatous polyp or early gastric carcinoma.

Mesenchymal neoplasms

Benign smooth muscle tumours are common tumours frequently observed at postmortem (Morson & Dawson 1979). They may be multiple, occur in both sexes, and increase in frequency with increasing age. These and the other mesenchymal gastric tumours are intramural or submucosal and as such are seen radiologically projecting into the gastric lumen forming a right or obtuse angle with the gastric wall. The surface of the tumour is often smooth with preservation of the overlying gastric mucosa, although central, 'bull's eye' ulceration is common, particularly with the larger tumours. Occasionally smooth muscle tumours become pedunculated. Symptoms are rare in small tumours less than 3 cm in size, but almost inevitable in lesions larger than 6 cm in diameter (Graffe et al 1960), and are usually secondary to ulceration. Patients characteristically present with acute upper gastrointestinal bleeding.

The vast majority of these tumours are benign and clearly so histologically. In cases where the appearances are less certain histologically, the size of the lesion is one of the best indices to predict malignant behaviour. Lesions less than 5 cm in size are rarely associated with metastases but 60% of tumours greater than 10 cm in size behave in a malignant fashion. Other features of malignancy include an irregular lobulated surface and extensive ulceration. Biopsy of the lesion often only reveals normal surface gastric epithelium although this may be helpful to exclude an epithelial neoplasm.

Other uncommon mesenchymal tumours include neurogenic tumours and glomus tumours which simulate leiomyomas radiologically.

Eosinophillic granulomatous polyps are rare and may be inflammatory or neurogenic in origin. Haemangiomas and lymphangiomas are also very rare. The features of aberrant pancreatic rests are well known; the subject was reviewed by Clements et al (1983).

Malignant neoplasms

Primary carcinomas

Carcinoma of the stomach is still one of the commonest malignant disorders in man despite a falling incidence in recent years. Formerly more common in males, the falling incidence has been more marked in the male population and now the male:female ratio approaches 1:1 (Antonioli 1984). The mean age of diagnosis in two large series since 1950 has been in the early sixties (Paulino & Roselli 1979, Green et al 1981). The large variation in the incidence in different geographical locations is a result of environmental factors rather than a genetic predisposition.

The vast majority of gastric carcinomas are adenocarcinomas; primary squamous and adenosquamous carcinomas are rare.

The common presenting symptoms include anorexia, weight loss, anaemia and epigastric pain with or without dyspepsia. Unfortunately the symptoms are often only trivial in the early stages and in the majority of cases the neoplasm has reached an advanced stage at presentation, partly explaining the very poor prognosis. The overall 5-year survival is 5–15% and there has been little improvement in the prognosis over the past 25 years (Adashek et al 1979). In Japan where the incidence of gastric carcinoma is very high, routine radiology and endoscopy screening programmes have been introduced in an attempt to detect the disease in the early stages. Large studies generated from such screening programmes have led to the concept of 'early gastric cancer' which has a much more favourable prognosis than the advanced disease, with a 5-year survival of over 90%. A 5-year survival of nearer 70% for early gastric cancer is quoted in several Western publications (Fielding et al 1980, Green et al 1981, Gold et al 1984). The treatment for gastric carcinoma is surgical, radiotherapy and chemotherapy being of only very limited palliative value.

Carcinoma of the stomach is most common in the prepyloric region, gastric antrum and on the lesser curve. Morson and Dawson (1979) recorded the following distribution; 47% in the antrum and pyloric region, 23% in the body of the stomach, 21% in the cardia, 2% in the fundus and 7% linitis plastica. In their series they referred to the unusually high incidence of neoplasms of the cardia and Antonioli (1984) believes that neoplasms in this region are becoming relatively more common, as demonstrated by several recent published series.

Early gastric cancer

Early gastric carcinoma (EGC) is defined as being localized to the mucosa or submucosa regardless of the presence or absence of lymph node involvement. Figure 6.4 shows the morphological classification of early gastric cancer. The prognosis for all types is favourable, particularly for those neoplasms localized to the mucosa sparing the submucosa. Certain morphological features and hence radiological appearances may indicate a more favourable lesion.

Radiological appearances. Shirakabe (1983) reviewed the radiology of EGC and reports an incidence of 74% depressed lesions (type IIc or III), 24% protuberant (type I or IIa) and 2% flat (type IIb). Type I lesions are similar radiologically to adenomas, and any pedunculated lesion greater than 2 cm in size or any broad-based sessile polyp greater than 1 cm should be suspected as a carcinoma. Occasionally type I lesions are massive. Type III lesions are also relatively easy to detect radiologically as a deep ulcer crater is present. This may be demonstrated on the double contrast phase of the examination or using single contrast techniques with profile views and en face compression studies. The distinction between the benign and malignant ulcer is, however, less straightforward. Type II lesions are often very subtle as the elevated or depressed components, if present, are very small. The mucosal pattern must be closely

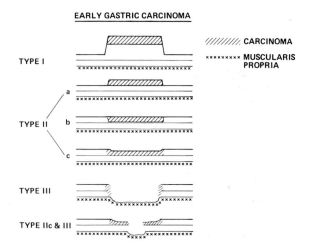

Fig. 6.4 Classification of early carcinoma.

scrutinized, as radiologically only a minor irregularity or granularity is apparent. These
features are best appreciated on good double contrast views (Fig. 6.5). Most type II EGC are
around 2 cm in diameter when detected (Green et
al 1981, Gold et al 1984) although lesions involving
large areas have been described. Any single lesion
may show a combination of the features of the different types in the classification (Fig. 6.4).
Multiple lesions in EGC occur in 8–32% of cases
(Green et al 1981, Montesi et al 1982, Shirakabe
1983). Five out of 12 cases of EGC reported by
Montesi et al (1982) were multifocal but the 21
satellite foci of EGC were very small with a
diameter of less than 5 mm. Some EGCs may be
missed on double contrast studies but detected on
endoscopy. Four out of 21 cases reported by Gold
et al (1984) appeared benign at endoscopy but
biopsies showed malignancy.

The sensitivity of barium studies in detecting
early gastric cancer varies between 43 and 66% in
recent series (Green et al 1981, Montesi et al 1982,
Gold et al 1984). In a large number of false negative cases, some abnormality was seen but thought
to be benign and the correct diagnosis was
achieved on endoscopy. In the series by Montesi
et al where the sensitivity was 66%, 33% were not
seen prospectively but an abnormality was identified on retrospective viewing, suggesting that as
experience increases the sensitivity may be expected to improve.

Advanced gastric carcinomas

Like oesophageal carcinoma, the majority of
gastric carcinomas present late and have reached
an advanced stage when first detected. These
tumours are nodular (44%), ulcerating (40%),
fungating or polypoid (7%), linitis plastica (7%)
or superficial (2%), the latter better considered as
early gastric carcinoma (Morson & Dawson 1979).

Radiological appearances. These advanced
gastric carcinomas are usually clearly demonstrated radiologically. Nodular carcinomas are
seen projecting into the gastric lumen with an irregular surface of numerous discrete or confluent
nodules, often with an angular shelf at the
perimeter and a relatively well-defined edge. Areas
of ulceration within the nodular mass are common.
Ulcerative carcinomas are predominantly crater
forming. The edge of the crater frequently appears
nodular with a sharp zone of transition between
the abnormal area and the normal gastric wall, as
compared with the gradual zone of transition surrounding the acute peptic ulcer due to the halo of
oedematous tissue frequently seen both pathologically and radiologically. Malignant ulcers tend to
be greater in width than depth, and the floor of
the crater lies within the gastric lumen and does
not project beyond the anticipated contour of the
normal gastric wall. The floor of a malignant ulcer
may show evidence of nodularity when viewed in
profile or en face although filling defects may also
be apparent in the floor of benign ulcers due to
adherent blood clot. The contour of the surrounding mucosal folds may be disturbed with tapering,
clubbing, fusion or abrupt termination. In benign
ulceration the mucosal folds may be seen reaching
the edge of the ulcer crater although when acutely
inflamed, oedematous mucosa may obliterate the
folds near the crater edge. Carman's meniscus sign
may be apparent with malignant ulcers located on

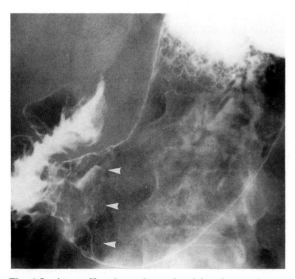

Fig. 6.5 A type II early carcinoma involving the gastric
antrum with a subtle granular and nodular appearance. The
approximate upper border (arrowheads) is not clearly seen.
Biopsies obtained at a subsequent endoscopy showed
evidence of carcinoma. The stomach appeared normal when
palpated at operation. When it was opened, however, the
mucosa appeared abnormal and an extensive mucosal
carcinoma was confirmed on histological examination of the
resected specimen.

the lesser curve due to apposition of the rolled edges of the neoplasm (Carman 1921). Some malignant ulcers will diminish in size with medical therapy for peptic ulceration, particularly the type III early gastric carcinomatous ulcers. Sakita et al (1971) demonstrated frequent healing of malignant ulcers and recommended that all patients with apparent benign gastric ulceration should be carefully followed up. Many workers believe that all gastric ulcers should be inspected endoscopically and an adequate number of biopsies taken, although Thompson G et al (1983) demonstrated that certain radiological criteria can reliably predict the benign nature of a gastric ulcer.

Fungating or polypoid lesions are less common and are characterized by a predominant large intraluminal component (Fig. 6.6). The surface of such neoplasms is frequently irregular with areas of ulceration and the appearances may be difficult to distinguish from leiomyosarcoma.

Scirrhous carcinomas of the stomach produce the linitis plastica appearance due to extensive submucosal infiltration. An intense fibrotic response to the neoplasm produces marked narrowing of the gastric lumen and a tube-like appearance. Disruption of the normal fold pattern is usual and areas of nodularity and ulceration are not uncommon. The limited distensibility of the stomach is best demonstrated using large quantities of barium after intravenous smooth muscle relaxants (Fig. 6.7).

Occasionally gastric carcinomas show extensive

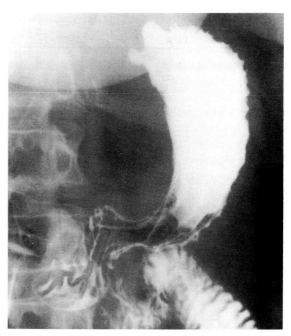

Fig. 6.7 Linitis plastica seen as a small volume stomach.

calcification, most easily appreciated on plain radiographs and usually secondary to a colloid-secreting adenocarcinoma.

Differential diagnosis

The differential diagnosis of gastric carcinoma will depend on the manifestations of the particular case in question. The diagnosis of polypoid lesions is discussed in a previous section. Type II early gastric cancer may be simulated by areas of atypical gastric epithelium usually resulting from intestinal metaplasia. As mentioned earlier, benign gastric ulcers may be difficult to differentiate from gastric carcinoma and endoscopic biopsies are required. Malignant degeneration of a previously benign gastric ulcer remains a contentious subject and is difficult to prove or disprove but even if accepted, it is agreed that its contribution to the incidence of gastric carcinoma is small.

More advanced lesions may be confused with lymphoma, lymphosarcoma and carcinoid tumours. Linitis plastica appearances may also be produced by corrosive damage, radiotherapy, Crohn's disease and eosinophilic gastroenteritis.

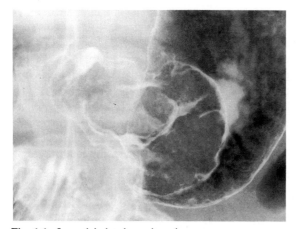

Fig. 6.6 Large lobulated antral carcinoma.

Spread and staging of gastric carcinoma

Direct spread

Direct spread through the gastric wall tends to occur early and depending on the site of the primary neoplasm may involve the spleen, pancreas, liver, left kidney and transverse colon via the greater omentum. Once the neoplasm has spread through the gastric serosa transperitoneal dissemination commonly occurs, producing peritoneal metastases with involvement of distant organs such as the ovaries and giving rise to a Krukenburg tumour. Direct infiltration across the gastro-oesophageal junction is common in carcinomas involving the region of the cardia and often such neoplasms present with dysphagia simulating an oesophageal primary. Direct invasion across the pylorus into the duodenum is unusual but not as rare as stated in many textbooks (Morson & Dawson 1979).

Lymphatic spread

Lymph node metastases are common and are found in 90% of cases of gastric carcinomas coming to postmortem and 70% of cases treated surgically. Lymph node metastases may be found in early gastric carcinoma, although they are rare (3.3%) in small lesions limited to the mucosa but become more frequent with lesions of larger area and with an extensive submucosal involvement (Kodama et al 1983).

The prognosis of early gastric carcinoma, although worsened by lymph node involvement, remains relatively good (Antonioli 1984). The perigastric lesser curve nodes are most frequently involved, followed by greater curve, coeliac and porta hepatis groups. Supradiaphragmatic nodal metastases are also well recognized and may spread to involve the supraclavicular and mediastinal groups, the latter resulting in lymphangitis carcinomatosis in some patients.

Blood stream spread

Blood-borne metastases are most commonly found in the liver but may also occur in the lungs, skin, ovaries, adrenals and bone. Bone metastases are often sclerotic.

Staging

The imaging modalities currently available to stage gastric carcinoma include conventional radiography, ultrasonography, radionuclide scintigraphy and CT. The rôle of endoscopic ultrasound of the stomach has not yet been fully evaluated. The chest radiograph is required to exclude pulmonary and mediastinal lymph node deposits. Ultrasonography is widely used to image the liver and detect or exclude hepatic metastases; it may also show subdiaphragmatic nodal enlargement and demonstrate ascites which may accompany hepatic involvement or peritoneal deposits. Ultrasound may also be used to assess gastric carcinoma and direct invasion into adjacent viscera (Derchi et al 1983). Other workers have also described the ultrasonic appearance of gastric carcinoma (Yek & Rabinowitz 1981, Derchi et al 1983). Although ultrasound in no way replaces or competes with contrast radiology as a primary imaging modality to demonstrate a gastric lesion, the recognition of gastric wall thickening and/or mass lesion may be helpful to direct further investigation towards the stomach in patients referred for abdominal ultrasound with non-specific upper abdominal symptoms due to an underlying gastric carcinoma.

CT is the most accurate modality currently available to stage carcinoma of the stomach and is able to demonstrate gastric wall thickening and/or mass effect of the primary neoplasm, direct extension into adjacent viscera, nodal involvement, hepatic and adrenal metastases and ascites (Lee et al 1979). Small pulmonary metastases, not visible on a chest radiograph, may also be shown by CT. Moss et al (1981b) describe the techniques and appearances in abdominal CT of gastric carcinoma, analysing the appearances of the primary neoplasm, evidence of direct extension into the spleen, pancreas, colon, oesophagus, duodenum or liver and the presence of hepatic and adrenal metastases. In those patients who came to surgery, the surgical and pathological findings showed good correlation with the CT appearances and they concluded that the high accuracy of CT staging may avoid unnecessary laparotomy.

Some of the difficulties encountered when staging gastric carcinomas with CT are similar to those seen with oesophageal tumours. Lack of intraperitoneal fat may cause problems making it difficult to assess direct invasion into adjacent viscera. The stomach is, however, relatively mobile and thus scans taken in the decubitus or prone position may help to discriminate between uninvolved viscera simply lying adjacent to the tumour and those with invasion. On repositioning, the uninvolved viscera may separate away from the tumour whereas those invaded by the tumour will remain in contact. In adenocarcinomas lymph node metastases are frequently found in normal-sized nodes and are thus missed at CT. This is similar to the situation at the gastro-oesophageal junction (Thompson W M et al 1983). Artefacts caused by air/contrast interfaces may degrade some images and require repeat sections.

There remains some debate regarding the rôle of radiological staging of gastric carcinoma, as the only effective curative or palliative treatment available is surgical (McFee & Aust 1981). Even if one accepts the argument that all cases of gastric carcinoma require explorative laparotomy, CT can provide useful preoperative information.

A recent study indicated that the main limitation of CT for staging gastric carcinoma is that it is unreliable for demonstrating local lymph node involvement and invasion of adjacent organs (Kleinhaus & Militianu 1988). Six out of seven patients in whom direct pancreatic involvement was documented surgically were misdiagnosed on CT. As CT is more sensitive than ultrasound (Derchi et al 1983), the rôle of ultrasound remains uncertain and Derchi and colleagues concluded that its value in preoperative staging is limited to those cases where CT is not available.

Endoscopic ultrasonography can be used to visualize the structures of the gastric wall (Heyder 1987, Shorvon et al 1987) and has a potential rôle in the case of small tumours of the gastric wall (Heyder 1987). Unlike the oesophagus, the regional lymph nodes of the stomach cannot be completely investigated.

Lymphomas

Gastric lymphoma accounts for 2–5% of all gastric malignancy. The stomach is the most common site of gastrointestinal involvement, seen in about 50% of cases (Brady & Asbell 1980, Herrmann et al 1980). The majority of cases of gastrointestinal tract involvement are due to non-Hodgkin's lymphoma. A review of a large series (813 cases) of non-Hodgkin's lymphoma cases (Herrmann et al 1980) showed that 71 patients presented as a primary gastrointestinal tract lymphoma, 31 showed secondary symptomatic involvement and a large proportion of cases coming to postmortem showed occult gastrointestinal tract involvement (156 out of 366). The average age of presentation is between the age of 50 and 60 (Brady & Asbell 1980, Herrmann et al 1980) and the incidence is slightly higher in males.

Symptoms of the disease include epigastric pain which may be diffuse and non-specific or ulcer-like in nature, weight loss, anorexia, nausea and vomiting. Anaemia is frequently observed and haematemesis and melaena are not uncommon.

Radiological appearances

Gastric lymphoma most commonly occurs in the antrum and body of the stomach. The lesion is characteristically large at presentation; 70% were greater than 10 cm in size in a series of 72 patients reported by Sherrick et al (1965). The lymphoma tends to occur in a submucosal and intramural location and gives rise to a diffuse thickening of the gastric wall with a lobulated surface and thickening and nodularity of the mucosal folds. The surfaces of the mucosal folds are relatively smooth, in contrast to the generalized irregularity found in widespread carcinoma, particularly of the linitis plastica type. Function of the abnormal stomach lining is disturbed leading to absent or diminished peristalsis. The volume of the stomach is, however, preserved and unlike infiltrating carcinoma, the lymphomatous stomach retains its distensibility.

In some patients with gastric lymphoma the major radiological manifestation is ulceration (Fig. 6.8). Such ulcers are often large and may be multiple and associated with a mass lesion. Less commonly, a large, frequently ulcerated polyp is seen and occasionally multiple polyps are seen, usually on a background of thickened and distorted folds. Hodgkin's disease accounts for about one-sixth of all gastric lymphoma and is usually secondary to involvement elsewhere (Marshak et al

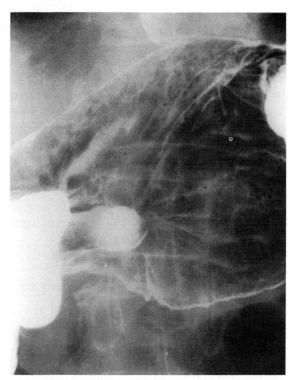

Fig. 6.8 Gastric lymphoma. A large ulcer is seen in the body of the stomach. This proved to be an ulcerating gastric lymphoma.

1983). It often appears radiologically similar to non-Hodgkin's lymphoma (Portmann et al 1954), but not infrequently produces a linitis plastica type appearance (Marshak et al 1983).

Lymphoma of the stomach may infiltrate across the gastro-oesophageal junction. Martin commonly demonstrated infiltration across the pylorus into the duodenum (Martin 1936) although Sherrick et al did not see this appearance in any of their 72 cases and concluded that it is unusual (Sherrick et al 1965).

The radiological manifestations are thus many and varied and lymphoma should be considered in the differential diagnosis of a number of conditions. Most important, it should be considered in cases of probable advanced gastric carcinoma, for biopsy revealing a diagnosis of lymphoma greatly improves the prognosis. Five-year survival is around 50% for stage I or II gastric lymphoma (Herrmann et al 1980). Gastric lymphoma may mimic a giant benign ulcer, or occasionally a large polyp or multiple polyps. It should also be considered in the differential diagnosis of thickened gastric folds including hypertrophic gastritis, Menetrier's disease, gastric varices, pseudolymphoma and eosinophilic gastroenteritis. Once the diagnosis is established appropriate staging should be undertaken.

Carcinoid tumours

Carcinoid tumours are rare and account for only 2–3% of all gastrointestinal tract carcinoids and about 0.3% of all gastric neoplasms. They occur equally in males and females, usually over the age of 40. Most are non-functioning and those that are may produce an atypical carcinoid syndrome with post-prandial flushing and peptic ulceration. Symptoms of non-functioning tumours are often non-specific; ulceration with consequent bleeding is not uncommon.

Radiological features

Gastric carcinoids occur throughout the stomach but are least common in the proximal region (Pochaczevsky & Sherman 1959). An intramural lesion protruding into the gastric lumen is seen in about two-thirds of cases and is easily mistaken for a smooth muscle neoplasm. Commonly they are about 2 cm in diameter, usually well defined with a smooth surface of preserved normal gastric mucosa, although ulceration is seen in about 40% of cases. In the absence of ulceration, mucosal biopsy at endoscopy is frequently normal. A less common manifestation of gastric carcinoid is that of multiple, small, usually sessile polyps which may occur throughout the stomach or in clusters (Marshak et al 1983). This pattern appears radiologically and endoscopically similar to other types of multiple polyposis and again superficial biopsy is unhelpful, a definitive diagnosis requiring polypectomy. Other unusual appearances of carcinoid tumours include fungating or large polypoid lesions or large malignant ulcers, in both cases radiologically indistinguishable from a primary adenocarcinoma (Pochaczevsky & Sherman 1959).

All carcinoid tumours are malignant; 15–35% have metastases at presentation and nearly all of those greater than 2 cm in size show local invasion and nodal metastases. Hepatic metastases are common. Both the primary neoplasm and the secondary deposits grow slowly and a long survival may be achieved by surgical resection of the primary tumour and metastases, if accessible. Palliation of symptoms due to hepatic metastases may be achieved by hepatic artery embolization (Odurny & Birch 1985). Osteoblastic bone metastases are well recognized.

Secondary neoplasms

Secondary neoplastic involvement of the stomach may result from direct spread of primary neoplasms in adjacent viscera or be due to distant blood-borne metastases. Invasion by adenocarcinomas of the lower oesophagus is not uncommon although unusual with primary squamous carcinoma. The stomach may also be involved by pancreatic carcinoma, carcinoma of the transverse colon infiltrating along the greater omentum, and carcinoma of the left kidney or left adrenal. Metastases to the stomach from distant sites are usually melanomas and breast carcinomas although examples of lung, kidney, thyroid and testicular neoplasms have been described (Willis 1973). Melanoma deposits characteristically occur in the submucosa and produce an intraluminal polypoid mass which frequently shows central, 'bull's eye' ulceration (Meyers & McSweeney 1972). Breast carcinomas like melanomas, involve the submucosa and they may produce submucosal nodules or plaques. Such lesions are usually asymptomatic and are most often described in postmortem studies. The most frequent manifestation seen radiologically is due to diffuse submucosal infiltration producing a linitis plastica type appearance (Jaffe 1975). The gastric mucosa is usually intact although it may develop a serrated or nodular configuration, pseudoulceration or true ulceration. This linitis plastica type appearance is usually symptomatic and hence prompts investigation.

THE DUODENUM

Benign neoplasms

Adenomas, an uncommon finding in the duodenum, behave similarly to those found elsewhere in the gastrointestinal tract and therefore carry a risk of malignant transformation. In a review of the literature Hessler & Braunstein (1978) found the reported rate of malignant transformation in 46 villous adenomas to be about 36%. They also reported a case of carcinoma of the duodenum arising in a previously benign villous adenoma. Multiple adenomatous polyps may be seen in the duodenum in familial polyposis coli (Yonemoto et al 1969). On barium examination adenomatous polyps have a similar appearance to those seen elsewhere in the gastrointestinal tract. Other benign duodenal neoplasms include Brunner's gland adenomas, leiomyomas, lipomas, neurogenic tumours and hamartomas.

Malignant neoplasms

Primary carcinomas

Most primary malignant neoplasms of the duodenum are carcinomas (Bosse & Neely 1969). Primary duodenal carcinoma is rare and accounts for less than 0.4% of all gastrointestinal carcinomas (Kleinerman et al 1950, Spira et al 1977, Nix et al 1985). Even so the duodenum is, inch for inch, the most frequent location of carcinoma in the small intestine.

The aetiology of duodenal carcinoma is unknown (Cortese & Cornell 1972). A total of 71 cases reported in the literature during a 10-year period were reviewed by Spira et al (1977). They found the highest incidence in the sixth, seventh and eighth decades of life with an average of 59 years. The male to female ratio in most series is approximately 1:1 (Spira et al 1977, Nix et al 1985).

Duodenal carcinomas are usually adenocarcinomas and are commonest in the second and third parts of the duodenum. Carcinoma of the ampulla of Vater is not considered a primary duodenal carcinoma and is not included in this review. The majority of carcinomas occur in the infra-ampullary part of the duodenum (38.3%) with the periampullary area being the next most common site (32.4%) (Spira et al 1977). Only 7% are seen in the supra-ampullary area.

Patients usually present with obstructive symptoms such as abdominal pain, nausea, postprandial fullness, weight loss and vomiting (Cortese & Cornell 1972, Spira et al 1977, Nix et al 1985). Occasionally patients present with massive haemorrhage or jaundice.

The radiological appearances of carcinoma of the duodenum are similar to those of carcinoma elsewhere in the gastrointestinal tract (Bosse & Neely 1969). Features include polypoid filling defects, ulceration with mucosal destruction, rigidity and constriction of the intestinal lumen (Fig. 6.9). There may be evidence of obstruction with proximal dilatation (Spira et al 1977). Characteristic constricting lesions with mucosal destruction and shouldering of the margins are frequently seen.

A careful double contrast barium examination of the duodenum, using a tube to inject barium and insufflate air, is essential to detect some of the smaller lesions. Thomas et al (1971) reported a case involving the third part of the duodenum which was not adequately demonstrated on two barium meal examinations. The diagnosis was made on combined hypotonic duodenography and small bowel enema examination which showed an irregular stenotic lesion. Computed tomography is useful to evaluate the extent of tumour growth and to assess operability.

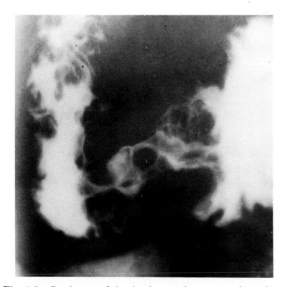

Fig. 6.9 Carcinoma of the duodenum shown as an irregular infiltrating polypoid lesion of the third part of the duodenum, with mucosal destruction, shouldering of the margins, and narrowing of the lumen.

Carcinoma of the duodenum carries a poor prognosis with a mean survival of 21 months (Nix et al 1985).

Leiomyosarcomas

Leiomyosarcomas are seen much less frequently in the duodenum than primary carcinoma. They develop in the subserous layer and grow extraluminally, displacing adjacent organs (Starzl et al 1960, Meyers 1971). They tend to outgrow their blood supply and are usually large when the diagnosis is made. Patients present with abdominal pain, weight loss, bleeding and jaundice. It is not normally possible to distinguish a leiomyosarcoma from a leiomyoma or carcinoma on radiological appearances.

Lymphomas

Involvement of the duodenum by lymphomas is uncommon, the more distal small intestine being a more frequent site. The duodenum is, however, frequently involved with lymphoma complicating immunosuppressive small intestinal disease (alpha-chain disease) (Khojasteh et al 1983). The radiological appearances in the duodenum are similar to those in other parts of the small intestine. Duodenal lymphomas carry a poor prognosis related in part to the technical difficulties of surgical removal (Dawson et al 1961).

CT is the technique of choice for assessing the extent of spread of primary or secondary involvement of the duodenum and should always be performed if surgical treatment is being considered.

Carcinoid tumours

Carcinoid tumours of the duodenum are rare, accounting for only 3–4% of duodenal neoplasms (Darling & Welch 1959, Charles et al 1963). The first part of the duodenum is the most common site of involvement. The radiological appearances include small submucosal polypoid lesions or ulcerating lesions in the duodenal bulb, and marked deformity of the second part of the duodenum with mass formation and ulceration (Clements & Roche 1984). In the six cases reported by Clements and Roche (1984) four had no metastases, one had evidence of local spread and the remaining patient developed overt liver metastases 25 years after the initial diagnosis. The primary duodenal lesion regressed following embolization of the liver metastases. Seymour et al (1982) reported a case with multiple sessile filling defects in the duodenal cap.

Secondary neoplasms

Secondary neoplasms of the duodenum frequently produce changes in the duodenum indistinguishable from primary carcinoma. The duodenum is involved by direct spread or by lymphatic or blood-borne metastases.

Carcinoma of the head of the pancreas frequently causes changes in the duodenum which can be detected radiologically. Widening, a double contour, irregularity of the inner margin, and occasionally the characteristic reversed '3' sign of Frostberg (1938) are well recognized features. Carcinoma of the body or tail of the pancreas may invade the fourth part of the duodenum and result in obstruction or bleeding.

Carcinoma of the right colon may invade the duodenum. In some patients the primary neoplasm will have been identified before duodenal invasion while in others the patient presents with duodenal symptoms. Radiologically, a constricting lesion with destruction of the mucosa (Fig. 6.10) or postbulbar ulceration with associated mucosal destruction are seen. CT is useful for identifying the extent of tumour infiltration (Diamond et al 1981) and should be performed if surgery is planned to assess whether the tumour is resectable.

Carcinoma of the right kidney may spread and involve the second part of the duodenum and occasionally the fourth part of the duodenum may be involved by lymphatic spread from a left renal carcinoma. As late as 14 years after primary renal cell carcinoma, these pathways may permit involvement of the duodenum, manifested by obstruction, bleeding or fistula formation (Khilnani & Wolf 1960, Veen et al 1976). Renal carcinoma invading the duodenum may produce changes indistinguishable from primary duodenal carcinoma (Lawson et al 1966, Meyers & McSweeney 1972).

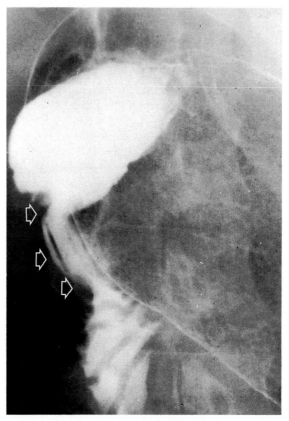

Fig. 6.10 Carcinoma of the colon infiltrating the duodenum causing marked symmetrical narrowing of the second part with destruction of the normal mucosal pattern (arrows). Carcinoma of an inverted caecum was found invading the duodenum at operation. (Reproduced from Nolan 1983 by kind permission.)

Carcinoma of the gall bladder or common bile duct may involve the duodenum with extensive infiltration, mucosal destruction and narrowing of the lumen. Radiological demonstration of metastatic melanoma in the duodenum is relatively uncommon. In patients dying from malignant melanoma 12% have metastases in the duodenum (Das Gupta & Brasfield 1964). They show characteristic appearance, being similar to primary carcinoma although sometimes they are seen as filling defects with ulceration or umbilication. Carcinoma of the breast and teratoma of the testes may spread to the duodenum (Shackleford et al 1942, Ngan 1970).

THE JEJUNUM AND ILEUM

Benign neoplasms

Benign neoplasms are an uncommon finding in the small intestine. The types encountered are similar to those found in other parts of the gastrointestinal tract and include leiomyomas, adenomas, hamartomas, lipomas, neuromas and inflammatory fibroid polyps.

Leiomyomas are the most common primary benign neoplasm, and patients characteristically present with acute bleeding. The leiomyoma may grow inwards into the lumen or outwards to form a mass on the serosal surface. Some grow in both directions to form a 'dumb-bell' type of tumour (Morson & Dawson 1979). An intraluminal leiomyoma is shown on barium examination as a round intraluminal filling defect (Miller & Lehman 1978). Angiography has proved to be the most reliable method for detecting leiomyomas of the small intestine and demonstrates the leiomyoma as a round or lobulated vascular mass (Fig. 6.11) (Boijsen & Reuter 1966, Forbes et al 1978).

Hamartomas are a developmental anomaly which may present in large numbers in the small intestine in patients with the Peutz–Jeghers syndrome (Dodds 1976).

Malignant neoplasms

The jejunum and ileum are uncommon sites for primary malignant neoplasms. Carcinoid tumours,

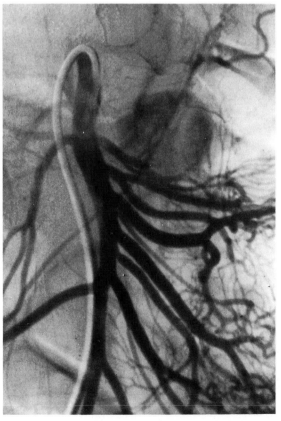

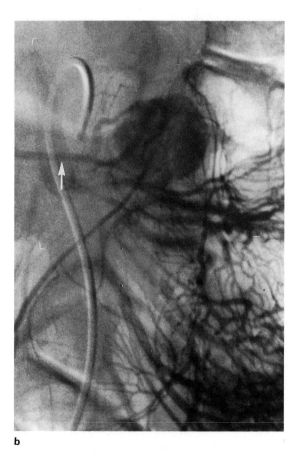

a   b

Fig. 6.11 Jejunal leiomyoma. Subtraction views of superior mesenteric arteriogram show (a) a round well-defined homogeneous vascular blush supplied mainly by the first jejunal branch. (b) An early draining vein can be seen in the late arterial phase (arrow). (Reproduced from Forbes et al 1978 by kind permission.)

primary lymphoma, carcinoma and leiomyosarcoma are the most common lesions.

Carcinoid tumours

The small intestine is the second most common site for carcinoid tumours and the most common site for malignant carcinoids (Boijsen et al 1974), the majority of which occur in the distal ileum (Bluth 1960, Jeffree et al 1984). Between 30 and 67% of gastrointestinal carcinoid tumours are invasive when discovered (Balthazar 1978). Most (75%) malignant carcinoid tumours originate in the ileum, the majority in the distal part (Silberman et al 1974, Grahame-Smith 1977, Jeffree et al 1984). No distinctive histological differences between benign and malignant carcinoid tumours are described and the neoplasm is considered to be malignant if there is local invasion or distant metastases. Neoplasms less than 1 cm in diameter are only occasionally malignant while those greater than 2 cm in diameter are consistently malignant. With time all will eventually enlarge, invade and metastasize (Balthazar 1978).

Patients present either with local manifestations of the neoplasm such as abdominal pain, diarrhoea and intermittent intestinal obstruction or with the carcinoid syndrome (Cope & Warwick 1974). Carcinoid tumours secrete 5-hydroxytryptamine (5-HT), kallikrein, bradykinin and sometimes histamine which are usually metabolized in the liver. When hepatic metastases are present these vasoactive substances may be released into the systemic circulation in significant quantities giving rise to the carcinoid syndrome (Grahame-Smith 1977). Flushing, particularly following alcohol, and diarrhoea are prominent manifestations. Other symptoms include asthma, peripheral oedema, cardiac lesions, peptic ulceration, malabsorption, abdominal pain and mental changes (Grahame-Smith 1977).

Radiology. In the absence of the carcinoid syndrome the diagnosis may be difficult. Conventional radiological investigation of the small intestine rarely leads to the detection of these neoplasms (Hermanutz et al 1974). This is because of the small size of most primary carcinoid tumours (Hermanutz et al 1974, Balthazar 1978).

Even when the neoplasm is observed on radiographs there may be difficulty in making the correct diagnosis. The small bowel enema (barium infusion, enteroclysis) is proving to be a valuable method for identifying primary carcinoid tumours and in our opinion is the investigation of choice in suspected cases (Schlangen 1976, Jeffree et al 1984, Jeffree & Nolan 1987). The radiological signs will reflect the pathological process and may be due to the primary lesion, to a mesenteric mass, to interference with the blood supply to the ileum by a secondary mass or to effects of fibrosis associated with the secondary mass. The most frequent radiological sign is an intramural (Fig. 6.12) or intraluminal filling defect in the ileum. Narrowing of a segment of ileum, sometimes showing an annular appearance, thickening of the valvulae conniventes, and separation of adjacent intestinal loops with rigidity and fixation may be seen. When fibrosis is associated with a secondary mass sharp angulation of a loop or loops may be observed.

Angiography has a very limited rôle in detecting the primary neoplasm. When angiography is being performed for therapeutic embolization a superior mesenteric angiogram may locate the ileal primary tumour if it has not already been found. A characteristic angiographic appearance is seen with a stellate arterial configuration, narrowing of deep

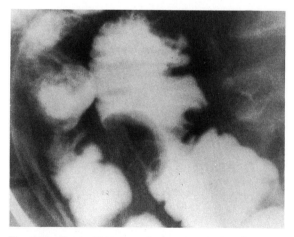

Fig. 6.12 Carcinoid tumour. A spot compression view showing an ileal carcinoid tumour as an intramural filling defect in the ileum. (Reproduced from Jeffree & Nolan 1987 by kind permission.)

mesenteric branches, poor to moderate accumulation of contrast medium in the neoplasm and non-filling of veins (Reuter & Boijsen 1966, Shimkin et al 1971, Claps et al 1972, Jeffree et al 1984).

Primary carcinoid tumours may be seen on CT as homogeneous soft tissue masses involving mesentery and intestinal wall, although in most cases the primary neoplasm is not visualized (McCarthy et al 1984, Hulnick 1986). By demonstrating the intestine, mesentery, lymph nodes and liver in a single examination CT is extremely useful in staging the neoplasms as well as in follow-up after surgery and chemotherapy. The characteristic changes are related to the desmoplastic response in the mesentery incited by the primary neoplasm. Although the primary neoplasm may not be seen its presence may be reflected by displacement or kinking of adjacent intestinal segments or a stellate radiation of mesenteric neurovascular bundles (Siegel et al 1980, McCarthy et al 1984, Picus et al 1984, Cockey et al 1985, Gould & Johnson 1986, Hulnick 1986). Mesenteric masses may reflect direct extension, metastases or local lymph nodes and occasionally are the only evidence of the disorder (Picus et al 1984). Malignant ascites may be present (McCarthy et al 1984). A rare finding is dystrophic calcification related to tumour necrosis in involved nodes as well as liver metastases (Siegel et al 1980, Cockey et al 1985). Liver metastases associated with marked hepatomegaly are a common finding at the time of CT diagnosis but are not always associated with the carcinoid syndrome. Liver metastases are usually hypodense and easily seen on precontrast scans but become isodense with hepatic parenchyma during the slow infusion of contrast medium, emphasizing the importance of non-contrast CT scans for evaluating liver metastases (McCarthy et al 1984, Hulnick 1986).

Surgical debulking of the primary tumour and liver metastases can help to reduce the severity and frequency of symptoms of the carcinoid syndrome (Ch'ng et al 1988). Therapeutic embolization at selective angiography has also been found to be a useful form of palliative treatment for hepatic metastases (Allison et al 1977, Allison 1988). With adequate pharmacological cover the technique is safe, effective, and relatively painless.

Lymphomas

Primary lymphoma is one of the most common neoplasms of the small intestine representing about 40% of primary malignant neoplasms (Good 1963). Intestinal lymphoma can be divided into two categories: those associated with previous immunological disturbance and consequent mucosal change and those which arise de novo in a previously normal intestine (Morson & Dawson 1979). It is difficult to define primary intestinal lymphoma and our definition is a modification of those suggested by Herrmann et al (1980) and Lewin et al (1978). Lymphomas are considered to be primary intestinal if the predominant lesion is in the intestine, the initial presenting symptoms are related to intestinal involvement and there is no evidence of a generalized or intestinal predisposing factor (Gourtsoyiannis & Nolan 1988).

Most patients present in the fourth to seventh decade of life with abdominal pain, intestinal obstruction, gastrointestinal bleeding, diarrhoea, weight loss and occasionally perforation (Rosenfelt & Rosenberg 1980, Gourtsoyiannis & Nolan 1988). There is frequently an abdominal mass on palpation. Conditions which predispose to intestinal lymphoma include coeliac disease (Gough et al 1962, Holmes et al 1976, Selby & Gallagher 1979, Swinson et al 1983), immunoproliferative small intestinal disease (alpha-chain disease) (Khojasteh et al 1983), and chronic lymphatic leukaemia (Gourtsoyiannis & Nolan 1988). Patients with coeliac disease who develop lymphoma are usually in the older age groups; most of the patients are over 50 (Swinson et al 1983, Cooper and Read 1985). Coeliac disease may be unmasked by the development of lymphoma (Cooper & Read 1985). Lymphoma complicating coeliac disease was originally classified on morphological and immunocytochemical grounds as malignant histiocytosis of the intestine (Isaacson & Wright 1978, Brunton & Guyer 1983). Recent evidence suggests, however, that it is of T-cell rather than histiocytic origin (Isaacson et al 1985).

Lymphomas originate in the lymphoid follicles of the submucosa and as these are more numerous in the ileum, the disorder is encountered more frequently in the ileum than in the jejunum. The exception is lymphoma complicating immunoproliferative small intestinal (alpha-chain) disease which usually affects the duodenum and proximal jejunum (Khojasteh et al 1983).

Radiology. The characteristic radiological patterns include polypoid masses, infiltration, ulceration, cavitation, thickened valvulae, multiple nodules, mesenteric masses and aneurysmal dilatation (Marshak et al 1961, Balikian et al 1969, Norfray et al 1973, Zornoza & Dodd 1980, Freeny 1983, Gourtsoyiannis & Nolan 1988). Small intestinal involvement is multifocal in 10–40% of cases (Zornoza & Dodd 1980).

Luminal narrowing including strictures is the most common finding. In some the narrowing is characteristic of malignancy with mucosal destruction whereas in others it is not (Gourtsoyiannis & Nolan 1988). Primary carcinoma, which is normally jejunal in location and solitary, can usually be differentiated from lymphoma.

Discrete, often multiple nodules which produce filling defects or bulbous enlargement of the mucosal folds may be seen (Gourtsoyiannis & Nolan 1988). Thickening of the valvulae conniventes is another characteristic finding.

The ulcers in lymphoma are characteristically broad-based. Large cavities secondary to central necrosis in a large neoplastic mass are highly characteristic (Fig. 6.13) (Sartoris et al 1984, Gourtsoyiannis & Nolan 1988) although similar findings are characteristic of leiomyosarcoma and are occasionally seen in metastases. Ileo-ileal fistulae may result from cavitation. Focal 'aneurysmal' dilatation is a well recognized but infrequent finding in small intestinal lymphoma (Cupps et al 1969, Gourtsoyiannis & Nolan 1988). The dilated part is seen as a long thick-walled aperistaltic segment filled with an amorphous collection of dilute barium and absence of mucosal markings. Proximal and distal to the aneurysmal dilatation the intestine is normal with no evidence of strictures or narrowing. The dilatation is presumed to be secondary to loss of muscle tone of the intestinal wall caused by extensive lymphomatous invasion and destruction of the muscle layers and neural plexi (Graves 1919, Ullman & Abeshouse 1932, Sartoris et al 1984).

The mesenteric form of intestinal lymphoma is

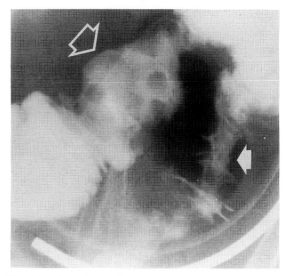

Fig. 6.13 Lymphoma of the small intestine shown on a spot compression view. There are two adjacent segments of involvement; the upper one shows a large cavity with a nodular pattern (open arrow) and the lower one concentric infiltration (closed arrow).

characterized by large extraluminal masses which extend into the retroperitoneum, displacing adjacent barium-filled loops of intestine (Marshak & Lindner 1976, Zornoza & Dodd 1980).

It may be difficult to differentiate intestinal lymphoma from Crohn's disease as similar radiological appearances may be seen in both conditions (Sartoris et al 1984, Gourtsoyiannis & Nolan 1988). When there is thickening of the valvulae conniventes with no other sign present it may be impossible to differentiate lymphoma from Crohn's disease or other conditions which cause thickening of the valvulae. The ulcers in lymphoma are broad-based, unlike the fissure ulcers, discrete ulcers or longitudinal ulcers seen in Crohn's disease (Nolan & Gourtsoyiannis 1980). Intestinal fistulae are seen in both conditions but in lymphoma the communication is usually through a large cavity.

CT can be used to show the extent of spread by demonstrating the size of the mass and evaluating the sites of neoplastic involvement of abdominal lymph nodes and solid viscera, allowing accurate staging in a single examination (Hulnick 1986). Delineation of the intestinal lumen with orally administered contrast medium is necessary for adequate recognition of intestinal wall thickening. The lymphoma may be seen as a large mass with only a small intraluminal component. There is only moderate enhancement of the lymphomatous mass after intravenous contrast medium. Central areas of irregular ulceration and cavitation may be seen (Pagani & Bernardino 1981, Megibow et al 1983, Hulnick 1986). Spread of the lymphoma into the mesentery may be demonstrated. Rarely calcification may be identified in the mass, usually after radiation or chemotherapy (Hulnick 1986).

Carcinoma

Primary carcinoma of the jejunum and ileum accounts for 15% of all small intestinal neoplasms (Good 1963, Ekberg & Ekholm 1980). Carcinomas are usually sited in the jejunum, less commonly in the ileum (Bridge & Perzin 1975, Bruneton et al 1983, Papadopoulos & Nolan 1985).

The aetiology of adenocarcinoma of the small intestine is unknown. Patients with primary adenocarcinoma have a high incidence of other primary neoplasms (Reyes & Talley 1970, Papadopoulos & Nolan 1985). Certain conditions are associated with a high risk of developing carcinoma. There is an increased incidence in patients with familial polyposis coli (Heffernon et al 1962) and coeliac disease. In a large population study adenocarcinoma of the small intestine was found in 19 patients with coeliac disease, compared with the 0.23 expected in the normal population (Swinson et al 1983). Patients with Crohn's disease of the small intestine also have an increased risk of developing carcinoma. Predisposing factors in patients with Crohn's disease include long duration of illness (15–20 years), chronic intestinal obstruction and excluded loops of small intestine associated with bypass operations (Greenstein et al 1978). Carcinoma complicating Crohn's disease is usually diagnosed at a late stage because the appearances are obscured by Crohn's disease.

Presenting symptoms of adenocarcinoma of the small intestine are non-specific and include abdominal pain, weight loss, anaemia, upper gastrointestinal bleeding, a palpable abdominal mass and intestinal obstruction.

The survival rate of patients with adenocarcinoma of the small intestine is poor with a 5-year survival of 15–23% (Wilson et al 1974, Mittal & Boczin 1980). Crohn's disease related carcinoma carries an even poorer prognosis (Collier et al 1985).

Radiology. The radiological features are similar to those of carcinoma of the colon. Characteristic appearances on barium examination include stricture formation with destruction of mucosa and shouldering of the margins, ulcerating lesions or polypoid masses (Papadopoulos & Nolan 1985).

Angiography and CT are useful for assessing operability. On angiography hypovascularity of the neoplasm is seen. Infiltration of arteries solely confined to the wall of the intestine indicates that the neoplasm has not invaded beyond the wall and that it can probably be radically resected (Ekberg & Ekholm 1980). Inoperability is usually the case when mesenteric artery branches of the first and second order are invaded.

Little information is available on the CT appearances of carcinoma of the small intestine (Hulnick 1986). When contrast medium outlines and distends the intestine the neoplasm can be identified as focal thickening of the intestinal wall with narrowing of the lumen either concentrically or asymmetrically (Hulnick 1986). There is moderate enhancement of the neoplasm following the intravenous administration of contrast medium. Associated bulky lymphadenopathy is less common than in lymphoma.

Leiomyosarcoma

Leiomyosarcomas rank with carcinoid tumours, lymphoma and carcinoma as one of the more common malignant neoplasms of the small intestine. Leiomyomatous neoplasms are intramural lesions arising from the circular or longitudinal muscle coats of the intestine, or more rarely, from the muscularis mucosae (Morson & Dawson 1979). With the exception of small symptomless growths it is impossible to separate them into benign and malignant lesions on histological appearances alone (Garvin et al 1979, Morson & Dawson 1979). The most important gross finding indicating whether the neoplasm is benign or malignant, apart from metastases, is the size (Starr & Dockerty 1955). The larger neoplasms are more likely to be malignant. The final diagnosis depends on the clinical behaviour of the neoplasm and the development of metastases.

Acute bleeding is the most common presenting symptom and massive gastrointestinal haemorrhage is frequent. Patients may, however, have intermittent melaena for several months or years (Starr & Dockerty 1955). Free perforation is an uncommon presentation (Golden & Stout 1941).

Surgical resection is the treatment of choice. Blood-vascular dissemination and peritoneal seeding are the routes of spread. Lymph nodes do not become involved and therefore extensive nodal dissection is unnecessary. Prolonged remission is frequent and large neoplasms which appear inoperable should be resected in order to offer the best possible opportunity of cure or prolonged remission (Starr & Dockerty 1955). Leiomyosarcomas differ from other malignant neoplasms of the small intestine in their greater tendency to bleed, to attain a large size without obstruction and to compatibility with long survival despite metastases (Dodds et al 1969).

Radiology. Plain radiographs are usually unhelpful although a leiomyosarcoma presenting as a mass containing calcification has been described (Ghahremani et al 1978). Leiomyosarcomas are often seen on barium studies as an abdominal mass and may be identified as a large extrinsic neoplasm displacing adjacent loops of intestine (Good 1963). This may be associated with an intraluminal filling defect and there may be destruction of adjacent mucosa and evidence of ulceration, cavitation or fistula formation (Martin 1955). The main feature is frequently a large cavity filled with barium and it may be difficult to identify the connection between the small intestine and the cavity.

The size and extent of the mass can be accurately demonstrated on CT (Hulnick 1986). Marked enhancement of the rim of the neoplasm around a well-defined cavity following intravenous contrast medium is a characteristic finding (Clark & Alexander 1982, McLeod et al 1984, Price et al 1988). Areas of central necrosis and liquefaction are identified within the primary neoplasm (Fig. 6.14) or liver metastes (Clark & Alexander 1982). A fluid level may be present in the cavity (Price et al 1988). Multiple homogeneous soft tissue masses throughout the abdomen indicate peritoneal metastases (Hulnick 1986).

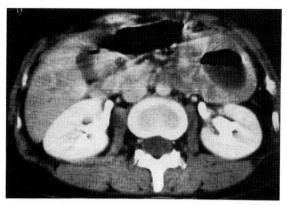

Fig. 6.14 Leiomyosarcoma. A contrast-enhanced CT scan shows a well circumscribed oval-shaped mass anterior to the left kidney. In the centre of the contrast-enhanced mass there is a well defined central cavity containing an air-fluid level. (Reproduced from Price et al 1988 by kind permission.)

Other primary neoplasms

Other primary neoplasms which may be encountered in the small intestine include Kaposi sarcoma, liposarcoma, angiosarcoma, fibrosarcoma and neurofibrosarcoma, although they are very uncommon (Walker 1987a).

Secondary neoplasms

Secondary neoplasms involve the small intestine by direct invasion from adjacent organs, lymphatic extension, peritoneal seeding and embolic metastases (Meyers & McSweeney 1972, Willis 1973, Meyers 1976, 1981). Characteristic radiological features may reflect the mode of spread and make it possible to indicate the primary site (Meyers 1981). More than one mechanism of spread may be encountered in a particular patient; this is most frequent with direct invasion and seeded metastases from intraperitoneal primaries (Meyers 1976).

Invasion of the small intestine is most common from primary neoplasms of the ovary, colon, prostate, uterus and kidney and indicates that an agressive neoplasm has broken through fascial planes (Khilnani et al 1966, Meyers & McSweeney 1972, Meyers 1976). The most characteristic radiological sign of a pelvic neoplasm directly invading the small intestine is that of a mass invading the adjacent intestine, often over a considerable length with mucosal destruction, narrowing of the lumen and obstruction (Meyers 1981). Tethering of the mucosal folds is often a conspicuous feature.

Spread via the lymphatics plays a minor rôle in the dissemination of secondary neoplasms to the small intestine (Meyers 1981). Carcinoma of the caecum spreading to the terminal ileum via the lymphatics is a classical example of this type of spread (Moffat & Gourley 1980).

Ascitic fluid flows preferentially in the peritoneal cavity along the route of the small intestinal mesentery towards the right lower quadrant. As a result, intraperitoneal seeding of abdominal neoplasms causes localization in the right lower quadrant at the lower end of the mesentery of the small intestine in over 40% of cases of intraperitoneal seeding (Meyers 1975). Stasis in the lower recess of the mesentery of the small intestine favours the deposition, fixation and growth of seeded metastases. Growth of the secondary deposits results in separation of the ileal loops in the right lower quadrant and angled tethering of the mucosal folds. The resulting narrowed loops may align in a parallel configuration described as 'palisading' (Meyers 1975).

Blood-borne metastatic spread to the small intestine from extra-abdominal sites is rare (Willis 1973, Garvin et al 1979, Walker 1987b). The commonest metastases are from malignant melanomas and primary carcinoma of the breast, lung, kidney and genital tract (Meyers & McSweeney 1972, Willis 1973, Walker 1987b). The metastases tend to be submucosal in location and the patients present clinically with obstruction, intussusception, bleeding or less frequently perforation.

Metastases should always be considered in the differential diagnosis of small intestinal neoplasms even if there is no known primary, as metastases may present before the primary lesion. Malignant melanoma is the most common neoplasm to metastasize to the small intestine (Walker 1987b) although frequently no symptoms are caused. In the report by Das Gupta and Brasfield (1964), the small intestine was the site of metastases in 54 out of 100 autopsies on patients who died from malignant melanoma whereas only 8 out of 1000 patients with known melanoma had small intestinal metastases confirmed at laparotomy.

Barium studies show metastatic melanoma characteristically as multiple submucosal polypoid lesions, frequently with central ulceration giving a 'bull's eye' or 'target' lesion (Pomerantz & Margolin 1962, Meyers & McSweeney 1972, Beckley 1974). Some metastatic melanomas are predominantly cavitating lesions. In a report by Goldstein and Zornoza (1978) of ten cases of cavitating metastases, seven were metastatic melanoma with one metastasis each from lung, rectum and endometrium. When multiple they may be confined to a segment of intestine, be within the field of a specific arterial distribution, or be widespread in the intestine (Meyers & McSweeney 1972). They tend to develop on the antimesenteric border and when multiple deposits are confined to a segment the nodules tend to be approximately the same size.

Carcinoma of the breast is probably the next most frequent neoplasm to metastasize to the small intestine but there is little information available regarding the radiological appearances. It is likely that breast metastases result in infiltration with narrowing and stricture formation (Tillotson & Douglas 1962, Rees et al 1976), sometimes with a linitis plastica appearance (Meyers & McSweeney 1972). Metastases to the intestine from carcinoma of the lung, an extremely uncommon finding, characteristically produce large mesenteric masses with infiltration of the intestinal wall, fixation and angulation of the intestine indistinguishable from other widespread intra-abdominal secondaries (Meyers & McSweeney 1972).

ACKNOWLEDGEMENTS

We are pleased to acknowledge support from the Oxford Regional Research Committee. We thank Miss Nicola Green for assisting us with the project and for preparing the manuscript. The photographic prints were prepared by the Department of Medical Illustration, John Radcliffe Hospital, Oxford.

REFERENCES

Adashek K, Sangel J, Longwire W 1979 Cancer of the stomach, a review of consecutive ten year intervals. Annals of Surgery 189: 6–10

Allison D J 1988 Embolization of liver tumours. In: Blumgart L H (ed) Surgery of the liver and biliary tract. Churchill Livingstone, Edinburgh, pp 1201–1217

Allison D J, Modlin I M, Jenkins W J 1977 Treatment of carcinoid liver metastases by hepatic artery embolization. Lancet 2: 1323–1325

Anderson M F, Harrell G S 1980 Secondary oesophageal tumours. American Journal of Roentgenology 135: 1243–1246

Antonioli D A 1984 Gastric cancer. In: Appleman H D (ed) Pathology of oesophagus, stomach and duodenum. Churchill Livingstone, Edinburgh, pp 121–144

Appleman H D 1984 Stromal tumours of the oesophagus, stomach and duodenum. In: Appleman H D (ed) Pathology of oesophagus, stomach and duodenum. Churchill Livingstone, Edinburgh, pp 195–242

Balikian J P, Nassar N T, Shamma'a M H, Shahid M J 1969 Primary lymphomas of the small intestine including the duodenum. A roentgenologic analysis of twenty-six cases. American Journal of Roentgenology 107: 131–141

Balthazar E J 1978 Carcinoid tumors of the alimentary tract. I. Radiographic diagnosis. Gastrointestinal Radiology 3: 47–56

Beckley D E 1974 Alimentary tract metastases from malignant melanoma. Clinical Radiology 25: 385–389

Berg J W 1958 Histological aspects of the relation between gastric adenomatous polyps and gastric cancer. Cancer 11: 1149–1155

Bleshman M H, Banner M P, Johnson R C, Deford J W 1978 The inflammatory oesophagogastric polyp and fold. Radiology 128: 589–593

Bluth I 1960 Gastrointestinal carcinoid tumours – roentgen features. Radiology 74: 573–580

Boijsen E, Reuter S R 1966 Mesenteric angiography in the evaluation of inflammatory and neoplastic disease of the intestine. Radiology 87: 1028–1036

Boijsen E, Kaude J, Tylen U 1974 Radiologic diagnosis of ileal carcinoid tumours. Acta Radiologica: Diagnosis (Stockholm) 15: 65–82

Bosse G, Neely J A 1969 Roentgenological findings in primary milignant tumors of the duodenum. American Journal of Roentgenology 107: 111–118

Brady L W, Asbell S O 1980 Malignant lymphoma of the gastrointestinal tract. Radiology 137: 291–298

Bridge M F, Perzin K H 1975 Primary adenocarcinoma of the jejunum and ileum. Cancer 36: 1876–1887

Bruneton J N, Drouillard J, Bourry J, Roux P, Lecomte P 1983 Adenocarcinoma of the small intestine. Current state of diagnosis and treatment. A study of 27 cases and a review of the literature. Journal de Radiologie et d'Electrologie 64: 117–123

Brunton F J, Guyer P B 1983 Malignant histiocytosis and ulcerative jejunitis of the small intestine. Clinical Radiology 34: 291–295

Carlson H C 1983 Carcinoma in the oesophagogastric junction. In: Marshak R H, Lindner A E, Maclansky D (eds) Radiology of the stomach. W B Saunders, Philadelphia, pp 172–204

Carman R D 1921 A new roentgen-ray sign of ulcerating gastric cancer. Journal of the American Medical Association 77: 990–992

Carnovale R L, Goldstein H M, Zornoza J, Dodd G D 1977 Radiological manifestations of oesophageal lymphoma. American Journal of Roentgenology 128: 751–754

Charles R N, Kelley M L, Campeti F 1963 Primary duodenal tumours. A study of 31 cases. Archives of Internal Medicine 111: 23–33

Ch'ng J L C, Polak J, Bloom S (1988) Endocrine aspects of liver tumours. In: Blumgart L H (ed) Surgery of the liver and biliary tract. Churchill Livingstone, Edinburgh, pp 1191–1199

Claps R J, Lande A, Lilienfeld R, Mieza M 1972 Angiographic demonstration of an ileal carcinoid. Radiology 103: 87–88

Clark R A, Alexander E S 1982 Computed tomography of gastrointestinal leiomyosarcoma. Gastrointestinal Radiology 7: 127–129

Clements J L Jr, Roche R R 1984 Carcinoid of the duodenum: a report of six cases. Gastrointestinal Radiology 9: 17–21

Clements J L, Torres W E, Ball T I 1983 Unusual benign lesions of the stomach. In: Marshak R H, Lindner A E, Maclansky D (eds) Radiology of the stomach. W B Saunders, Philadelphia, pp 460–497

Cockey B M, Fishman E K, Jones B, Siegelman S S 1985 Computed tomography of abdominal carcinoid tumor. Journal of Computer Assisted Tomography 9: 38–42

Collier P T, Turowski P, Diamond D L 1985 Small intestinal adenocarcinoma complicating regional enteritis. Cancer 55: 516–521

Cooper B T, Read A E 1985 Small intestinal lymphoma. World Journal of Surgery (New York) 9: 930–937

Cope V, Warwick F 1974 The role of radiology in the detection of endocrine tumours of the gastrointestinal tract. Clinics in Gastroenterology 3: 621–642

Cortese A F, Cornell G N 1972 Carcinoma of the duodenum. Cancer 29: 1010–1015

Cupps R E, Hodgson J R, Dockerty M B, Adson M A 1969 Primary lymphoma of the small intestine: problems of roentgenologic diagnosis. Radiology 92: 1355–1362

Darling R C, Welch C E 1959 Tumours of the small intestine. New England Journal of Medicine 260: 397–408

Das Gupta T K, Brasfield R D 1964 Metastatic melanoma of the gastrointestinal tract. Archives of Surgery 88: 969–973

Dawson I M P, Cornes J S, Morson B C 1961 Primary malignant lymphoid tumours of the intestinal tract. Report of 37 cases with a study of factors influencing prognosis. British Journal of Surgery 49: 80–89

Derchi L E, Biggi E, Rolland G A, Cicio G R, Neumaier C E 1983 Sonographic staging of gastric cancer. American Journal of Roentgenology 140: 273–276

Diamond R T, Greenberg H M, Boult I F 1981 Direct metastatic spread of right colonic adenocarcinoma to duodenum – barium and computed tomographic findings. Gastrointestinal Radiology 6: 339–341

Dodds W J 1976 Clinical and roentgen features of the intestinal polyposis syndromes. Gastrointestinal Radiology 1: 127–142

Dodds W J, Goldberg H T, Margulis A R 1969 Leiomyosarcoma of the small intestine. American Journal of Roentgenology 107: 142–149

Earlam R, Cunha-Melo J R 1980a Oesophageal squamous cell carcinoma. I. A critical review of surgery. British Journal of Surgery 67: 381–390

Earlam R, Cunha-Melo J R 1980b Oesophageal squamous cell carcinoma. II. A critical review of radiotherapy. British Journal of Surgery 67: 457–461

Ekberg O, Ekholm S 1980 Radiology in primary small bowel adenocarcinoma. Gastrointestinal Radiology 5: 49–53

Fielding W L, Ellis D J, Jones B G et al 1980 Natural

history of 'early' gastric cancer: results of a ten year regional survery. British Medical Journal 281: 965–968

Forbes W S C, Nolan D J, Fletcher E W L, Lee E 1978 Small bowel melaena: two cases diagnosed by angiography. British Journal of Surgery 65: 168–170

Freeny P C 1983 Lymphoma of the gastrointestinal tract: conventional radiography and computed tomography. In: Margulis A R, Golding C A (eds) Diagnostic radiology. University of California, San Francisco, pp 213–224

Frostberg N 1938 Characteristic duodenal deformity in cases of different kinds of peri-varterial enlargement of the pancreas. Act Radiologica (Stockholm) 19: 164–173

Garvin P J, Herrmann V, Kawinski D L, William V L 1979 Benign and malignant tumours of the small intestine. Current Problems in Cancer 3: 1–46

Ghahremani G G, Meyers M A, Port R B 1978 Calcified primary tumors of the gastrointestinal tract. Gastrointestinal Radiology 2: 331–339

Giulli R, Gignoux M 1980 Treatment of carcinoma of the oesophagus. Retrospective study of 2400 patients. Annals of Surgery 192: 44–52

Gold R P, Green P H R, O'Toole K M, Seaman W B 1984 Early gastric cancer – radiographic experience. Radiology 152: 283–290

Golden T, Stout A P 1941 Smooth muscle tumours of the gastrointestinal tract and retroperitoneal tissues. Surgery, Gynecology and Obstetrics 73: 784–810

Goldstein H M, Zornoza J 1978 Association of squamous cell carcinoma of the head and neck with cancer of the esophagus. American Journal of Roentgenology 131: 791–794

Good C A 1963 Tumours of the small intestine. American Journal of Roentgenology 89: 685–705

Gordon R, Laufer I, Kressel Y H 1980 Gastric polyps on routine double-contrast examination of the stomach. Radiology 134: 27–30

Gough K R, Read A E, Naish J M 1962 Intestinal reticulosis as a complication of idiopathic steatorrhoea. Gut 3: 232–239

Gould M, Johnson R J 1986 Computed tomography of abdominal carcinoid tumour. British Journal of Radiology 59: 881–885

Gourtsoyiannis N C, Nolan D J 1988 Lymphoma of the small intestine: radiological features. Clinical Radiology 39: 639–645

Gowing N F C 1962 Pathology of oesophageal tumours. In: Tanner N C, Smithers D W (eds) Tumours of the oesophagus. Livingstone, London, pp 91–135

Graffe W, Thorbjarnason B, Pearce J M, Beal J M 1960 Benign neoplasms of the stomach. American Journal of Surgery 100: 561–571

Grahame-Smith D G 1977 The carcinoid syndrome. In: Truelove S C, Lee E (eds) Topics in gastroenterology – 5. Blackwell Scientific, Oxford, pp 285–312

Graves S 1919 Primary lymphoblastoma of the intestines. Report of 3 cases: one with apparent recovery following operation. Journal of Medical Research 11: 415–431

Green P H R, O'Toole K M, Weinberg L M, Goldfarb J 1981 Early gastric cancer. Gastroenterology 81: 247–256

Greenstein A J, Sachar D, Pucillo A et al 1978 Cancer in Crohn's disease after diversionary surgery. A report of seven adenocarcinomas occurring in excluded bowel. American Journal of Surgery 125: 86–90

Halvorsen R A Jr, Magruder-Habib K, Foster W L,

Roberts L, Postlethwait R W, Thompson W M 1986 Esophageal cancer staging by CT – long term follow-up Radiology 161: 147–151

Hambraeus G M, Mercke C E, Hammar E, Landberg E, Wang-Anderson W 1981 Surgery alone or combined with radiation therapy in esophageal carcinoma. Cancer 48: 63–68

Heffernon E W, Metcalfe O, Schwarz H J 1962 Polyposis of the small and large bowel with carcinoma in a villous polyp of the jejunum. Gastroenterology 42: 60–62

Hermanutz K D, Bucheler E, Biersack H J 1974 The radiological diagnosis of carcinoids. Fortschritte auf dem Gebiete der Rontgenstrahlen und der Nuklearmedizin 121: 186–196

Herrmann R, Panahom A M, Barcos M P, Walsh D, Stutzman L 1980 Gastrointestinal involvement in non-Hodgkin's lymphoma. Cancer 46: 215–222

Hessler P C, Braunstein E 1978 Adenocarcinoma of the duodenum arising in a villous adenoma. Gastrointestinal Radiology 2: 355–357

Heyder N 1987 Endoscopic ultrasonography of tumours of the oesophagus and the stomach. Surgical Endoscopy 1: 17–23

Holmes G K T, Stokes P L, Sorahan T M, Prior P, Waterhouse J A H, Cooke W T 1976 Coeliac disease, gluten-free diet and malignancy. Gut 17: 612–619

Hulnick D H 1986 Small intestine. In: Megibow A J, Balthazar E J (eds) Computed tomography of the gastrointestinal tract. C V Mosby, St Louis, Missouri, pp 217–278

Isaacson P G, Wright D H 1978 Intestinal lymphomas associated with malabsorption. Lancet 1: 67–70

Isaacson P G, Spencer J, Connolly C E et al 1985 Malignant histiocytosis of the intestine: a T-cell lymphoma. Lancet 2: 688–691

Itai Y, Kogure T, Okuyama Y, Ariyama H 1978 Superficial esophageal carcinoma. Radiology 126: 597–601

Jacobson F 1962 The Paterson–Kelly syndrome and carcinoma of the oesophagus. In: Tanner N C, Smithers D W (eds) Tumours of the oesophagus. Livingstone, London, pp 53–60

Jaffe N 1975 Metastatic involvement of the stomach secondary to breast carcinoma. American Journal of Roentgenology 123: 512–521

Jeffree M A, Nolan D J 1987 Multiple ileal carcinoid tumours. Case report. British Journal of Radiology 60: 402–403

Jeffree M A, Barter S J, Hemingway A P, Nolan D J 1984 Primary carcinoid tumours of the ileum: the radiological appearances. Clinical Radiology 35: 451–455

Johnston O, James B, Theron C, MacDonald J R 1953 Smooth muscle tumours of the oesophagus. Thorax 8: 251–265

Kayima T, Morishita T, Asakura H, Miura S, Munakata Y, Tsuchiya M 1982 Long term follow-up study of gastric adenoma and its relation to gastric protruded carcinoma. Cancer 50: 2496–2503

Khilnani M T, Wolf B S 1960 Late involvement of the alimentary tract by carcinoma of the kidney. American Journal of Digestive Diseases 5: 529–540

Khilnani M T, Marshak R H, Eliasoph J, Wolf B S 1966 Roentgen features of metastases to the colon. American Journal of Roentgenology 96: 302–310

Khojasteh A, Hangshenass M, Haghighi P 1983

Immunoproliferative small intestinal disease. New England Journal of Medicine 308: 1401–1405

Kleinerman J, Yardumian K, Tamaki H T 1950 Primary carcinoma of the duodenum. Annals of Internal Medicine 32: 451–465

Kleinhaus U, Militianu D 1988 Computed tomography in the preoperative evaluation of gastric carcinoma. Gastrointestinal Radiology 13: 97–101

Kodama Y, Inkuchi K, Soejima K, Matsusaka T, Okamura T 1983 Growth patterns and prognosis in early gastric carcinoma. Cancer 51: 320–326

Kohler R E, Moss A A, Marguilis A R 1976 Early radiographic manifestations of carcinoma of the oesophagus. Radiology 119: 1–5

Lawson L J, Holt L P, Rooke H W 1966 Recurrent duodenal haemorrhage from renal carcinoma. British Journal of Urology 38: 133–137

Lawson T L, Dodds W J 1976 Infiltrating carcinoma simulating achalasia. Gastrointestinal Radiology 1: 245–248

Le Roux B T 1961 An analysis of 700 cases of carcinoma of the hypopharynx, the oesophagus and proximal stomach. Thorax 16: 226–255

Lee K R, Levine E, Moffat R E, Bigongiari L R, Hermreck A S 1979 Computed tomagraphic staging of malignant gastric neoplasms. Radiology 133: 151–155

Lewin K J, Ranchod M, Dorfman R F 1978 Lymphomas of the gastrointestinal tract. A study of 117 cases presenting with gastrointestinal disease. Cancer 42: 693–707

Marshak R H, Lindner A E 1976 Radiology of the small intestine, 2nd edn. W B Saunders, Philadelphia.

Marshak R H, Wolf B S, Eliasoph J 1961 The roentgen findings in lymphosarcoma of the small intestine. American Journal of Roentgenology 86: 682–692

Marshak R H, Lindner A E, Maklansky D 1983 Lymphoma of the stomach. In: Marshak R H, Lindner A E, Maclansky D (eds) Radiology of the stomach. W B Saunders, Philadelphia, pp 235–262

Martin J F 1955 Leiosarcoma of the small intestine: report of three cases and review of the literature. American Journal of Roentgenology 74: 1081–1088

Martin W C 1936 Lymphoblastoma of the gastrointestinal tract. American Journal of Roentgenology 36: 881–891

McCarthy S M, Stark D D, Moss A A, Goldberg H I 1984 Computed tomography of malignant carcinoid disease. Journal of Computer Assisted Tomography 8: 846–850

McFee A S, Aust J B 1981 Gastric carcinoma and the CAT scan. Gastroenterology 80: 196–198

McLeod A J, Zornoza J, Shirkhoda A 1984 Leiomyosarcoma: computed tomographic findings. Radiology 152: 133–136

Megibow A J, Balthazar E J, Naidich D P, Bosniak M A 1983 Computed tomography of gastrointestinal lymphoma. American Journal of Roentgenology 141: 541–547

Meyers M A 1971 Leiomyosarcoma of the duodenum. Clinical Radiology 22: 257–260

Meyers M A 1975 Metastatic seeding along the small bowel mesentery. American Journal of Roentgenology 123: 67–73

Meyers M A 1976 Clinical involvement of mesenteric and antimesenteric borders of small bowel loops. II. Radiologic interpretation of pathologic alterations. Gastrointestinal Radiology 1: 49–58

Meyers M A Intraperitoneal spread of malignancies and its effect on the bowel. Clinical Radiology 32: 129–146

Meyers M A, McSweeney J 1972 Secondary neoplasms of the bowel. Radiology 105: 1–11

Miller C 1962 Carcinoma of the thoracic oesophagus. British Journal of Surgery 49: 507–522

Miller R E, Lehman G 1978 Gastrointestinal haemorrhage from ileal leiomyoma. Utility of the complete reflux small bowel examination. Gastrointestinal Radiology 2: 367–369

Ming S C, Goldman H 1965 Gastric polyps. Cancer 18: 721–726

Minielly J A, Harrison E G Jr, Fontana R S, Payner W S 1967 Verrucous squamous cell carcinoma of the oesophagus. Cancer 20: 2078–2087

Mitros F A 1984 Pathology of the oesophagus, stomach and duodenum. In: Appleman H D (ed) Pathology of oesophagus, stomach and duodenum. Churchill Livingstone, Edinburgh, pp 1–35

Mittal V K, Boczin J H 1980 Primary malignant tumours of the small bowel. American Journal of Surgery 140: 396–399

Moffat R E, Gourley W K 1980 Ileal lymphatic metastases from cecal carcinoma. Radiology 135: 55–58

Monaco A P, Roth S I, Castleman B, Welch C C 1962 Adenomatous polyps of the stomach. A clinical and pathological study of 153 cases. Cancer 15: 456–467

Montesi A, Graziani L, Pesares A, De Nigris E, Bearzi I 1982 Radiologic diagnosis of early gastric cancer by routine double-contrast examination. Gastrointestinal Radiology 7: 205–215

Morson B C, Dawson I M P 1979 Gastrointestinal pathology, 2nd edn. Blackwell Scientific, Oxford.

Moss A A, Schnyder P, Candardjis G, Margulis A R 1980 Computed tomography of benign and malignant gastric abnormalities. Journal of Clinical Gastroenterology 2: 401–404

Moss A A, Schnyder P, Thoeni R F, Margulis A R 1981a Esophageal carcinoma: pretherapy staging by computed tomography. American Journal of Roentgenology 136: 1051–1056

Moss A A, Schnyder P, Marks W, Margulis A R 1981b Gastric adenocarcinoma: a comparison of the accuracy and economics of staging by computerized tomography and surgery. Gastroenterology 80: 45–50

Murata Y, Muroi M, Yoshida M, Ide H, Hanyu F 1987 Endoscopic ultrasonography in the diagnosis of esophageal carcinoma. Surgical Endoscopy 1: 11–16

Ngan H 1970 Involvement of the duodenum by metastases from tumours of the genital tract. British Journal of Radiology 43: 701–705

Nix G A, Wilson J H, Dees J 1985 Primary malignant tumours of the duodenum. Fortschritte auf dem Gebiete der Rontgenstrahlen und der Nuklearmedizin 142: 385–390

Nolan D J, Gourtsoyiannis N C 1980 Crohn's disease of the small intestine: a review of the radiological appearances in 100 consecutive patients examined by a barium infusion technique. Clinical Radiology 30: 597–603

Norfray J, Calenoff L, Zanon B Jr 1973 Aneurysmal lymphoma of the small intestine. American Journal of Roentgenology 119: 335–341

Odurny A, Birch S J 1985 Hepatic arterial embolization in patients with metastatic carcinoid tumours. Clinical Radiology 36: 597–602

Op den Orth J O, Dekker W 1981 Gastric adenomas. Radiology 141: 289–294

Pagani J J, Bernardino M E 1981 CT-radiographic correlation of ulcerating small bowel lymphomas. American Journal of Roentgenology 136: 998–1000

Papadopoulos V D, Nolan D J 1985 Carcinoma of the small intestine. Clinical Radiology 36: 409–413

Parnell S A, Peppercorn M A, Antonioli D A, Cohen M A, Joffe N 1978 Squamous cell papilloma of the esophagus. Report of a case after peptic esophagitis and repeated bougienage with a review of the literature. Gastroenterology 74: 910–913

Paulino F, Roselli A 1979 Early gastric cancer – a report of 25 cases. Surgery 15: 171–176

Picus D, Balfe D M, Kohler R E, Roper C L, Owen J W 1983 Computed tomography in the staging of esophageal carcinoma. Radiology 146: 433–438

Picus D, Glazer H S, Levitt R G, Husband J E 1984 Computed tomography of abdominal carcinoid tumours. American Journal of Roentgenology 143: 581–584

Pochaczevsky R, Sherman R S 1959 The roentgen appearance of gastric argentaffinoma. Radiology 72: 330–337

Poleyard G D, Marty A T, Birhaun W B, O'Reilly R R 1977 Adenocarcinoma in columnar lined oesophagus. Archives of Surgery 112: 997–1000

Pomerantz H, Margolin H N 1962 Metastases to the gastrointestinal tract from malignant melanoma. American Journal of Roentgenology 88: 712–717

Portmann V V, Dunne E F, Hazard J B 1954 Manifestations of Hodgkin's disease of the gastrointestinal tract. American Journal of Roentgenology 72: 772–787

Price J, McGuire L J, Chan M S Y 1988 Case of the month. Multiple mystifying melaenas. British Journal of Radiology 61: 521–522

Quint L, Glazer E M, Orringer M B, Cross B H 1985a Esophageal carcinoma. CT findings. Radiology 155: 171–175

Quint L E, Glazer G M, Orringer M B 1985b Esophageal imaging by MR and CT: study of normal anatomy and neoplasms. Radiology 156: 727–731

Raven R W 1948 Carcinoma of the oesophagus – a clinico-pathological study. British Journal of Surgery 36: 70–73

Rees B I, Okwonga W, Jenkins I L 1976 Intestinal metastases from carcinoma of the breast. Clinical Oncology 2: 113–119

Reuter S R, Boijsen E 1966 Angiographic findings in two ileal carcinoid tumours. Radiology 87: 836–840

Reyes E L, Talley R W 1970 Primary malignant tumours of the small intestine. American Journal of Gastroenterology 54: 30–43

Rosenfelt F, Rosenberg S A 1980 Diffuse histiocytic lymphoma presenting with gastrointestinal tract lesions. Cancer 45: 2188–2193

Sakita T, Ogura Y, Takasu S, Fukutomi H, Miwa T, Yoshimori M 1971 Observations on the healing of ulcerations in early gastric cancer. Gastroenterology 60: 835–844

Sartoris D J, Harell G S, Anderson M F, Zboralske F 1984 Small bowel lymphoma and regional enteritis: radiographic similarities. Radiology 152: 291–296

Schatzki R, Hawes E H 1942 The roentgenological appearances of extra mucosal tumours of the oesophagus. American Journal of Roentgenology 48: 1–5

Schlangen J T 1976 Radiology of carcinoid tumours of the small intestine. Radiologia Clinica (Basel) 45: 105–114

Schneeblock G, Terrier F, Fuchs W A 1983 Computed tomography in carcinoma of oesophagus and cardia. Gastrointestinal Radiology 8: 193–206

Selby W S, Gallagher N D 1979 Malignancy in a 19-year experience of adult coeliac disease. Digestive Diseases and Sciences 24: 684–688

Seymour E O, Griffin C N, Kurtz S M 1982 Carcinoid tumours of the duodenal cap presenting as multiple polypoid defects. Gastrointestinal Radiology 7: 19–21

Shackleford R T, Fisher A M, Firor W B 1942 Duodenal tumour of unusual character. Annals of Surgery 116: 864–873

Sherrick D W, Hodgson J R, Docherty M B 1965 The roentgenological diagnosis of primary gastric lymphoma. Radiology 84: 925–932

Shimkin P M, DeVita V T, Dopman J L 1971 Arteriography of an ileal carcinoid tumour. Journal of the Canadian Association of Radiologists 22: 259–269

Shirakabe H 1983 Early gastric carcinoma. In: Marshak R H, Lindner A E, Maclansky D (eds) Radiology of the stomach. W B Saunders, Philadelphia, pp 147–171

Shorvon P J, Lees W R, Frost R A, Cotton P B 1987 Upper gastrointestinal endoscopic ultrasonography in gastroenterology. British Journal of Radiology 60: 429–438

Siegel R S, Kuhns L R, Borlaza G S, McCormick T L, Simmons J L 1980 Computed tomography and angiography in ileal carcinoid tumor and retractile mesenteritis. Radiology 134: 437–440

Silberman H, Crichlow R W, Caplan H S 1974 Neoplasms of the small bowel. Annals of Surgery 180: 157–161

Spira I A, Ghazi A, Wolfe W I 1977 Primary adenocarcinoma of the duodenum. Cancer 39: 1721–1726

Sridhar C, Jay Zeshind H, Rising J A 1980 Verrucous squamous cell carcinoma. Radiology 136: 614

Starr G F, Dockerty M B 1955 Leiomyomas and leiomyosarcoma of the small intestine. Cancer 8: 101–111

Starzl T E, Bernhard V M, Heneger G C 1960 Two cases of leiomyosarcoma of the duodenum. Archives of Surgery 80: 528–532

Suzuki H, Kobayatki S, Fredo M, Nakayama K 1972 Diagnosis of early esophageal cancer. Surgery 71: 99–103

Swinson C M, Slavin G, Coles E C, Booth C C 1983 Coeliac disease and malignancy. Lancet 1: 111–115

Tanner N C, Smithers D W 1962 Tumours of the oesophagus. Livingstone, London.

Thomas E, Bowey R R, Hislop I G, O'Brien J A 1971 Duodenal carcinoma diagnosed by hypotonic duodenography and small bowel enema. Australasian Radiology 15: 343–345

Thompson G, Soners S, Stevenson G W 1983 Benign gastric ulcer: a reliable radiological diagnosis. American Journal of Roentgenology 141: 331–333

Thompson W M, Halvorsen R A, Foster W L, Williford M E, Postlethwait R W, Korobkin M 1983 Computed tomography for staging esophageal and gastroesophageal cancer. Re-evaluation. American Journal of Roentgenology 141: 951–958

Thorpe R P, Neiman B 1950 Rhabdomyosarcoma of the oesophagus. Journal of Thoracic and Cardiovascular Surgery 21: 77

Tillotson P M, Douglas R G 1962 Metastatic tumor of the small intestine. Three cases presenting unusual clinical and roentgenographic findings. American Journal of Roentgenology 88: 702–706

Tomasulo J 1971 Gastric polyps. Cancer 27: 1346–1355

Toreson W E 1944 Secondary carcinoma of the esophagus as a cause of dysphagia. Archives of Pathology 38: 82–84

Ullman A, Abeshouse B S 1932 Lymphosarcoma of the small and large intestines. Annals of Surgery 95: 878–915

Veen H F, Oscarson J E A, Malt R A 1976 Alien cancers of the duodenum. Surgery, Gynecology and Obstetrics. 143: 39–42

Walker M J 1987a Sarcomas of the small intestine. In: Nelson R L, Nyhus L M (eds) Surgery of the small intestine. Appleton-Century-Crofts, East Norwalk, Connecticut, pp 243–255

Walker M J 1987b Tumors that metastasize to the small intestine. In: Nelson R L, Nyhus L M (eds) Surgery of the small intestine. Appleton-Century-Crofts, East Norwalk, Connecticut, pp 257–262

Willis R A 1973 The spread of tumours in the human body, 3rd edn. Butterworth, London.

Wilson J M, Melvin D B, Gray G F 1974 Primary malignancies of the small bowel: a report of 96 cases and a review of the literature. Annals of Surgery 180: 175–180

Witzel L, Halter F, Gretillat P A, Scheurer V, Keller M 1976 Evaluation of specific value of endoscopic biopsies and brush cytology for malignancies of the oesophagus and stomach. Gut 17: 375–377

Yamada A 1979 The radiologic assessment of resectability and prognosis in esophageal carcinoma. Gastrointestinal Radiology 4: 213–218

Yek H-C, Rabinowitz J E 1981 Ultrasound and computed tomography of gastric wall lesions. Radiology 141: 147–155

Yonemoto R H, Slyback J B, Byron R L, Rosen R B 1969 Familial polyposis of the entire gastrointestinal tract. Archives of Surgery 99: 427–434

Zornoza J, Dodd G D 1980 Lymphoma of the gastrointestinal tract. Seminars in Roentgenology 15: 272–287

Zornoza J, Lindell M M 1980 Radiological evaluation of small oesophageal carcinoma. Gastrointestinal Radiology 5: 107–111

7. The Rectum

J. Beynon   N. J. McC. Mortensen   J. Virjee

INTRODUCTION

Surgery remains the best radical form of treatment for rectal cancer, survival being dependent on local tumour invasion, lymph node spread and surgical technique (Phillips et al 1984a,b, Williams et al 1985a).

The surgical management of rectal cancer has changed in recent years particularly with the introduction of per-anal local excision (PLE) (Lock et al 1978, Whiteway et al 1985) and also sphincter saving procedures (SSR) (Nicholls et al 1979, El liot et al 1982, Anderberg et al 1983, Heald & Ryall 1986, Hojo 1986), either in the form of low anterior resection using the stapling gun or colo-anal anastomosis. These techniques in a large number of cases have replaced the more ablative operation of abdomino-perineal excision (APE), although the proportion of patients receiving either form of treatment varies in reports from different centres.

The choice of operation is most commonly governed by a number of factors including the mobility, accessibility and size of the tumour as judged by digital examination and a similar assessment of the presence of involved retrorectal lymph nodes. The results of digital examination are highly subjective and related to surgical experience. Minor variations in the extent of tumour spread are difficult to recognize, while gross variations such as confinement to the rectal wall or spread beyond can be more confidently predicted with an accuracy of around 75% (Nicholls et al 1982). Digital rectal examination still remains the cornerstone of preoperative staging in rectal cancer despite these criticisms, probably because the newer radiological techniques are not freely available at present to the majority of surgeons. However, only the lower third and the lower part of the middle third of the rectum are amenable to digital examination.

Histological grading may also influence the decision. The presence of a poorly differentiated lesion will sometimes exclude PLE or SSR in favour of a more radical method of treatment. However, this histological assessment based on preoperative biopsies only reflects the differentiation of the resected specimen in 50–60% of cases, the differences being due to observer variation and also problems in sampling (Thomas et al 1983).

A reduction in the incidence of recurrent disease and prolongation of survival time are the two major objectives in the treatment of rectal carcinoma. Local recurrence occurs with an incidence which varies between 3 and 30% (average 14%). The incidence of local recurrence following SSR and APE varies between reports (Elliot et al 1982, Phillips et al 1984a,b, Williams et al 1985a, Heald & Ryall 1986) and there is still a continuing debate as to whether an adequate excision of the tumour and associated mesorectal nodes is achieved by SSR for middle and lower third tumours when compared to APE. Better patient selection could improve the results for these individual procedures. Two further factors may also give a better outcome: firstly an improvement in surgical technique with meticulous dissection of the mesorectum (Heald & Ryall 1986), and secondly the inclusion of some form of adjuvant therapy, in particular radiotherapy (MRC Third Report 1984, Papillon 1984, Pahlman et al 1985, Cummings 1984, 1986). Trials of preoperative, sandwich and postoperative radiotherapy are currently in progress and may show some advantage but it seems likely that only patients with advanced local disease will benefit. The correct identification of these patients preoperatively would ensure that only those at high risk of local recurrence would be included in these trials.

Locally recurrent rectal cancer is invariably detected late when no further surgical treatment can be offered. It has its maximal incidence at 9–18 months following surgery (Phillips et al 1984a, b). Two patterns of recurrent disease are recognized: extraluminal recurrence and suture line recurrence. Exfoliated and viable cancer cells may implant at the site of an anastomosis or be spilled into the operative field (Rosenberg 1979, Umpleby et al 1984). An inadequate excision of the mesorectum will also give rise to pelvic recurrence (Heald & Ryall 1986). Routine postoperative sigmoidoscopy should detect suture line recurrence. Extraluminal recurrence, although sometimes manifesting itself as suture line recurrence, usually escapes detection until well advanced. In the case of patients treated by APE, it is unlikely at present that locally recurrent rectal cancer will be detected until well advanced since most centres do not advocate routine radiological review of the pelvis unless indicated by the appearance of symptoms.

There are thus three main areas in the management of rectal cancer where surgical decision making could benefit from more precise information which is not always available from careful digital examination. These are:

1. The assessment of local invasion and perirectal lymph node involvement so as to guide more accurately the choice of individual surgical procedures.

2. The definition of those patients who would be suitable for adjuvant therapy.

3. The earlier detection of locally recurrent disease, in particular that arising in the pelvis following APE and also extrinsic to the rectal lumen in patients treated by SSR.

A number of radiological techniques are available which are applicable in this field and it is the purpose of this review to discuss their relative merits.

The diagnosis of rectal cancer is based on a good clinical history and examination, rectal examination, rectoscopy and barium enema to detect synchronous lesions which are present in up to 5% of cases. Following referral to a specialist practice with suggestive symptomatology, diagnosis seldom presents a problem so these aspects of this disease will not be discussed any further. The presence of liver metastases will also affect the management; their detection is discussed elsewhere.

STAGING OF RECTAL CANCER

The accuracy of any radiological technique has to be compared with the 'gold standard' of histological staging.

The Dukes' classification (Dukes 1932, Fitzgerald 1982, Zinkin 1983) is the most commonly used method and divides tumours into three stages:

A – Carcinoma limited to the wall of the rectum.
B – Spread of carcinoma into extrarectal tissues but no nodal involvement.
C – Lymph node involvement.

This latter group was later subdivided (Gabriel et al 1935) into C1 and C2 to indicate the involvement of either local or apical nodes respectively. In addition a grade 'D' was introduced (Turnbull et al 1967) to allow the classification of tumours with distant metastatic spread or those with involvement of an adjacent organ. The prognosis and likelihood of local recurrence can be closely related to the Dukes' stage for whatever position in the rectum.

More recently the UICC have introduced a TNM staging (UICC TNM Atlas 1982), T referring to the tumour, N the nodes and M the distant metastatic disease. In this classification the tumour growth is subdivided into the groups T1–T4 (Fig. 7.1) as follows:

T1 – Tumour confined to the mucosa and/or submucosa.
T2 – Tumour confined to muscularis propria and/or serosa.
T3 – Tumour extending into the perirectal tissues.
T4 – Tumour involving an adjacent organ.

Nodal assessment is denoted N0 or N1 to indicate either the absence or presence of involved nodes. Similarly, metastatic disease is designated M0 or M1.

The effectiveness of these techniques has usually

UICC STAGING OF RECTAL CANCER

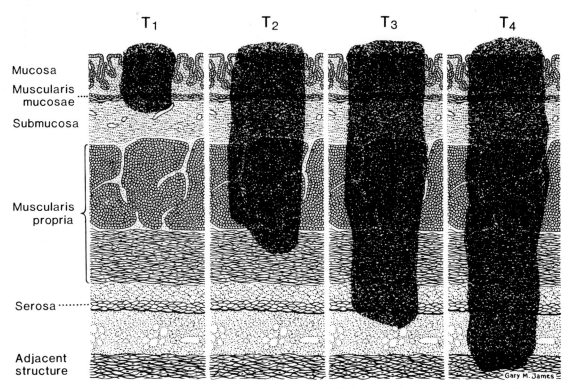

Fig. 7.1 UICC grading of local invasion in rectal cancer (reproduced with the permission of the British Journal of Surgery).

been expressed in the form of the accuracy, sensitivity, specificity, positive predictive value (PPV) and negative predictive value (NPV) with respect to prediction of invasion beyond the rectal wall. These parameters are calculated in the following way:

Accuracy = TP + TN/ TP + TN + FP + FN
Sensitivity = TP/ TP + FN
Specificity = TN/ TN + FP
PPV = TP/ TP + FP
NPV = TN/ TN + FN
TP = true positive
FP = false positive
TN = true negative
FN = false negative

COMPUTED TOMOGRAPHY (CT)

Since its introduction into clinical practice CT has been used in the assessment of primary rectal can-

cers and also for the evaluation of patients with locally recurrent disease.

The assessment of invasion in primary rectal cancer

One of the first reports on the effectiveness of CT in assessing local invasion came from St Mark's Hospital (Dixon et al 1981). Taking 1.3 cm thick slices from the anal verge to the rectosigmoid with both oral and rectal contrast, they found that CT could confidently identify patients with extensive extrarectal spread (89%), while it proved no more accurate than digital examination (Nicholls et al 1982) in the identification of patients with other degrees of spread. However, no definition of what was meant by extensive extrarectal spread was given in this report. CT also identified 4 out of 14 patients with involved perirectal nodes (sensitivity 28%), compared with the two specialist clinicians in the study who had sensitivities of 27% and 58%.

Since then there have been varying reports on the effectiveness of CT in the staging of rectal cancer. Theoni et al (1981) examined 39 patients taking 1.0 cm, and in certain areas 0.5 cm thick sections. Their overall accuracy of staging was 92%; however, they compared their radiological assessment with the Dukes' staging despite having five different radiological degrees of spread. These were:

Stage I – intraluminal polypoid mass without thickening of the bowel wall.
Stage II – thickening of the bowel wall (>0.5 cm) without invasion of the surrounding tissue.
Stage IIIA – invasion of surrounding tissue but no extension to the pelvic side walls.
Stage IIIB – extension to the pelvic side walls.
Stage IV – pelvic tumour and distant metastases.

They emphasized in their report that CT could not distinguish between extension of tumour to or through the muscularis propria or serosa. Additionally, a large number of patients in their study had advanced disease with 24 classified as either stage C or stage D. No comment on the effectiveness of CT in the assessment of lymph node metastases was made but they commented that in their experience CT was less accurate than lymphangiography.

Zaunbauer et al (1981) prospectively examined 11 patients with primary rectal cancers and were able to classify them according to the UICC method. They implied that the T1 stage was represented by endoluminal thickening of the rectal wall, an intact serosa and preservation of the perirectal fat planes. T2 was represented by extension into the muscular and serosal layers and T3 by extension into the perirectal fat planes indicated by increased density and partial obliteration of the contours. The presence of T4 disease was noted if any adjacent organs were involved. Using these criteria they correctly identified 1 patient in each of the T1 and T2 groups, 2 in the T3 group and 7 in the T4 group; this reflected a bias in the distribution of the patients towards those with advanced local disease. They noted that an increase in size of lymph nodes above 1.5 cm transverse diameter suggested malignant infiltration; this was observed in 50% of their cases but the accuracy of the observation when compared to histopathology is not recorded.

Clark et al (1984) also found that CT imaged the extramural extension of tumour well, and that using simultaneous intravenous contrast could demonstrate ureteric involvement as well.

Work from the Manchester group (Zheng et al 1984) has confirmed the usefulness of CT in the assessment of local invasion in rectal cancer. They compared their preoperative scans (1.0 cm thick contiguous sections) with surgical observations at the time of laparotomy. CT correctly identified 19 out of 20 patients with extrarectal spread of tumour whilst it overstaged 7 patients in whom no evidence of extension could be observed. CT detected 6 out of 10 patients with extension to the pelvic side wall and also 11 patients with obliteration of the presacral fat plane, only 7 of whom were found to have compatible findings at laparotomy. Additionally, 2 patients with obliteration of the presacral fat plane were not detected by CT. Zheng and colleagues reported good correlation between CT findings and surgery when there was extension of tumour to involve adjacent organs. Perirectal lymph nodes of greater than 1 cm diameter were demonstrated in 8 patients, 7 of whom were shown to have metastatic disease. Conversely, 14 patients were detected with lymph nodes less than 1 cm diameter but only 4 of these had metastatic spread. 2 patients with lymph node spread were not detected by CT. Regional node assessment was only correct in 1 out of 8 cases.

More recently Williams et al (1985b) using 1.2 cm thick CT sections classified local extension of tumour into two basic categories, either present or absent. If present, they then designated it as either minimal (reaching the outer margin of the rectal wall and just into the perirectal fat), moderate (established spread into the extrarectal tissues) and extensive when other organs were involved. Although they did not record their reporting criteria they correctly identified 16 out of 17 patients with malignant extension (94%). In addition, 26 out of 28 patients (93%) without spread were correctly identified. The sensitivity, specificity and accuracy of pelvic CT in detecting local malignant extension was 94, 90 and 93% respectively, although again there was a definite bias in the patients examined, with nearly two-thirds having no extension and thus being Dukes' A carcinomas, which in most series would only account for approximately 15% of patients.

Rifkin and Wechsler (1986) examined 71 primary rectal cancers. They found that the lesion was identified in 50 of their cases, and noted that perirectal fat infiltration was correctly predicted in 16 out of 29 cases. There were 9 false positives where CT predicted fat infiltration. 33 patients were accurately identified with normal fat. Their sensitivity and specificity for predicting perirectal fat infiltration were therefore 55% and 79% respectively while the PPV was 64% and the NPV 72%. Lymph node involvement on CT was predicted in 3 out of 13 cases giving a sensitivity of 23%, specificity of 100%, positive predictive value of 100% and negative predictive value of 83%.

Kramann and Hildebrandt (1986) classified 29 tumours according to the UICC into groups T1–T4, taking 4 mm thick CT sections. Five of the group considered to be T2 were found to have been understaged. Out of 23 cases classified as T3, 5 were overstaged. They have not, however, as with some other authors (Romano et al 1985) described their criteria for defining the individual degrees of invasion. Lymph nodes were only confirmed as malignant if greater than 1 cm in diameter and 3 out of 4 were correctly identified.

Our own experience is similar (Beynon et al 1986a,b,c). We have taken 0.8 cm thick sections of the pelvis following the administration of both rectal and intravenous contrast. With two consultant radiologists reporting all scans prior to surgery, later comparisons were made directly with histopathology. Only three degrees of invasion could confidently be reported (Figs 7.2, 7.3, 7.4). Criteria for this reporting were the presence of a thickened rectal wall (compared to adjacent normal rectum), minimal irregularity of the outer margin of the wall with no fat encroachment (equivalent to the pathological grades T1 and T2) or irregularity of the outer margin of the rectal wall with fat encroachment or involvement of another organ (equivalent to the grades T3 and T4 respectively). In the 44 patients we have studied to date the overall accuracy of CT was 82% while invasion beyond the rectal wall was predicted with a sensitivity of 86%, specificity of 62%, positive

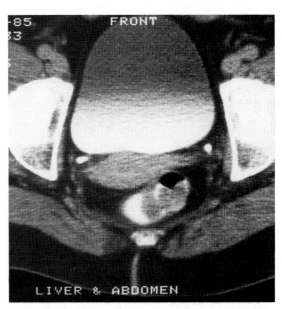

Fig. 7.2 CT scan of a rectal tumour showing confinement to the wall.

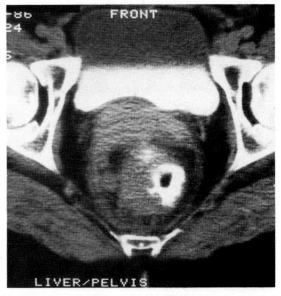

Fig. 7.3 CT scan of the rectum showing invasion out into the adjacent tissues with a small involved perirectal node.

predictive value of 91% and negative predictive value of 50%.

Overall we have been disappointed with the identification of lymph nodes which have only clearly been identified in 3 out of 13 patients with

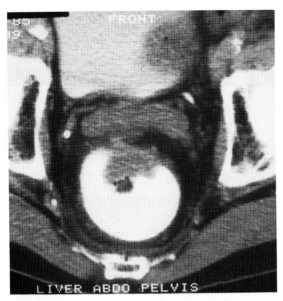

Fig. 7.4 CT scan of the rectum showing a rectal tumour invading anteriorly into the seminal vesicles.

involved nodes. Our results confirm those of other authors that at this stage only nodes of 1 cm or greater diameter can be identified. Node size is, of course, no indication of involvement with tumour and may just represent reactive changes.

Summary

In summary there seems little doubt that preoperative CT can accurately predict invasion beyond the rectal wall or confinement to it, and in doing so gives additional information to the surgeon with which to plan management. We remain sceptical that CT can resolve the degree of invasion sufficiently to grade tumours according to the UICC classification and it seems that little is added to the information gained by digital examination except that tumours of the middle and upper third of the rectum can be assessed. In addition CT is expensive and time consuming and there may be scheduling difficulties in busy departments. Lymph node assessment is also disappointing.

CT in the detection of distant metastatic spread

CT is an accurate method for detecting overt

hepatic metastatic disease but recently its effectiveness in the detection of so-called occult hepatic metastases (OHM) has been reported (Finlay & McArdle 1983, 1986). In their study presumptive diagnoses of the presence of OHMs were made in one-third of patients undergoing a curative resection of colorectal cancer, and subsequent follow-up has confirmed their observations. Patients in their study underwent routine scanning perioperatively and at least twice in the subsequent year. Their results showed that in a large proportion of these patients the disease is systemic from the outset, and that the survival curves for the other patients approximate to each other despite differing Dukes' grades. If all patients were similarly aggressively assessed prior to surgery it would take many years for us to assess the results of treatment on those patients without systemic disease at presentation – quite a daunting prospect.

The detection and assessment of recurrent rectal cancer

Locally recurrent rectal cancer may be difficult to detect clinically, particularly if extrarectal in those treated by SSR and in patients who have been treated by APE. Once suspected, the course of events should include clinical examination, rectoscopy and biopsy, examination under anaesthetic and radiological assessment of the extent of both local and distant disease. CT is extensively used in this situation to aid both the detection and assessment of recurrent rectal cancers.

Lee et al (1981) noted that postoperative fibrosis and recurrent tumour have the same density though they tend to differ in CT appearance. The presence of fibrosis may show no detectable abnormality or minimal streaky densities while recurrence is suggested by the presence of a globular mass; the size of this mass to be significant must be greater than 1.5 cm in diameter. These findings on CT can of course be confirmed by the use of percutaneous biopsy as suggested by Zelas et al (1980).

Zaunbauer et al (1981) noted that recurrent rectal cancers have the same density characteristics as primary tumours (absorption values of 40–50 Hounsfield units). They noted that CT was the ideal technique for the demonstration of recurrent rectal malignancy, especially following APR. In this study 32 out of 34 patients with recurrence were identified while only 15 out of 22 cases were identified in those patients who had previously been treated by anterior resection. Zaunbauer and colleagues did not share the optimism of the previous authors and recommended the use of biopsy to differentiate between fibrosis and recurrence.

Summary

There appears to be one outstanding area in the management of rectal cancer where CT has a distinct advantage, that is in the identification of possible local recurrence in patients who have undergone APE. Recurrence suggested by new symptomatology or rising carcinoembryonic antigen (CEA) should be followed by CT scan. The interpretation of the postoperative pelvis is by no means easy, however, and discrete lesions should then be biopsied percutaneously under CT control for histological diagnosis.

ENDORECTAL SONOGRAPHY

Endosonography (ES) of the rectum was first introduced by Wild, Reid and Foderick (1950, 1956, 1978a,b). Using a primitive probe they examined both normal and abnormal tissue and demonstrated the first recurrent rectal cancer. Technical limitations, however, meant that this type of imaging remained only an intriguing possibility until reintroduced into clinical practice by Dragsted and Gammelgaard (1983). Using a rigid rotating endosonic probe initially designed for prostatic ultrasound, they assessed 13 primary rectal cancers and correctly predicted the degree of invasion in 11 cases when compared to histopathology.

Interpretation of the image

Further studies seem to have confirmed the promise of this technique. The fundamental problem is an accurate understanding of the normal ultrasonographic anatomy of the rectal wall. Various authors have reported five, seven, nine and even 11 ultrasonic layers in the gastrointestinal wall (Aibe 1984a,b, Caletti et al 1984, Tanaka et al 1984, Fukuda 1985, Konishi et al 1985, Saitoh et al 1986), although most authors agree that five basic layers can be clearly identified both in vivo and in vitro. Since an accurate prediction of the degree of invasion depends upon a correct interpretation of these layers the problem is of some importance. The five layers from the luminal aspect outwards are a first hyperechoic layer, a second hypoechoic, a third hyperechoic, a fourth hypoechoic and lastly another hyperechoic layer (Fig. 7.5). Whether or not these represent the anatomical layers of the rectal wall where there are also five histological layers, or are ultrasonic interfaces which do not coincide with the anatomy remains controversial.

There does seem to be agreement between most authors that the fourth hypoechoic layer corresponds to the morphological entity which is the muscularis propria. In Bristol we have examined fresh operative specimens of rectum and colon in the laboratory and identified the five basic layers (Beynon et al 1986d). By sharp dissection we have then removed firstly the mucosa and muscularis mucosae and then in addition the submucosa, repeating the scan on each occasion to see which layers remain. We observed that if the mucosa and muscularis mucosae were removed three layers were left which the histologists identified as submucosa, muscularis propria and perirectal fat with serosa when it is present. Secondly, if the

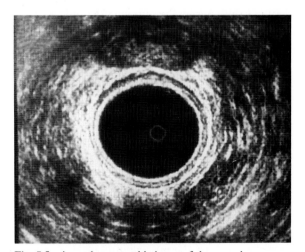

Fig. 7.5 An endosonographic image of the normal rectum showing a five-layered structure.

submucosa was also removed then two ultrasonic layers remained which were identified as muscularis propria and perirectal fat with serosa when present. It thus appears from our laboratory work that the five basic ultrasonic layers correspond essentially to the five histological layers of the rectal wall.

In essence the first hyperechoic layer is the boundary echo produced by the mucosa, the second hypoechoic layer is made up of the mucosa and the signal produced by the muscularis mucosae combined, the third hyperechoic layer is the submucosa, the fourth hypoechoic layer is the muscularis propria and the last layer is produced by perirectal fat and serosa when present.

Konishi et al (1985) using a 5 MHz probe were not able in their examination of this problem to differentiate the mucosa from the submucosa. Saitoh et al (1986), however, have like us defined the third hyperechoic layer as submucosa. Others believe that the submucosa and mucosa cannot be differentiated and that the third layer is only an interface between mucosa/submucosa and the muscularis propria (Boscaini et al 1986, Hildebrandt et al 1986). Some of the evidence for these interpretations is taken from in vitro work on polyethylene membranes (Boscaini et al 1986). Using this technique the axial resolution for their equipment (IVB 505 S Toshiba with 4.5 and 5 MHz probes) was found to be 1000 microns. Since the axial resolution was greater than the combined thicknesses of the submucosa/mucosa, they concluded that the submucosa could not be resolved as a morphological entity, but only as an interface. The muscularis propria with a thickness of 1500–1800 microns can therefore be resolved as an independent layer. Our results were obtained using transducers of 5.5 and 7.0 MHz with resolutions of 600 and 400 microns respectively. With this improved axial resolution, we believe our evidence shows we have been able to resolve the submucosa as an independent layer and that the complete image produced represents the morphological layers of the rectum, with the exception of the muscularis mucosae which gives a combined image with the mucosa. Hildebrandt et al (1986) have used the same transducer as ourselves but have not removed the mucosa/muscularis mucosae and submucosa as distinct entities. Whichever interpretation is finally adopted, it is the disruption of the interfaces/layers which matters in the assessment of local invasion.

Endosonography in the staging of primary rectal cancer

The initial results of Dragsted & Gammelgaard (1983) using a 3.5 MHz Bruel and Kjaer transducer have already been discussed. The early promise has been confirmed by Hildebrandt and Fiefel (1985) who successfully staged 23 out of 25 patients with the same equipment. In this group of 25 patients, 8 tumours were beyond the reach of digital examination and of the 17 palpable tumours 15 were correctly assessed prior to surgery by the examining finger and 2 patients were overstaged. They suggested that the UICC system for staging should be adopted for use in ultrasonic staging by the use of the prefix 'u' i.e. uT1–uT4. Two problems were encountered in this initial report: the distinction between T1 and T2 tumours using the 4 MHz probe and the examination of stenotic tumours. Hildebrandt and Fiefel have now reported a total of 76 cases with later examinations being performed with a 7.0 MHz transducer. In this series they have overstaged 8 tumours and understaged 1.

Konishi et al (1985) compared a 5.0 MHz linear array (SSD-256 Aloka) and a 3.5 MHz radial chair type scanner (ASU 8MC Aloka, Japan). In their experience with the radial scanner 18 out of 21 cases were visualized (88.7%) while with the linear array all of the 38 tumours assessed were visualized. This reflects the intrinsic problem in using a chair-mounted probe where the transducer is essentially limited to the same area of the rectum as the examining finger. They classified the depth of invasion as either confinement within or extension beyond the layer they identified as the muscularis propria. With the linear array they overstaged 3 cases and understaged 1. Two cases could not be staged: one was shown histologically to be confined to the rectum, whilst the other extended beyond the muscularis propria. The radial scanner overstaged 1 case, with 9 being non-classified, 1 showing confinement to the mucosa/submucosa, 3 with invasion into the muscularis propria and 5 with extrarectal invasion. They concluded that the radial scanner was inferior to the linear array. This may have been because the longer, more mobile instrument could more easily be manoeuvred into a suitable position for the best imaging.

Using an Olympus-Aloka ultrasonic endoscope (GF UM1, UM2, 7.5 MHz and Aloka probes of 7.5 MHz and 5.0 MHz) Saitoh et al (1986) described three degrees of invasion broadly comparable to Dukes' histological staging:

Group 1 – confinement to the rectal wall.
Group 2 – invasion beyond the muscularis propria.
Group 3 – invasion of another organ.

11 of their 99 patients could not be examined sufficiently because of severe stenosis. In the remaining 88 cases diagnostic accuracy rates were 82.9% in group 1, 91.9% in group 2 and 75% in group 3. Eight patients were overstaged and 1 understaged.

Rifkin & Wechsler (1986) have used radial (Bruel and Kjaer 1846 and/or 1849, or Aloka 520) and linear (Toshiba SAL50A, Aloka 280 SL, Kramed, GE RT3000) scanners. They identified the tumour in 79 out of 85 patients with 2 failures of examination. They again classified their patients ultrasonically into those with or without confine-ment to the rectal wall. 25 patients with invasion into the perirectal fat were correctly identified but 8 were overstaged. In addition, they identified correctly 43 patients with no invasion into the fat but understaged 5 patients. Thus their prediction of fat infiltration had a sensitivity of 83%, specificity of 84%, PPV of 76% and NPV of 90%.

In Bristol we have two year's experience in preoperative staging of rectal cancer (Beynon et al 1986a,b,c,e). We have used an 1846 scanner (Bruel and Kjaer, Denmark) with at first a 5.5 but now a 7.0 MHz transducer. This equipment consists of a rotating rod over which is placed a metallic overtube (Fig. 7.6). The transducer is placed at the end of the rod and is covered with a latex balloon which is inflated with degassed water following insertion into the rectum. We have overcome the problem of examining stenotic tumours in three ways; (a) by using a sheath with a plastic nose cone, so protecting the transducer from snagging against the stenotic lesion, (b) by using a 60° forward-looking transducer instead of the usual 90° so that a forward view can be obtained; and (c) by using a specially constructed rectoscope which can be guided up to or beyond the lesion under direct vision and allows the endoprobe to be inserted

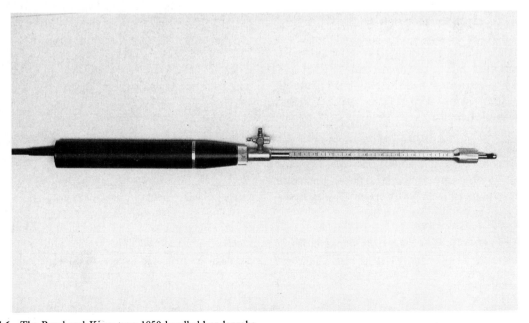

Fig. 7.6 The Bruel and Kjaer type 1850 handheld endoprobe.

through it to the exact location of the tumour. Though in some of these situations the whole length of the tumour cannot be visualized, the more distal portion can give useful though not always complete images with which to stage a tumour. Using these modifications we have experienced no problems since the formal start of our study.

We classified invasion in the same way as Hildebrandt and Fiefel (1985) and have adopted their suggestion for the ultrasonic staging (uT1–uT4). In the 82 patients studied to date 7 cases were T1, 11 cases T2, 58 cases T3 and 6 cases T4 (Figs 7.7, 7.8). These assessments when compared to postoperative histopathology had a coefficient of correlation of 0.88 ($p < 0.001$ Rank Spearman). The overall accuracy of ultrasound in preoperative staging was 92%, and invasion beyond the muscularis propria was predicted with a sensitivity of 97%, specificity of 94%, PPV of 98% and NPV of 89%. Endoluminal ultrasound (ES) could also predict confinement to the wall or spread beyond with an accuracy of 95% (Table 7.1).

Can the assessment of lymph node involvement be improved using this technique? Hildebrandt et al (1986) have reported that since using a 7 MHz transducer lymph node metastases have been identified. In the 27 patients they have scanned 12 were preoperatively thought to have metastatic involvement of perirectal lymph nodes. However, following resection this was confirmed in only 6 cases, while the other 6 showed reactive changes. They reported 1 false negative result. Rifkin and Wechsler (1986) identified 10 out of 13 patients with positive nodes, with 6 false positives in the remaining 66 patients. This gave an overall sensitivity of 67%, specificity of 91%, PPV of 63% and NPV of 92%.

Saitoh et al (1986) had an accuracy of 73.2% for the node positive group and 82.3% for the node negative group (19 false positives and 3 false nega-

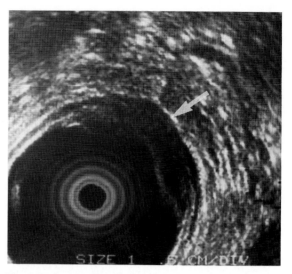

Fig. 7.7 An ultrasonic T_2 tumour of the rectum. This scan shows invasion of the tumour into the echopoor muscularis propria with an intact echogenic interface between the muscle and fat (arrowed).

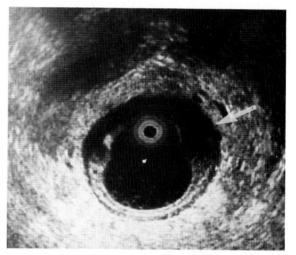

Fig. 7.8 An ultrasonic T_3 tumour of the rectum. The tumour in this scan has disrupted the interface between the muscle and the perirectal fat indicating invasion (arrowed).

Table 7.1 Ultrasonic prediction of invasion beyond the muscularis propria

Study	No. of patients	Accuracy (%)	Sensitivity (%)	Specificity (%)	PPV (%)	NPV (%)
Rifkin & Wechsler 1986	79	84	83	84	76	90
Beynon et al 1986a	82	92	97	94	98	89
Hildebrandt et al 1986	76	88	100	81	87	100

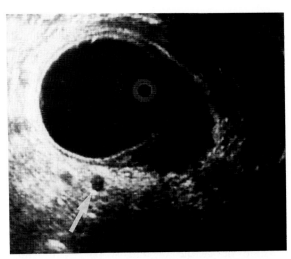

Fig. 7.9 An ultrasonic T₃ tumour of the rectum with adjacent involved perirectal lymph node (arrowed).

tives), though they noted that metastatic and non-metastatic nodes as small as 5 mm in diameter could be detected.

In our own experience involved lymph nodes appear echopoor (Fig. 7.9), though we have observed false positives with the same appearance (Fig. 7.10). The nodes are usually observed within 1 cm of the tumour. Overall accuracy for predicting lymph node involvement is 81% while

correlation of ultrasonic assessments with histological data shows a correlation coefficient of 0.62 ($p < 0.001$). The sensitivity of the investigation is 85%, the specificity 77%, the PPV 76% and the NPV 86%. We have investigated the reasons for the false positive diagnoses in two ways: firstly by assessing the individual histological appearances of the lymph nodes lying within 1 cm of the rectal wall, and secondly by looking at the sizes of these nodes. This data has then been compared with false positive, false negative, true positive and true negative ultrasonic scan reports. Using a multivariant analysis we have been unable to show any obvious histological architectural reason accounting for the incorrect assessments.

Endosonography or computed tomography?

Romano et al (1985) have made a comparison of ES and CT. With CT tumours were graded according to the UICC classification. In their study ultrasound correctly staged 20 out of 23 tumours while CT correctly assessed 19 out of 23.

Rifkin and Wechsler (1986) have also compared the two techniques and found ES to be far more accurate in predicting perirectal fat involvement (Table 7.2).

We have performed a comparative study of ES, CT and digital rectal examination in the assessment of local invasion in rectal cancer. In our group of 44 cases to date, the overall accuracy of digital examination was 68% and this fell to 52% if all the non-palpable tumours were included. Invasion beyond the muscularis propria was predicted with a sensitivity of 68%, specificity of 83%, PPV of 100% and NPV of 46%. ES in the same patients had an accuracy of 91%, sensitivity of 94%, specificity of 87%, PPV of 97% and NPV of 78%. CT, in contrast, could not define the same four levels of invasion (UICC) we had used for the digital and ultrasonic assessments, and as we have already discussed could only define

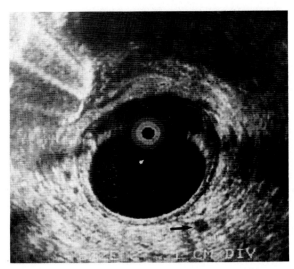

Fig. 7.10 An ultrasonic T₃ tumour of the rectum with adjacent lesion (arrowed) misinterpreted as an involved perirectal lymph node.

Table 7.2 Perirectal fat infiltration (Rifkin & Wechsler 1986)

	No.	Sensitivity (%)	Specificity (%)	PPV (%)	NPV (%)
ES	79	83	84	76	90
CT	71	55	79	64	72

Table 7.3 Prediction of invasion beyond the muscularis propria (Beynon et al 1986a)

	No. of patients	Accuracy (%)	Sensitivity (%)	Specificity (%)	PPV (%)	NPV (%)
Digital palpable	34	68	68	83	100	46
Digital total	44	52				
CT	44	82	86	62	91	50
Endosonography	44	91	94	87	97	78

confinement to the wall, spread beyond, or involvement of an adjacent organ. The overall accuracy for CT in doing this was 82% while invasion beyond the muscularis propria was predicted with a sensitivity of 86%, specificity of 62%, PPV of 91% and NPV of 50% (Table 7.3). If our results for ES are put in the same context as the CT results then the accuracy of ultrasound in predicting either confinement or spread of tumour beyond the wall was 95%.

Summary

It is thus apparent from our own and other studies that ES is more accurate than either CT or digital examination and can predict invasion of tumour layer by layer in the rectal wall. The advantage of this degree of accuracy in staging may have important implications for the management of rectal cancer enabling the more precise planning of surgical treatment, particularly in defining those patients suitable for local excision and restorative surgery. It may also play an important rôle in trials of preoperative radiotherapy defining both those patients who would benefit and those whose survival or risk of local recurrence would not be improved.

Locally recurrent rectal cancer

ES can be used per rectum following restorative resection (SSR) or per vaginum in female patients after APE. Hildebrandt et al (1986) detected 22 recurrences but only 6 of these were noted with ultrasound alone. The other cases had either elevated carcinoembryonic antigen (CEA) or endoscopic evidence of recurrence or both.

Romano et al (1985) detected 8 local recurrences confirmed by various means in their follow-up group of 42 patients. They also had 2 false posi-

tives, the diagnosis of postoperative fibrosis being confirmed by percutaneous biopsy.

We have examined 85 patients for evidence of recurrence of their rectal carcinomas (Beynon et al 1989); of 22 recurrences only 3 were detected by ultrasound alone, all the other lesions being either palpable or visible on endoscopic examination (Fig. 7.11).

The routine use of ES in this way may be a better method of follow-up, especially when combined with conventional methods of clinical examination and rectosigmoidoscopy. Detection of these early extraluminal lesions, however, is not diagnostic of recurrence and confirmatory biopsy can be performed under ultrasound control via the perineum.

The identification of recurrence at an earlier stage would undoubtedly allow greater scope for

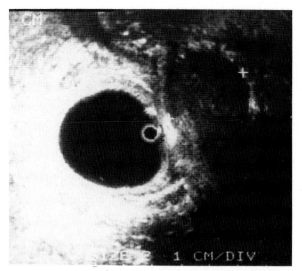

Fig. 7.11 An extrarectal recurrence on the left anterior wall of the rectum with no clinical mucosal disruption. Measured at 3.1 cm diameter.

both surgeon and radiotherapist in the planning of subsequent management.

MAGNETIC RESONANCE IMAGING (MRI)

Magnetic resonance imaging (MRI) is a relatively new technique in the staging of rectal cancer and there is as yet little published data on its value. The technique employs radio frequency radiation in the presence of a static magnetic field to generate signals from naturally occurring nuclei in biological tissues. The information in MR images can be obtained from these signals in any orthogonal plane. Image contrast is dependent on the interaction of proton density, relaxation times of the proton following radio frequency disturbance (T_1, T_2) and the timing parameters of the radio frequency pulse sequences employed.

MRI has advantages over CT in pelvic imaging due to its greater contrast resolution and ability to scan directly in the coronal and saggital planes. Butch et al (1986) compared MRI and CT in 16 patients and concluded that both techniques were similar in their ability to assess local invasion. Neither technique could distinguish normal lymph nodes from involved nodes.

Hodgman et al (1986) have recently compared CT and MRI. 34 patients were examined, 30 by CT, 27 by MRI and 23 by both. MRI scans were performed on a Picker 0.15 Tesla resistive magnet using several different inversion recovery (IR) and spin echo (SE) pulse sequences. CT sections were taken through the pelvis at 1 cm intervals after oral and rectal contrast administration. 24 out of 30 (80%) were staged correctly by CT (staged according to the Theoni classification for comparison with the Astler Coller pathological stage). 3 cases were understaged and 3 overstaged. 16 out of 27 (59%) were correctly staged by MRI: 7 cases were understaged and 4 overstaged.

Of those examined by both techniques, CT staged 18 out of 23 cases correctly (78%) and MRI 14 out of 23 (61%). CT overstaged 2 cases and understaged 3. MRI by comparison overstaged 4 cases and understaged 5.

For the detection of lymph node metastases, Hodgman and colleagues found that CT was equally specific but more sensitive than MRI

Table 7.4 Lymph node metastases (after Hodgman et al 1986)

	Number of cases (%)	
	CT	MRI
Accuracy	15/23 (65)	9/23 (39)
Sensitivity	6/15 (40)	2/15 (13)
Specificity	9/10 (90)	7/8 (88)
False positive	1/23 (4)	1/23 (4)
False negative	7/23 (30)	13/23 (57)

(Table 7.4). They comment that the detection of lymph nodes with either technique depends on the identification of nodes of diameter 1.5 cm or greater.

In this latter study CT was superior to MRI in the staging of rectal carcinoma though it must be remembered that MRI is a new technique which has yet to be fully evaluated. The authors pointed out that with experience through the period of the study the quality of the MRI images improved due to technical refinements.

The Manchester group (Johnson et al 1987a)

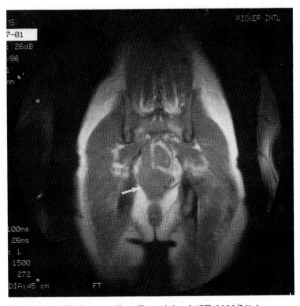

Fig. 7.12 MR intermediate T_1 weighted (SE 1100/26) image of the rectum showing a primary rectal carcinoma extending to the pelvic side wall on the right and involving the levator ani muscle (arrowed). (We are grateful to Dr R. Johnson for the MR images.)

have compared MRI (Picker superconducting whole body imaging system operating at 0.26 Tesla) and CT in new patients with advanced local disease (tumour extending through the wall) and also in patients with biopsy-proven recurrent rectal cancer. The two techniques compared favourably in assessing the extent of the disease, though MRI was better for the delineation of the disease, mainly as a result of the images obtained in both saggital and coronal planes (Figs. 7.12, 7.13). The introduction of air or particulate iron oxide (Saini et al 1986) can help in determining the extent of intramural tumour though this is of doubtful clinical usefulness.

What of the detection of recurrent rectal cancer? Johnson et al (1987b) have approached the problem by looking at tissue characterization to see whether MRI can differentiate recurrence from fibrosis or infection. They have studied patients with recurrent rectal cancer ($n=28$), primary rectal cancer ($n=2$) and fibrotic pelvic mass ($n=7$). The primary patients or those with recurrence were chosen for study after the demonstration of a mass greater than 5 cm in diameter on CT. Their initial

studies have shown that in patients with tumour bulk or a fibrotic mass greater than 5 cm in diameter there is a significant difference in the T_1 relaxation times (Table 7.5).

They have also studied patients with recurrent rectal carcinoma and primary malignancies undergoing radiotherapy. Initial results suggest a correlation between clinical response, changes in the size of tumour seen on MR images and the measured relaxation time.

Summary

It appears that at present there is little extra to be offered by MRI that cannot be determined by CT in the staging of primary rectal cancer. MRI is,

Table 7.5 Carcinoma of the rectum and fibrosis: mean relaxation times $\pm$ SE (after Johnson et al 1987b)

	No. of cases	T_1 (ms)	T_2 (ms)
Carcinoma of the rectum	30	*817 $\pm$ 29	69 $\pm$ 3
Fibrosis	7	*458 $\pm$ 67	58 $\pm$ 3

*$p<0.001$

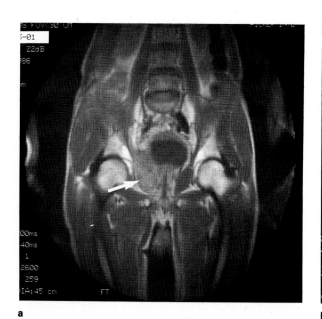 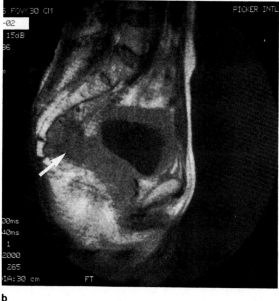

a   b

Fig. 7.13 (a) MR coronal T_2 weighted image (SE 1200/40) showing a recurrent rectal carcinoma on the right pelvic side wall (arrowed) inseparable from the prostate and right lateral wall of the bladder. (b) A sagittal scan of the same patient. A T_1 weighted image (SE 600/40) illustrates the recurrent tumour mass in the sacral hollow (arrowed) extending anteriorly to involve the prostate and bladder.

however, in an early stage of assessment and further studies are necessary.

The most promising development in the application of MRI to the rectum is undoubtedly in the detection of recurrence and particularly in the differentiation of this from fibrosis (*see* Ch. 2).

LYMPHOSCINTIGRAPHY AND CARCINOMA OF THE RECTUM

The involvement of local lymph nodes in carcinoma of the rectum is of great prognostic significance and is associated with increased risk of local recurrence and decreased survival (Phillips et al 1984a,b). The preceding techniques all have their limitations in the identification of involved lymph nodes and this has rekindled interest in lymphoscintigraphy.

Interstitial radiocolloid lymphoscintigraphy has been used to determine whether pelvic lymphatics and nodes can be visualized with the same accuracy as breast lymphatics. Ege and Cummings (1980) have performed a large study on 184 patients with varying pelvic malignancies and reported a good correlation between observed patterns of lymph node involvement and disease states. However, there was no correlation in this study with the 'gold standard' of histopathology. In contrast, Reasbeck et al (1984) investigated 18 patients with rectal carcinoma, 20 controls and 4 patients with inflammatory bowel disease, performing lymphoscintigraphy on each and subjecting the resected specimens of the rectal carcinomas to detailed histopathological assessment. They concluded that whatever radionuclide they used (^{99m}Tc-dextran or ^{99m}Tc-antimony sulphide colloid) no reliable imaging of mesorectal lymph nodes involved by metastatic colorectal carcinoma could be obtained.

Simple lymphoscintigraphy is unlikely to be of use in the routine management of rectal cancer, but with the advent of monoclonal antibodies the position of monoclonal immunoscintigraphy is yet to be established (Finan et al 1986).

CONCLUSION

The rôles of the individual methods in the routine management of primary and recurrent rectal cancer are yet to be fully established. They undoubtedly offer a degree of accuracy both in staging and diagnosis which has not been possible before.

At present CT has the edge over MRI in the staging of primary rectal cancer, but this may just be due to greater experience with the technique. The encouraging results from the Manchester group seem to indicate a promising rôle in the future for MRI in the diagnosis and assessment of patients with recurrent rectal carcinoma. However, neither CT nor MRI is likely to be able to assess accurately the involvement of local lymph nodes. We would advocate CT or MRI as the radiological method of choice at present for the investigation of patients following APE, though there is undoubtedly a place for ES in the follow-up of female patients treated this way who can be scanned transvaginally.

The high degree of variability in the pelvic lymphatics does not ensure a healthy future for plain lymphoscintigraphy since correlation between preoperative scans and postoperative histopathology is poor. Monoclonal immunolymphoscintigraphy is as yet in its infancy and many problems need to be overcome before reproducible data will be forthcoming. The technique is an attractive one, however, and there are many potential applications in the field of oncology.

ES is having an increasing impact on both the radiological and surgical community. There is good evidence now from many sources around the world to show that this is an accurate and reproducible technique for the preoperative staging of rectal cancer. It offers additional information regarding the status of perirectal lymph nodes though it has certain limitations in this area, and also provides a simple method for assessing the pelvis in patients who have undergone SSR and in females who have been treated by APE.

In our opinion ES is the method of choice for the staging of primary rectal cancer and when combined with other routine methods of follow-up provides the most effective method at present available for the early detection and assessment of recurrence. It will take some years and the more widespread use of ES before we will be able to assess fully its effect, if any, on the incidence of local recurrence and also survival.

REFERENCES

Aibe T 1984a A study on the structure of layers of the gastrointestinal wall visualized by means of the ultrasonic endoscope. I. The structure of layers of the gastric wall. Gastroenterological Endoscopy 26: 1447–1464

Aibe T 1984b A study on the structure of layers of the gastrointestinal wall visualized by means of the ultrasonic endoscope. II. The structure of layers of the oesophageal wall and the colonic wall. Gastroenterological Endoscopy 26: 1465–1473

Anderberg B, Enbald P, Sjodahl R, Wetterfors J 1983 Recurrent rectal carcinoma after anterior resection and rectal stapling. British Journal of Surgery 70: 1–4

Beynon J, Mortensen N J McC, Foy D M A, Channer J L, Virjee J, Goddard P 1986a Endorectal sonography: Laboratory and clinical experience in Bristol. International Journal of Colorectal Disease 1: 212–215

Beynon J, Roe A M, Foy D M A, Channer J L, Goddard P, Virjee J, Mortensen N J McC 1986b Transrectal ultrasound or computed tomography for the assessment of local invasion in rectal cancer. Surgical Forum 37: 199–201

Beynon J, Mortensen N J McC, Foy D M A, Channer J L, Virjee J, Goddard P 1986c Preoperative assessment of local invasion in rectal cancer: digital examination, endoluminal sonography or computed tomography? British Journal of Surgery 73: 1015–1017

Beynon J, Foy D M A, Channer J L, Temple L N, Virjee J, Mortensen N J McC 1986d The ultrasonographic anatomy of the normal colon and rectum. Diseases of the Colon and Rectum 29: 810–813

Beynon J, Foy D M A, Roe A M, Temple L N, Mortensen N J McC 1986e Endoluminal ultrasound in the assessment of local invasion in rectal cancer. British Journal of Surgery 73: 474–477

Beynon J, Mortensen N J McC, Foy D M A, Channer J L, Virjee J 1989 The detection and evaluation of locally recurrent rectal cancer with rectal endosonography. Diseases of the Colon and Rectum 32: 509–517

Boscaini M, Masoni L, Montori A 1986 Transrectal ultrasonography: Three years' experience. International Journal of Colorectal Disease 1: 208–211

Butch R J, Stark D D, Wittenberg J et al 1986 Staging rectal cancer by MR and CT. American Journal of Radiology 146: 1155–1160

Calletti G, Bolondi L, Labo G 1984 Ultrasonic endoscopy – the gastrointestinal wall. Scandinavian Journal of Gastroenterology 19 (suppl 102): 5–8

Clark J, Bankoff M, Carter B, Smith T J 1984 The use of computerized tomography scan in the staging and follow-up study of carcinoma of the rectum. Surgery, Gynaecology and Obstetrics 59: 335–342

Cummings B J 1984 Adjuvant radiation therapy for rectal adenocarcinoma. Diseases of the Colon and Rectum 27: 826–836

Cummings B J 1986 A critical review of adjuvant preoperative radiation therapy for adenocarcinoma of the rectum. British Journal of Surgery 73: 332–338

Dixon A K, Fry I K, Morson B C, Nicholls R J, York Mason A 1981 Preoperative computed tomography of carcinoma of the rectum. British Journal of Radiology 54: 655–659

Dragsted J, Gammelgaard J 1983 Endoluminal ultrasonic scanning in the evaluation of rectal cancer. Gastrointestinal Radiology 8: 367–369

Dukes C 1932 The classification of cancer of the rectum. Journal of Pathology 35: 323–332

Ege G N, Cummings B J 1980 Interstitial radiocolloid iliopelvic lymphoscintigraphy: technique, anatomy and clinical application. International Journal of Radiation Oncology, Biology and Physics 6: 1483–1490

Elliot M S, Todd I P, Nicholls R J 1982 Radical restorative surgery for poorly differentiated carcinoma of the mid-rectum. British Journal of Surgery 69: 273–274

Finan P J, Ritson A, Ware F et al 1986 Monoclonal immunoscintigraphy for the detection of primary colorectal cancers: a prospective study. British Journal of Surgery 73: 177–179

Finlay I G, McArdle C S 1983 Effect of occult hepatic metastases on survival after curative resection for colorectal carcinoma. Gastroenterology 85: 596–599

Finlay I G, McArdle C S 1986 Occult hepatic metastases in colorectal carcinoma. British Journal of Surgery 73: 732–735

Fitzgerald R H 1982 What is the Dukes' system for carcinoma of the rectum? Diseases of the Colon and Rectum 25: 474–477

Fukuda M 1985 Endoscopic ultrasonography. World Federation of Ultrasound in Medicine and Biology 1985: 13–16

Gabriel W B, Dukes C E, Bussey H J 1935 Lymphatic spread in cancer of the rectum. British Journal of Surgery 23: 395–413

Heald R J, Ryall R D H 1986 Recurrence and survival after total mesorectal excision for rectal cancer. Lancet 1 1479–1482

Hildebrandt U, Fiefel G 1985 Preoperative staging of rectal cancer by intrarectal ultrasound. Diseases of the Colon and Rectum 1986 28: 42–46

Hildebrandt U, Fiefel G, Schwarz H P, Scherr O 1986 Endorectal ultrasound: Instrumentation and clinical aspects. International Journal of Colorectal Disease 1: 203–207

Hodgman C G, MacCarty R L, Wolff B G et al 1986 Preoperative staging of rectal carcinoma by computed tomography and 0.15 T magnetic resonance imaging. Diseases of the Colon and Rectum 29: 446–450

Hojo K 1986 Anastomotic recurrence after sphincter-saving resection for rectal cancer. Diseases of the Colon and Rectum 29: 11–14

Johnson R J, Jenkins J P R, Isherwood I 1987a Magnetic resonance imaging in oncology. In: Bleehen N (ed) Investigation techniques in oncology. Springer-Verlag, Berlin, pp 125–150

Johnson R J, Jenkins J P R, Isherwood I, Jamer R D, Schofield P F 1987b Quantitative magnetic resonance imaging in rectal cancer. British Journal of Radiology 60: 761–764

Konishi F, Muto T, Takahashi H, Itoh K, Kanazawa K, Morioka Y 1985 Transrectal ultrasonography for the assessment of invasion of rectal carcinoma. Diseases of the Colon and Rectum 28: 889–894

Kramann B, Hildebrandt U 1986 Computed tomography versus endosonography in the staging of rectal carcinoma: a comparative study. International Journal of Colorectal Disease 1: 216–218

Lee J K T, Stanley R J, Sagel S S, Levitt R G, McClennan B L 1981 CT apperance of the pelvis after abdomino-perineal resection for rectal carcinoma. Radiology 141: 737–741

Lock M R, Cairns D W, Ritche J K, Lockhart-Mummery H E 1978 The treatment of early colorectal cancer by local excision. British Journal of Surgery 65: 346–349

Nicholls R J, Ritche J K, Wadsworth J, Parks A G 1979 Total excision or restorative resection for carcinoma of the middle third of the rectum. British Journal of Surgery 66: 625–627

Nicholls R J, York Mason A, Morson B C, Dixon A K, Kelsey Fry I 1982 The clinical staging of rectal cancer. British Journal of Surgery 69: 404–409

Pahlman L, Glimelius B, Graffman S 1985 Pre- versus postoperative radiotherapy in rectal carcinoma: an interim report from a randomized multicentre trial. British Journal of Surgery 72: 961–966

Papillon J 1984 New prospects in the conservative treatment of rectal cancer. Diseases of the Colon and Rectum 27: 695–700

Phillips R K S, Hittinger R, Blesovsky L, Fry J S, Fielding L P 1984a Large bowel cancer: surgical pathology and its relationship to survival. British Journal of Surgery 71: 604–610

Phillips R K S, Hittinger R, Blesovsky L, Fry J S, Fielding L P 1984b Local recurrence following 'curative' surgery for large bowel cancer: 1. The overall picture. British Journal of Surgery 71: 12–16

Reasbeck P G, Manktelow A, McArthur A M, Packer S G K, Berkeley B 1984 An evaluation of pelvic lymphoscintigraphy in the staging of colorectal carcinoma. British Journal of Surgery 71: 936–940

Rifkin M D, Wechsler R J 1986 A comparison of computed tomography and endorectal ultrasound in staging rectal cancer. International Journal of Colorectal Disease 1: 219–223

Romano G, De Rosa P, Vallone G, Rotondo A, Grassi R, Santangelo M L 1985 Intrarectal ultrasound and computed tomography in the pre- and postoperative assessment of patients with rectal carcinoma. British Journal of Surgery September suppl: S117–S119

Rosenberg I L 1979 The aetiology of colonic suture-line recurrence. Annals of the Royal College of Surgeons of England 61: 251–257

Saini S, Sullivan J, Ferruci J T, Stark D D, Wittenberg J 1986 Particulate iron oxide (magnetite) as a potential bowel contrast agent for MRI. Magnetic Resonance Imaging 4: 179–180

Saitoh N, Okui K, Sarashina H, Suzuki M, Arai T, Nunomura M 1986 Evaluation of echographic diagnosis of rectal cancer using intrarectal ultrasonic examination. Diseases of the Colon and Rectum 29: 234–242

Tanaka Y, Yasuda K, Aibe T et al 1984 Anatomical and pathological aspects in ultrasonic endoscopy for GI tract. Scandinavian Journal of Gastroenterology 19 (suppl 94): 43–50

Theoni R F, Moss A A, Schnyder P, Margulis A R 1981 Detection and staging of primary rectal cancer by computed tomography. Radiology 141: 135–138

Third report of an MRC working party – The evaluation of low dose pre-operative radiotherapy in the management of operable rectal cancer; results of a randomly controlled trial. British Journal of Surgery (1984) 71: 21–25

Third report of the MRC trial: Clinico-pathological features of prognostic significance in operable rectal cancer in 17 centres in the UK. British Journal of Cancer (1984) 50: 435–442

Thomas G D H, Dixon M F, Smeeton N C, Williams N S 1983 Observer variation in the histological grading of rectal carcinoma. Journal of Clinical Pathology 36: 385–391

Turnbull R B Jr, Kyle K, Watson F R, Spratt J 1967 Cancer of the colon: the influence of the no-touch isolation technique on survival rates. Annals of Surgery 166: 420–427

UICC TNM Atlas 1982 Spiessel B, Schiebe O, Wagner G (eds). Springer-Verlag, New York

Umpleby H C, Fermor B, Symes M O, Williamson R C N 1984 Viability of exfoliated colorectal carcinoma cells. British Journal of Surgery 71: 659–663

Whiteway J, Nicholls R J, Morson B C 1985 The rôle of surgical local excision in the treatment of rectal cancer. British Journal of Surgery 72: 694–697

Wild J J 1950 The use of ultrasonic pulses for the measurement of biologic tissues and the detection of tissue density changes. Surgery 27: 183–188

Wild J J, Foderick J W 1978a The feasibility of echometric detection of cancer in the lower gastrointestinal tract I. American Journal of Proctology, Gastroenterology and Colon and Rectal Surgery Jan–Feb: 16–25

Wild J J, Foderick J W 1978b The feasibility of echometric detection of cancer of the lower gastrointestinal tract II. American Journal of Proctology, Gastroenterology and Colon and Rectal Surgery Mar–Apr: 11–20

Wild J J, Reid J M 1956 Diagnostic use of ultrasound. British Journal of Physical Medicine 19: 248–257

Williams N S, Durdey P, Johnston D 1985a The outcome following sphincter saving resection and abdomino-perineal resection for low rectal cancer. British Journal of Surgery 72: 595–598

Williams N S, Durdey P, Quirke P et al 1985b Pre-operative staging of rectal neoplasm and its impact on clinical management. British Journal of Surgery 72: 868–874

Zaunbauer W, Haertel M, Fuchs W A 1981 Computed tomography in carcinoma of the rectum. Gastrointestinal Radiology 6: 79–84

Zelas P, Haaga J R, Lavery I C, Fazio V W 1980 The diagnosis by percutaneous biopsy with computed tomography of a recurrence of carcinoma of the rectum in the pelvis. Surgery, Gynecology and Obstetrics 151: 525–527

Zheng G, Johnson R J, Eddleston B, Schofield P F, James R D 1984 Computed tomographic scanning in rectal cancer. Journal of the Royal Society of Medicine 77: 915–920

Zinkin L D 1983 A critical review of the classifications and staging of colorectal cancer. Diseases of the Colon and Rectum 26: 37–43

8. The liver, biliary system and pancreas

D. F. Martin

INTRODUCTION

Until recently malignant disease of the hepato-biliary system and pancreas was diagnosed at laparotomy or at post mortem examination. With the advent of high quality real time ultrasound (US), computed tomography (CT), direct cholangiography (PTC and ERCP) and, to a lesser extent selective angiography, accurate preoperative diagnosis of these tumours is now possible, particularly when the techniques are supplemented by image-guided biopsy. Similarly, it is possible to make a reasonably accurate preoperative assessment of the operability of lesions and therefore to tailor surgical management for individual patients, particularly whether to undertake a curative procedure or palliation only. In addition, for patients who have inoperable tumours, palliative non-surgical techniques such as endoscopic stenting have been developed. When considering the rôle of radiological staging of hepatobiliary and pancreatic malignancy, it is important to keep a few simple points in mind. Firstly, most patients present clinically when the tumour is already unresectable. Secondly, most patients are elderly, and may have poor nutritional status and concomitant medical conditions which will influence postoperative morbidity and mortality. Thirdly, surgical treatment frequently involves an extensive procedure, e.g. Whipple's procedure for carcinoma of the pancreas, and appropriate surgical expertise is necessary.

The radiologist must be aware of the clinical situation of each patient presenting for staging and has two major responsibilities: firstly, to be clear in reporting on the inoperability of lesions in order to prevent inappropriate surgery being attempted,

and secondly, not to over-interpret radiological findings which would preclude an attempt at a curative procedure.

With these thoughts in mind it is obviously difficult to draw up hard and fast guidelines regarding the radiological management of patients with hepatobiliary or pancreatic malignancy. This chapter describes the clinical features, prognosis, treatment options and radiological management of each type of malignancy.

DIAGNOSTIC AND THERAPEUTIC TECHNIQUES COMMONLY USED IN THE MANAGEMENT OF HEPATOBILIARY AND PANCREATIC MALIGNANCY

Dynamic incremental contrast-enhanced computed tomography

The aim of this procedure is to opacify visceral arteries, portal vein, hepatic veins and inferior vena cava during CT examination to demonstrate more precisely the anatomical location of malignant lesions and their involvement of vascular structures.

Following plain CT examination of the liver and pancreas, a 19 gauge butterfly needle is inserted into an antecubital fossa vein. 100–200 ml of contrast medium with an iodine concentration of between 240 and 300 mg of iodine/ml is injected using a pump injector at the rate of 2 ml/s. For ideal opacification of all vessels, including the hepatic veins, a delay of 50–60 s after the start of infusion should be used before scanning commences. Because of the need for a long delay, the larger volume of 200 ml of contrast is preferable where possible. Contiguous 1 cm sections are performed as rapidly as possible with reconstruction of the images being delayed until the full batch of scans is complete. Normally 3–4 slices can be obtained during each suspended respiration. With this technique, high quality angiographic CT images can be obtained.

Endoscopic retrograde cholangiopancreatography (ERCP) and endoprosthesis (stent) insertion

Endoscopic examination is performed on a fluoroscopy table with the patient fairly heavily sedated with a combination of a benzodiazepine and an opioid analgesic. Patients should be starved for at least six hours prior to the procedure and intravenous prophylactic antibiotics which can be secreted into bile should be given. Diagnostic ERCP is performed using a standard diagnostic duodenoscope. The bile duct is cannulated with a 5 French ERCP catheter which will, if necessary, accept an 0.035 inch guide-wire. Low density contrast medium (Urografin 150) is best for opacifying the biliary system and sufficient contrast should be injected to make a complete assessment of the malignant stricture and the biliary system proximal to the stricture. Once the extent of the lesion has been defined, endoscopic sphincterotomy using a specially constructed wire loop-containing catheter and surgical diathermy can be performed if considered necessary, although in our experience this is rarely indicated for the insertion of endoprostheses. The standard endoscope is replaced by another which has a 4.2 mm operating channel and is capable of accepting endoprostheses up to 12 French in diameter. The bile ducts are cannulated using a combination of a 6 French catheter over an 0.035 inch Teflon-coated, straight guide-wire and the tumour is negotiated with this combination. A 10 or 12 French stent is then passed down through the operating channel of the endoscope, pushed onward over the catheter and guide-wire assembly by a 10 French pusher tube. Once the endoprosthesis is satisfactorily positioned, the guide-wire can be removed, and cholangiography can be performed through the 6 French catheter in order to ensure adequate positioning. Once this is achieved, the 6 French catheter and the endoscope are removed.

The use of the large channel endoscope, which is a difficult instrument to manoeuvre freely in the duodenum, occasionally makes re-entry into the bile duct system difficult. If this is felt to be likely during the initial ERCP examination, a 0.035 inch guide-wire can be passed through the 5 French injection cannula and positioned within the bile ducts above the tumour. The 5 French catheter is then replaced with a 6 French pigtail catheter and the endoscope is removed, leaving the catheter and guide-wire assembly within the bile ducts. The large channel endoscope can then be inserted into the duodeum over the catheter and guide-wire assembly and the endoprosthesis can be positioned over the 6 French catheter (Martin 1988).

Percutaneous transhepatic cholangiography (PTC) and endoprosthesis insertion

PTC is performed in the standard manner. Its use in our experience is confined to those patients in whom ERCP has failed to demonstrate the full extent of tumour involvement, or in whom endoprosthesis insertion is not possible using the endoscopic route. Once PTC has been performed, an 0.035 inch guide-wire is inserted into the biliary system, either using a 1-stick system, which enables exchange of a 22 gauge fine needle over an 0.018 inch guide-wire for a 6 French catheter, which will take the 0.035 inch wire, or by a separate puncture using an 18 gauge needle. The guide-wire is negotiated into the common duct through the tumour, into the duodenum, using a catheter/wire combination. Rather than insert a large diameter endoprosthesis through the liver, a procedure accompanied by significant risk of bleeding or biliary leak, we choose to position a guide-wire in the duodenum and then grasp this guide-wire through an endoscope. The wire is withdrawn up the biopsy channel of the endoscope and a 10 or 12 French endoprosthesis is then inserted endoscopically over the wire. The wire is withdrawn up through the endoscope, leaving the stent in position. If considered necessary, a 6 French catheter can be left within the intrahepatic ducts to allow temporary intrahepatic duct drainage and repeat cholangiography can be performed 24 hours after the procedure.

If at the initial attempt it is not possible to

negotiate the tumour and pass a guide-wire into the duodenum, percutaneous drainage can be undertaken for two to three days to allow decompression of the duct system, and a second attempt at passing a guide-wire into the duodenum is normally successful. If this is not successful, then long term percutaneous biliary drainage can be used and the catheter replaced if necessary.

Whipple's procedure

This is the most commonly performed curative surgical technique for lesions involving the distal common duct, the papilla of Vater and the head of the pancreas. It involves removal of the antrum of the stomach, the head of the pancreas and the duodenal loop. Enteric continuity is established using a gastroenterostomy and both the pancreatic duct and bile duct are also anastomosed to jejunum. The most common complication of the procedure is leakage of the pancreaticojejunal anastomosis, and because of this it has been proposed that total pancreatectomy is a suitable alternative procedure. However, it has yet to be shown that total pancreatectomy offers better long term survival and the metabolic consequences of total pancreatectomy can be difficult to manage. Whipple's procedure involves a prolonged, meticulous dissection of retroperitoneal structures and may fail at a late stage because of involvement of the superior mesenteric or portal veins by tumour. For this reason adequate preoperative investigation is helpful in defining those patients in whom Whipple's procedure would be futile.

TUMOURS OF THE GALL BLADDER

The most common tumour to arise within the gall bladder is adenocarcinoma, although less common tumours such as squamous carcinoma, carcinoid, primary sarcoma, melanoma and lymphoma are described. Gall bladder carcinoma is the commonest primary malignancy of the biliary apparatus and is the fifth most common gastrointestinal cancer. It usually occurs in the eighth decade of life and is approximately three times more common in women than in men. The female preponderance reflects the association of gall bladder carcinoma with gallstones which are present in approximately 75% of cases. Other apparent risk factors are a previous clinical episode of cholecystitis, porcelain gall bladder and possibly familial polyposis coli. It spreads by direct invasion of adjacent structures including the liver parenchyma, the extra- and intrahepatic bile ducts, the duodenum and the hepatic flexure of the colon. Local lymphatic spread occurs relatively early but haematogenous spread is late.

Clinical features

Patients with gall bladder carcinoma usually present when the tumour is advanced, and frequently with bile duct obstruction. Occasionally a tumour is discovered incidentally during cholecystectomy or at ultrasound examination.

Prognosis

The prognosis seems to depend upon the mode of presentation. The majority of patients have evidence of local invasion such as obstructive jaundice, ascites or intestinal obstruction, and the tumours are inoperable. Those in whom the tumour is discovered only on pathological examination of the gall bladder may already have had curative surgery.

Treatment options

When tumour is discovered incidentally at operation for cholecystectomy, the extent of surgery will be determined by the surgical findings. For tumours confined to and not penetrating the gall bladder wall, simple cholecystectomy may be all that is necessary (Bergdahl 1980), although some have suggested (Bismuth et al 1982) that more extensive resection, taking the local lymph nodes and even resection of the liver, may improve survival. Where tumour penetrates the gall bladder or involves local lymph nodes, then radical surgery appears indicated (Nevin et al 1976), although survival is poor. When the tumour has spread to involve the liver, extensive surgery including hepatic resection may be undertaken, although it is unlikely that this has significant benefit (Bismuth & Malt 1979, Nevin et al 1976).

For those patients whose tumour is found

incidentally at ultrasound examination, the treatment options are essentially the same as those indicated above, although more precise information regarding the extent of tumour should be obtained before surgery is contemplated.

Most patients are inoperable but in those with jaundice for whom palliation is desirable the choice lies between surgical bypass, particularly to the left intrahepatic duct system, or endoprosthesis insertion.

Chemotherapy and radiotherapy have been used in advanced disease but at present do not offer significant palliation.

Radiology

Staging

When the tumour is discovered at operation, intra-operative ultrasound can be used to identify hepatic metastases not evident surgically and to assess the extent of local invasion of the liver; the findings will direct the extent of surgery. The frequency with which gall bladder carcinoma is discovered incidentally at operation should decline with the use of ultrasound as a primary diagnostic procedure for gall bladder disease.

In the majority of carcinomas oral cholecystography demonstrates a non-functioning gall bladder (Vattinen 1970), but ultrasound can detect a tumour complicating gallstones with a high degree of accuracy (Dalla Palma et al 1980, Weiner et al 1984) and identify associated features such as lymphadenopathy, bile duct obstruction, direct hepatic invasion and metastases. CT can compliment US in the assessment of extent. Like US, CT can demonstrate the primary lesion, hepatic invasion (Fig. 8.1) and metastases, local lymphadenopathy and hepatic artery and portal vein involvement. Both US and CT are accurate in assessing extensive disease but each technique is less accurate in the assessment of early disease. A combination of the two may stage potentially resectable tumours more accurately.

Angiography is occasionally performed, mainly to ascertain involvement of the hepatic artery or portal vein. If present, the chances of successful surgical clearance are reduced. Similar information can probably be obtained using US or CT, both non-invasive procedures.

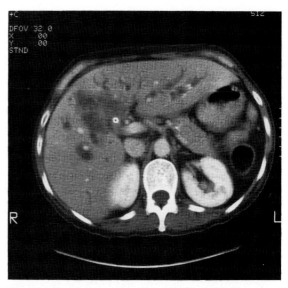

Fig. 8.1 Dynamic contrast-enhanced CT section in a patient with gall bladder carcinoma demonstrating dilated bile ducts and tumour invasion into the left and right lobes of the liver. An endoprosthesis for biliary drainage has been inserted.

Direct cholangiography may give helpful information regarding the extent of disease, even in patients without obstructive jaundice (Ogoshi & Niwa 1977). The most common finding, although non-specific, is non-filling of the gall bladder but this is common during ERCP in patients with gall bladder stones (Martin & Tweedle 1987). It gives no information regarding local lymph node involvement or extension into the liver unless there are ductal abnormalities in the right and left lobar segments immediately adjacent to the gall bladder fossa. However, where there is encroachment into the intrahepatic ducts or into the common duct, these features indicate that simple cholecystectomy and regional lymph node clearance will not be curative and that hepatic resection with a choledocho-enteric anastomosis will be required. Where there is involvement of the second degree intrahepatic biliary radicles involving both lobes, the tumour is unresectable.

Treatment

Fluoroscopy-guided insertion of a prosthesis to bypass malignant obstruction is best achieved endoscopically as the morbidity and mortality is lower than with the percutaneous transhepatic route. However, in a small proportion of patients it is not possible to pass a guide-wire through the stricture from below and a percutaneous approach and combined procedure should be used. In addition, if both hepatic ducts are involved, then ideally an endoprosthesis should be positioned in each lobe of the liver in order to avoid cholangitis developing in the undrained segment. This is difficult using an endoscopic approach, and again a combined approach may be effective. Because stents have a relatively limited lifespan of approximately eight months, it is our policy to change stents prospectively at six-monthly intervals provided the patient's condition allows.

BILE DUCT MALIGNANCY

Bile duct tumours are rare compared with other malignant tumours involving the biliary system. The most common tumour is cholangiocarcinoma; there are a few reports of other neoplasms such as carcinoid. Cholangiocarcinomas consist of three types: firstly, a polypoid type which is commoner in the lower common duct; secondly a nodular or localized type which occurs in the mid or upper common duct — some of these lesions are soft and fleshy but others can be schirrhous; and thirdly, a diffuse schirrhous type which occurs most commonly in the upper common duct or at the confluence of the hepatic ducts (Klatskin tumour). Tumours may be multiple, particularly the polypoid type, although this is infrequent, occurring in less than 10% of cases. Whilst there is no clear link between gallstone disease and cholangiocarcinoma, the two conditions can coexist and common duct stones and cholangiocarcinoma are occasionally seen. Interestingly the stones usually lie distal to the malignant obstruction. Predisposing factors which have been suggested include ulcerative colitis, perhaps because of an association with unrecognized sclerosing cholangitis, choledochal cyst and, in the Far East, chronic biliary infestation with liver flukes.

Clinical features

Most bile duct carcinomas present with obstructive jaundice which is usually progressive, although on occasion, particularly with the polypoid type, it can be intermittent. Patients may suffer a long prodromal illness with malaise and weight loss although specific features such as right upper quadrant pain are uncommon. Occasionally bile duct carcinoma is discovered during the investigation of an incidental finding of elevated serum alkaline phosphatase.

Prognosis

Most patients do not survive for a year after diagnosis and die from chronic biliary obstruction or sepsis due to progressive local disease. It has been suggested that with aggressive surgery even the most difficult cholangiocarcinomas at the confluence of the hepatic ducts can be treated and mean survival extended to approximately two years (Benjamin & Blumgart 1979, Hadjis et al 1985). Metastases to local lymph nodes, liver and omentum are uncommon.

Treatment options

Possible methods of treatment for bile duct tumours include curative or palliative surgery and surgical or non-surgical intubation. Preoperative percutaneous bile duct drainage was in vogue for a period (Hatfield et al 1982) but whilst it seems theoretically reasonable to operate on a patient whose jaundice has subsided and in whom the metabolic consequences of biliary obstruction have improved, the consequences of infection complicating preoperative catheter drainage seem to outweigh the advantages. There now seems to be general agreement that preoperative drainage is not routinely indicated. Indeed, Blumgart et al (1984) have proposed that the subsequent operative mortality in patients in whom preoperative drainage has been performed is higher than in patients where such procedures have not been undertaken.

Treatment options depend upon the site of the lesion. For distal common duct tumours, primary resection or more commonly pancreaticoduodenectomy (Whipple's procedure) are undertaken as curative procedures in patients fit enough to withstand surgery. Whipple's procedure carries a significant postoperative mortality but in experienced hands this can be 10% or less (Lerut et al 1984, Jones et al 1985). The 5-year survival rate for distal common duct. tumours treated by Whipple's procedure is better than for pancreatic carcinoma but is still only about 15% (Alexander et al 1984). For distal common duct tumours palliative choledocho-enteric bypass is usually a simple surgical technique with low·operative mortality, but long term survivors are few. Mid to upper common duct tumours can similarly be managed by local resection or by Whipple's procedure and similar results to those for distal common duct lesions can be expected. In cholangiocarcinoma at the confluence of the hepatic ducts the situation is less clear. Traditionally most surgeons, even specialists in hepatobiliary surgery, have felt that the majority of these lesions are inoperable or carry such a high operative mortality as to prohibit attempts at primary resection. However, Blumgart et al (1984) have been strong proponents of an aggressive approach to hilar cholangiocarcinoma, undertaking liver resection, meticulous choledocho-enteric anastomosis and even vascular reconstruction where necessary. As part of this aggressive approach they propose extensive preoperative investigation to assess resectability. Approximately 30% of patients in their series were suitable for resection and of those considered suitable, only 60% actually underwent resection. Those who were considered resectable but not treated in this way were unfit for major surgery or were found to have more extensive disease at laparotomy. Even with radical resection local recurrence is common and the mean survival is approximately two years. Intubation techniques (intraoperative, percutaneous or endoscopic) are clearly only palliative procedures and will do little to lengthen the life expectancy of the patient with cholangiocarcinoma at any site.

Radiotherapy with external radiation or using percutaneously or endoscopically placed intraluminal iridium sources has been reported (Fletcher et al 1981) and perhaps offers some palliation without significant side-effects, particularly now that high intensity microsources which can be passed down fine catheters are available.

Radiology

Staging

The diagnosis of malignant obstruction is generally simple. Ultrasound examination will demonstrate the presence and often the level of bile duct obstruction. The malignant nature of the obstructing lesion is usually best demonstrated by ERCP although for proximal tumours PTC, occasionally with separate right and left duct punctures, may be necessary. Histological confirmation of cholangiocarcinoma can be difficult and in many reported series relating to management, histological confirmation was not available. Staging of the tumour to assess technical resectability is more difficult. Initial investigations such as a chest radiograph and ultrasound examination of the liver may demonstrate metastatic disease which precludes curative surgery. Blumgart et al (1986) have suggested that resectability depends upon the extent of involvement of intrahepatic bile ducts, portal vein, hepatic artery and inferior vena cava. Others have suggested (Beazley et al 1984) that apparent vascular involvement on preoperative investigation may be due to tumour compression rather than tumour invasion. This may be a semantic argument because it seems that with cholangiocarcinoma, compression of vascular structures may not allow removal of tumour from the vessel due to associated fibrotic reaction (Voyles et al 1983).

Ultrasound examination can be helpful in demonstrating regional lymphadenopathy and can allow guided percutaneous aspiration biopsy of the nodes; their presence does not necessarily preclude resection. Invasion or compression of the portal vein should also be demonstrable (Fig. 8.2). CT, particularly with dynamic intravenous contrast enhancement, allows assessment of invasion or compression of the portal vein and to some extent the hepatic artery and inferior vena cava. Blumgart et al (1984) believe that preoperative evaluation is not complete unless angiography is performed. Involvement of the hepatic artery and portal vein and their branches is more likely to be demonstrated by angiography than by CT, but as yet there is no comparative study which demonstrates the superiority of angiography for staging.

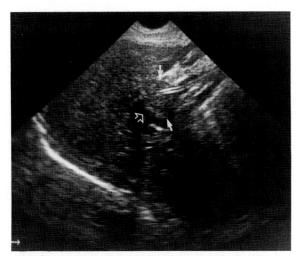

Fig. 8.2 Longitudinal ultrasound demonstrating a mass at the proximal end of the common duct (straight arrows), displacing the portal vein posteriorly (open arrow). An endoprosthesis is in position through the tumour within the bile ducts.

Direct cholangiography seems of limited value in assessing resectability of cholangiocarcinoma except in tumours involving the bifurcation of the hepatic ducts. When tumour involves only the main hepatic ducts then resection is possible. However, more extensive tumours involving intrahepatic duct radicles are less likely to be resectable (Fig. 8.3).

Our own approach is to exclude the presence of overt metastases by chest radiography and liver ultrasound and then go on to assess involvement of the vessels by ultrasound and contrast-enhanced CT in patients who are free of metastatic disease and considered physically fit for surgery. If these investigations suggest an operable lesion then laparotomy is performed.

Treatment

Radiological management of cholangiocarcinoma is essentially confined to insertion of biliary endoprostheses (stent), either percutaneously or endoscopically, although the insertion of catheters for iridium wire internal radiotherapy can also be accomplished. For common bile duct tumours endoscopic insertion is preferable. A single 10 or 12 French stent can be successfully inserted in 80–

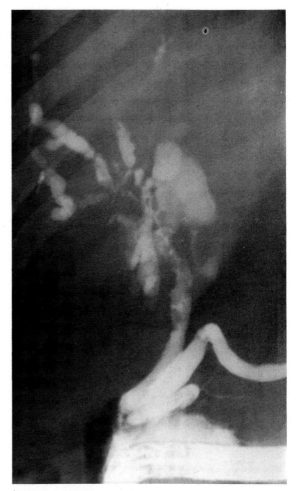

Fig. 8.3 ERCP demonstrating a polypoid tumour involving the common hepatic duct and the first and second degree intrahepatic duct radicles. The extent of involvement indicates inoperable tumour.

90% of patients and should allow adequate drainage. The endoscopic management of strictures involving the hepatic ducts is more difficult. A single stent can be inserted in the majority of cases but cholangitis developing in the undrained segment is a significant complication and drainage of both lobes of the liver is preferable (Fig. 8.4). This can only be achieved in about 30% of cases even in the most experienced hands (Huibregtse & Tytgat 1984).

Blocking of these biliary stents is also common, as described above, and we routinely change all

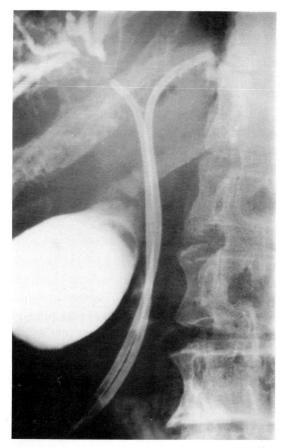

Fig. 8.4 ERCP examination in a patient with inoperable hilar cholangiocarcinoma, demonstrating endoscopically inserted endoprostheses in the right and left hepatic ducts. The gall bladder is well opacified.

large bore stents after six months in an effort to avoid the complications of blockage.

TUMOURS OF THE PAPILLA OF VATER

Information on tumours of the papilla of Vater is complicated by the fact that peripapillary tumours of the common bile duct and those of the head of the pancreas are often included in this group when surgical treatment and prognosis are considered. It has been increasingly recognized that primary malignancy of the papilla itself is not uncommon and has the best overall prognosis of all tumours of the biliary apparatus. In addition to primary adenocarcinoma the papilla may be involved by duodenal adenocarcinoma, carcinoid or leiomyo-sarcoma. Malignancies involving the papilla of Vater have no obvious predisposing factor but there does appear to be an increased incidence of papillary neoplasms in familial polyposis coli and in Gardener's syndrome. Men and women are equally affected, neoplasms increasing in frequency with age.

Clinical features

Patients with carcinoma of the papilla of Vater classically present with obstructive jaundice, which can be relapsing, and is occasionally associated with anaemia, gastrointestinal bleeding and steatorrhoea. These last two features may give rise to the so-called 'silver stool' said to be characteristic of malignant papillary obstruction. However, in our experience this is exceedingly rare. Most commonly tumours of the papilla present with progressive painless obstructive jaundice.

Prognosis

Whilst the 5-year survival of patients with, periampullary pancreatic adenocarcinoma is approximately 5%, the 5-year survival of patients with adenocarcinoma of the papilla is as high as 50% following surgery (Tarazi et al 1986).

Treatment options

The optimum surgical approach to carcinoma of the papilla is uncertain. Many surgeons believe that Whipple's pancreato-duodenectomy is the treatment of choice but others (Tarazi et al 1986, Knox & Kingston 1986) have demonstrated that long term survival can be achieved by local resection and cite the relatively high post operative mortality of Whipple's procedure as an indication that extensive surgery is not necessarily required.

Endoscopic management of papillary tumours can be achieved by endoscopic sphincterotomy which temporarily relieves jaundice in the majority of patients. In those in whom an adequate sphincterotomy is not possible, or in whom tumour extension causes restenosis, an endoscopic stent can be inserted to relieve obstruction.

Radiology

Ultrasound is the preferred initial investigation in patients presenting with obstructive jaundice and in those with carcinoma of the papilla of Vater it will normally demonstrate dilated bile ducts down to the level of the papilla. A mass involving the distal common duct may be detected but will not be distinguishable from other causes of malignant distal bile duct obstruction. Ultrasound may demonstrate regional lymphadenopathy or liver metastases although these are late features and are uncommon at presentation. ERCP allows direct inspection of the papilla which may be obviously involved by tumour but in a proportion of patients may simply appear bulbous. Biopsies can be obtained to confirm the diagnosis. If the papilla looks frankly neoplastic, biopsy should be obtained before endoscopic sphincterotomy as artefacts due to diathermy may make histological interpretation difficult. Where the papilla is bulbous, endoscopic sphincterotomy will allow drainage and biopsies may be taken following this. In view of the difficulties of interpreting such biopsies repeat biopsy may be wise after one month. When the papilla is bulbous it is occasionally difficult to perform endoscopic cholangiography and sphincterotomy and a pre-cut papillotomy using a needle-knife cutting directly into or immediately above the tumour is a useful technique (Martin & Tweedle 1984).

In our experience patients treated by endoscopic sphincterotomy obtain good relief of jaundice and can expect to remain symptom free for some months. However, slow but steady growth of the tumour will eventually cause reobstruction and further 'sphincterotomy' may then be difficult. Primary endoscopic stenting may avoid the complications of restenosis. However, as patients with a papillary carcinoma have a relatively good prognosis repeated endoscopic stent changes may be necessary and it is our policy, in patients who have no demonstrable metastatic disease and are fit, to perform either local resection of the neoplasm or Whipple's procedure.

MALIGNANT PANCREATIC TUMOURS

A large number of epithelial, mesenchymal and endothelial tumours can affect the pancreas, pancreatic ductal adenocarcinoma being the most common. Of importance to the radiologist from the standpoint of both diagnosis and treatment is the presence or absence of hormonal activity. For this reason pancreatic neoplasms will be discussed under two broad headings: firstly, non-endocrine tumours, particularly adenocarcinomas, and secondly endocrine tumours.

PANCREATIC ADENOCARCINOMA

Adenocarcinoma of the pancreas appears to be increasing in incidence and is now the second most common gastrointestinal malignancy, accounting for approximately 10% of all such neoplasms. Adenocarcinoma occurs most frequently in the head of the pancreas, between 50 and 70% of the tumours occurring at this site. Although close proximity to the bile duct leads to biliary obstruction and hence relatively early presentation, the majority of the tumours are inoperable when the patient is first seen. Most patients die within 12 months of diagnosis and even those patients selected for radical surgery have a 5-year survival of 10% or less. Until recently postoperative mortality for extensive resection procedures has been prohibitively high. These factors have led to the development of non-operative palliative procedures, both radiological and endoscopic, for the management of such patients. Because of the ease with which these procedures can be performed, it is important that radiological staging is performed in patients who are sufficiently fit to withstand surgery: only in this way can the small number of patients who may have resectable tumours be allowed to achieve long term survival.

Clinical features

Jaundice due to biliary obstruction is the commonest presenting feature. Involvement of the common duct by direct extension from carcinoma in the head of the gland is almost invariable but can also occur in patients with carcinoma of the body or tail, although more commonly it is due to metastatic lymphadenopathy at the porta hepatis. Weight loss is a similarly common symptom and may be profound. Carcinoma of the body or tail of the gland may present in the early stages with epigastric pain, characteristically radiating through to the back. Diabetes mellitus may be present although this is not always of recent onset. Other symptoms such as diarrhoea, abdominal bloating, nausea and vomiting may occur, and vomiting in particular raises the possibility of duodenal obstruction.

Prognosis

The prognosis for the patient with pancreatic carcinoma is poor. That for tumours of the head of the gland is slightly better than for the body or the tail and this probably relates to the delay in diagnosis which may occur in patients with tumours outside the head. In the past staging of pancreatic carcinoma was performed at laparotomy and the extent of surgery dictated by the findings. Thus patients who are not fit for surgery have the worst prognosis and few survive six months. Those in whom surgical intubation or a biliary bypass procedure is possible survive a little longer, but rarely beyond 18 months. Patients found to have a resectable tumour undergo either Whipple's procedure or, occasionally, total pancreatectomy. In the past both of these procedures had high postoperative mortality rates, figures of 10–20% being common and 5-year survival rarely being more than 10%. More recently some centres have reported postoperative mortality of 3–4% for Whipple's procedure and although long term data are lacking, it may be that the 5-year survival rate is improving (Trede 1987).

Treatment options

In the patient presenting with obstructive jaundice due to pancreatic carcinoma there are essentially three treatment options:

1. Whipple's procedure: described in a previous section.
2. Bypass procedure: in patients with inoperable tumour, biliary bypass may be performed by cholecystjejunostomy or choledochojejunostomy. Although cholecystjejunostomy is the simpler procedure it is often difficult to be confident that the cystic duct is not involved with tumour. Choledochojejunostomy is technically more difficult for the surgeon but offers better biliary decompression. If duodenal involvement is present at operation gastroenterostomy is necessary. In approximately 15% of patients who do not demonstrate duodenal obstruction at the time of surgery this will occur before death, and some surgeons advocate a pre-emptive gastroenterostomy at the time of biliary bypass.

3. Bile duct intubation: ideally transtumoral intubation at surgery should never be necessary. Patients in whom preoperative radiology indicates inoperable tumour can undergo endoscopic or transhepatic intubation. In those patients in whom preoperative radiology suggests that the neoplasm is operable but this is not found to be so at surgery, biliary-enteric bypass can usually be performed. The choice between percutaneous transhepatic or endoscopic intubation is a vexed one but will depend to a large degree upon the availability of local expertise. The relative merits of the techniques are discussed in the following sections.

Radiology

Staging

Most patients with pancreatic adenocarcinoma will be inoperable at the time of presentation. The tumour is likely to have spread beyond the pancreas and may have involved the duodenum, local vascular structures and lymph nodes. In addition a proportion of patients will have liver or lung metastases.

Initial investigations include a chest radiograph and ultrasound examination of the upper abdomen to exclude overt metastases. Suspect lesions within the liver can be biopsied, as can the primary lesion, under US guidance. The sensitivity of fine needle biopsy of the pancreas is approximately 70–80% (Luning et al 1985, Hall-Craggs & Lees 1986) and therefore a negative biopsy does not exclude disease.

As the majority of patients present with obstructive jaundice, direct cholangiography, usually ERCP, will be the next diagnostic procedure. Endoscopy has the advantage over percutaneous cholangiography of demonstrating direct invasion of the duodenum or papilla and thereby allowing biopsy. If the duodenum is directly involved then surgery with gastroenterostomy and biliary-enteric bypass is probably the most sensible course of action. Although there has been debate as to the specificity of ERCP in the diagnosis of pancreatic carcinoma, in general the differentiation of chronic pancreatitis from carcinoma is straightforward. In pancreatic carcinoma, both the pancreatic duct and bile duct usually show a short segment of stenosis at the same level. The pancreatic ducts downstream from the obstructing lesion are normal whilst the duct system upstream from the neoplasm shows uniform dilatation (Fig. 8.5). In chronic pancreatitis the pancreatic duct system is more likely to show widespread abnormality and the bile duct stricture associated with chronic pancreatitis is usually longer and smoother than in pancreatic carcinoma. However, these radiological features are not absolute and there are cases when the diagnosis is difficult, particularly when pancreatic carcinoma occurs in a patient with pre-existing chronic pancreatitis. Endoscopic biopsy

from within the bile duct or the pancreatic duct or guided aspiration biopsy may help clarify these cases. The size of the tumour at ERCP can give an indication of the likelihood of resectability. Nix et al (1984) showed that tumours less than 4 cm in diameter were resectable in 77% of cases, tumours between 4.5 and 6 cm were resectable in 24%, whilst those over 7 cm in diameter were resectable in only 9%. In patients considered fit for surgery and with no evidence of metastases, in whom the ERCP demonstrates a small tumour, further investigation is warranted.

Factors which influence curative resection are the presence of tumour in local lymph nodes, invasion of the transverse mesocolon and involvement of the superior mesenteric vessels or the portal vein. Whilst some (Moossa & Lavelle-Jones 1988) believe that coeliac axis and superior mesenteric angiography are necessary in the staging of pancreatic carcinoma, not all workers accept this (Braasch 1988). Visceral angiography can provide a valuable road map for the surgeon, particularly with regard to the common variants of origin of the hepatic artery, but these should be apparent to the surgeon at the time of laparotomy and angiography may be avoidable. More important is the demonstration of encasement or involvement of vessels. However, this information can be equally well obtained by dynamic incremental, contrast-enhanced CT scanning (Jafri et al 1984, Freeny et al 1988). Ultrasound examination may also demonstrate involvement of the splenic vein or portal vein (Garra et al 1987) although it is probably less accurate than CT or angiography. CT may also demonstrate peripancreatic lymphadenopathy (Zeman et al 1985) and may occasionally demonstrate liver and lung base metastases not previously identified. Magnetic resonance imaging of the pancreas does not as yet provide comparable information to CT (Tscholakoff et al 1986, Jenkins et al 1987). It is our policy to perform dynamic contrast-enhanced CT in patients under consideration for curable resection. Clinical examination, chest radiography and upper abdominal ultrasound will not have demonstrated metastases and ERCP will have shown a small neoplasm. If CT suggests that the neoplasm is resectable then the patient proceeds to laparotomy and Whipple's procedure.

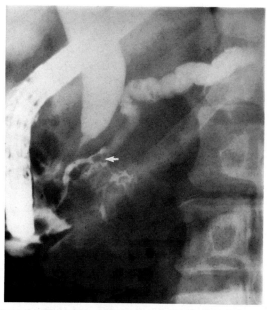

Fig. 8.5 ERCP in a patient presenting with obstructive jaundice with a small tumour in the head of the pancreas. The pancreatic duct downstream from a polypoid filling defect (arrow) is normal, whilst the duct system upstream from the defect is dilated. The bile duct is obstructed at the same level.

Treatment

If the tumour is unresectable then biliary endo-prosthesis (stent) insertion offers the simplest approach to palliation. No randomized study comparing surgical biliary bypass with biliary stenting is available to assess postprocedure complications, morbidity and mortality. However, biliary stenting gives effective palliation, avoids the need for a laparotomy with its attendant risk of wound and chest infection and requires the patient to be in hospital for a shorter period.

Percutaneous transhepatic external biliary drainage is relatively easy to perform but procedure-related complications such as haemorrhage, biliary peritonitis, pleural collections and cholangitis occur in up to 15% of patients. Early metabolic complications due to sodium and water depletion can be troublesome and longer term complications of cholangitis and subcutaneous sepsis are frequent (Carrasco et al 1984). One of the major problems with percutaneous external drainage is the presence of a tube which some patients find distressing and may remove. Because of these complications percutaneous stent insertion was developed. 12 gauge French or larger stents can be inserted percutaneously through the liver substance and provide good palliation. However, the immediate complication rate may approach 20% (Mueller et al 1982) and late complications due to stent migration or obstruction can be difficult to treat. In addition the procedure may cause considerable distress to the patient and require general anaesthesia. Also the procedure may take some time and the radiologist can receive a significant radiation dose (Mendez et al 1984).

Endoscopic insertion of a 10 or 12 French gauge stent can be achieved in over 90% of cases (Huibregtse & Tytgat 1984) and has a lower immediate complication rate than the percutaneous route. In addition, endoscopy allows direct inspection of the duodenum and papilla. The main long term complication of endoscopic stenting is blocking of the endoprosthesis producing recurrent jaundice or cholangitis. The replacement of the stent is easier endoscopically than percutaneously. It is our policy to insert a biliary stent wherever possible at initial ERCP performed for diagnosis. If subsequent CT indicates that the lesion is in-operable then palliative drainage has already been performed.

Failure to insert a biliary stent endoscopically occurs in about 10% of patients with pancreatic carcinoma. In this situation, a combined percutaneous and endoscopic procedure may allow a stent to be positioned across the tumour.

In patients with inoperable pancreatic adenocarcinoma, particularly involving the body of the gland, severe pain can be controlled by coeliac axis blockade. This can be achieved using alcohol or phenol injected under CT guidance, and the procedure can be repeated if necessary.

Whilst the use of chemotherapy and radiotherapy have been ineffective in the past, regimens are developing which may be beneficial. As a number of the chemotherapeutic agents used are excreted in bile, biliary decompression is necessary prior to commencement of chemotherapy. Although no long term results are yet available we have experienced some promising results with this approach, even to the extent of being able to remove the biliary stent without recurrence of jaundice.

PANCREATIC ENDOCRINE TUMOURS

Introduction

Although islet cell tumours only comprise 3–4% of all pancreatic tumours they are of particular importance to the radiologist. Small tumours can cause disabling symptoms and, as the majority are benign and solitary, surgical removal is curative. The radiologist has two rôles, firstly to demonstrate the presence and site of the tumour, and secondly to demonstrate whether the tumour is solitary, multiple or metastatic.

Clinical features

Diagnosis of islet cell tumour is made clinically and biochemically. The characteristic features of individual cell tumours are indicated in Table 8.1. Although most present in middle age, some occur at the extremes of age. Insulinoma is the commonest islet cell tumour, comprising 80% of all tumours. Whilst pancreatic adenocarcinoma occurs most commonly in the head of the gland, islet

Table 8.1 Characteristic features of pancreatic endocrine tumours

Tumour	Age	Sex	Clinical feature	Site	Extra-pancreatic	Single/multiple	Histology	Comment
Insulinoma	Middle age mainly	M = F	Whipple's triad Hypoglycaemia Related symptoms corrected by i.v. dextrose	Head = body > tail	1% (99% within pancreas)	90% solitary	90% benign	Commonest sporadic tumour 75–80% of all endocrine tumours in pancreas 10% occur in MEN★
Gastrinoma	Middle age	M > F 65–35	Zollinger–Ellison syndrome Peptic ulcer Diarrhoea	Tail > body > head	15% outside pancreas In stomach or duodenum wall usually solitary	Most benign tumours are multiple	60% malignant	Commonest tumour in MEN but 75% are sporadic
Vipoma	Middle age	F > M 65–35	Pancreatic cholera Watery diarrhoea Achlorhydria Hypochlorrhydria Hypokalaemia	Tail > body > head	Mostly pancreatic, other tumours phaeo. Ganglioneuro-blastoma can secrete VIP★ especially in children	Rarely multiple	50% malignant	Rare in MEN
Somatostinoma	Middle age	M = F ?	Diabetes mellitus Weight loss Steatorrhoea Gastric hyposecretion Diarrhoea Gallstones	Tail = body > head	Rare	Solitary, often > 3 cm	90% malignant	Sporadic
Glucagonoma	Middle age	M = F	Hyperglycaemia Skin rash (necrotic migratory erythema)	Tail = body > head	Rare	Solitary	75% malignant	Sporadic
Non-Functioning	Middle age	M = F	Mass, compression bleeding	Tail = body > head	Rare	Solitary	Most benign	Can be sporadic or familial

★VIP = vasoactive intestinal polypeptide
★MEN = multiple endocrine neoplasia

cell tumours are more common in the body and the tail. Some tumours, particularly gastrinoma, occur outside the pancreas, usually in the gastric or duodenal wall but occasionally at other sites within the abdomen. Although most tumours are discrete neoplasms, hypersecretion of insulin, gastrin or vasoactive intestinal polypeptide (VIP) can occur because of islet cell hyperplasia in approximately 10% of cases. All islet cell tumours can occur in hereditary multiple endocrine neoplasia (MEN) syndromes. The commonest to do so is gastrinoma, although 70% of these tumours appear sporadically. 10% of insulinomas occur in hereditary endocrine neoplasia.

Histologically it is difficult to determine the activity of pancreatic islet cell tumours and the only reliable evidence of malignancy is the presence of metastatic disease.

Prognosis

The outlook for patients with islet cell tumours, even malignant lesions, is considerably better than for those with pancreatic adenocarcinomas. Nevertheless, prognosis does depend upon the histology and endocrine activity of the tumour and the ability of the surgeon to resect the lesion.

Treatment options

Treatment depends upon the extent and activity of the tumour. Benign solitary lesions such as insulinoma are best dealt with by surgical enucleation which is curative. Multiple or metastatic lesions are not usually resectable although surgical debulking may reduce symptoms. In the Zollinger–Ellison syndrome symptoms can usually be prevented by H_2 antagonists although where this fails total gastrectomy may be necessary. Medical therapy with somatostatin, streptozotocin or other chemotherapeutic agents may help. Embolization techniques may also be helpful in reducing the severity of symptoms, particularly in patients with liver metastases.

Radiology

Staging

The extent to which information regarding the

site, number and presence of metastases should be sought depends on tumour type. For example, insulinoma is usually benign, solitary and arises within the pancreas. Gastrinoma, on the other hand, is far more likely to be multiple, malignant and arise outside the pancreas. Initial radiological investigations should include a chest radiograph and upper abdominal ultrasound. Gunther et al (1985) and Gorman et al (1986) have demonstrated that meticulous preoperative ultrasound can demonstrate between 50 and 60% of pancreatic islet cell tumours. Detectable tumours are either hyper- or hypoechoic compared with the pancreatic parenchyma. Isoechoic lesions do occur and have been detected by the presence of a hypoechoic halo around the lesions. In addition to the primary tumour, regional lymphadenopathy and hepatic metastases should be detectable. When ultrasound is negative or gives insufficient information then pre- and postcontrast-enhanced dynamic incremental scanning is necessary. Pancreatic tumours 1 cm or more in diameter can be detected in this way (Fig. 8.6). The tumours are most commonly isodense on the non-contrast scan but enhance uniformly on the dynamic postcontrast images. Calcification, heterogeneity and cyst formation rarely occur. CT may also

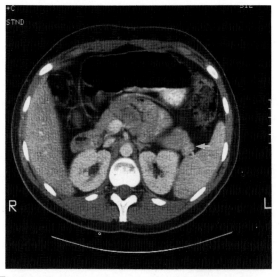

Fig. 8.6 Dynamic contrast-enhanced CT demonstrating a surgically proven 1.5 cm insulinoma at the tip of the tail of the pancreas (arrow).

demonstrate regional lymphadenopathy, hepatic metastases and the occasional extra-pancreatic tumour.

Superselective visceral angiography has always been a gold standard for the localization of islet cell tumour. Reported successful localization is variable but Dodds et al (1985) state that a detection rate of 70% should be expected and 100% specificity has been reported (Collen et al 1984). Lesions as small as 0.5 cm can be detected as opacified homogeneous lesions. The tumours are normally well circumscribed but only in larger lesions is there evidence of neovascularity or of early venous shunting. The visceral vessels are usually of normal calibre, except in vipoma where the vessels may be significantly dilated and in gastrinoma where the gastric vessels may be dilated. Involvement of the peripancreatic veins and visceral arteries can be demonstrated in both benign and malignant tumours (Bok et al 1984). Occasionally ultrasound, CT and angiography fail to detect the lesion. Whilst the surgeon would maintain that bimanual palpation of the pancreas at laparotomy will localize most tumours (Carter 1987), other radiological techniques may be useful. Selective venous sampling along the splenic vein, from the pancreatic veins and then along the portal vein may localize the lesion and although this is the most invasive investigation performed in these patients, it appears to be the most accurate (Gunther et al 1985).

Both endoscopic and intraoperative ultrasound allow the use of high frequency transducers for evaluation of the pancreas and it seems likely that these techniques may detect tumours which are otherwise radiologically undetectable and indeed some which are surgically undetectable (Gorman et al 1986).

Treatment

In patients with metastatic, hormonally active malignancy surgical debulking of the tumour may be beneficial. Similar benefit may be obtained by hepatic artery embolization (Allison 1982) where a reduction in tumour bulk as well as a reduction in hormonal output can be achieved.

Embolization techniques have the advantage that treatment can be repeated if necessary. By the adjunctive use of embolization with medical therapy, including chemotherapy, many years of relatively symptom-free life can be obtained.

LIVER

LIVER METASTASES

Metastases are the commonest form of hepatic malignancy and are a frequent feature of almost all malignant diseases particularly those arising from the gastrointestinal tract. Three clinical situations exist in practice:

1. Clinically evident liver metastases.
2. Metastases not evident clinically in patients being staged or reassessed for a primary tumour outside the liver.
3. Characterization of a focal lesion within the liver found incidentally in patients not known to have primary tumour. This last group will be discussed more fully in the section on primary malignant tumours of the liver.

Clinically evident metastases

Clinical features

Weight loss, anorexia, right upper quadrant discomfort and tenderness and a palpable epigastric mass, often with ascites, are features of hepatic metastases. Often this is an incidental feature of terminal illness and does not warrant investigation. However, occasionally treatment may be indicated because of a favourable histology or in order to manage a distressing symptom such as pain.

Prognosis

Gross metastases to the liver from primary tumours such as breast, lung, stomach and pancreas are associated with a poor prognosis and an anticipated survival time of only a few months from diagnosis. Some patients with slow growing metastases may have a better prognosis.

Treatment options

It is sometimes necessary to define the radiological extent of metastatic involvement of the liver. A simple descriptive classification fulfils most clinical requirements. Metastases should be described as solitary or multiple (Fig. 8.7), as involving the right, left or both lobes and as occupying more than or less than 50% of the liver volume.

Surgery. When metastases involve both lobes of the liver, surgery is not a treatment option. With less extensive disease surgery may be useful, particularly in colorectal carcinoma, and this will be discussed in the following sections.

Radiotherapy. Some patients with a poor prognosis and distressing symptoms due to tumour bulk may obtain symptomatic relief with palliative radiotherapy.

Chemotherapy. Most current information regarding chemotherapy of liver metastases relates to the management of colorectal carcinoma. The response rate to intravenous chemotherapy is disappointing with no evidence of complete responses and only 20% of patients experiencing any benefit. Complex regimens with multiple agents may improve responses but can also be expected to increase toxicity.

Hepatic arterial occlusion. The majority of patients treated by hepatic artery occlusion have had metastases from primary colorectal neoplasia; it is considered that the response rates are more favourable in these patients. Because the major blood supply to hepatic metastases is arterial whereas the predominant supply to the liver itself is portal, attempts have been made for a number of years to treat metastases by hepatic arterial ligation at surgery and more recently by transcatheter occlusion. Surgical ligation of the hepatic artery does not appear to prolong survival although it offers palliation of pain due to tumour bulk. Almersjo et al (1972) have concluded that even extensive dearterialization by ligation of the hepatic vessels does not significantly prolong survival.

Percutaneous transcatheter hepatic artery embolization has been reported using particulate matter such as Ivalon, Gelfoam, Sterispon or lyophilized dura mater, usually in combination with steel spring coils (Chuang & Wallace 1981, Powell-Tuck et al 1984). Most studies have demonstrated some benefit in terms of reduction of tumour size or improvement of symptoms but have not shown prolongation of survival. Allison (1988) concludes that embolization may have a marginal effect upon improving survival. In hepatocellular carcinoma Nakao et al (1986) and Kinoshita et al (1986) have demonstrated the benefit of regional portal vein occlusion in addition to hepatic arterial embolization. No reports of this method of treatment for hepatic metastases are available but it may be expected to offer some benefit to patients with localized metastases where segmental portal vein embolization can be undertaken.

Miller et al (1984) reported that EOE 13 (ethiodized oil emulsion) was taken up predominantly by tumour rather than by normal liver when injected intra-arterially. Others have used lipiodol together with chemotherapeutic agents administered as a slow infusion into the hepatic artery, and have demonstrated that targeting of the chemotherapy to malignant tissue can be achieved (Konno et al 1984). Kobayashi et al (1987) have demonstrated some response in terms of reduction in size of tumour using this technique.

Transcatheter management of hepatic metastases can result in complications. In addition to the procedural problems of arteriography and embolization, which include inadvertent embolization of extrahepatic structures, a postembolization syndrome with nausea, pain, fever and leukocytosis occurs in about 50% of patients.

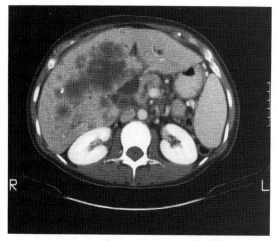

Fig. 8.7 Dynamic contrast-enhanced CT from a patient with primary pancreatic carcinoma demonstrating multiple liver metastases and peripancreatic lymph node involvement.

Other complications such as cholecystitis, gall bladder infarction, bile duct necrosis and stricture have been reported (Kuroda et al 1983, Makuuchi et al 1985, Clark & Gallant 1987). In addition, during chemotherapy jaundice can occur due to chemical hepatitis, which in one series (Anderson et al 1986) occurred in 54% of patients. Although intrahepatic gas formation following embolization appears to be common (Allison 1988), hepatic abscess is relatively uncommon.

Radiology

Diagnosis. Macroscopic liver metastases of the order of 1 cm diameter or larger can be demonstrated by hepatic scintigraphy, ultrasound, CT, angiography or magnetic resonance imaging (MRI). Each method of imaging is imperfect, having approximately 80% accuracy. Reported studies rank each imaging method differently, but in the UK ultrasound is generally performed first because of its ready availability and improved specificity over radio-isotope imaging using technetium-labelled colloid. CT scanning, particularly with dynamic incremental contrast enhancement is more accurate, as is MRI, but as access to MRI is limited contrast-enhanced CT is the current imaging gold standard (Ferrucci et al 1988). In most patients in whom liver metastases are clinically apparent, ultrasound or radio-isotope imaging supplemented if necessary by CT scanning will readily confirm the diagnosis. If histological confirmation is necessary image-guided biopsy is straightforward. If in the presence of clinically evident metastases radiological investigations are negative or equivocal then a simple Tru-cut biopsy of the right lobe of the liver may provide the answer. Occasionally more extensive investigation is required and this is discussed in the following sections.

Detection of liver metastases not clinically apparent

Occasionally in order to stage malignant disease arising outside the liver or in an attempt to improve long term survival in patients in whom metastases to the liver are common, it is necessary to attempt to detect metastases at an early stage.

Radiological staging in this way is of increasing importance in the management of a number of primary tumours including testicular, lung, breast, ovarian tumours and malignant melanoma. Most of the information currently available relates to the detection of metastases from colorectal neoplasms.

When a primary colorectal neoplasm has been excised the presence of hepatic metastases is the most important factor determining survival. Prognosis depends upon the number and extent, being worse for patients with multiple metastases involving both lobes of the liver and best for patients with a solitary metastasis. In this latter group a 5-year survival of 16% has been recorded without treatment (Wood 1984). In view of this some surgeons are keen to detect solitary lesions at an early stage and remove them, and this has been achieved with encouraging results (Taylor 1985). Clinical examination and biochemical investigations are unhelpful in detecting early disease and radiology is the mainstay of diagnosis.

Treatment options

Surgery. Although surgery is not a treatment option in patients with extensive metastases, resection or partial hepatectomy is an option in patients with lesions confined to one lobe. The primary colorectal carcinoma should have been completely excised and there should be no evidence of local recurrence or extrahepatic metastases. Preoperative investigation should demonstrate tumour confined to a single lobe without invasion of the portal vein or vena cava and there should be no evidence of cirrhosis (Taylor 1985). Although it is generally considered that metastases should be confined to one lobe, others (Iwatsuki et al 1986, Bradpiece et al 1987) have reported major hepatic resection for patients with tumour involving both lobes. After surgery the prognosis depends on the degree of liver resection undertaken. Localized wedge resection for solitary metastasis has a better prognosis than if extensive hepatic resection is performed for multiple lesions. This may be because undetectable micrometastases are present in the remaining liver and at other sites. The clear margin of liver removed adjacent to the metastasis also effects prognosis, being best if this is at least 2 cm in diameter (Rajpal et al 1982).

Fortner et al (1984) have established that only about 5% of patients with colorectal cancer could possibly benefit from liver resection and Taylor (1985) estimates that fewer than 20% of patients with hepatic metastases are suitable for surgery. In patients with solitary lesions or lesions confined to one lobe surgery appears to be the most effective option, but where disease is more extensive then radiotherapy, chemotherapy or hepatic arterial occlusion as described above are options worth considering.

Radiology

Whilst ultrasound and CT are the principal techniques used to identify liver metastases it is difficult to discover from published series how accurate either technique is in detecting a solitary metastasis. Unfortunately a significant number of metastases are not detected by ultrasound, CT or angiography (Lundstedt et al 1987). Attempts have been made to increase the sensitivity of ultrasound examination using contrast agents such as prefluoro chemicals (Mattrey et al 1987) or carbon dioxide microbubbles (Matsuda & Yabuuchi 1986). It seems likely that CT arteriography using water-soluble contrast medium (Stack et al 1984) and more particularly lipiodol (Matsui et al 1987) can improve the sensitivity of CT in the detection of metastases but this is an invasive procedure and therefore not suitable for routine staging. Reports of delayed hepatic CT scanning some 4–6 hours after intravenous injection of iodine indicate that it may be useful in detecting and defining metastases if initial plain and contrast-enhanced scans are equivocal or if better assessment of size is necessary (Bernadino et al 1986). Leveson et al (1985) using hepatic flow scintigraphy have concluded that this technique is capable of detecting occult metastases which lead to a derangement of hepatic arterial and portal venous supply. However, it has yet to be shown that improved survival is possible when treatment is given on the basis of an abnormal hepatic perfusion index. Reinig et al (1987) have suggested that MRI with specifically chosen pulse sequences compares favourably with EOE 13-enhanced CT and propose that MRI should be the investigation of choice for the identification of early liver metastases. Recently Stark et al (1988) have proposed that MRI images after an intravenous injection of super-paramagnetic ferrite particles allow detection of liver metastases as small as 3 mm in diameter.

Carcinoembryonic antigen (CEA) is a tumour-associated antigen secreted in some patients with colorectal carcinoma. The detection of rising CEA levels following treatment of the primary tumour usually indicates local recurrence or metastatic disease or both, but it is not yet clear whether or not treatment based upon monitoring of the serum CEA allows prolongation of survival. However, monoclonal and polyclonal antibodies have been raised to CEA and labelled with iodine-131 or indium-111 to allow gamma camera imaging (Begent et al 1982). At present the technique is relatively insensitive but it will continue to develop and no doubt improve. The possibility also exists that targeted radiotherapy using monoclonal antibodies can be undertaken in the management of colorectal metastases.

MALIGNANT TUMOURS OF THE LIVER

The discovery of a single liver lesion can cause diagnostic problems. When on ultrasound examination the lesion is cystic the problem is relatively simple, further management being guided by the clinician's suspicions of the presence of a simple cyst, a pyogenic abscess or a hydatid cyst. Benign and malignant hepatic neoplasms are rarely cystic. When the focal liver lesion is solid then a significant problem arises. Should the lesion be biopsied? Thompson et al (1985) have pointed out the risks of biopsy, particularly haemorrhage, and the fact that biopsy at an early stage does not always make a significant difference to management. These authors devised an algorithm for the investigation of the focal liver lesion based on ultrasound, CT, angiography, inferior vena cavography and laparoscopy in an attempt to avoid early and possibly risky biopsy of incidental lesions, particularly haemangiomas. However, Thompson et al and others (Reading et al 1988) also point out that the classical features of hepatic haemangiomas are not always present, particularly in larger lesions, and the temptation therefore is to biopsy when the diagnosis is uncertain in an attempt to avoid overlooking malignant lesions at a stage where cure is possible. This is obviously a complex clinical problem where it is difficult to lay down firm guidelines for investigation. The management of focal liver disease should be guided by clinical factors such as the age of the patient and the presenting clinical features as well as the radiological features. A young woman who is not taking oral contraceptives who has an incidentally discovered solitary well-defined echodense lesion can be assumed to have a hepatic haemangioma. The lesion should not change in appearance on follow-up investigation (Reading et al 1988). However, a middle-aged or elderly patient with a lesion of similar radiological appearances is not a candidate for such expectant management as the risks of overlooking primary or secondary hepatic malignancy are significantly greater.

Primary liver neoplasms are usually hepatocellular carcinoma and less commonly angiosarcoma, fibrosarcoma and, in children, hepatoblastoma. With the exception of hepatoblastoma the clinical features and management of rare tumours are similar to those for hepatocellular carcinoma.

There is considerable geographical variation in incidence of the hepatocellular carcinoma. In the UK and USA the incidence is low whilst it is considerably higher in black Africans, particularly from Mozambique, and in the Chinese. It most commonly occurs in patients with chronic liver disease, particularly cirrhosis, or in those who are chronic hepatitis B carriers. Hepatitis B infection is thought to account for the wide geographical variation in the incidence of the tumour. Hepatocellular carcinoma occurs approximately three times more frequently in males than in females, probably a reflection of hepatitis B infection and chronic liver disease. In areas where the tumour is common it tends to present at around 40 years of age, whereas in areas where the tumour is infrequent the peak incidence is in much older patients. Whilst the vast majority of hepatocellular carcinomas occur in relation to chronic hepatitis B infection or cirrhosis, other aetiological factors have also been implicated. These include aflatoxin, a fungal toxin from aspergillus flavus, iron accumulation in the liver, particularly in primary haemochromatosis, chronic venous obstruction, androgens, oestrogens and vinylchloride. Anabolic steroids, initially used in the management of aplastic anaemia but more recently used as a performance-enhancing agent by athletes, have also been implicated. Although the risk of hepatic adenomas developing in women on oral contraceptives is well recognized, there does appear to be a small but definite risk of hepatocellular carcinoma with these agents. Vinylchloride monomer is implicated in the development of angiosarcoma of the liver but there also appears to be an increased risk of hepatocellular carcinoma in exposed individuals.

Clinical features

In patients with established chronic liver disease the development of hepatocellular carcinoma is usually associated with the deterioration in biochemical liver function or the appearance of fever, ascites or abdominal discomfort. In patients without cirrhosis the clinical presentation is usually with upper abdominal pain, a palpable mass, weight loss, anorexia and malaise. The serum alpha fetoprotein is significantly elevated in the majority of patients, although less commonly in the UK and USA than in African patients. Alpha fetoprotein levels do not correlate with the extent of disease. However, in patients with chronic liver disease repeated estimation of serum alpha fetoprotein may indicate the development of hepatocellular carcinoma or its recurrence after treatment.

Prognosis

The prognosis in hepatocellular carcinoma depends upon a number of factors:

1. The histological type of tumour
2. Multiplicity of tumours
3. Extent of liver involvement
4. Presence of cirrhosis
5. Venous involvement
6. Bile duct involvement
7. Metastases.

Each of the factors listed above has an effect on the surgeon's ability to remove the whole of the tumour which offers the only hope of cure.

From a practical point of view hepatocellular

carcinoma is divided into three macroscopic types; nodular, massive and diffuse. The nodular type is the most common, usually occurs in cirrhosis and tends to be multifocal although the lesions may be confined to one lobe of the liver. The massive type is slightly less common and tends to be a solitary, large lesion, usually in the right lobe of the liver although there may be a number of small tumour nodules immediately adjacent to the main neoplasm. The massive type occurs in patients without cirrhosis and in younger patients and is therefore the most common type reported in surgical series. The diffuse type occurs in the cirrhotic liver and is usually widely infiltrative and may only be detectable on liver biopsy. Two other types are worthy of mention; a clear cell hepatocellular carcinoma, which may be associated with a better prognosis, and the fibrolamellar hepatocellular carcinoma which tends to occur in younger patients, particularly women, and occasionally contains calcification. This type occurs particularly in the left lobe and is said to have a better prognosis than other hepatocellular carcinomas (Fig. 8.8).

The presence of cirrhosis affects prognosis not only because of its association with particular types of hepatocellular carcinoma but also because of the effects of limited hepatic function on the surgeon's ability to resect the liver. When there is no cir-

rhosis the minimal residual functioning hepatic mass necessary to maintain liver function after surgery is approximately 25–30% but in patients with cirrhosis the necessary residual liver mass is much greater. The extent of safe resection will obviously vary between individuals depending upon the state of the functioning liver. However, removal of half of the liver, particularly a right hepatectomy, is associated with a significant risk of postoperative liver failure, a complication which is usually fatal (Mimura et al 1986).

Venous involvement in hepatocellular carcinoma is common and is evident at autopsy in the portal vein in approximately 60% and in the hepatic vein in approximately 25% of patients. Intrahepatic portal venous spread has been demonstrated in 20% of patients undergoing surgery (Ong 1977). Involvement of the inferior vena cava and right atrium occur, but less commonly. Bile duct involvement leading to obstructive jaundice is usually a late feature (Lee et al 1984).

Local lymphadenopathy is relatively uncommon but pulmonary metastases are more frequent.

The most favourable situation with regard to curative surgery is when a solitary massive hepatocellular carcinoma occurs in a non-cirrhotic patient without involvement of major venous structures and confined to one lobe (Fig. 8.9). As the majority of hepatocellular carcinomas occur in cirrhotic patients only a minority are resectable, and overall fewer than 30% of patients with hepatocellular carcinoma undergo successful resection. With fibrolamellar hepatomas the situation is slightly different and Nagorney et al (1985) have demonstrated that 75% can be resected. Data on long term survival after hepatic resection is difficult to obtain but 5-year survival following resection in patients without cirrhosis is approximately 25%.

Treatment options

Surgical resection offers the only hope of cure for the patient with hepatocellular carcinoma and the factors which govern surgical resectability are discussed in the previous sections. For patients in whom surgery is not possible or feasible the outlook is very poor; fewer than 10% of patients can be expected to survive one year from initial

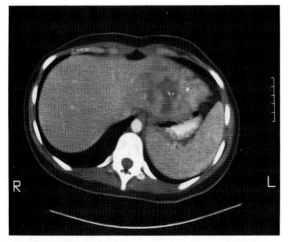

Fig. 8.8 Fibrolamellar hepatocellular carcinoma occurring in the left lobe of the liver in a young woman. Note the calcification within the lesion.

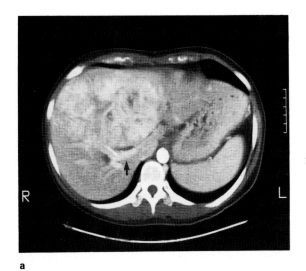 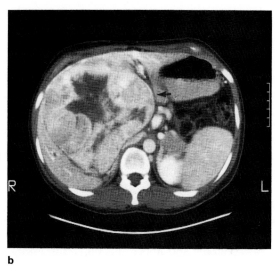

a   b

Fig. 8.9 (a) Large hepatocellular carcinoma in hepatitis B positive Chinese patient. The tumour involves the anterior segment of the right lobe of the liver, evidenced by its close proximity to the posteriorly displaced right branch of the portal vein (arrow). (b) A section 5 cm below demonstrates that this large tumour also involves the medial segment of the left lobe, where it is seen to abut the falciform ligament (arrow).

presentation. Numerous non-operative methods of treatment have been attempted including hepatic artery ligation with and without systemic or local chemotherapy, portal vein ligation, embolization and radiotherapy but from reported studies it seems unlikely that any of these therapeutic modalities offers an improvement in survival (Lai et al 1986). However, for the palliation of symptoms due to tumour mass and for control of bleeding hepatic artery embolization (Chuang & Wallace 1981) may be useful and can be repeated if necessary.

Radiology

Diagnosis and staging

There are three principal questions asked of the radiologist in the management of hepatocellular carcinoma: firstly, in the patient clinically suspected of having hepatocellular carcinoma, how can the diagnosis best be confirmed? Secondly, in the patient known to have hepatocellular carcinoma how can the extent of the disease be best demonstrated preoperatively? Thirdly, in patients who are at risk of developing hepatocellular carcinoma, can regular radiological screening con-

tribute to early diagnosis and treatment with improved survival?

1. Diagnosis of hepatoma when clinically suspected. Generally the diagnosis of clinically suspected hepatoma by imaging methods is straightforward. Ultrasound, CT, hepatic scintigraphy and MRI are probably equal in their ability to demonstrate an abnormality. A range of sensitivity and specificity is reported for each imaging modality but a sensitivity of about 80% can be expected. Ultrasound is probably the best initial method: lesions not evident with one method of imaging may be apparent with another and therefore in the situation where a tumour is suspected ultrasound should be followed by CT with contrast enhancement. The degree of sensitivity of each modality depends upon the degree of sophistication employed in that examination. For instance, dynamic contrast-enhanced CT will be more sensitive than plain CT, and CT with hepatic artery infusion with water-soluble contrast or with lipid contrast will be more sensitive than standard contrast-enhanced CT. SPECT (single photon emission computed tomography) will be more sensitive than simple gamma camera isotope imaging. Of course, the demonstration of an abnormality on imaging is not histologically specific and biopsy is necessary to prove the presence of hepatocellular carcinoma. Histological interpretation of biopsy specimens can be difficult but a combination of imaging methods with biopsy in the relevant clinical setting can be expected to give a positive diagnosis in the majority of patients.

2. Staging of patients with proven hepatocellular carcinoma. Hepatocellular carcinoma spreads locally, compressing and invading adjacent liver. There may be satellite nodules in the massive type or multiple tumours in the nodular type. Venous involvement, particularly of the hepatic and portal veins, is common. Local lymphadenopathy is rare but widespread metastases can occur. Initial investigations should include a chest radiograph and upper abdominal ultrasound in an attempt to evaluate these factors. If ultrasound gives insufficient information then CT with contrast should be the next step and has been shown to be superior to ultrasound in the evaluation of venous involvement (Mathieu et al 1988) (Fig. 8.10). Contrast CT can also demonstrate lymphadenopathy in hepatocellular carcinoma (Araki et al 1988) and CT using intra-arterial lipiodol has been shown to be superior to arteriography in the demonstration of multifocal tumour (Hayashi et al 1987) although this latter study also demonstrated that intraoperative ultrasound is sup-

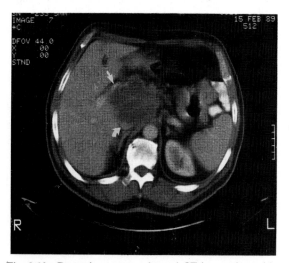

Fig. 8.10 Dynamic contrast-enhanced CT in a patient with hepatocellular carcinoma involving the caudate lobe, demonstrating compression and displacement of a portal vein (straight arrow) and the inferior vena cava (curved arrow).

erior to both CT and arteriography. It appears that the more diligent and sophisticated the method of searching for spread of neoplasm the more likely it is to be found. The extent of preoperative radiological investigations will be influenced by factors such as the age of the patient, presence or absence of chronic liver disease and the availability of radiological expertise. Our own practice is to rely on clinical features, biochemical findings and liver biopsy to determine the presence of chronic liver disease. Chest radiography, ultrasound and dynamic contrast-enhanced CT evaluate the extent of the lesion, and where the tumour appears resectable laparotomy is performed. The decision about whether to operate for hepatocellular carcinoma in patients with cirrhosis is difficult. When preoperative investigation indicates that the tumour can be removed by wedge resection then this is likely to be associated with low postoperative mortality and little risk of liver failure as adequate functioning residual liver will remain. Where more extensive hepatic resection is necessary, Mimura et al (1986) has demonstrated that assessment of hepatic blood flow using gold colloid correlates well with the risk of postoperative liver failure and death.

3. Can hepatocellular carcinoma be detected in high risk patients? As a group of patients likely to develop hepatocellular carcinoma can be identified (hepatitis B carriers and cirrhotics) and as the majority of hepatocellular carcinomas are not resectable at presentation, it is tempting to develop a screening programme for early tumour detection when surgery may be curative. Serum alpha fetoprotein is a biochemical marker for hepatocellular carcinoma but is not elevated in all patients, particularly in Europe and the USA. For a screening test to be appropriate it has to be minimally invasive and safe. Ultrasound, scintigraphy, CT and MRI are therefore probably appropriate screening methods but angiography is not acceptable. Ultrasound has been most widely used and the results of early studies (Sheu et al 1985, Kanematsu et al 1985, Tanaka et al 1986a) are promising. Ultrasound can be complemented by fine needle aspiration biopsy as in one study (Tanaka et al 1986b) and has been reported as being more accurate than scintigraphy, CT or angiography. Kudo et al (1986) have confirmed ultrasound as being more accurate than scintigraphy or CT in the detection of tumours of less than 5 cm in diameter whilst others (Hosoki et al 1984, Matsui et al 1985) propose that contrast-enhanced CT is better. MRI also has its proponents (Ebara et al 1986). However, none of the reported studies has addressed the two most important problems in any screening programme: firstly, the incidence of false positive findings and secondly the effect of treatment of small hepatocellular carcinoma on survival.

Finally worthy of particular mention is the histological and apparently clinical entity of fibrolamellar hepatocellular carcinoma. This tumour, usually large in size at presentation, occurs most commonly in adolescent and young adult female patients. The serum alpha fetoprotein is always normal and there are none of the risk factors normally present in other histological types. Patients present with features typical of hepatocellular carcinoma – anorexia, upper abdominal discomfort, weight loss, malaise and a palpable upper abdominal mass. Haemorrhage into the tumour is an occasional mode of presentation. On plain radiographs many of these tumours are seen to contain calcification and this is also apparent in an additional number on CT. Ultrasound normally demonstrates the heterogeneous, fairly well-defined lesion. CT similarly demonstrates a well-defined lesion with poor or little enhancement. Venous involvement is common as in other types of hepatocellular carcinoma. Successful resection and improved prognosis is reported with this neoplasm, which may be due in part to the age of the patients and the presence of an otherwise normal liver (Friedman et al 1985, Adam et al 1986, Francis et al 1986).

Treatment

Lai et al (1986) in a controlled study compared surgical hepatic dearterialization; hepatic artery ligation and cannulation for infusion chemotherapy; hepatic artery ligation and portal vein infusion chemotherapy; and external radiation in the management of unresectable hepatocellular carcinomas and concluded that none of these treatments offered any benefit in terms of survival and symptomatic palliation.

Despite the negative results of this controlled study, others believe that radiological methods are of help in the management of specific problems in hepatocellular carcinoma. Yamada et al (1983) have evaluated the rôle of hepatic artery embolization, repeated if necessary, in 120 patients with unresectable hepatocellular carcinoma and found a cumulative 1-year survival of 44% with demonstrable reduction in tumour vessels at arteriography and a reduction in tumour bulk. Nakao et al (1987) report the successful management of obstructive jaundice in hepatocellular carcinoma with hepatic artery embolization and Kobayashi et al (1987) have reported a 55% survival rate at one year in patients with advanced hepatocellular carcinoma after treatment with hepatic arterial injection of lipiodol combined with adriamycin or mitomycin C. Kinoshita et al (1986) have used preoperative segmental portal vein embolization in addition to hepatic artery embolization and believe that this technique is useful in reducing spread of the tumour within the liver and as an adjunct to curative surgery. A number of authors (Livraghi et al 1986, Shiina et al 1987, Sheu et al 1987, Livraghi et al 1988) have reported the preliminary results of percutaneous alcohol injection of liver neoplasms and most conclude that this may be a valuable technique which causes tumour necrosis and a reduction in the vascularity of hepatocellular carcinoma. It seems likely that further development of techniques such as hepatic artery and portal vein embolization, targeting of chemotherapy and alcohol injection will occur but refinement of techniques and their indications together with long term studies will be necessary before the place of each of these techniques in the management of hepatocellular carcinoma can be ascertained.

REFERENCES

Adam A, Gibson R N, Soreide O, Hemingway A P, Carr D H, Blumgart L H, Allison D J 1986 The radiology of fibrolamellar hepatoma. Clinical Radiology 37: 355–358

Alexander F, Rossi R L, O'Bryan M, Khettriy U, Braasch J W, Watkins E 1984 Biliary carcinoma: a review of 109 cases. American Journal of Surgery 147: 503–509

Allison D J 1982 The non-surgical management of metastatic endocrine tumours to the liver. In: Wilkins R A, Viamonte M (eds) Interventional radiology. Blackwell Scientific, Oxford, ch 14, pp 191–208

Allison D J 1988 Embolisation of liver tumours. In: Blumgart L H (ed) Surgery of the liver and biliary tract. Churchill Livingstone, Edinburgh, ch 94

Almersjo O, Bengmark S, Rudenstam C M, Hafstrom L O, Nilsson L A V 1972 Evaluation of hepatic dearterialization in primary and secondary cancer of the liver. American Journal of Surgery 124: 5–9

Anderson S D, Holley H C, Berland L L, Van Dyke J A, Stanley R J 1986 Causes of jaundice during hepatic artery infusion chemotherapy Radiology 161: 439–442

Araki T, Hihara T, Karikomi M, Kachi K, Uchiyama G 1988 Hepatocellular carcinoma: metastatic abdominal lymph nodes identified by computed tomography. Gastrointestinal Radiology 13: 247–252

Beazley R M, Hadjis N, Benjamin I S, Blumgart L H 1984 Clinicopathological aspects of high bile duct cancer, experience with resection and bypass surgical treatments. Annals of Surgery 199: 623–626

Begent R H J, Keep P A, Green A J et al 1982 Liposomally entrapped second antibody improves tumour imaging with radiolabelled (first) antitumour antibody. Lancet 2: 739–742

Benjamin I S, Blumgart L H 1979 Biliary bypass and reconstruction. In: Wright R, Alberti K G, Karran S, Millward-Sadler G D T (eds) Liver and biliary disease: pathophysiology, diagnosis, management. Sanders, London, ch 54

Bergdahl L 1980 Gallbladder carcinoma first diagnosed at microscopic examination of gallbladders removed for presumed benign disease. Annals of Surgery 191: 19–22

Bernardino M E, Erwin B C, Steinberg H V, Baumgartner B R, Torpes W E, Gedgaudas-McClees R U 1986 Delayed hepatic CT scanning: increased confidence and improved detection of hepatic metastases. Radiology 159: 71–74

Bismuth H, Malt R 1979 Carcinoma of the biliary tract. New England Journal of Medicine 301: 704–706

Bismuth H, Houissin D, Castaing D 1982 Major and minor segmentectomies 'reglees' in liver surgery. World Journal of Surgery 6: 10–24

Blumgart L H, Hadjis N S, Benjamin I S, Beazley R M 1984 Surgical approaches to cholangiocarcinoma at confluence of hepatic ducts. Lancet 1: 66–70

Blumgart L H, Bengmark S, Launois B 1986 Liver resection in high bile duct tumours. In: Bengmark S, Blumgart L H (eds) Liver surgery, Clinical Surgery International 12. Churchill Livingstone, Edinburgh

Bok E L, Cho K J, Williams D M, Brady T M, Weiss C A, Forrest M E 1984 Venous involvement in islet cell tumours of the pancreas. American Journal of Roentgenology 142: 319–322

Braasch J W 1988 Periampullary and pancreatic cancer. In: Blumgart L H (ed) Surgery of the liver and biliary tract. Churchill Livingstone, Edinburgh, ch 66

Bradpiece H A, Benjamin I S, Halevy A, Blumgart L H 1987 Major hepatic resection for colorectal liver metastases. British Journal of Surgery 74: 324–326

Carrasco C H, Zornoza J, Bechtel W J 1984 Malignant biliary obstruction: complications of percutaneous biliary drainage. Radiology 152: 343–346

Carter D C 1987 Pancreatic endocrine tumours. British Medical Journal 294: 593-594

Chuang V P, Wallace S 1981 Arterial infusion and occlusion in cancer patients. Seminars in Roentgenology 16: 13–25

Clark R A, Gallant T E 1987 Bile duct strictures associated with hepatic arterial infusion chemotherapy. Gastrointestinal Radiology 12: 148–151

Collen M J, Doppman J L, Krudy A G et al 1984 Assessment of the ability of angiography to localize gastrinoma in patients with Zollinger–Ellison syndrome. Gastroenterology 86: 1051

Dalla Palma L, Rizzatto G, Pozzi-Mucelli R S, Bazzocchi M 1980 Grey scale ultrasonography in the evaluation of carcinoma of the gallbladder. British Journal of Radiology 53: 662–667

Dodds W J, Wilson S D, Thorsen M K, Stewart E T, Lawson T L, Foley W D 1985 MEN 1 syndrome and islet cell lesions of the pancreas. Seminars in Roentgenology 20: 17–63

Ebara M, Ohto M, Wanatabe Y et al 1986 Diagnosis of small hepatocellular carcinoma: Correlation of MR imaging and tumour histologic studies. Radiology 159: 371–378

Ferrucci J T, Freeny P C, Stark D D et al 1988. Advances in hepatobiliary radiology. Radiology 168: 319–338

Fletcher M S, Dawson J L, Wheeler P G, Brinkley D, Nunnerley H, Williams R 1981 Treatment of high bile duct carcinoma by internal radiotherapy with iridium-192 wire. Lancet 2: 172–174

Fortner J G, Silva J S, Golbey R B, Cox E B, MacLean B J 1984 Multivariate analysis of a personal series of 247 consecutive patients with liver metastases from colorectal cancer: 1. Treatment by hepatic resection. Annals of Surgery 199: 306–316

Francis I R, Agha F P, Thompson N W, Keren D F 1986 Fibrolamellar hepatocarcinoma: Clinical radiologic and pathologic features. Gastrointestinal Radiology 11: 67–72

Freeny P C, Marks W M, Ryan J A, Traverso L W 1988 Pancreatic ductal adenocarcinoma: diagnosis and staging with dynamic CT. Radiology 166: 125–133

Friedman A C, Lichtenstein J E, Goodman Z, Fishman E K, Siegelman S S, Dachman A H 1985 Fibrolamellar hepatocellular carcinoma. Radiology 157: 583–587

Garra B S, Shawker T H, Doppman J L, Sindelar W F 1987 Comparison of angiography and ultrasound in the evaluation of the portal venous system in pancreatic carcinoma. Journal of Clinical Ultrasound 15: 83–93

Gorman B, Charboneau J W, James E M et al 1986 Benign pancreatic insulinoma: Pre-operative and intra-operative sonographic localization. American Journal of Roentgenology 147: 929–934

Gunther R W, Klose K J, Ruckert K, Beyer J, Kuhn F P, Klotter H J 1985 Localization of small islet cell tumours. Pre-operative and intra-operative ultrasound. Computed tomography, arteriography, digital subtraction angiography and pancreatic venous sampling. Gastrointestinal Radiology 10: 145–152

Hadjis N S, Collier N A, Blumgart L H 1985 Malignant masquerade at the hilium of the liver. British Journal of Surgery 72: 659–661

Hall-Craggs M A, Lees W R 1986 Fine-needle aspiration biopsy: pancreatic and biliary tumours. American Journal of Roentgenology 147: 399–402

Hatfield A R W, Terblanche J, Fataar S et al 1982 Preoperative external biliary drainage in obstructive jaundice. Lancet 2: 896–899

Hayashi N, Yamamoto K, Tamaki N et al 1987 Metastatic nodules of hepatocellular carcinoma; detection with angiography, CT and US. Radiology 165: 61–63

Hosoki T, Toyonaga Y, Araki Y, Mori S 1984 Dynamic computed tomography of isodense hepatocellular carcinoma. Journal of Computer Assisted Tomography 8: 263–268

Huibregtse K, Tytgat G W T 1984 Endoscopic placement of biliary prosthesis. In: Salmon P (ed) Advances in gastrointestinal endoscopy vol 1. Chapman & Hall, London, pp 219–231

Iwatsuki S, Esquivel C O, Gordon R D, Starzl T E 1986 Liver resection for metastatic colorectal cancer. Surgery 100: 804–810

Jafri S Z H, Aisen A M, Glazer G M, Weiss C A 1984 Comparison of CT and angiography in assessing resectability of pancreatic carcinoma. American Journal of Roentgenology 142: 525–529

Jenkins J P R, Braganza J M, Hickey D S, Isherwood I, Machin M 1987 Quantitative tissue characterisation in pancreatic disease using magnetic resonance imaging. British Journal of Radiology 60: 333–341

Jones B A, Langer B, Taylor B R, Girotti M 1985 Periampullary tumours: which ones should be resected? American Journal of Surgery 149: 46–51

Kanematsu T, Sonoda T, Takenaka K, Matsumata T, Sugimachi K, Inokuchi K 1985 The value of ultrasound in the diagnosis and treatment of small hepatocellular carcinoma. British Journal of Surgery 72: 23–25

Kinoshita H, Sakai K, Hirohashi K, Igawa S, Yamasaki O, Kubo S 1986 Preoperative portal vein embolisation for hepatocellular carcinoma. World Journal of Surgery 10: 803–808

Knox R A, Kingston R D 1986 Carcinoma of the ampulla of Vater. British Journal of Surgery 73: 72–73

Kobayashi H, Inoue H, Shimada J, Yano T, Maeda T, Oyama T, Shinohara S 1987 Intra-arterial infection of adriamycin/mitomycin C lipiodol suspension in liver metastases. Acta Radiologica 28: 275–280

Konno T, Meada H, Iwai K, Maki S, Tashiro S, Uchida M, Migauchi Y 1984 Selective targeting of anti-cancer drug and simultaneous image enhancement of solid tumours by arterially administered lipid contrast medium. Cancer 54: 2367–2374

Kudo M, Hirasa M, Takakuwa H et al 1986 Small hepatocellular carcinomas in chronic liver disease: Detection with SPECT. Radiology 159: 697–703

Kuroda C, Iwasaki M, Tanaka T et al 1983 Gallbladder infarction following hepatic transcatheter arterial embolisation. Radiology 149: 85–89

Lai E C S, Choi T K, Tong S W, Ong G B, Wong J 1986 Treatment of unresectable hepatocellular carcinoma: Results of a randomised controlled trial. World Journal of Surgery 10: 501–509

Lee N W, Wong K P, Siu K F, Wong J 1984 Cholangiography in hepatocellular carcinoma with obstructive jaundice. Clinical Radiology 35: 119–123

Lerut J P, Gianello P R, Otte J B, Kestens P J 1984 Pancreaticoduodenal resection – surgical experience and evaluation of risk factors in 103 patients. Annals of Surgery 199: 432–437

Leveson S H, Wiggins P A, Giles G R, Parkin A, Robinson P J 1985 Deranged liver blood flow patterns in the detection of liver metastases. British Journal of Surgery 72: 128–130

Livraghi T, Festi D, Monti F, Salmi A, Vettori C 1986 US-guided percutaneous alcohol injection of small hepatic and abdominal tumours. Radiology 161: 309–312

Livraghi T, Salmi A, Bolondi L, Marin G, Arienti V, Monti F, Vettori C 1988 Small hepatocellular carcinoma: percutaneous alcohol injection – results in 23 patients. Radiology 168: 313–317

Lundstedt C, Ekberg H, Lunderquist A, Tranberg K G 1987 Site and number of liver tumours recorded at angiography and computed tomography compared with the findings at laparotomy and of resected liver specimens. Acta Radiologica 28: 153–160

Luning M, Kursawe R, Schopke W, Lorenz D, Menzel A, Hoppe E, Meyer R 1985 CT guided percutaneous fine-needle biopsy of the pancreas. European Journal of Radiology 5: 104–108

Makuuchi M, Sukigara M, Mori T et al 1985 Bile duct necrosis: complication of transcatheter hepatic arterial embolization. Radiology 156: 331–334

Martin D F 1988 Catheter and wire guided endoscope exchange for biliary stents. Lancet 2: 542–543

Martin D F, Tweedle D E F 1984 The value of pre-cut papillotomy at ERCP and endoscopic sphincterotomy. Gut 25: A549

Martin D F, Tweedle D E F 1987 Endoscopic management of common duct stones without cholecystectomy. British Journal of Surgery 74: 209–211

Mathieu D, Guinet C, Bouklia-Hassane A, Vasile N 1988 Hepatic vein involvement in hepatocellular carcinoma. Gastrointestinal Radiology 13: 55–60

Matsuda Y, Yabuchi I 1986 Hepatic tumours: US contrast enhancement with CO_2 microbubbles. Radiology 161: 701–705

Matsui O, Takashima T, Kadoya M et al 1985 Dynamic computed tomography during arterial portography: the most sensitive examination for small hepatocellular carcinoma. Journal of Computer Assisted Tomography 9: 19–24

Matsui O, Takashima T, Kadoya M et al 1987 Liver metastases from colorectal cancers: Detection with CT during arterial portography. Radiology 165: 65–69

Mattrey R F, Strich G, Shelton R E et al 1987 Perfluorochemicals as US contrast agents for tumour imaging and hepatosplenography: preliminary clinical results. Radiology 163: 339–343

Mendez G, Russell E, LePage J R, Guerra J J, Posniak R A, Trefler M 1984 Abandonment of endoprosthetic drainage technique in malignant biliary obstruction. American Journal of Roentgenology 143: 617–622

Miller D L, Schneider P D, Willis M, Vermess M, Doppman J L 1984 Intraarterial administration of EOE-13 for the CT evaluation of hepatic artery infusion chemotherapy. Journal of Computer Assisted Tomography 8: 332–334

Mimura H, Takakura N, Opino Y et al 1986 Determination of the extent of feasible hepatic resection from hepatic blood flow. World Journal of Surgery 10: 302–310

Moossa A R, Lavelle-Jones M 1988 Whipple pancreaticoduodenumectomy. In: Blumgart L H (ed) Surgery of the liver and biliary tract. Churchill Livingstone, Edinburgh, ch 67

Mueller P R, Van Sonnenberg E, Ferrucci J T 1982 Percutaneous biliary drainage; Technical and catheter-related problems in 200 procedures. American Journal of Roentgenology 138: 17–23

Nagorney D M, Adson M A, Weiland L H, Knight C D, Smalley S R, Zinsmeister A R 1985 Fibrolamellar hepatoma. American Journal of Surgery 149: 113

Nakao N, Miura K, Takahashi H, Ohinishi M, Miura T, Okamoto E, Ishikawa Y 1986 Hepatocellular carcinoma: Combined hepatic, arterial and portal venous embolisation. Radiology 161: 303–307

Nakao N, Ishikura R, Miura T, Takahashi H 1987 Transcatheter arterial embolisation in hepatoma complicated with obstructive jaundice. Cardiovascular and Interventional Radiology 10: 40–42

Nevin J E, Moran T J, Kay S, King R 1976 Carcinoma of the gallbladder. Cancer 37: 141–148

Nix G A J J, Schmitz P I M, Wilson J H P, Van Blankenstein M, Groeneveld C F M, Hofwijk R 1984 Carcinoma of the head of the pancreas: Therapeutic implications of endoscopic retrograde cholangiopancreatography findings. Gastroenterology 87: 37–43

Ogoshi K, Niwa M 1977 The diagnostic evaluation of ERCP in pancreatic and biliary carcinoma. Gastroenterologia Japonica 12: 218–223

Ong G B 1977 Techniques and therapies for primary and metastatic liver cancer. In: Hickey R C (ed) Current problems in cancer, 2. Year Book, Chicago, pp 1–48

Powell-Tuck J, McIvor J, Reynolds K W, Murray-Lyon I M 1984 Prediction of early death after therapeutic hepatic arterial embolisation. British Medical Journal 288: 1257–1259

Rajpal S, Dasmahapatra K S, Ledesma E J, Nittelman A 1982 Extensive resections of isolated metastasis from carcinoma of the colon and rectum. Surgery, Gynecology and Obstetrics 155: 813–816

Reading N G, Forbes A, Nunnerley H B, Williams R 1988 Hepatic haemangioma: A critical review of diagnosis and management. Quarterly Journal of Medicine 67: 431–445

Reinig J W, Dwyer A J, Miller D L et al 1987 Liver metastasis detection: comparative sensitivities of MR imaging and CT scanning. Radiology 162: 43–47

Sheu J-C, Sung J-L, Chen D-S et al 1985 Early detection of hepatocellular carcinoma by real-time ultrasonography. A prospective study. Cancer 56: 660–666

Sheu J-C, Huang G-T, Chen D-S et al 1987 Small hepatocellular carcinoma: intratumour ethanol treatment using new needle and guidance systems. Radiology 163: 43–48

Shiina S, Yasuda H, Muto H et al 1987 Percutaneous ethanol injection in the treatment of liver neoplasms. American Journal of Roentgenology 149: 949–952

Stack J, Legge D, Behan M 1984 Computed tomographic arteriography in the pre-surgical evaluation of hepatic tumours. Clinical Radiology 35: 189–192

Stark D D, Weissleder R, Elizondo G et al 1988 Superparamagnetic iron oxide: Clinical application as a contrast agent for MR imaging of the liver. Radiology 168: 297–301

Tanaka S, Kitamura T, Ohshima A et al 1986a Diagnostic accuracy of ultrasonography for hepatocellular carcinoma. Cancer 58: 344–347

Tanaka S, Kitamura T, Kasugai H, Okano Y, Tatsuta M, Okuda S 1986b Early diagnosis of hepatocellular carcinoma: Usefulness of ultrasonically guided fine-needle aspiration biopsy. Journal of Clinical Ultrasound 14: 11–16

Tarazi R Y, Hermann R E, Vogt D P et al 1986 Results of surgical treatment of periampullary tumours: a 35-year experience. Surgery 100: 716–723

Taylor I 1985 Colorectal liver metastases — to treat or not to treat? British Journal of Surgery 72: 511–516

Thompson J N, Gibson R, Czerniak A, Blumgart L H 1985 Focal liver lesions; a plan for management. British Medical Journal 290: 1643–1645

Trede M 1987 Treatment of pancreatic carcinoma: the surgeon's dilemma. British Journal of Surgery 74: 79–80

Tscholakoff D, Hricak H, Thoeni R, Winkler M L, Margulis A R 1986 MR imaging in the diagnosis of pancreatic disease. American Journal of Roentgenology 148: 703–709

Vattinen E 1970 Carcinoma of the gallbladder; a study of 390 cases diagnosed in Finland 1953–67. Annales Chirurgiae et Gynaecologiae Supplementum 59: 7–81

Voyles C R, Bowley N J, Allison D J, Benjamin I S, Blumgart L H 1983 Carcinoma of the proximal extrahepatic biliary tree. Radiological assessment and therapeutic alternatives. Annals of Surgery 197: 188–193

Weiner S N, Koenisberg M, Morehouse H, Hoffman J 1984 Sonography and computed tomography in the diagnosis of carcinoma of the gallbladder. American Journal of Roentgenology 142: 735–739

Wood C B 1984 Natural history of liver metastases. In: Van de Velde C J H, Sugarbaker P H (eds) Liver metastases. Martinus Nijhoff, Amsterdam, pp 47–54

Yamada R, Sato M, Kawabata M, Nakatsuka H, Nakamura K, Takashima S 1983 Hepatic artery embolisation in 120 patients with unresectable: hepatoma. Radiology 148: 397–401

Zeman R K, Schiebler M, Clark L R, Jaffe M H, Paushter D M, Grant E G, Choyke P L 1985 The clinical and imaging spectrum of pancreaticoduodenal lymph node enlargement. American Journal of Roentgenology 144: 1223–1227

9. The kidney, bladder and prostate

D. Rickards C. R. Chapple

INTRODUCTION

Malignant neoplasms of the urinary tract involving the prostate, bladder and kidney are a common and important group of tumours. Carcinoma of the prostate can be regarded as a disease associated with ageing, being rare before the age of 60 and with a reported incidence of up to 40% in men aged 70–79 years, but with a likely subclinical incidence far higher than this (Rullis et al 1975). Carcinoma of the bladder is the second most common genitourinary tumour, accounting for 2% of all malignant disease; it forms a major part of the urologist's workload. Despite a marked increase in our knowledge, survival of patients with this disease has changed little in 40 years (McCorron & Marshall 1979). Renal tumours, the majority of which are adenocarcinomas of the kidney (86%), comprise 2–3% of all neoplasms, carry a high mortality and are increasing in incidence. A feature of urinary tract malignant neoplasms is that they are often clinically silent until a fairly advanced stage in their natural history. With the exception of carcinoma of the prostate a definitive diagnosis cannot usually be made on clinical grounds alone, and accurate investigation in the majority of patients relies upon radiological techniques. In view of the large diagnostic armamentarium now available, it is important in each individual patient to tailor the investigative approach not only to the diagnostic resources available but bearing in mind the relevance of any such information obtained to the subsequent clinical management of that patient.

RENAL TUMOURS

Clinico-pathological aspects of renal parenchymal malignancy

Although renal tumours may be considered histologically to be benign or malignant, in clinical practice this subdivision is often of more theoretical than practical importance. With the exception of cysts, lipomas and angiomyolipomatas (Totty et al 1981) which are amenable to accurate radiological diagnosis, the remainder of benign renal tumours often cannot be differentiated from carcinomas. Indeed, even at the time of histological examination, adenomas and oncocytomas cannot be differentiated with certainty from a well-differentiated adenocarcinoma and often have to be considered to be malignant. (Bennington & Beckwith 1975, Mostofi 1979, Lieber et al 1981).

Malignant renal tumours may be primary or secondary. Metastatic renal deposits result from primary carcinomas of the lung, breast and uterus (Abeshouse et al 1941). They are radiologically poorly visualized, ill-defined lesions and usually present at a late stage in the natural history of the disease when the patient's prognosis is poor.

Although any constituent tissue of the kidney may be involved in neoplastic transformation, mesenchymal sarcomas are rare. They are treated by primary surgery. Leiomyosarcoma is the commonest of this group, which overall have a poor prognosis with the exception of liposarcomas which can present clinically when large, but despite this carry a good prognosis. The commonest malignant tumours of the kidney are renal adenocarcinomas in adults and nephroblastomas in children.

Renal adenocarcinoma

Adenocarcinoma of the kidney accounts for 80% of all malignant tumours of the renal parenchyma (Smith D R 1981) and is an under-diagnosed condition. Well-differentiated adenocarcinomas cannot be distinguished histologically from benign adenomas in the majority of cases. The designated distinction between benign and malignant is on the basis of size. Tumours less than 3 cm in diameter are regarded as benign, whilst those greater than 3 cm are treated as malignant. Reported post mortem series have demonstrated a high incidence of small renal parenchymal adenomas (Bennington & Beckwith 1975).

There is a rare genetic tendency to develop these tumours in patients with cerebellar or retinal angiomas (Greene & Rosenthal 1951) and case reports of sporadic indicence in other families have been reported. The rôle of environmental factors in their aetiology is undecided (Bloom 1967, Pavone-Macalusco 1967). Recent reports suggest that the incidence of tumour is increasing (Davies 1985). Looking at the latest statistics, the death rate from this tumour reported in the 1986 United Kingdom statistics was male 1382, female 847 (OPCS unpublished).

Although the classical triad of haematuria, loin pain and a palpable mass is described, the simultaneous occurrence of all three at presentation is rare with the cardinal symptom being haematuria (Best 1987). Systemic effects (Chisholm & Roy 1971) include pyrexia (Rawlins et al 1970), anaemia (Bowman & Martinez 1968), polycythaemia (Hammond & Winnick 1974), altered liver function tests (Fletcher et al 1981), hypertension (Hollifield et al 1975) and hypercalcaemia (Jung et al 1976, Altaffer & Chenault 1979). Although in many of these situations the aetiology is unclear, the high prevalence of these and other rarer systemic side-effects appears to be related to the propensity of these tumours to produce endocrine substances (Woodhouse et al 1985). As with any tumour, which may remain occult for a long period of its natural history, these tumours can present with metastases to the lungs,

bone or brain. Local disease extension blocking the renal vein may produce a varicocoele (most likely on the left side).

Tumour staging (Fig. 9.1 and Table 9.1). Although tumour staging has an important bearing on individual patient prognosis, preoperative radiological staging can be difficult and is often inaccurate. In addition, in the absence of evidence of metastatic disease most clinicians will opt for surgical intervention wherever technically possible, which includes all tumour stages apart from T4. Of particular importance in management is the actual diagnosis of a solid space-occupying renal lesion. The decision as to whether this is benign or malignant and the true nature of such a lesion may not be apparent until formal histologi-

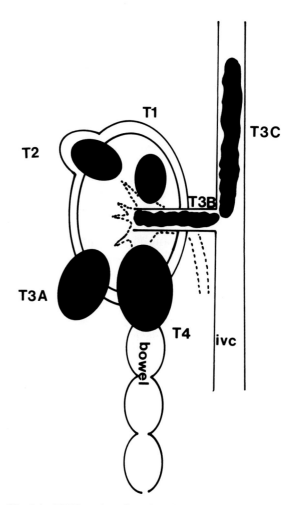

Fig. 9.1 TNM staging of renal carcinoma.

Table 9.1 TNM classification for staging primary renal tumours (UICC 1978)

Category T

T0	No tumour
T1	Small tumour, no renal enlargement. There is limited calyceal distortion or deformity and circumscribed vascular deformities surrounded by renal parenchyma
T2	Large tumour producing distortion or enlargement of the kidney and calyceal or pelvic involvement
T3A T3B T3C	Spread of tumour into the peripelvic or perinephric fat or hilar renal vessels
T4	Extension of tumour into neighbouring organs or the abdominal wall

Category N

N0	No regional lymph node involvement
N1	Involvement of single ipsilateral regional lymph nodes
N2	Involvement of contralateral, bilateral or multiple regional lymph nodes
N3	Fixed regional lymph node involvement
N4	Extension into juxtaregional lymph nodes

Category M

M0	No evidence of metastatic spread
M1	Distant metastatic spread

cal examination of the surgical specimen has been carried out.

Tumour behaviour and prognosis. It is of interest to note that the kinetics of tumour growth are such that the average diameter of a renal adenocarcinoma at nephrectomy is 7.5 cm, representing a growth phase which has encompassed 90% of the natural history of the lesion (Bloom 1967). The chief incidence of these tumours is in the fifth to seventh decades of life with a reported male of female ratio of 1.5–2 to 1. The incidence reported for the United Kingdom in 1983 was 1575 male to 935 female cases (OPCS 1986).

The long term prognosis of patients should be guarded since these lesions often do not present until a late stage in their natural history, when there is already widespread dissemination of the disease which is often occult. The unpredictable nature of renal adenocarcinoma has also been attributed to the part played by host immune factors, which may well provide the explanation for the wide variance in the reported 5-year survival rates (McDonald 1982): 56–82% with disease confined to the kidney, 8–50% with renal vein or caval involvement and 0–3% for patients with

metastases on presentation. Conversely, 74% of patients presenting with metastases are dead within one year (Patel & Lavengood 1978) — a figure to be borne in mind when considering the rare but well publicized incidence of spontaneous and usually transient regression (0.8%) (Middleton 1980).

In addition, approximately one-third of patients who develop tumour regression eventually die of disseminated disease (Fairlamb 1981). It is to be expected that the incidence of metastases should correlate with tumour size. Indeed, 8% of patients with a tumour less than 5 cm in diameter have metastatic disease, compared with 80% of those with a tumour over 10 cm in diameter (Bracken & Johnson 1979).

Treatment options. The optimum treatment for renal adenocarcinoma is radical excision. Careful preoperative staging to tumour spread is therefore important, particularly in the context of demonstrating if the renal vein or inferior vena cava is involved as this allows for a planned surgical approach. Invasion of the main renal vein or its major tributaries occurs in up to 30% of patients (Myers et al 1968). Adjuvant pre- or postoperative radiotherapy does not help to reduce local tumour recurrence in cases where there is local extrarenal disease. Preoperative renal arterial embolization, although having theoretical advantages, is not without its dangers and has failed to achieve widespread acceptance. Hormonal therapy with a variety of agents (in particular progestogens) is the most successful form of systemic therapy and can occasionally induce significant responses (up to 11% in a large series: Bloom & Hendry 1982). Currently attention is directed at the systemic use of interferon.

Nephroblastoma

Nephroblastoma of the kidneys is a highly malignant tumour occurring with considerable variation in histological composition and differentiation. Tumour staging differs from that of adenocarcinoma, tumours being classified as follows by the National Wilms' Tumour Study Group (D'Angio et al 1976):

Stage 1 – Tumour limited to kidney (complete resection)

Stage 2 – Tumour extending beyond kidney, complete resection

Stage 3 – Residual tumour left in abdomen

Stage 4 – Haematogenous metastases

Stage 5 – Bilateral tumours.

Tumour behaviour and prognosis. The degree of differentiation of the tumour correlates closely with patterns of metastatic spread (Beckwith & Palmer 1978). It is almost exclusively confined to children under 4 years of age, although there are reported cases in adults (Babaian et al 1980). It is considered to be a congenital or embryomal tumour and 6% are present at birth. It has an incidence of 1 in 10 000 live births. The tumours are usually large at presentation when a mass is the most noticeable feature. They are associated with congenital anomalies and associated biochemical abnormalities have been reported, namely hyper-secretion of renin, erythropoietin and mucopoly-saccharide.

Treatment options. Nephroblastomas are amenable to cure using a combined therapeutic approach encompassing surgery, radiotherapy and chemotherapy. At an early stage 80–90% cure rates can be expected, and even if pulmonary metastases are present cure can be expected in 50% of patients (Smith D R 1981). Preoperative staging of these lesions is of limited importance since although it allows for the tailoring of the combined therapeutic approach, the fundamental step in treatment is surgical debulking and peroperative staging of the tumour.

Clinico-pathological aspects of urothelial neoplasia, renal pelvis and ureter

The urinary tract has a uniform urothelial lining which under the influence of environmental carcinogens may undergo field change with the subsequent development of neoplasms in any part of the urothelium (Melicow 1945). Renal pelvic and ureteric transitional cell carcinomas (TCC) are rare. Their incidence is placed in perspective if one relates it to that of bladder transitional cell carcinoma, namely one case of renal pelvic and one case of ureteric carcinoma for every 64 (Williams & Mitchell 1973a) and 51 (Williams & Mitchell 1973b) cases of bladder transitional cell carcinoma

respectively. Tumours of the renal pelvis occur predominantly in male patients and comprise approximately 10% of all renal tumours. Similarly, malignant tumours of the ureter occur most commonly in men and two-thirds arise in the distal ureter (Smith D R 1981).

Tumour staging

The staging of upper tract urothelial tumours is as follows:

Stage A – Mucosal infiltration only

Stage B – Involvement of mucosa and superficial muscle layer

Stage C – Invasion of renal pelvic muscle, renal substance or penetration through ureteric wall

Stage D – Peri-ureteric involvement or peri-pelvic, peri-renal or hilar vessel involvement.

The diagnosis of upper tract TCC relies largely on the use of upper urinary tract imaging by intravenous urography, supplemented by cytological investigation of the urine. These lesions can be extremely difficult to visualize and may not present until a late stage in their natural history. A patient may be misdiagnosed as having a simple idiopathic renal pelvi-ureteric junction obstruction, and it is not until later that the underlying TCC becomes evident.

Tumour behaviour and prognosis

Transitional cell carcinomas (TCC) are slow growing neoplasms which usually spread by local invasion: blood-borne metastases occur later in natural history. Patient prognosis is therefore strongly influenced by the stage at which the tumour first presents. The survival figures are largely dependent upon whether there is muscle invasion at the time of first diagnosis.

Treatment options

Optimal treatment of renal pelvic or ureteric TCC is by radical surgical excision. Radiotherapy should be reserved for cases where there is local spillage of tumour at the time of surgery or for palliation. Systemic chemotherapy has not been shown to be beneficial. Even if comprehensive preoperative investigation is carried out, accurate staging of these lesions is usually only available after histological examination of the surgical specimen.

Radiological diagnosis and staging

Introduction

Over the past decade the newer imaging techniques, in particular CT, have had an enormous impact on both the diagnosis and staging of renal tumours. Radiological investigation is usually conducted as a consequence of symptoms, but renal carcinoma is increasingly diagnosed as an incidental finding (Ueda & Mihara 1987).

Radiological techniques for the detection of tumour follow a traditional route of excretory urography (EU), retrograde pyelography and ultrasound (US), all of which provide some infor-

mation on tumour staging. The staging of the tumour requires CT and possibly magnetic resonance imaging (MRI), in some cases enhanced with venography and angiography. Therapeutic possibilities other than surgery involve transcatheter tumour embolization and percutaneous tumour ablation. Follow-up studies of the tumour itself or the site of surgery are predominantly the province of CT.

Diagnostic and 'T' staging

EU remains the backbone of the investigation of the patient with suspected upper tract urological malignancy. EU may detect renal masses (Fig. 9.2), but determination of nature and extent requires other techniques. Without tomography tumours of 4 cm or less may be missed (Curry et al 1986), and despite good tomography small tumours originating on the anterior or posterior

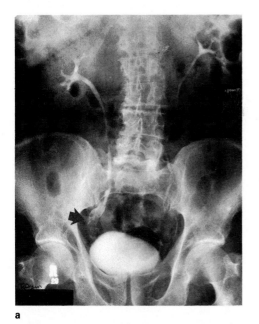
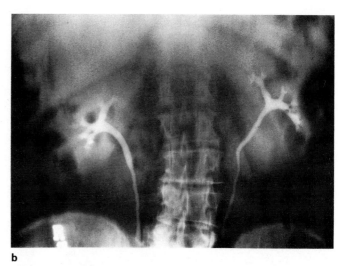

a   b

Fig. 9.2 (a) Full length EU film at 10 min in a man with haematuria. There is a lesion involving the right lower ureter (arrow). It is expanding the ureter, is irregular and predominantly a filling defect. Such lesions are more likely to be transitional cell tumours than other causes of ureteric filling defects. Because transitional cell tumours may be multicentric, a careful search for other lesions is important. Note the displacement of the left lower pole. (b) Tomogram of the kidneys. The right pelvicalyceal system appears normal. There is displacement of the left lower pole calyces and a mass lesion in the lower pole. US showed a solid lesion and biopsy confirmed a renal adenocarcinoma. The classical treatment for the right ureteric lesion is nephroureterectomy and that for the left is nephrectomy. In this patient, a left nephrectomy and right ureterectomy were performed together with a transverse uretero-ureterostomy anastomosing the normal left ureter to the normal right renal pelvis.

aspect of the kidney causing no distortion of the renal outline or displacement of the pelvicalyceal system are likely to be overlooked (Lloyd et al 1978, Cronan et al 1982). With this in mind it becomes impossible to exclude a renal tumour with a normal EU (Demos et al 1985). In the patient with clinical signs of urological malignancy, a normal EU and cystoscopic examination, further imaging is mandatory.

Occasionally the plain film may show calcification related to a renal mass. The type of calcification is less important than its position in determining whether it is related to malignant or benign disease. Calcification within a mass is more probable in malignant tumours (Daniel et al 1972). A renal mass detected on EU is statistically more likely to be benign, usually a simple renal cyst. Such lesions require further investigation even if a renal tumour is not suspected as cysts can mimic tumours. Occasionally simple cysts coincide with tumour and in the absence of any other cause of the patient's symptoms, such cysts need aspirating and the aspirant sent for cytology. A blood clot within the renal pelvis, ureter or bladder associated with a mass on EU is highly suggestive of malignancy (Fig. 9.3). In any event, abnormality detected on EU suggestive of a mass lesion necessi-

tates further investigation. To treat purely on the information provided by the urogram is inappropriate.

EU provides little information about tumour staging. The loss of fat planes between the kidney and liver or spleen is not diagnostic of local extension of tumour. It is usual with adenocarcinomas of the kidney that some renal function is identified and that displaced or abnormal calyces be seen, irrespective of tumour size. This is not necessarily the case with transitional cell tumours. Large pelvic tumours may cause obstruction to the upper tract with loss or considerable delay of renal function, or focal caliecstasis should tumour obstruct an infundibulum.

EU is sensitive for small transitional cell tumours within the collecting system, but requires good radiographic technique (Fig. 9.4). Any doubt

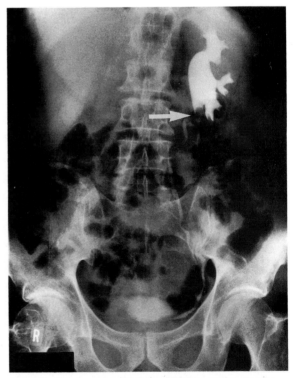

Fig. 9.4 Routine annual full length follow-up 10 min film in a man who has previously undergone right nephroureterectomy for transitional cell carcinoma. There is a well-defined filling defect in the left proximal ureter (arrow) which proved to be a recurrent transitional cell tumour. No other lesions were found. Surgery involved local excision of the tumour and end-to-end ureteric anastomosis.

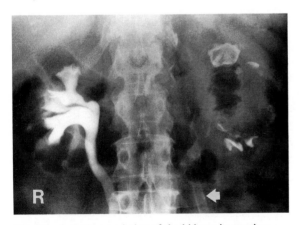

Fig. 9.3 A 5 min coned view of the kidneys in a patient with gross haematuria. The right pelvicalyceal system is normal. On the left, there is distortion of the pelvis and calyceal system by a centrally located mass lesion associated with a linear filling defect in the proximal ureter (arrow). The association of a renal mass and such filling defects is highly suggestive of an actively bleeding renal carcinoma producing blood clots within the ureter.

about the integrity of the upper tracts at EU requires further imaging. Retrograde pyelography, although invasive, is a small extension to cystoscopy which patients with haematuria will be subjected to. Dilute contrast in small doses under fluoroscopic control will localize the vast majority of small upper tract transitional tumours. The ureter is normally only partly opacified at EU and is best imaged by retrograde pyelography.

Both US and CT have recently proven to be sensitive techniques for the detection and characterization of renal masses and enhance the information provided by EU. US allows for rapid, non-invasive differentiation between solid and cystic renal masses in 95–98% of cases. Renal carcinomas may be echodense, echolucent or isoechoic with the renal parenchyma (Coleman et al 1980, Charboneau et al 1983). Up to 40% of tumours have cystic spaces within them due to necrosis, haemorrhage or tumour vascularity. The tumour may be sharply marginated or be an irregular mass infiltrating normal renal parenchyma. Extracapsular spread of tumour is difficult to detect on US, but extension into the liver with the loss of the interface between the liver and the right kidney is more readily identified. US is valuable in detecting venous extension of tumour into the renal vein and inferior vena cava (IVC) (Fig. 9.5), thus differentiating T1 from T3 and T4 tumours (Walzer et al 1980, Thomas & Bernardino 1981). The extent of renal vein involvement is both a prognostic factor and alters the potential surgical approach. More aggressive renal tumours are more likely to involve the IVC, especially when the tumour is right-sided because of the shorter renal vein (Schwerk et al 1985). Involvement of the renal vein and IVC in the absence of nodal disease does not preclude surgical intervention or long term survival (Smith R B 1981). Tumour extension into the renal vein occurs in up to 30% of cases, but represents a significant problem in 5–10% when the inferior vena cava is involved (Clayman et al 1980, Webb et al 1987). Tumour thrombus may extend as far as the right heart and completely block the IVC, but more typically a sliver of tumour thrombus is found lying free within the IVC with no evidence of infiltration of the vessel wall. Tumour extension into the intrahepatic IVC or the right heart is best seen with

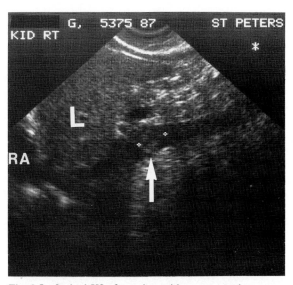

Fig. 9.5 Sagittal US of a patient with proven renal adenocarcinoma. There is a mass within the lumen of the inferior vena cava (IVC) (arrow between calipers) due to endovenous tumour extension. The right atrium (RA) and upper vena cava are clear (L = liver). The lesion is T3.

echocardiography. Enlargement of the renal vein to more than 1.5 cm is due to either tumour thrombus or increased blood flow (Thomas & Bernardino 1981). Doppler flow spectrum analysis will distinguish between the two and will indicate the vascularity of the lesion, useful information prior to angiography or embolization (Dubbins & Wells 1986).

Small transitional cell tumours (1–4 mm) lying within the normally echodense renal sinus and collecting system are difficult if not impossible to detect on US. Slightly larger tumours are within the spatial resolution of modern ultrasound machines and appear as echopoor masses within the collecting system causing displacement. US is operator dependent and the search for upper tract urothelial lesions requires great expertise; even then small lesions will be missed. In the ureter, US has little to offer. The proximal and distal few centimetres can be imaged, but again small lesions are easily missed and are best imaged by either EU or retrograde studies.

CT has largely replaced angiography and venography as diagnostic and staging techniques in renal cell carcinoma (Weyman et al 1980, Wadsworth et al 1982). Upper abdominal CT can show

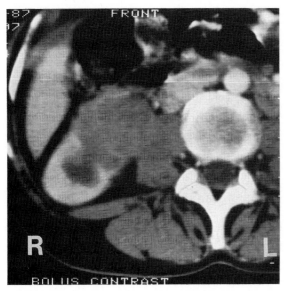

Fig. 9.6 Dynamic CT scan of the right kidney. There is a right renal carcinoma infiltrating the right psoas muscle. The inferior vena cava at this level is normal. The lesion is T4.

simultaneously direct tumour spread (Fig. 9.6), enlarged lymph nodes, venous involvement and hepatic metastatic disease. Carcinomas on CT are usually heterogeneous, have attenuation values less than those for normal renal parenchyma and transiently enhance following intravenous contrast. Dynamic CT immediately following a bolus of 50–100 ml of contrast provides more information than does conventional CT, especially about endovenous tumour extension, and should be routine in all cases (Lang 1984). Tumours are sharply demarcated or have no discernable interface with normal renal parenchyma. Three types of renal growth pattern as seen on CT are described: solid, cystic and papillary.

The association of renal cyst and carcinoma has been a subject of discussion for many years (Murphy & Marshall 1980). On any form of imaging there is a range of cystic renal lesions which can be separated from each other in order that the most appropriate form of imaging and treatment is employed. Most cysts found on US or CT are clearly benign, but cystic renal carcinomas account for 10% of tumours and appear similar on imaging to a necrotic tumour and to a tumour arising in a cyst wall. Distinction between these entities is

usually possible on CT (Bosniak 1986). Simple benign cysts appear as a homogeneous water density mass with an attenuation value of $-10/+10$ Hounsfield units (HU). They do not enhance and have no detectable wall thickness. Occasionally, simple cysts may not meet these criteria because of partial volume effects, patient movement artefact or beam enhancement. If these criteria are met, no further investigation is needed. If a cyst does not have an attenuation value of water density or is heterogeneous, has a detectable wall and septae running through it or forms an irregular interface with surrounding renal parenchyma, it is a complex one which needs further investigation. The differential diagnoses include a complicated simple cyst, infected cyst, cystic nephroma, abscess and cystic malignancy. Hyperdense renal cysts, 40–70 HU, are due to increased iron content in the cyst following haemorrhage, protein or calcium (Zirinsky et al 1984, Parienty et al 1985). Aspiration biopsy under CT or US control may rapidly resolve the situation. Even in the presence of tumour, clear fluid may be aspirated (Khorsand 1965, Marshall 1980). Bloodstained fluid is more indicative of malignancy and will be found in 30% of cases (Lang 1966). Cystic necrotic tumour may have a low attenuation centre which may enhance, a thick wall and an irregular interface with surrounding parenchyma (Fig. 9.7a). Multilocular cystic nephroma is a type of hamartoma with multiple well-defined cysts and septae. It is not a diagnosis usually made preoperatively.

Papillary adenocarcinomas are characterized clinically by their slower growth, lower stage at presentation and better prognosis than other types of adenocarcinoma (Mancilla-Jimenez et al 1976). 80% of patients with papillary tumours will be stage T1 or T2 at presentation compared with 50% of non-papillary tumours. Calcification, necrosis and cystic degeneration are commonly seen in papillary tumours and they are hypovascular, enhancing poorly (Press et al 1984). Such observations on CT should suggest papillary carcinoma, an important finding if partial nephrectomy is being considered.

There are occasions when biopsy of a renal mass is needed; this is performed under US or CT guidance. A 18 gauge trucut biopsy using the

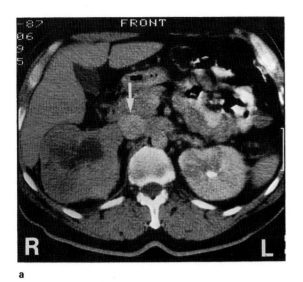
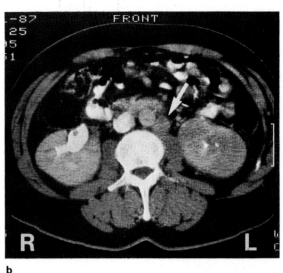

Fig. 9.7 (a) Dynamic CT scan at the level of the renal hilum in a patient with adenocarcinoma of the right kidney. There is a partly cystic carcinoma not infiltrating the liver or the inferior vena cava (arrow). The tumour is T2. (b) Dynamic CT in the same patient at a lower level. There is para-aortic lymphadenopathy (arrow) and distortion of the left renal outline. The right lower pole appears normal. The patient has bilateral renal adenocarcinomas and evidence of retroperitoneal lymphadenopathy, N1.

Bioty gun invariably supplies adequate tissue for histological diagnosis. Seeding of tumour in the tract has been reported, but is a rare phenomenon and the risks of seeding outweigh the benefits of an accurate histological diagnosis (Nadel et al 1986).

CT is able to distinguish between all the 'T' stages in renal carcinoma. The perinephric fat and Gerota's fascia are well defined on CT except in thin patients and children who have little intra-abdominal fat content. Apparent invasion of the perinephric fat by tumour can be due to collateral vessels or coexisting inflammatory disease, but in most cases CT is able to distinguish between T1 and T2 tumours and is certainly more accurate than angiography in this respect (Johnson et al 1987). Involvement of the renal vein (T3) as evidenced by enlargement of the vein, perinephric extension of the tumour and retroperitoneal lymphadenopathy (Fig. 9.7a and b) all support the diagnosis of renal carcinoma. Dynamic CT is accurate in detecting endovenous tumour thrombus except in cases where a large bulky tumour distorts the renal hilum to such an extent that the vein cannot be found. Thrombus within the vena cava may enlarge the vena cava or produce low at-

tenuation filling defects following contrast enhancement. To facilitate vena caval enhancement, contrast is given via a foot vein while dynamic scanning, remembering that apparent filling defects may be due to unopacified venous blood entering the cava. Incomplete occlusion of the cava, collaterals or an enlarged azygous system may be identified. The upper extent of tumour thrombus needs to be identified so that the most appropriate surgical approach is employed. If CT fails to define this, US, echocardiography or superior venacavography can be performed (Fig. 9.8).

Urothelial tumours within the collecting system and ureter can be staged by CT. The crucial factor is to assess whether the tumour has infiltrated renal parenchyma or periureteric tissues (stage C) or is localized to the mucosa or lamina propria (stage A and B). Tumours on CT appear as intraluminal filling defects, as an infiltrating mass or thickening of the ureteric wall. Thin section (3 or 5 mm) CT scans will improve the detection rate by increasing the spatial resolution. Baron et al (1982) in their series of 24 patients were able to differentiate between stage B and stage C or D tumours in 23, but were unable to distinguish

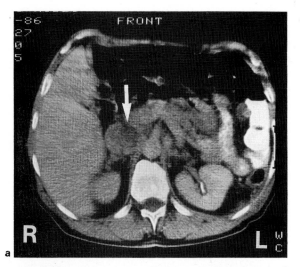

between stage A and stage B lesions. With stage A and stage B tumours a sharp demarcation was present between the tumour and adjacent fat. Their attenuation value is similar to renal parenchyma and they enhance poorly.

There are few diagnostic or staging indications for angiography if CT is available (Mauro et al 1982). If CT or US fail to provide sufficient information or if they contradict each other, angiography can be performed and the findings in adenocarcinoma are characteristic (Fig. 9.9). The main renal artery is enlarged and there is neovascularity within the tumour mass associated with early venous filling. Extension of the tumour to involve contiguous structures is evidenced by neovascularity to these structures, usually not from

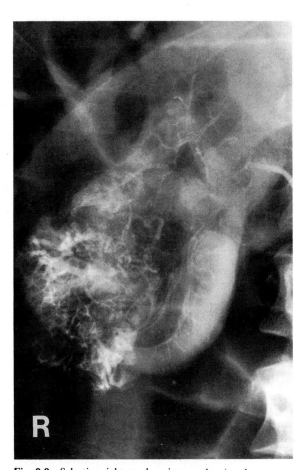

Fig. 9.8 (a) Dynamic CT scan in a patient with known right renal adenocarcinoma. There is an irregular filling defect in the inferior vena cava consistent with endovenous tumour extension (arrow). The upper limit of the tumour thrombus could not be clearly identified by either CT or US. (b) Superior vena cavogram in the same patient. Contrast is seen in the right atrium and upper portion of the inferior vena cava (IVC). The filling defects (arrow) are due to endovenous tumour extension which does not extend to the right atrium (RA). This would permit a more conservative surgical approach. The lesion is T3.

Fig. 9.9 Selective right renal angiogram showing the classical appearance of renal adenocarcinoma. Neovascularity extends beyond the renal outline and there is distortion of the lower pole. The lesion is T3.

the renal artery. Angiography is a prelude to embolization. Transitional cell and papillary tumours are hypovascular.

There are insufficient reports to date to determine whether MRI is superior to CT in the diagnosis and staging of renal tumours. Early experience with MRI showed that it provided similar information to CT (Choyke et al 1984) and as early as 1983 it was being proposed as the primary imaging modality of choice for the investigation of renal masses (Hriack et al 1983b). Sadly, MRI has not yet been shown to produce accurate tissue characterization for renal masses, the overlap between inflammatory, neoplastic and benign lesions being too great (Leung et al 1984). The MR characteristics of renal cell carcinoma are not consistent except that there is a relatively long T_1 compared to normal renal parenchyma on SE sequences. Hriack et al (1985) in a recent study correctly staged 26 out of 27 tumours compared with surgical staging. MRI correctly diagnosed the tumours in all cases, was able to identify retroperitoneal lymphadenopathy and direct invasion into adjacent organs, and evaluated endovenous extension well, distinguishing thrombus from reduced blood flow on T_2 weighted sequences. Thus, MRI was specifically useful in staging T3A, T3B, T3C and T4 tumours, those requiring detailed imaging of the renal vein and vena cava. MRI is also capable of distinguishing tumour thrombus which infiltrates the vein wall from that which does not.

Urothelial tumours are difficult to detect unless they are large or infiltrative (stage C). On inversion recovery (IR) sequences, urothelial lesions are isodense with normal parenchyma, but on spin echo (SE) sequences the signal intensity was increased (Hriack et al 1985, Papanicolaou et al 1986).

'N' staging

CT is accurate for defining lymph node enlargement in the retroperitoneum and retrocrural space, areas which should be covered during renal CT (Fig. 9.7b). CT is unable to distinguish tumour in normal-sized nodes and nodes greater than 1 cm in diameter are presumed to be invaded. The sensitivity and accuracy of CT in detecting nodal disease is 80% (Johnson et al 1987). MRI is capable of detecting enlarged lymph nodes, but like CT is unable to identify tumour in nodes of normal size.

'M' staging

Renal tumours classically metastazise to the lungs. The only effective method of detecting parenchymal deposits is by contiguous section CT through the chest, but in practice plain film radiographs are performed. Parenchymal deposits may be mimicked by tumour emboli secondary to endovenous extension. If doubt exists as to the aetiology of a specific lesion, fine needle aspiration biopsy will usually resolve the situation. Deposits which can be identified on plain film chest radiology can be followed up on serial films. Osseous involvement is assessed by radioisotope studies enhanced by plain film techniques.

Therapeutic radiology

Although not frequently used, radiology does offer therapeutic measures for the treatment of renal tumours or the symptoms associated with tumour. Three main techniques are used:

1. Tumour embolization
2. Transcatheter regional chemotherapy
3. Percutaneous tumour ablation.

Rendering renal tumours avascular prior to surgery was in vogue in the late 1970s and early 1980s following Lalli's initial report (Lalli et al 1969). However, the efficacy of the procedure remains in doubt despite large series, mainly because no controlled trials have been undertaken. There are four indications for embolization:

1. To achieve avascularity prior to surgery
2. To induce the production of tumour antibodies
3. To control haematuria
4. To control pain.

The technique requires selective catheterization of the renal artery followed by its embolization with various embolic materials. Gelfoam particles followed by stainless steel coils are the most commonly used (Fig. 9.10). Gelfoam, causes

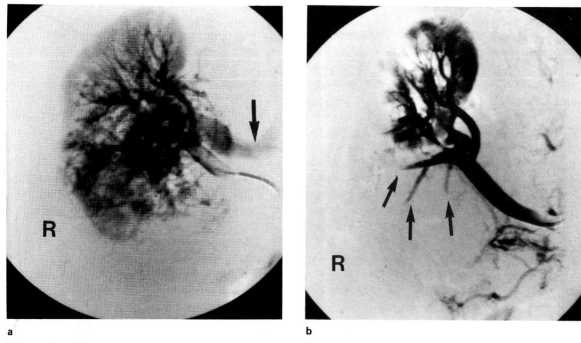

a   b

Fig. 9.10   (a) DSA of the right kidney in a patient with renal adenocarcinoma. There is neovascularity predominantly involving the lower pole and early venous filling (arrow). The patient had gross haematuria and pulmonary parenchymal metastatic disease. Definitive surgery was not considered an option. (b) Following selective embolization of the lower pole vessels (arrows) with Gelfoam particles and Gianturco coils: the lower pole is successfully embolized and the patient's bleeding stopped. Interestingly, there was some regression in the size of the pulmonary metastases, but this was short-lived lasting less than 8 weeks.

embolization of the peripheral vasculature whilst steel coils are used for the main renal arteries or their branches. Embolization leads to a non-functioning kidney, but also to easier surgery in an avascular field (Ekelund et al 1981).

Since most urological surgeons are confident that they can remove large and vascular tumours without undue difficulty, embolization to produce avascularity is not often used. Should embolization be carried out, it is performed 5–6 days prior to surgery, but is usually associated with complications. Following embolization, most patients complain of loin pain, develop a fever, are nauseated and have an ileus for up to five days, hardly the best preparation for major surgery. The use of ethanol as an embolic material is reported to decrease the postembolization syndrome considerably, the reason for which is not known (Ellman et al 1981). Embolic material may escape into the general circulation away from the target organ leading to unintentional embolization of other ves-

sels. Coils have ended up in the femoral and internal iliac artery requiring embolectomy (Chuang 1979). Infarction of both large and small bowel may occur secondary to ethanol embolization (Cox et al 1982). In the light of these complications, the use of embolization to make the surgeon's task easier seems in doubt. In those patients with gross haematuria whose condition does not permit radical surgery or in patients with inoperable tumours, embolization is useful to minimize or stop haemorrhage. It is likely that recurrent bleeding will occur due to collaterals forming and revascularizing the tumour. Pain associated with inoperable tumours is eventually reduced following embolization.

Renal carcinomas are immunogenic. Embolization induces the release of tumour antigens which may in turn precipitate an antitumour reaction and produce regression or ablation of metastatic disease. It appears unlikely in the present state of knowledge that this significantly affects prognosis.

Embolization with radioactive iodine seeds to downstage advanced tumours prior to surgery has been reported (Lang et al 1983). This produces a much higher dose to the tumour than can be achieved with external beam radiation, with a transcatheter dose of 160 Gy. Regional transcatheter chemotherapy offers another therapeutic approach: few reports are available and no comparative studies with intravenous chemotherapy are reported (Wiley et al 1975, Kato et al 1981).

The technique applied to percutaneous stone removal has been extended for the staging and treatment of upper tract urothelial tumours (Woodhouse et al 1986). Although upper tract transitional cell tumours are uncommon, the classic treatment of them is nephroureterectomy. Should recurrent tumours occur in the contralateral kidney, surgical choices are limited to partial nephrectomy or percutaneous treatment. Similarly, the development of tumour in a solitary kidney or synchronous bilateral tumours, which can occur in 2% of cases, produces a therapeutic dilemma (Mazeman 1976). Percutaneous inspection of the pelvicalyceal system permits accurate staging. If the tumour is confined to the urothelium, percutaneous ablation with diathermy is performed and the tract into the kidney irradiated with an iridium wire to forestall tumour cell implantation (Fig. 9.11). This technique can

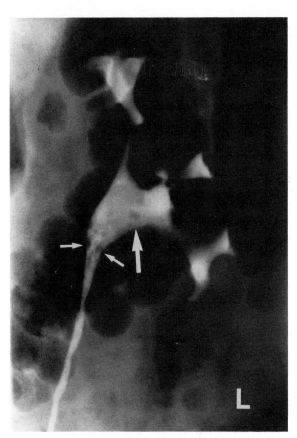

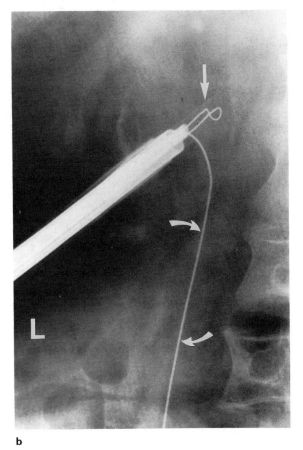

a   b

Fig. 9.11 (a) Coned view of the left kidney in a patient who has previously had a right nephroureterectomy for transitional cell carcinoma and now has recurrent disease in the left kidney (arrows). The bladder and left ureter were normal. (b) The patient is prone. The left collecting system has been punctured and a tract dilated up to 26 French over a guide wire (curved arrow). The urothelial lesions were resected under direct vision with a resectoscope (arrow). All the tumours were removed and a follow-up EU 2 months later was essentially normal.

be compared to the treatment given for similar lesions in the bladder.

Less common renal tumours

Although Wilms' tumours are the most common renal neoplasm in children, they are rare in adults accounting for 0.5% of all renal tumours (Jagasia & Thurman 1965). The tumours in adults tend to be large on presentation, but otherwise have no specific characteristics on imaging which would separate them from renal adenocarcinomas. They tend to have areas of necrosis and haemorrhage within them and are relatively hypovascular, enhancing poorly on CT (Fig. 9.12). At presentation they have often infiltrated retroperitoneal structures and have ill-defined margins. The prognosis of such tumours is poor (Kumar et al 1984).

Fat within a tumour mass is characteristic of a benign hamartoma, but can occur in malignant liposarcomas of the kidney. As previously mentioned, these tumours can grow to a huge size before presentation and carry a good prognosis. Renal haemangiopericytomas are usually localized to the capsule of the kidney and are associated with hypoglycaemia (Bennington & Beckwith 1975).

Suggested staging protocol

Once the diagnosis of renal tumour has been made, the recommended staging modality is CT of the kidneys, liver and retroperitoneum. Dynamic CT to detect endovenous tumour extension is needed. If CT or US fails to image the veins satisfactorily, inferior and perhaps superior vena cavography should be performed. Angiography is rarely indicated except as a prelude to interventional techniques. Equivocal chest deposits are resolved by CT. MRI is likely to surpass CT for the staging of renal tumours.

Follow-up

The follow-up of patients with renal carcinoma depends upon treatment. In the case of total nephrectomy, follow-up is directed towards the search for possible metastatic disease and recurrence of tumour in the postnephrectomy bed

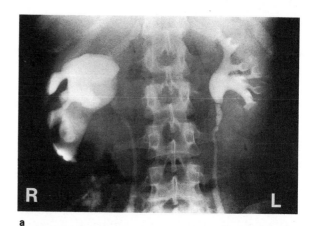

a

b

Fig. 9.12 (a) A 10 min EU film of an 18-year-old female with pain in the right loin. There is distortion and dilatation of the right collecting system. The left kidney is normal. (b) Dynamic CT scan. There is a partly cystic mass lesion expanding the right kidney, the solid element of which enhances poorly. The low attenuation areas are due to necrosis and haemorrhage. The fascial plane between the tumour and liver is preserved and the retroperitoneum is normal. Histologically, this was an adult Wilms' tumour. There are no characteristic features which differentiate this tumour from a hypernephroma.

(Forbes et al 1978). Following nephrectomy, clinical suspicion of local recurrence is best validated with CT. Loops of bowel fall into the vacated renal bed and can become stuck down and immobilized due to adhesions. Unopacified loops of bowel can mimic tumour recurrences so adequate bowel preparation is needed. Enhanced scans rarely help as the recurrent disease is usually hypovascular.

In those patients in whom nephrectomy was not an option either to the patient or to the clinician, the response of the tumour mass to non-surgical treatment can be monitored with either CT, US or MRI.

Irrespective of treatment, all patients need regular chest radiographs to search for pulmonary metastatic disease.

BLADDER CARCINOMA

Clinico-pathological aspects

The urothelium lining the urinary tract is uniform: it provides a watertight barrier which prevents reabsorption yet can adapt to luminal expansion. This is of particular importance when considering the bladder. As discussed previously, tumours of the urothelium, lining the renal pelvis, ureter, bladder and urethra have important features in common. The majority are transitional cell carcinomas (over 90%). Truly benign adenomas are rare (approximately 2%) (Miller et al 1969, Foss 1975). Bladder tumours are the second most common of all genitourinary neoplasms surpassed only by prostatic carcinoma: in the UK in 1983 6683 males and 2564 females were diagnosed as new cases (OPCS 1986). The epidemiological data available suggests that the genesis of these tumours is strongly influenced by environmental factors, such as smoking and occupational exposure to chemicals (Morrison 1984).

A well recognized but poorly understood variant of the urothelial carcinoma is carcinoma in situ. This will often present insiduously with a history of frequency and dysuria in the absence of demonstrable infection. Carcinoma in situ (CIS), unless considered in the differential diagnosis, is notoriously difficult to diagnose and may only be evident on the basis of abnormal urine cytology and histological examination of random biopsy specimens. CIS has an unpredictable natural history since up to 50% of patients develop invasive carcinoma within three years (Riddle et al 1976). Transitional cell carcinoma accounts for 90% of bladder tumours. The remaining 10% of neoplasms are predominantly of two types: squamous carcinoma which complicates chronic irritative conditions including schistosomiasis, and primary adenocarcinoma which most commonly occurs on the anterior wall of the bladder and is thought to arise from urachal remnants. Adenocarcinomas can also involve the bladder by the direct spread of carcinoma from adjacent structures.

Tumour behaviour

Transitional cell carcinoma of the bladder is most common in men with a male to female ratio of 4 to 1. It affects an older age group, over the age of 50. At the time of first presentation this tumour is most common on the posterior or lateral walls of the bladder, particularly near the ureteric orifices (Melicow 1974). Recurrent tumour can occur in more anterior parts of the bladder suggesting possible seedling implantation of exfoliated tumour cells at the time of initial surgical treatment (Page et al 1978). Despite a wealth of collated information on this subject the overall survival has remained relatively static over the last 40 years (McCorron & Marshall 1979). Prediction of tumour behaviour from routine histopathological examination of the primary tumour can be difficult, particularly with well-differentiated lesions. Recent work has demonstrated that cytogenetic analysis of tumour chromosomes can be an accurate means of investigation, but this is time consuming and not universally available. Similar but less detailed information on tumour ploidy which provides useful prognostic information can be provided by the technique of urinary flow cytometry.

Transitional cell carcinomas are usually slow growing neoplasms which initially spread by local invasion. Once they have invaded the perivesical fat they spread to local lymph nodes or beyond in 84% of cases (Jewett & Strong 1946). Blood-borne spread is usually a terminal event. Patient prognosis is therefore directly related to the extent of tumour spread and accurate staging should be carried out whenever possible.

Tumour staging (Fig. 9.13 and Table 9.2)

The diagnosis of bladder cancer is usually made at the time of cystoscopy. Clinical staging of a bladder carcinoma is inaccurate since in up to two-thirds of patients (Richie et al 1975),

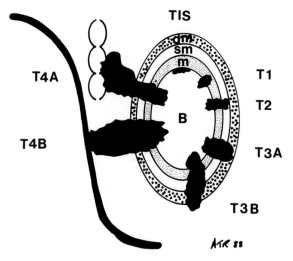

Fig. 9.13 TNM staging of bladder carcinoma. m = mucosa; sm = superficial muscle; dm = deep muscle; B = bladder.

Table 9.2 TNM classification for staging bladder carcinoma (UICC 1978)

Category T	
Tis	Preinvasive carcinoma (carcinoma in situ)
TA	Papillary non-invasive carcinoma
T0	No evidence of primary tumour
T1	Tumour does not extend beyond the lamina propria and if a mass is palpable it is freely mobile and should disappear after complete transurethral resection of the tumour
T2	Tumour involves the superficial muscle. Mobile bladder induration which disappears after complete transurethral resection
T3	Tumour invades into deep muscle. Palpable induration or mass which is mobile, but persists after complete transurethral resection of tumour
T3A	Invasion of deep muscle alone
T3B	Extension of tumour through bladder wall
T4	Tumour fixed or extending into neighbouring structures
T4A	Infiltrating into prostate, uterus or vagina
T4B	Tumour fixed to pelvic or abdominal wall

The suffix (m) is added to indicate multiple tumours, e.g. T1 (m)

Category N	
N0	No involved regional lymph nodes
N1	Involvement of single ipsilateral lymph node
N2	Involvement of contralateral, bilateral or multiple regional lymph nodes
N3	Fixed regional lymph nodes with a free space between them and the tumour
N4	Extension into juxtaregional lymph nodes

Category M	
M0	No distant metastases
M1	Distant metastases

particularly those with deeply invasive neoplasms, there is a tendency to understage the tumours (Schmidt & Weinstein 1976).

Treatment options and prognosis

As mentioned previously, patient prognosis relies heavily on the tumour behaviour which in turn is an expression of the interrelated factors of tumour grade and the stage of a tumour at the time of first presentation. 5-year survival of patients with superficial tumours (T1, T2) of the bladder is between 50–80% as opposed to 6–23% in the presence of deeper invasion (T3, T4) (Grossman 1979, Pilepich & Perez 1982). The accurate staging of a bladder cancer is extremely important since it is vital in determining subsequent patient management. Low grade, low stage tumours will tend to be amenable to local resection with regular endoscopic follow-up of the bladder. At the other end of the spectrum, high grade, high stage tumours will require radical cystourethrectomy either combined with or as an alternative to radiotherapy. Intravesical chemotherapy has been advocated for local control of seedling implantation but has not been as successful as initially forecast on theoretical grounds. The rôle of parenteral chemotherapy is as yet undecided. In view of the unpredictable nature of carcinoma in situ many would tend to opt for early radical surgery if there is any doubt as to the progression of the disease process.

Radiological diagnosis and staging of bladder carcinoma

Despite the dramatic advances in radiology, cystoscopy is the essential procedure for the diagnosis and histological grading of bladder tumours. The rôle of radiology is to assess the normality of the upper tracts, stage the bladder tumour as accurately as possible and monitor the effects of treatment. In the majority of bladder tumours, very little radiology is required at all on the patient's initial presentation and no radiology in the follow-up of tumour. The patient presenting with haematuria will have an EU, not to diagnose a bladder tumour but to examine the upper tracts. Even if on the EU there is a possible cause of the patient's haematuria attributable to the upper tracts, a cystoscopy will be performed which with histological findings can assess bladder muscle wall involvement, but cannot diagnose the full thickness of bladder wall involvement or spread into perivesical fat. If at cystoscopy a bladder tumour appears as TIS or T1, resection of the tumour is performed until normal muscle is seen. Evidently it is the surgeon's experience which dictates whether a tumour seen at cystoscopy is likely to be amenable to transurethral resection. If there is doubt about the stage of the tumour or if it is obviously an infiltrating lesion, staging needs to be done. The crucial factor in all staging modalities is differentiation of T2 from T3A lesions, i.e. those involving the deep layer. At cystoscopy, the distinction between T2 and T3A lesions cannot accurately be made. T2 lesions are treated endoscopically and T3A by cystectomy and/or radiotherapy: accurate pretreatment staging therefore dramatically changes treatment options. Radiotherapy is the treatment of choice for T4 lesions. If the tumuor recurs after radical radiotherapy then palliative cystectomy is the only treatment option and will only be carried out if there is no evidence of extensive perivesical spread or metastases.

Until recently, US and CT were the only imaging techniques which gave worthwhile information for staging bladder tumours, but both have their limitations. The advent of MRI in recent times has already made an impact on bladder tumour staging and may become the imaging modality of choice.

'T' staging

The cystographic phase of the EU has little to offer in either the diagnosis or staging of bladder tumours, only large tumours being seen (Hillman et al 1981). EU is sensitive to the diagnosis of associated urothelial lesions in the ureter and pelvicalyceal system and for that reason alone needs to be done in all patients with suspected or proven bladder tumour. Upper tract obstruction, acquired and congenital lesions will be identified. Combining EU with the information derived from cystoscopy and bimanual examination under anaesthesia understages 50% of bladder tumours (Schmidt & Weinstein 1976). Double and triple contrast cystography, angiography and lymphangiography have been used to stage bladder tumours. Angiography performed with both intravesical and perivesical gas insufflation has a high degree of staging accuracy (95%), but is highly invasive and requires considerable operator skill.

Vesical US can be performed endoscopically or via the suprapubic, transabdominal approach. Endoscopic transurethral US is invasive and usually performed at the time of cystoscopy. The 7.5 or 10 MHz probes used are dedicated to bladder US, are expensive and as yet not perfected. Endoscopic transrectal bladder US is less invasive, but with currently available probe technology is limited to imaging the inferior aspect of the bladder. With the development of multiplanar probes this approach may prove more useful and reliable. Suprapubic bladder US can be performed with any modern US machine with either sector or linear array 3.5 or 5 MHz probes (Fig. 9.14). The normal distended bladder appears as a uniform structure, smooth in outline and having a uniform

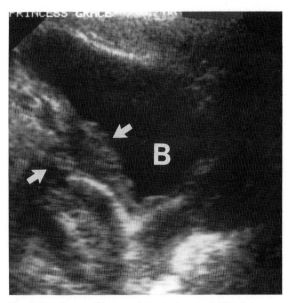

Fig. 9.14 Suprapubic-transabdominal sagittal US of the bladder. There is a mass (arrows) involving the bladder wall and extending beyond it. The US diagnosis is of a T3B bladder tumour.

echogenic pattern. It is not possible to distinguish between the deep and superficial muscle layers and the mucosa. Tumours appear as echopoor masses. T1 lesions do not cause any interruption of the underlying bladder wall (Fig. 9.15). T2 lesions show superficial infiltration of the echodense bladder wall by the echopoor tumour and may locally thicken the bladder wall. T34 tumours cause distortion of the bladder wall and the whole thickness of the bladder wall is involved by the echopoor tumour mass (Fig. 9.16). Perivesical extension in the T3B lesions may also be seen.

A high degree of accuracy has been claimed for both transurethral and transabdominal techniques (McLaughlin et al 1975, Nakamura & Niijima 1980, Singer et al 1981, Jeager et al 1985). Using transurethral scanning, Devonec et al (1987) reported an 80% correlation between US and pathological staging in 50 patients. Abu-Yousef & Narayana (1982a) correctly staged by transabdominal US all 12 patients in their series who had been adequately pathologically staged. Denkhaus et al (1985) reported their experience of suprapubic scanning in 61 patients with bladder tumours and reported a staging accuracy of 83%, overstaging the tumour in 10% of cases and understaging it in 7%. There are problems with interpretation common to all techniques. Tumours

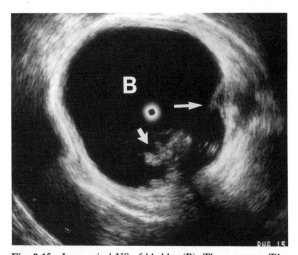

Fig. 9.15 Intravesical US of bladder (B). There are two T1 bladder tumours (arrows). The apparent defect in the normally echogenic bladder wall associated with the larger lesion is artefactual due to air introduced during cystoscopy trapped between the tumour and the bladder wall.

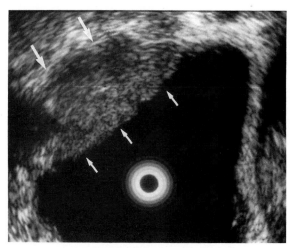

Fig. 9.16 Intravesical US of bladder. There is a T3 bladder tumour involving the normally echogenic bladder wall and infiltrating the deep layers (arrows).

in the dome of the bladder may be obscured due to shadowing from adjacent bowel gas. Large tumours can be associated with calcification, the acoustic shadow of which will obscure the underlying bladder wall. The air bubble in the anterior aspect of the bladder introduced during cystoscopy prior to transurethral US causes artefacts which can result in tumours being missed. This is easily avoided if the operating table is tilted at various angles to move the air bubble around. Bladder wall oedema associated with catheterization and chronic cystitis or a hypertrophied bladder wall cannot be differentiated from a solid bladder tumour (Abu-Yousef & Narayana 1982b). A trabeculated bladder mimics multilocular tumour (Denkhaus et al 1985). Overall, non-invasive suprapubic US gives similar results to invasive urethral US for staging bladder tumours. For large tumours, T3A, T3B and T4, the suprapubic approach gives better results because of the better tissue penetration afforded by the lower frequency probes used.

CT is unable to distinguish stages lower than T3A from each other, all showing localized or generalized thickening of the bladder wall with clear definition of the bladder wall against the perivesical fat. If this definition is lost the tumour is staged as T3B (Fig. 9.17) and if adjoining structures of the pelvic side walls are involved the

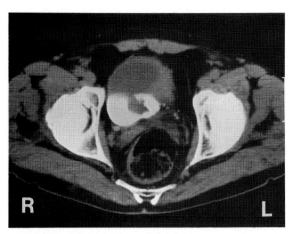

Fig. 9.17 CT of pelvis following IV contrast. There is a T3B lesion on the left lateral wall.

tumour is T4. CT is able to distinguish T3B from T4 lesions in 80–83% of cases (Kellett et al 1980, Vock et al 1982, Salo et al 1985). Both CT and US are very useful in those patients who harbour tumours in large vesical diverticulae: such lesions are difficult to find on cystoscopy.

Although CT has been the single most effective modality for staging bladder tumours, reports are now emerging which show that MRI is as accurate, if not more so (Amendola et al 1986, Lee & Rholl 1986, Johnson 1987). Attention has been focused on the areas in which CT has been shown to be inaccurate: the differentiation between T2 and T3A lesions and the presence of metastatic disease in normal-sized nodes.

Like CT, MRI is not able to distinguish T1 from T2 lesions. T3A lesions cannot be distinguished from T2 lesions if only small focal areas of the bladder wall are involved. If extensions into the deep muscular layers involve the entire wall, MRI will differentiate T2 from T3A. Bladder wall hypertrophy is clearly distinguishable from tumour on MRI (Hriack et al 1983a). Although transverse axial images locate most tumours, those located near the bladder base or in the dome of the bladder are better defined with sagittal or coronal sections. Lesions on the postero-lateral walls may be over-staged on transverse images alone while sagittal or coronal images may show an intact bladder wall. To assess tumour extensions into adjacent organs, the prostate and rectum, sagittal

images are again needed. MRI images with T_1 weighting define the intravesical extent of tumour and the perivesical extension in T3B lesions. Involvement of the bladder wall itself is best imaged on T_2-weighted sequences.

'N' staging

Lymphangiography should be accurate in assessing lymph node involvement as the bladder lymphatics drain into the external iliac chain. This has not, however, been the case: a correlation with pathological examination of 48% has been reported (Farrah & Cerny 1978), although accuracies of up to 96% have been recorded (Jing et al 1982). CT and MRI are unable to identify involved normal-sized nodes.

'M' staging

Transitional cell tumours classically metastasize to the lungs, liver and skeleton. A normal chest radiograph to all intents excludes secondary pulmonary deposits, but should there be suspicion about the radiograph, CT should be undertaken. The liver is best screened by US which is more accurate than isotope scanning. Skeletal metastases are best assessed with isotope scanning.

Follow-up

The patient with a TIS or T1 tumour will have regular cystoscopy to ensure localized recurrence of tumour does not occur. It is probably unnecessary to check the upper tracts unless there is evidence that the patient has vesicoureteric reflux. There is an established association between treated lower tract tumours and the appearance of upper tract lesions between 2 and 16 years after adequate treatment (Affre et al 1981). The authors suggest that there is a place for periodic EU especially if reflux occurs, which is more common after transurethral ablation of bladder tumours.

In those patients with T2 and T3 lesions who have undergone cystectomy, follow-up is directed at the site of the excised tumour and to imaging of urinary diversions. The identification of recurrence at the site of surgery is the province of CT; small bowel loops within the pelvis make US unsatisfactory. Good results for detecting recurrence in postcystectomy cases are reported (Lee et al 1981). A mass of any kind seen in the pelvis in the adequately prepared patient is suspicious of recurrence and should be confirmed by needle aspiration or biopsy under CT control. The detection of early recurrence will prolong patients' survival. CT is more difficult to interpret in those patients who have had radiotherapy or partial cystectomy. Thickening and fibrosis of the soft tissue and bladder wall due to surgery and/or radiotherapy can simulate recurrence. Following cystectomy, some form of urinary diversion has to be fashioned. Many types of diversionary procedures are described, but most common are an ileal loop or percutaneous ureterostomy. Ileal loops can be complicated by poor drainage due to stenoses

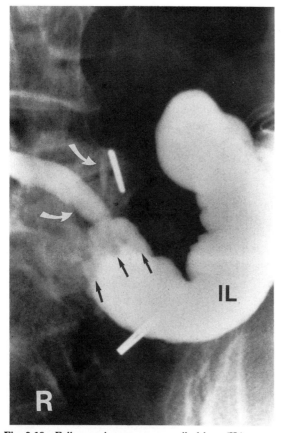

Fig. 9.18 Follow-up loopogram on an ileal loop (IL) following total cystectomy. There is an irregular filling defect (straight arrows) at the anastomosis with the ureters (curved arrows) due to recurrent tumour.

at the uretero-conduit anastomosis or due to stenoses within the loop. Recurrent tumours at the anastomosis are well described, as is metastatic disease to other parts of the loop (Amis et al 1981) (Fig. 9.18). Recurrent upper tract tumours can also be seen on loopograms where enterovesical reflux occurs and, loop fistulae and leaks can also occur. All these potential complications are demonstrated by loopography using a small Foley's catheter in the loop and the injection of contrast under flouroscopic control.

Inoperable T4 lesions which are treated with chemotherapy or radiotherapy may be followed up with CT or MRI.

Therapeutic radiology

In the event of intractable bleeding from the bladder secondary to inoperable T3 or T4 lesions, transcatheter embolization of the internal iliac arteries can be performed as an alternative to surgical ligation or palliative radiotherapy to control haemorrhage (Fig. 9.19). Embolization should be limited if possible to the anterior division if the internal iliac artery. Occlusion of the posterior division can lead to severe gluteal pain and buttock claudication. Sciatic nerve damage can occur due to embolization of the arteria comitans nervi ischiadicis, a branch of the anterior division which supplies the sciatic nerve. If tumour is localized to one lateral aspect of the bladder, embolization of the ipsilateral internal iliac arteries will suffice, but in the extent of an extensive tumour both will have to be embolized. Gelfoam is the embolic material of choice. A success rate for satisfactory control of haemorrhage can be expected in 90% of cases (McIvor et al 1982).

Transcatheter regional chemotherapy using actinomycin D infused via the internal iliac artery has been shown to downgrade tumours. This occurred in 4 out of 12 patients with T2 and T3 lesions and in 4 out of 5 patients with T4 lesions reported by Ogata et al (1973). Unfortunately complication rates were high, over 25% getting skin necrosis and 10% sciatic neuritis, and the technique has not gained acceptance.

Bladder tumours which arise near the vesico-ureteric junction or those which are extensive may cause renal failure secondary to obstruc-

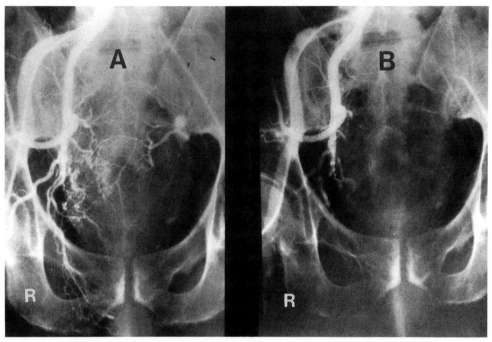

Fig. 9.19 Angiogram of an inoperable T4 bladder tumour which was associated with persistent haemorrhage requiring repeated blood transfusion (**A**). The right internal iliac vessel has been embolized (**B**) with good result.

tion. Decompression of the upper tract by percutaneous nephrostomy is technically simple and will certainly relieve obstruction. Similarly, the strictured distal ureter can be stented or dilated. The decision to treat at all may be a difficult one. Ureteric obstruction usually occurs late in the disease process or with advanced disease, and may be that a ureamic death is more appropriate than a death from disseminated metastatic disease in a patient with normal renal function following diversion. Postradiotherapy strictures causing obstruction can be treated more vigorously and may well respond to dilatation (Fig. 9.20). Dilatation or stent insertion is done via an antegrade approach, as the ureteric orifices will be difficult if not impossible to see at cystoscopy.

Suggested staging protocol

Cystoscopy remains the technique of choice for initial staging of bladder tumours. If at cystoscopy the lesion is T1 or T2, endoscopic resection is performed and the upper tracts screened by excretory urography. If the lesion is evidently unresectable at cystoscopy, the tumour needs to be staged. To assess the extent of muscle wall involvement i.e. to distinguish T2 from T3A and T3B lesions, both intravesical US and MRI can be carried out. The rôle of CT is limited as it is unable to differentiate lesions lower than T3A from each other. T4 tumours can be imaged by both CT and MRI.

PROSTATIC MALIGNANCY

Clinico-pathological aspects

This neoplasm is the sixth commonest in the UK being the most common cancer of the male genitourinary tract (Chisholm 1985). In 1983, 9127 new cases were diagnosed (OPCS 1986) and there were 6910 deaths (OPCS unpublished). In the USA it is the second commonest cause of cancer death in men (Klein 1979). The tumour does carry a significant morbidity and mortality. Carcinoma of the prostate is rare before the age of 60, but

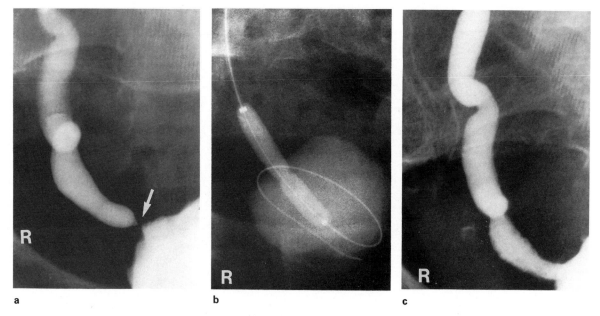

a   b   c

Fig. 9.20   (a) A tight ureteric stricture (arrow) causing obstruction to the patient's only kidney following radiotherapy for a T3 bladder tumour. Cystoscopy revealed no residual active tumour. The obstruction was initially treated with a percutaneous nephrostomy to decompress the upper tract. (b) The stricture has been bypassed with a guide wire following an antegrade approach and the stricture dilated with a balloon catheter. (c) Follow-up nephrostogram 7 days later shows considerable resolution of the stricture and some residual oedema of the urothelium following dilatation.

increases in frequency thereafter with a reported prevalence of up to two-thirds in one post mortem series with a mean presenting age of 80 years (Rullis et al 1975).

Periurethral glandular hyperplasia (prostatic hyperplasia (BPH)) is so common that it can be considered to be an inevitable consequence of puberty. Not surprisingly, benign and malignant prostatic disease often coexist, but the relationship between BPH and adenocarcinoma of the prostate appears to be coincidental (Armenian et al 1974). Although both conditions appear to be under the trophic influence of testosterone, carcinoma of the prostate usually originates in the peripheral zone of the prostate in the compressed prostate otherwise known as the surgical capsule. Carcinoma may, however, arise in any part of the prostate gland. It usually becomes symptomatic late in its natural history with symptoms which may be a consequence of bladder outflow obstruction or related to bony metastases. The diagnosis of carcinoma of the prostate can be suspected from a rectal examination, but is often and incidental finding at histological examination of a surgical resection.

Malignant neoplasms of the prostate are usually adenocarcinomas containing a variable proportion of epithelial and schirrous elements within them. Other rarer neoplasms include transitional cell carcinoma arising in prostatic ducts, lymphoma and squamous cell carcinoma. The prostate is a major site for the production of the enzyme acid phosphatase; this can be used as a serum marker for adenocarcinoma, bearing in mind that only 70% of patients with metastatic disease have elevated levels. Recent work has reported the usefulness of prostate specific antigen as an additional tumour-specific marker (Allhoff et al 1983). It must, however, be remembered that elevated serum levels of these 'markers' cannot be regarded to be pathognomic of the presence of prostatic cancer since it is well recognized that the elevation of enzyme can follow prostatic massage in the presence of benign prostatic disease.

Tumour behaviour

Adenocarcinoma of the prostate spreads via the perineural lymphatics, and early haematogenous spread is common via the prostatic venous plexus and vertebral veins to the bones of the pelvis, lumbar sacral spine and femurs.

Transitional cell carcinoma of the prostatic ducts is well recognized but is much less common that adenocarcinoma. It often occurs in association with other urothelial neoplasia but is a highly malignant condition carrying a poor prognosis and is best treated by early radical radiotherapy. Squamous carcinoma is rare (Mott 1979); and lymphomas in the prostate have also been reported.

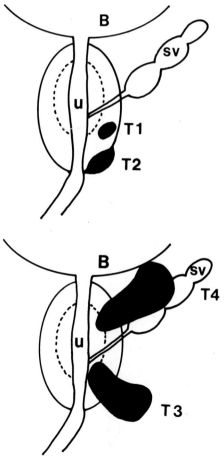

Fig. 9.21 TNM staging of prostate carcinoma. B = bladder; sv = seminal vesicle; u = urethra.

Tumour staging (Fig. 9.21 and Table 9.3)

The most widely used staging system for carcinoma of the prostate is based on the TNM classification.

The management of adenocarcinoma of the prostate is largely dependent on the stage of the tumour. Traditionally, staging has depended on clinical appraisal of the prostate gland by rectal examination.

Treatment options and prognosis

T0 and T1 adenocarcinoma of the prostate diagnosed as incidental pathological findings are best treated by surveillance, particularly if second-look transurethral resection of the prostate demonstrates no residual tumour. Local radiotherapy is used for the primary treatment of other early stage tumours confined to the prostate. A considerable divergence of opinion exists spanning the Atlantic as to the management of the T1, T2 group of patients. In North America and parts of Europe radical prostatectomy is favoured (Correa et al 1977, Hodges et al 1979), but it is rarely practiced in this country. Work contrasting these two therapeutic approaches suggests that radical surgery may carry a significant advantage over radiotherapy (Paulson et al 1982), but this still remains to be proven.

Table 9.3 TNM classification for staging prostatic carcinoma (UICC 1978)

Category T

T0	Incidental carcinoma found on histology
T1	Intracapsular carcinomatous nodule with a normal glandular outline
T2	Intracapsular carcinoma deforming the gland
T3	Carcinoma invading beyond the prostatic capsule
T4	Tumour fixed to adjacent organs

Category N

N0	No evidence of regional lymph node involvement
N1	Single ipsilateral lymph node
N2	Contralateral, bilateral or multiple regional lymph nodes
N3	Fixed regional lymph nodes
N4	Extension to juxtaregional lymph nodes

Category M

M0	No evidence of distant metastatic spread
M1	Distant metastases

The majority of patients have either locally advanced or metastatic disease at the time of first presentation. In one study 76 out of 100 consecutive patients had T2–T4 tumours and 61% of these had evident metastatic disease at the time of diagnosis (Chisholm 1981). This factor plays an important rôle in determining the ultimate prognosis of this condition. A significant proportion of adenocarcinomas of the prostate are sensitive to hormonal manipulation, which is the treatment of choice for locally advanced or metastatic disease. Hormonal manipulation involves a reduction in serum levels of testosterone by chemical or surgical means. The results of systemic chemotherapy are disappointing, although a combination of a nitrogen mustard and oestrogen (estramustine) can occasionally be beneficial. Palliative radiotherapy can be very helpful in the management of bone pain. Recent work has reported encouraging results from the implantation of radioactive gold grains or iridium wire into the prostate gland, producing high local levels of radioactivity (Fowler et al 1979). This raises important therapeutic potential for the accurate localization of these implants using radiological techniques.

Adenocarcinoma of the prostate is predominantly a disease of the elderly which presents late in its natural history. Considerable scope exists for earlier diagnosis which should have wide ranging effects in determining both treatment and the ultimate prognosis.

Radiological diagnosis and staging

Until US and CT were in common usage, there was no radiological method of imaging the prostate itself. EU indirectly gave some indication of prostatic size by the degree of elevation of the bladder base on the cystographic phase. Angiography played no rôle. Clinical staging consisting of digital rectal examination, per-rectal biopsy and bimanual examination is accurate in experienced hands as long as the tumour lies in the posterior lobe of the gland, but is not considered sufficiently accurate to determine the most appropriate treatment (Catalona & Stein 1982). Because clinical assessment is inaccurate, imaging techniques are being extensively studied to ascertain whether they can accurately detect and stage tumours, and can differentiate those confined to the prostate from those which are not. Prostate tumour is associated with obstructive lower tract symptoms and radiology plays a rôle in assessing the dynamic effect this may have on the bladder. The detection of nodal disease is facilitated by cross-sectional imaging, but lymphangiography is still performed. Osseous prostatic metastatic disease requires both plain films and isotope studies.

'T' staging

Traditionally, the prostate was divided anatomically into four lobes: posterior, middle, anterior and lateral. This concept of the prostate is now defunct. The prostate is divided into two separate components, the peripheral or posterior zone and the central or internal zone. The peripheral zone occupies the posterior, lateral and apical part of the gland and normally has a homogenous, isoechoic echo pattern on US. On CT, the peripheral zone is homogeneous and not discernible from the central zone. MRI with T_2-weighted sequences shows the peripheral zone as a high intensity structure, again homogeneous. The remainder of the prostate is the central part of the gland; it is glandular in nature and includes the urethra and the periurethral glands. On US, the central zone is heterogeneous and hyperechoic. It is heterogeneous on T_2-weighted MR images, though of lower signal intensity than the peripheral zone. Running between the peripheral and central zones is the corpora amylacea in which run the ejaculatory ducts. Calcification often occurs within the ducts and represents the apparent surgical capsule of the prostate down to which urologists resect during transurethral resection. Tumour commonly though not exclusively arises in the posterior part of the gland whilst benign hyperplasia originates in the central zone.

Patients with clinically suspected prostatic malignancy warrant an excretory urodynamogram which combines the EU with a flow rate which provides both anatomical and limited urodynamic assessment of the urinary tract (Turner-Warwick et al 1979). Upper tract dilatation complicating prostatomegaly may have a number of aetiological factors: elevation of the vesicoureteric junction and secondary obstruction to the distal ureters is one cause. The ureters as they pass between the seminal vesicles and the posterior bladder wall may be invaded by T4 prostatic tumours causing obstruction. Lastly, outflow tract obstruction can give rise to high pressure bladders which in turn may cause dilatation of the upper tracts. The degree of outflow obstruction can only be adequately assessed with full urodynamic studies, but the addition of a flow rate with the EU gives a rough idea of the efficiency of bladder emptying when combined with an immediate postmicturition film. Some information as to the anatomy of the bladder will also be seen on EU. The degree of bladder wall thickening, the presence of diverticulae which may be large and other complications of outflow tract obstruction, e.g. stones, will be seen. Prostate tumours commonly originate in the posterior aspect of the gland well away from the prostatic urethra. Small posteriorly situated tumours are unlikely to be associated with prostatic symptoms unless tumour coincides with benign prostatic hypertrophy which originates in the central part of the gland. Overall, EU has no real application in staging prostatic tumour or in detecting the tumour itself.

To distinguish non-invasively between T2 and the more extensive T3 and T4 lesions, US and CT have undergone extensive study (Van Engelshoven & Kreel 1979, Golimbu et al 1981, Kohri et al 1981). US probe technology has advanced rapidly. The prostate can be imaged using widely available sector or linear array probes via the suprapubic-transabdominal route using the full bladder as an acoustic window (Abu-Yousef & Narayana 1982b). There have been conflicting reports as to the accuracy of staging using this technique. One study suggested it was of no value (Greenberg et al 1982) whilst in another US compared favourably with pathological staging (Denkhaus et al 1983). The most recently published report studied 18 patients with prostatic carcinoma (Abu-Yousef & Narayana 1985). Tumour was accurately diagnosed in 95% and staged in 83% as opposed to accuracy in clinical staging of 56%. Carcinomas appeared as echogenic foci within the peripheral zone in all patients, with associated echolucent foci in 20%. Involvement of the seminal vesicles and bladder wall and capsular defects could be identified, permitting accurate staging.

Despite the reported accuracy of the non-invasive suprapubic approach, it has not attracted much attention and indeed the published series supporting its use as a staging method have been small. In contrast, transrectal US has been extensively studied following Watanabe's original report (Watanabe et al 1971). The echo pattern of prostatic carcinoma has been a source of confusion. The earliest cadaver studies by Brooman et al (1981) correctly diagnosed 6 cases of prostatic carcinoma in 35 specimens of rectum, bladder and prostate removed en bloc, but the echo patterns were not described. From the same group in a review article (Peeling & Griffiths 1984) prostate carcinoma was described as being exclusively echogenic and indistinguishable from intraprostatic calcification and prostatic inflammatory disease (Kohri et al 1981). The theory that all carcinomas may not be purely echogenic was first mooted by Rifkin et al (1983) who found that tumours were of mixed echogenicity in nearly 25% of their cases. It was stated, however, that tumours were never seen as echopoor areas. More recent studies have cast considerable doubt on this early work. Lee et al (1986) biopsied under transrectal US control 32 echopoor lesions in the peripheral zone of the gland to find that 22 of them proved to harbour tumour. The histological findings of 8 hyperechoic lesions fulfilling all the previously held criteria for tumour proved that these cases were benign disease. These findings were confirmed in a study of 44 prostate glands in vitro in which tumour was echopoor in 54%, slightly hypoechoic in 22% and not definable in 24% (Dahnert et al 1986): again no case of echogenic tumour was seen. The worry here is that 24% of tumours are isoechoic with normal peripheral zone echotexture.

In view of these conflicting reports, certain deductions can be made. Firstly, there is almost certainly a considerable overlap between the echo patterns of benign and malignant disease. It would seem that the newer US machines and recent probe technology may be partly responsible for the

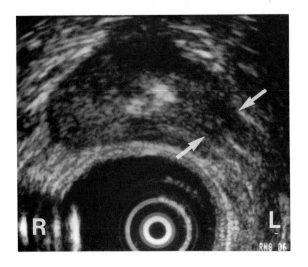

a

confusion. Whilst early reports suggested that tumour was echogenic, later reports suggest the opposite, perhaps because of the increased spatial resolution of the newer machines. The ability to detect small tumours has increased and it is these which appear as echopoor lesions. Once tumours enlarge they tend to become more echogenic (Rifkin et al 1986). Secondly, if in doubt a US-guided biopsy should be performed (Fig. 9.22). There is controversy as to the best method. The perineal approach under linear array transrectal US guidance is simple to perform. Initial infiltration of local anaesthetic under guidance with a 22 gauge needle down to the prostate capsule is followed by an 18 gauge trucut biopsy. The technique can be performed on an outpatient basis and may be complicated by transient

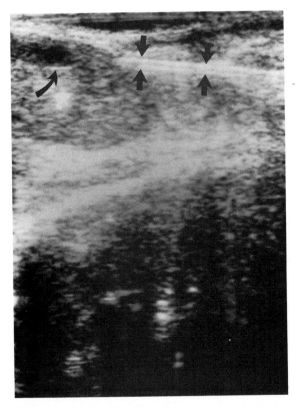

b

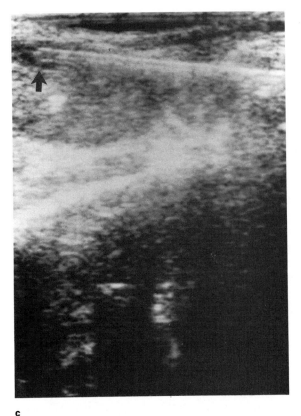

c

Fig. 9.22 (a) Transverse axial TRUS. There is an echopoor lesion in the left peripheral zone (arrows). (b) Sagittal TRUS confirming the presence of the echopoor lesion (curved arrow). The biopsy needle is seen approaching the lesion (straight arrows). (c) The tip of the biopsy needle is within the echopoor lesion after taking the biopsy. The lesion proved to be a poorly-differentiated adenocarcinoma.

haematuria. There is a move to perform transrectal biopsies under US guidance using special guides attached to the probe. This technique is more cumbersome than the perineal route and has more attendant complications, specifically infection. Thirdly, transrectal US is going to miss a significant number of tumours irrespective of the skill of the operator. This casts doubt on the use of the technique as a screening test for early carcinoma.

The ability of transrectal ultrasound to stage prostatic tumour is limited. T1 tumours can be differentiated from T2 tumours which deform the gland with the capsule intact. The strength of ultrasound is its ability to distinguish T2 from T3 tumours (Fig. 9.23), i.e. to detect those breaching the prostatic capsule with local extension into the seminal vesicles or bladder base. There is doubt that US is more accurate than CT in this respect (Rickards et al 1983), although minor degrees of capsular invasion do not appear to affect survival significantly (Sanders et al 1987). Seminal vesicle invasion is often difficult to discern by the transrectal route and may be more evident on suprapubic scanning. Certainly the high frequency probes used in transrectal scanning have limited depth penetration.

CT is unable to distinguish between benign and malignant disease confined to the prostate and so has no rôle in the staging of T1 or T2 tumours. Extracapsular spread into the periprostatic fat, seminal vesicles or bladder base or pelvic lymph node disease indicate T3 disease on CT (Fig. 9.24), but there are problems. Invasion of the seminal vesicle is important as it is associated with microscopic nodal involvement and hence a worse prognosis (Lange & Narayana 1983). CT was considered to be accurate in detecting seminal vesicle invasion, but Platt et al (1987) in a recent study demonstrated that filling in of the seminal vesicle angle was a poor sign of invasion. 23 observations of seminal vesicle involvement on CT were not confirmed by examination of the surgical specimens. Local invasion into the periprostatic fat was more accurate, but still had a low specificity (60%). Of all the signs analysed, CT was most accurate in the detection of involved lymph nodes, predominantly because of a high specificity (96%). Overall, CT has little rôle to

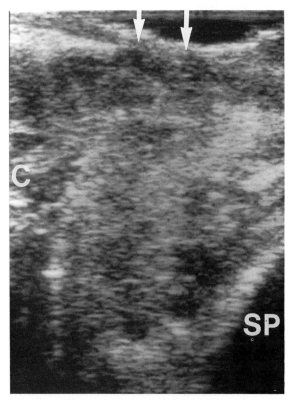

Fig. 9.23 TRUS of a T3 prostatic malignancy. The prostate is enlarged and there is infiltration of the anterior rectal wall (arrows). (SP = symphysis pubis; C = cranial).

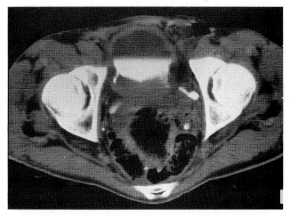

Fig. 9.24 CT scan of pelvis following IV contrast. There is infiltration of the posterior aspect of the bladder wall and involvement of the rectal wall. On CT, this prostatic tumour is T4.

play in the staging of prostatic tumour and is probably only useful in detecting unsuspected nodal involvement. It is useful in radiotherapy planning (see Ch. 18).

Of all imaging modalities, MRI is emerging as the single most accurate method for staging local disease extent and may indeed prove to be more accurate than transrectal US in diagnosing tumour confined to the prostate itself. It is evident that an extensive MRI protocol is needed encompassing T_1 and T_2-weighted images obtained in several planes. Such a protocol would take up to an hour to perform, making MRI a technique wholly inappropriate for the diagnosis of prostatic malignancy. There have been reports discussing tissue characterization by MRI and the concensus is that its rôle is limited (Bryan et al 1983, 1986, Ling et al 1986). There have been many reports on the staging ability of MRI and more criteria are employed for the diagnosis of extracapsular tumour spread, T3 lesions, than are used for CT. The periprostatic venous plexus appears as a high intensity linear structure on T_2-weighted images postero-laterally on each side of the gland. If this structure is not symmetrical or is of lower signal intensity than fat on T_2-weighted images, it is considered to be involved and to represent T3 disease. If the periprostatic fat differs in any way on any pulse sequence from subcutaneous fat, it is indicative of extracapsular spread. The seminal vesicles have a signal intensity similar to that of muscle on T_1-weighted images and similar to fat on T_2 sequences. If the seminal vesicles are enlarged or have a signal intensity lower than that of fat on T_2 images, they are considered to be involved. Using these criteria, Biondetti et al (1987) in a study of 29 patients with clinical stage T2 prostatic malignancy found abnormalities of the periprostatic venous plexus to be the most sensitive indicator for detecting extracapsular spread and periprostatic fat involvement to be the least sensitive. Overall, they found that MRI had an accuracy of 89% in differentiating T2 from T3 or T4 tumours. MRI has been compared to clinical and CT staging in a recent study of 46 patients who had undergone radical prostatectomy permitting accurate pathological staging (Hriack et al 1987). Of the 46 patients studied, 26 were confirmed to have T2 disease and 20 T3 disease. Clinical staging

achieved an accuracy of 61%. Using just T_1-weighted transverse sequences, MRI achieved an accuracy exactly comparable to clinical staging. When supplemented with T_2-weighted transverse and sagittal or coronal images, the accuracy rose to 83%. With the expanding MRI technology including the use of surface and intrarectal coils, MRI may prove to be the most accurate imaging modality for the staging of prostatic malignancy.

'N' staging

Lymphangiography is still performed in many centres for assessing nodes. The prostate is drained by two chains of nodes which in turn drain into the external iliac chain and these are generally accepted to be the first nodes involved in prostatic malignancy (Flocks et al 1959). They are opacified following bipedal lymphangiography (Zingg et al 1974). Defects within the nodes greater than 1 cm in diameter are highly reliable indicators of metastatic nodal disease, but nodal defects smaller than 5 mm in diameter will not be seen. If the lymphangiogram is equivocal due to areas of unilateral non-opacification suspicious of total nodal replacement, defects less than 1 cm in diameter or nodes with irregular outlines, then aspiration biopsy under radiological control with a 22 gauge Chiba needle is valuable (Dan et al 1982).

Lymphangiography is able to detect metastatic involvement in normal-sized nodes, unlike CT or MRI where the nodes are deemed to be involved if enlarged. For prostatic cancer, bipedal lymphangiography has a specificity of 92% and an overall accuracy of 78% (Spellman et al 1977). CT has been reported to have a specificity of 88% and an accuracy of 70–90% (Golimbu et al 1981, Morgan et al 1981). There are as yet no figures for MRI.

'M' staging

Prostate tumour metastasizes predominantly to bone; isotope scanning is discussed elsewhere.

Suggested staging protocol

The diagnosis of prostatic tumour is often made clinically or on examination of the chippings following transurethral resection for bladder outflow obstruction. If suspected clinically, transrectal US and a biopsy of any suspicious area should be carried out. If the tumour grade is low and the acid phosphatase normal, the patient needs a bone scan and a chest X-ray only. If there is US or clinical evidence that the tumour is likely to be T3 or worse, then the patient needs staging with a CT scan of the abdomen and pelvis, or if available an MRI scan. Lymphangiography should be performed if the CT scan is negative to ensure that the nodes are clear of metastatic involvement. If lymphangiography is equivocal a percutaneous aspiration biopsy can be done.

REFERENCES

Abeshouse B S, Goldstein A E 1941 Metastatic malignant tumours of the kidney – a review of the literature and report of 23 cases. Urologic and Cutaneous Review 45: 163–186

Abu-Yousef M M, Narayana A S 1982a Urinary bladder tumours studied by cystosonography. Radiology 153: 227–231

Abu-Yousef M M, Narayana A S 1982b Transabdominal ultrasound in the evaluation of prostatic size. Journal of Clinical Ultrasound 10: 275–278

Abu-Yousef M M, Narayana A S 1985 Prostatic carcinoma: detection and staging using suprapubic US. Radiology 156: 175–180

Abu-Yousef M M, Narayana A S, Brown R C 1984 Cystosonography in the evaluation of bullous cystitis: a catheter induced reaction. Radiology 151: 471–473

Affre J, Michel J R, de Peyronnet R, Deltour F, Moreau J F 1981 Secondary foci of primary tumours of the bladder in the upper urinary tract. Urologic Radiology 3: 7–12

Allhoff E P, Proppe K H, Chapman C M, Lin C W, Prout G R Jr 1983 Evaluation of prostate specific acid phosphatase and prostate specific antigen in the identification of prostatic cancer. Journal of Urology 129: 315–318

Altaffer L F, Chenault W 1979 Paraneoplastic endocrinopathies associated with renal tumours. Journal of Urology 122: 573–577

Amendola M A, Glazer G M, Grossman H B, Aisen A M, Francis I R 1986 Staging of bladder carcinoma: MRI–CT–surgical correlation. American Journal of Radiology 146: 1179–1183

Amis E S, Cronan J J, Pfister R C 1981 Filling defects in small bowel urinary conduits. American Journal of Radiology 137: 787–792

Armenian K H, Lilienfeld A M, Diamond E L, Brass I D J 1974 Relations between benign prostatic hyperplasia and cancer of the prostate. Lancet 2: 115–117

Babaian R J, Skinner D G, Waisman J 1980 Wilms' tumour in the adult patient. Diagnosis, management and review of the world medical literature. Cancer 45: 1713–1719

Baron R L, McLennan B L, Lee J K T, Lawson T L 1982 Computed tomography of the renal pelvis and ureter. Radiology 144: 125–130

Beckwith J B, Palmer N F 1978 Histopathology and prognosis of Wilms' cancer. Cancer 41: 1937–1948

Bennington L F, Beckwith J B 1975 Tumours of the kidney, renal pelvis and ureter. Atlas of tumour pathology, 2nd series, Fascicle 12. Armed Forces Institute of Pathology, Washington, pp 94–99

Best B G 1987 Renal carcinoma: a ten-year review, 1971–80. British Journal of Urology 60: 100–102

Biondetti P R, Lee J K T, Ling D, Catalona W J 1987 Clinical stage B prostatic carcinoma: staging with MR imaging. Radiology 162: 325–329

Bloom H J G 1967 The kidney. In: Raven R, Roe F J C (eds) The prevention of cancer. Butterworths, London, pp 220–235

Bloom H J G, Hendry W F 1982 Influence of hormones on the kidney. In: Chisholm G D, Williams D I (eds) Scientific foundations of urology. Heinemann, London, pp 684–690

Bosniak M A 1986 The current radiological approach to renal cysts. Radiology 158: 1–10

Bowman H S, Martinez E J 1968 Fever, anaemia and hyperhaptoglobinaemia, an extra-renal trail of hypernephroma. Annals of Internal Medicine 68: 613–620

Bracken B, Johnson K 1979 How accurate is angiographic staging of renal carcinoma? Urology 14: 96–99

Brooman P J, Peeling W B, Griffiths G J, Roberts B, Evans K 1981 A comparison between digital examination and per-rectal ultrasound in the evaluation of the prostate. British Journal of Urology 53: 617–620

Bryan P J, Butler H E, LiPuma J P 1983 NMR scanning of the pelvis: initial experience with a 0.3 T system. American Journal of Radiology 141: 111–118

Bryan P J, Butler H E, Nelson A D et al 1986 Magnetic resonance imaging of the prostate. American Journal of Radiology 146: 543–546

Catalona W J, Stein A J 1982 Staging errors in clinically localised prostatic cancer. Journal of Urology 127: 452–456

Charboneau J W, Hattery R R, Ernst E C, James E M, Williamson B, Hartman G W 1983 Spectrum of sonographic findings in 125 renal masses other than benign renal cysts. American Journal of Radiology 140: 87–94

Chisholm G D 1981 Perspectives and prospects. In: Dunkin W (ed) Recent results in cancer research, prostate cancer. Springer-Verlag, Heidelberg, 78: 173–184

Chisholm G D 1985 Carcinoma of the prostate. In Whitfield H N, Hendry W F (eds) Textbook of genitourinary surgery. Churchill Livingstone, Edinburgh, pp 1001–1018

Chisholm G D, Roy R R 1971 Systemic effects of malignant renal tumours. British Journal of Urology 43: 687–700

Choyke P L, Kressel H Y, Pollack H, Arger P M, Axel L, Mamourian A C 1984 Focal renal masses: magnetic resonance imaging. Radiology 152: 471–477

Chuang V P 1979 Non-operative removal of Gianturco coils from abdominal aorta. American Journal of Radiology 132: 996–997

Clayman R V, Gonzalez R, Fralay E E 1980 Renal cell cancer invading the inferior vena cava. Clinical review and anatomical approach. Journal of Urology 123: 157–163

Coleman B G, Arger P H, Mulhern C B, Pollack H M,

Banner M P, Arenson R L 1980 Gray scale ultrasonic spectrum of hypernephromas. Radiology 137: 757

Correa R J Jr, Gibbons R P, Cummings K B, Mason J T 1977 Total prostatectomy for Stage B carcinoma of the prostate. Journal of Urology 117: 328–329

Cox G G, Rak Lee K, Price H J 1982 Colonic infarction following ethanol embolisation for renal carcinoma. Radiology 145: 343–345

Cronan J J, Zeman R K, Rosenfeld A T 1982 Comparison of computed tomography, ultrasound and angiography in the detction of renal cell carcinoma. Journal of Urology 127: 712–714

Curry N S, Schabel S I, Betsill W L 1986 Small renal neoplasms: Diagnostic imaging, pathological features and clinical course. Radiology 158: 113–117

Dahnert W F, Hamper U M, Eggleston M D, Walsh P C, Sanders R C 1986 Prostatic evaluation by transrectal sonography with histological correlation: the echopenic appearance of early carcinoma. Radiology 158: 97–102

Dan S J, Efremidis S C, Train J S, Cohen B A, Mitty H A 1982 Equivocal lymphogram and lymph node aspiration: importance in staging carcinoma of the prostate. Urologic Radiology 4: 215–219

D'Angio G J, Evans A E, Breslow N et al 1976 The treatment of Wilm's tumour. Results of the national Wilm's tumour study. Cancer 38: 633–646.

Daniel W W, Hartman G, Witten D M, Farrow G M, Kelasis P P 1972 Calcified renal masses: a review of 10 years' experience at the Mayo clinic. Radiology 103: 503–508

Davies J M 1985 Incidence of urological tumours. In: Whitfield H N, Hendry W F (eds) Textbook of genitourinary surgery. Churchill Livingstone, Edinburgh, vol 2, pp 885–890

Demos C T, Schiffer M, Love L 1985 Normal excretory urography in patients with primary kidney neoplasms. Urologic Radiology 7: 75–79

Denkhaus H, Dierkopf W, Grabbe E, Donn F 1983 Comparative study of suprapubic sonography and computed tomography for staging of prostatic carcinoma. Urologic Radiology 5: 1–9

Denkhaus H, Crone-Munzebrock W, Huland H 1985 Non-invasive ultrasound in detecting and staging bladder carcinoma. Urologic Radiology 7: 121–131

Devonec M, Chapelon J Y, Codas H, Dubernard J M, Revillard J P, Cathignol D 1987 Evaluation of bladder cancer with a miniature high frequency transurethral ultrasonography probe. British Journal of Radiology 59: 550–553

Dubbins P A, Wells I 1986 Renal carcinoma: Duplex Doppler evaluation. British Journal of Radiology 59: 231–236

Ellman B A, Parkill B J, Curry T S 1981 Ablation of renal tumours with absolute ethanol: a new technique. Radiology 141: 619–626

Ekelund L, Karp W, Mansson W, Olsson R 1981 Palliative embolisation of renal tumours: follow-up of 19 cases. Urologic Radiology 3: 13–18

Fairlamb D J 1981 Spontaneous regression of metastases of renal cancer. Cancer 37: 2102–2106

Farrah R N, Cerny J C 1978 Lymphangiography in staging patients with carcinoma of the bladder. Journal of Urology 119: 40–41

Fletcher M S, Packham A D, Pryor J P, Yates Bell A J 1981 Hepatic dysfunction in renal carcinoma. British Journal of Urology 53: 533–536

Flocks R H, Culp D, Porto R 1959 Lymphatic spread from prostatic cancer. Journal of Urology 81: 194–196

Forbes W S C, Isherwood I, Fawcitt R A 1978 Computed tomography in the evaluation of the solitary or unilateral nonfunctioning kidney. Journal of Computer Assisted Tomography 2: 389–394

Foss L G 1975 Tumours of the urinary bladder. Atlas of tumour pathology, 2nd series, Fascicle 2 Armed Forces Institute of Pathology, Washington

Fowler J E Jr, Barrell W, Hilaris B S, Whitmore W F 1979 Complications of ^{125}I implantation and pelvic lymphadenectomy in the treatment of prostatic cancer. Journal of Urology 121: 447–451

Golimbu M, Morales P, Al-Askari S, Shulman Y 1981 CAT scanning in staging of prostatic cancer. Urology 18: 305–308

Greenberg M, Nieman H L, Vogelzang R, Falkowski W 1982 Ultrasonic features of prostatic carcinoma. Journal of Clinical Ultrasound 10: 307–312

Greene L F, Rosenthal M H 1951 Multiple hypernephroma of the kidney in association with Lindom's disease. New England Journal of Medicine 244: 633–634

Grossman H B 1979 Current therapy of bladder carcinoma. Journal of Urology 121: 1–7

Hammond D, Winnick S 1974 Paraneoplastic erythrocytosis and ectopic erythropoietins. Annals of the New York Academy of Science 230: 219–227

Hillman B J, Silvert M, Cook G et al 1981 Recognition of bladder tumours by excretory urography. Radiology 138: 319–323

Hodges C V, Pearce H D, Stille L 1979 Radical prostatectomy for carcinoma: 30-year experience and 15-year survivals. Journal of Urology 122: 180–182

Hollifield J W, Page D L, Smith C, Michelakis A M, Staab E, Rhamy R 1975 Renin secreting clear cell carcinoma of the kidney. Archives of Internal Medicine 135: 859–864

Hriack H, Alpers C, Crooks L E, Sheldon P E 1983a Magnetic resonance imaging of the normal female pelvis: initial experience. American Journal of Radiology 141: 1119–1128

Hriack H, Williams R D, Moon K L et al 1983b Nuclear magnetic resonance imaging of the kidney: Renal masses. Radiology 147: 765–772

Hriack H, Demas B E, Williams R D et al 1985 Magnetic resonance imaging in the diagnosis and staging of renal and perirenal neoplasms. Radiology 154: 709–715

Hriack H, Dooms G C, Jeffrey R B et al 1987 Prostatic carcinoma: staging by clinical assessment, CT and MR imaging. Radiology 162: 331–336

Jeager N, Radeke H W, Vahlensieck W 1985 Diagnosis of urinary bladder cancer by transurethral sonography. Urology and Nephrology 78: 323–329

Jagasia K H, Thurman W G 1965 Wilms' tumour in the adult. Archives of Internal Medicine 115: 322–325

Jewett H J, Strong G H 1946 Infiltrating carcinoma of the bladder: relation of depth of penetration of the bladder wall to incidence of local extension and metastases. Journal of Urology 55: 366–372

Jing B, Wallace S, Zornoza J 1982 Metastases of the retroperitoneum and pelvic lymph nodes. Computed tomography and lymphangiography. Radiological Clinics of North America 20: 511–530

Johnson C D, Dunnick N R, Cohan R J, Illescas F F 1987 Renal adenocarcinoma: CT staging of 100 tumours. American Journal of Radiology 148: 59–63

Johnson R J 1987 Magnetic resonance imaging in carcinoma of the bladder. British Journal of Radiology 60: 946

Jung A, Schneider P H, Miller R, Walton R J 1976 Hypercalcaemia and parathyroid hyperplasia associated with renal adenocarcinoma. Postgraduate Medical Journal 52: 106–108

Kato T, Memoto R, Mori H, Takahashi M, Tamakawa T 1981 Transcatheter arterial chemoembolisation of renal cell carcinoma with microencapsulated mitomycin C. Journal of Urology 125: 19–24

Kellett M J, Oliver R T D, Husband J E, Kelsey Fry I 1980 Computed tomography as an adjunct to bimanual examination for staging bladder carcinoma. British Journal of Urology 52: 101–106

Khorsand D 1965 Carcinoma with solitary renal cysts. Journal of Urology 93: 440–444

Klein L A 1979 Prostatic carcinoma. New England Journal of Medicine 300: 824–833

Kohri K, Kaneko S, Akiyama T, Yachiku S, Kurita T 1981 Ultrasonic evaluation of prostatic carcinoma. Urology 17: 214–217

Kumar R, Amparo E G, David R, Fagan C J, Morettin L B 1984 Adult Wilms' tumour: clinical and radiographic features. Urologic Radiology 6: 164–169

Lalli A F, Petersen N, Bookstein J J 1969 Roentgen-guided infarction of the kidneys and lungs. A potential therapeutic technique. Radiology 93: 434–435

Lang E K 1966 The differential diagnosis of renal cysts and tumours. Radiology 87: 883–888

Lang E K 1984 Comparison of dynamic and conventional computed tomography, angiography and ultrasonography in the staging of renal cell carcinoma. Cancer 54: 2205–2214

Lang E K, Sullivan J, DeKernion J B 1983 Work in progress: transcatheter embolisation of renal cell carcinoma with radioactive infarct particles. Radiology 147: 413–418

Lange P H, Narayana P 1983 Understaging and undergrading of prostatic cancer. Urology 21: 113–118

Lee J K T, Rholl K S 1986 MRI of the bladder and prostate. American Journal of Radiology 147: 732–736

Lee J K T, McClennan B L, Stanley R J, Levitt R G, Sagel S S 1981 Utility of CT in evaluation of post-cystectomy patients. American Journal of Radiology 136: 483–487

Lee F, Gray J M, McCleary R D et al 1986 Prostatic evaluation by transrectal sonography: criteria for diagnosis of early carcinoma. Radiology 158: 91–95

Leung A W L, Bydder G M, Steiner R E, Bryant D J, Young I R 1984 Magnetic resonance imaging of the kidneys. American Journal of Radiology 143: 1215–1227

Lieber M M, Tomera K M, Farrow G M 1981 Renal oncocytoma. Journal of Urology 125: 481–485

Ling D, Lee J K T, Heiken J P, Balfe D M, Glazer H S, McClennan B L 1986 Prostatic carcinoma and benign prostatic hyperplasia: inability of MR imaging to distinguish between the two diseases. Radiology 158: 103–107

Lloyd L K, Witten D M, Bueschen A T, Daniel W 1978 Enhanced detection of asymptomatic renal masses with routine tomography during excretory urography. Urology 11: 523–528

Mancilla-Jimenez R, Stanley R J, Blath R A 1976 Papillary renal cell carcinoma. Cancer 38: 2469–2480

Marshall F F 1980 The rôle of selective exploration in ambiguous renal cystic lesions. Urological Clinics of North America 7: 689–695

Mauro M L, Wadsworth D E, Stanley R J, McLennan B L 1982 Renal cell carcinoma: angiography in the CT era. American Journal of Radiology 139: 1135–1138

Mazeman E 1976 Tumours of the upper tract calyces, renal pelvis and ureter. European Urology 2: 120–128

McCorron J P, Marshall V F 1979 The survival of patients with bladder tumours treated by surgery: comparative results of an old and recent series. Journal of Urology 122: 322–324

McDonald M W 1982 Current therapy for renal cell carcinoma. Journal of Urology 127: 211–217

McIvor J, Williams E, Southcott R D C 1982 Control of severe vesicle haemorrhage by therapeutic embolisation. Clinical Radiology 33: 561–567

McLaughlin I S, Morley P, Deanne R F, Barnett E, Graham A G, Kyle K F 1975 Ultrasound in the staging of bladder tumours. British Journal of Urology 47: 51–56

Melicow M M 1945 Tumours of the urinary drainage tract: urothelial tumours. Journal of Urology 54: 186–193

Melicow M M 1974 Tumours of the bladder: a multivocal problem. Journal of Urology 112: 467–478

Middleton, A W Jr 1980 Indications for and results of nephrectomy for metastatic renal cell carcinoma. Urological Clinics of North America 7: 711–717

Miller A, Mitchell J P, Brown N J 1969 The Bristol bladder tumour registry. British Journal of Urology 41 (suppl): 1–64

Morgan C L, Calkins R F, Cavalcanti E J 1981 Computed tomography in the evaluation, staging and therapy of carcinoma of the bladder and prostate. Radiology 140: 751–761

Morrison A S 1984 Advances in the aetiology of urothelial cancer. Urological Clinics of North America 11: 4: 557–566

Mostofi F K 1979 Tumours of the renal parenchyma. In: Churg J (ed) Kidney disease – present status. International Academy of Pathology Monograph vol 20. Williams and Wilkins, Baltimore, pp 356–412

Mott L J M 1979 Squamous cell carcinoma of the prostate. Report of two cases and a review of the literature. Journal of Urology 121: 833–835

Murphy J B, Marshall F F 1980 Renal cyst versus tumour: a continuing dilemma. Journal of Urology 123: 566–569

Myers J H Jr, Fehrenbaher L G, Kelalis P P 1968 Prognostic significance of renal vein invasion by hypernephroma. Journal of Urology 100: 420–423

Nadel N, Baumgartner B R, Bernardino E 1986 Percutaneous renal biopsies: accuracy, safety and indications. Urologic Radiology 8: 67–71

Nakamura S, Niijima T 1980 Staging of bladder cancer by ultrasonography: a new technique by transurethral intravesical scanning. Journal of Urology 124: 341–344

Office of Population Censuses and Surveys. Cancer statistics – registrations England and Wales for 1983: 1986, Series MBI 15. HMSO, London

Office of Population Censuses and Surveys. Mortality statistics, England and Wales for 1986: 1987 Unpublished data. HMSO, London

Ogata J, Migita N, Nakamura T 1973 Treatment of carcinoma of the bladder by the infusion of the anti-cancer agent (mitomycin D) via the internal iliac artery. Journal of Urology 110: 667–670

Page B H, Levison V B, Curwen M P 1978 Site of recurrence of non-infiltrating bladder tumours. British Journal of Urology 50: 237–242

Papanicolaou N, Hahn P F, Edelman R et al 1986 Magnetic

resonance imaging of the kidney. Urologic Radiology 8: 139–150

Parienty R A, Pradel J, Parienty I 1985 Cystic renal cancers. CT characteristics. Radioloy 157: 741–744

Patel N P, Lavengood R W 1978 Renal cell carcinoma: natural history and results of treatment. Journal of Urology 119: 722–726

Paulson D F, Lin G H, Hinshaw W, Stephani S and the Uro-Oncology Research Group 1982 Radical surgery versus radiotherapy for adenocarcinoma of the prostate. Journal of Urology 128: 502–504

Pavone-Macalusco M 1967 Aetiology of kidney tumours. In: King J S (ed) Renal neoplasia. Little Brown, Boston, pp 247–300

Peeling W B, Griffiths G J 1984 Imaging of the prostate by ultrasound, review article. Journal of Urology 132: 217–224

Pilepich M V, Perez C A 1982 Does radiotherapy alter the course of genitourinary cancer? In: Paulson D F (ed) Genitourinary cancer. Martinus Nijhoff, Boston, pp 215–238

Platt J F, Bree R L, Schwab R E 1987 The accuracy of CT in the stanging of carcinoma of the prostate. American Journal of Radiology 149: 315–318

Press G A, McClennan B L, Melson G L, Weyman P J, Mauro M A, Lee J K T 1984 Papillary renal cell carcinoma: CT and sonographic evaluation. American Journal of Radiology 143: 1005–1009

Rawlins M D, Luff R H, Cranston W I 1970 Pyrexia in renal carcinoma. Lancet 1: 1371–1373

Richie J P, Skinner D G, Kaufmann J J 1975 Carcinoma of the bladder. Treatment by radical cystectomy. Journal of Surgical Research 18: 271–278

Rickards D, Gowland M, Brooman P, Mamtora H, Blacklock N J, Isherwood I 1983 Computed tomography and transrectal ultrasound in the diagnosis of prostatic disease: a comparative study. British Journal of Urology 55: 726–732

Riddle P R, Chisholm G D, Trott P A, Pugh R C B 1976 Flat carcinoma in situ of the bladder. British Journal of Urology 47: 829–833

Rifkin M D, Kurtz A B, Choi H Y, Goldberg B B 1983 Endoscopic ultrasonic evaluation of the prostate using a transrectal probe: prospective evaluation and acoustic characterisation. Radiology 149: 265–271

Rifkin M D, Friedland G W, Shortliffe L 1986 Prostatic evaluation by transrectal endosonography: detection of carcinoma. Radiology 158: 85–90

Rullis I, Schaeffer J A, Lilien O M 1975 Incidence of prostatic carcinoma in the elderly. Urology 6: 295–297

Salo J O, Kivisaari L, Lehtonen T 1985 CT in determining the depth of infiltration of bladder tumours. Urologic Radiology 7: 88–93

Sanders R C, Hamper U M, Dahnert W F 1987 Update on prostatic ultrasound. Urologic Radiology 9: 110–118

Schmidt J D, Weinstein S H 1976 Pitfalls in the clinical staging of bladder tumours. Urological Clinics of North America 3: 107–127

Schwerk W B, Schwerk W N, Rodeck G 1985 Venous renal tumour extension: A prospective ultrasound evaluation. Radiology 156: 491–495

Singer D, Itzchak Y, Fischelovitch Y 1981 Ultrasonographic assessment of bladder tumours. II Clinical staging. Journal of Urology 126: 34–36

Smith D R 1981 Tumours of the genitourinary tract. In:

Smith D R (ed) General urology. Lange Medical Publications, California, pp 271–353

Smith R B 1981 Long term survival of a vena caval recurrence of renal cell carcinoma. Journal of Urology 125: 575–578

Spellman M C, Castellino R A, Ray G R 1977 An evaluation of lymphography in localised carcinoma of the prostate. Radiology 125: 639–645

Totty W G, McLennan B L, Nelson G L, Patel R 1981 Relative value of computerised tomography and ultrasonography in the assessment of renal angiomyolipoma. Journal of Computer Assisted Tomography 5: 173–178

Thomas J L, Bernardino M E 1981 Neoplastic-induced renal vein enlargement: sonographic detection. American Journal of Roentgenology 136: 75–79

Turner-Warwick R T, Whiteside C G, Milroy E J G, Pengelly A W, Thompson D T 1979 The intravenous urodynamogram. British Journal of Urology 51: 15–18

Ueda T, Mihara Y 1987 Incidental detection of renal carcinoma during radiological imaging. British Journal of Urology 59: 513–515

Urine Internationale Contre Cancer (UICC) 1978 TNM classification of malignant tumours. UICC, Geneva

Van Engelshoven J M A, Kreel L 1979 Computed tomography of the prostate. Journal of Computer Assisted Tomography 3: 45–51

Vock P, Haertel M, Fuchs W A, Karrer P, Bishop M C, Singg E J 1982 Computed tomography in staging carcinoma of the urinary bladder. British Journal of Urology 54: 158–163

Wadsworth D E, McClennan B L, Stanley R J 1982 CT of the renal mass. Urologic Radiology 4: 85–94

Walzer A, Werner S N, Koenigsberg M 1980 The ultrasound appearance of tumour extension into the left renal vein and inferior vena cava. Journal of Urology 123: 945–946

Watanabe H, Kaiho H, Tanaka M, Terasawa Y 1971 Diagnostic applications of ultrasonotomography to the prostate. Investigations in Urology 8: 548–559

Webb J A W, Murray A, Bary P R, Hendry W F 1987 The accuracy and limitations of ultrasound in the assessment of venous extension in renal carcinoma. British Journal of Urology 60: 14–17

Weyman P L, McClennan B L, Stanley R J, Levitt R G, Sagel S S 1980 Comparison of computed tomography and angiography in the evaluation of renal cell carcinoma. Radiology 137: 417–424

Wiley A L, Wirtanan G W, Joo P et al 1975 Clinical and theoretical aspects of the treatment of surgically unresectable retroperitoneal malignancy with combined intra-arterial actinomycin D and radiotherapy. Cancer 36: 107–122

Williams C B, Mitchell J P 1973a Carcinoma of the renal pelvis – a review of 43 cases. British Journal of Urology 45: 370–376

Williams C B, Mitchell J P 1973b Carcinoma of the ureter – a review of 54 cases. British Journal of Urology 45: 377–387

Woodhouse C R J, Hendry W F, Blood H J G 1985 Renal carcinoma. In: Whitfield H N, Hendry W F (eds) Textbook of genitourinary surgery. Churchill Livingstone, Edinburgh, pp 945–961

Woodhouse C R J, Kellett M J, Bloom H J G 1986

Percutaneous renal surgery and local radiotherapy in the management of renal pelvic transitional cell carcinoma. British Journal of Urology 58: 245–249

Zingg B J, Fuchs W A, Heritier P, Gothlin J 1974 Lymphography in carcinoma of the prostate. Journal of

Urology 46: 549–554

Zirinsky K, Auh Y H, Rubenstein W A, Williams J J, Pasmantier M W, Kaxman E 1984 CT of the hyperdense renal cysts: sonographic correlation. American Journal of Radiology 143: 151–156

10. The testes

J. E. Husband

INTRODUCTION

Evaluation of patients with testicular tumours is an exciting and rewarding area of oncology and one which is a considerable challenge to the radiologist. Although rare, these tumours are important because they predominantly affect young men at a time of heavy responsibility and cure can be achieved in a high proportion of patients. Dramatic improvements in treatment results are mainly due to the introduction of effective chemotherapeutic agents but accurate methods of assessing disease with the use of serum markers and imaging techniques have also made a striking impact.

The radiologist's assessment is critical to appropriate management and he/she must have a detailed knowledge of the pattern of tumour spread and of the advantages and limitations of the techniques employed for tumour detection. Better understanding of tumour behaviour and treatment response has led to an appreciation of the importance of tumour volume as a prognostic indicator (Tyrrell & Peckham 1976, Einhorn & Donohue 1977). In patients with small volume metastatic disease – stages IM, IIA, IIB, IIIA, IIIB, IVAL1, IVAL2, IVBL1 and IVBL2 as defined by the MRC Working Party on testicular tumours (1985), see Table 10.2 – cure rates approaching 100% are obtained whereas in those patients with bulky advanced disease the prognosis is less favourable (Peckham et al 1979, Ball et al 1982, Peckham et al 1983). The major responsibility of the radiologist is, therefore, to identify small volume metastases at the earliest opportunity, but even in those patients with obvious advanced spread accurate information regarding extent of disease is also essential. Following initial staging radiology plays an integral rôle in follow-up, not only to document treatment response but also to determine operability following chemotherapy in selected patients and to identify relapse.

The incidence of testicular tumours varies considerably in different parts of the world. They are most frequently seen in Northern Europe and the white population of the United States where approximately 4–5/100 000 of the population are affected. In the United Kingdom the incidence is about 2.5/100 000 (Muir & Nectoux 1979). The aetiology of these tumours remains obscure but testicular maldescent is a known predisposing factor in about 5–10% of patients (Mostofi & Price 1973). Other abnormalities linked with testicular tumours include congenital abnormalities of the urinary tract. Thus, not infrequently, initial staging investigations reveal renal abnormalities such as a horseshoe kidney, or congenital pelviureteric junction obstruction which was previously unrecognized.

The histology of testicular cancer varies as does the age at presentation and sensitivity to drugs and irradiation. The majority of tumours are of germ cell origin. These include seminomas which are the most common histological type, accounting for 40.2% of the British Testicular Tumour Panel Series, teratomas accounting for 31.4% and combined tumours with seminomatous and teratomatous elements accounting for 14.3%. Yolk sac tumours of childhood are also considered to be of germ cell origin but are rare. Other rare tumours arising from the testis include malignant lymphoma, Sertoli cell tumours, Leydig (interstitial) cell tumours and paratesticular embryonal sarcomas of childhood (Pugh 1976).

Malignant teratomas may arise from stem cells or from true differentiated cells and are therefore subclassified according to cell type. The British Testicular Tumour Panel nomenclature used in this text is shown in Table 10.1 together with the American classification.

The radiology of the most common tumours, seminoma and malignant teratoma, is discussed in this text. Seminomas differ from malignant teratomas in several ways. The peak age at presentation of seminoma is 35 to 40 years whereas malignant teratoma presents earlier, most frequently between 25 and 30 years. Seminomas tend to present at an early stage of disease and more than 70% of patients are stage I at the time of orchidectomy (Kademian et al 1976, Calman et al 1979). Malignant teratomas present either with early or advanced disease; approximately 50% of patients with malignant teratomas are stage I at presentation (Peckham 1981).

Seminomas are very radiosensitive which explains the excellent results of radiotherapy for early stage disease. Before the advent of chemotherapy the prognosis of patients with Stage III and IV disease was extremely poor. However, increasing improvements are now being made with the use of platinum-based combination chemotherapy (Peckham et al 1985, van Oosterom et al 1986).

Malignant teratoma may produce the serum markers human chorionic gonadotrophin (βHCG)

and alphafetoprotein (AFP). These markers are highly sensitive indicators of the presence of active tumour and are produced by metastases as well as by the primary tumour. Raised levels of AFP are more frequently seen than raised levels of βHCG. In patients with raised markers prior to orchidectomy and no metastatic disease the serum marker levels rapidly return to normal following surgery. In patients with metastases, however, serum markers often remain elevated, only falling when disease is under control. Since not all teratomas produce serum markers they are only of value in about 80% of these patients.

Testicular teratomas are less radiosensitive than seminomas. Treatment options include combination chemotherapy for all stages of metastatic disease and radiotherapy for early stage tumours, and in some centres radical lymphadenectomy is undertaken at the time of staging. At the Royal Marsden Hospital, combination chemotherapy (incorporating cis-platin or carbo-platin) is now used for all stages of metastatic disease with increasingly effective results and long term survival is achieved in 75–90% of all patients (Peckham et al 1983, Einhorn et al 1985). In the USA staging lymphadenectomy is frequently performed for patients with testicular teratomas (Johnson et al 1976). However, the procedure carries high morbidity and in the majority of patients who have no metastases in the retroperitoneal nodes it has no therapeutic value.

In the group of patients considered to have Stage I disease by clinical staging methods, approximately 20–30% harbour microscopic deposits in the retroperitoneal nodes (Kademian & Wirtanen 1977). Until recently all stage I patients received radiotherapy at the Royal Marsden Hospital but since chemotherapy is curative in patients with small volume disease a surveillance policy has been introduced whereby treatment is only given to those patients who relapse following orchidectomy alone (Peckham et al 1982). Stringent criteria for entering into such a surveillance policy are observed and radiology plays an essential rôle in observation of these patients.

Table 10.1 Classification of testicular tumours

British Testicular Tumour Panel	American
Seminoma	Seminoma
Teratoma	
Teratoma differentiated (TD)	Teratoma
Malignant teratoma intermediate (MTI)	Teratocarcinoma
Malignant teratoma undifferentiated (MTU)	Embryonal carcinoma
Malignant teratoma trophoblastic (MTT)	Choriocarcinoma
Combined tumour	
Yolk sac tumour (orchioblastoma)	

Other: Sertoli cell
      Leydig cell
      Lymphoma	

PATTERN OF TUMOUR SPREAD

Testicular teratomas may spread by direct infiltration of adjacent tissues but this is uncommon since the tunica provides an effective barrier against direct extension unless scrotal surgery has been undertaken. Spread from the primary site predominantly occurs by way of the lymphatic system and by the haematogenous routes.

Lymphatic spread occurs via four to eight effluent lymphatic vessels which pass from the mediastinum of the testis along the spermatic cord to the internal inguinal ring. From here the lymphatics follow the spermatic blood vessels to the point where they cross the ureters. The lymphatics then spread out and enter the retroperitoneal lymph nodes. Right-sided tumours spread to the interaortic/caval nodes, the precaval, para-aortic, paracaval and then to the right common iliac and right external iliac nodes. Approximately 20% of patients show crossover with involvement of left-sided nodes (Ray et al 1974, Dixon et al 1986, Bradey et al 1987). Left-sided tumours rarely show crossover and primarily spread to the left para-aortic nodes, the pre-aortic nodes and then to the left common iliac and left external iliac nodes. The upper para-aortic nodes just below the renal vessels are more commonly involved than the lower para-aortic nodes in left-sided tumours, but in right-sided tumours nodes may be seen any-where between the renal hilum and the aortic bifurcation (Figs. 10.1 and 10.2).

In addition to these sites spread may occur directly to the so-called 'echelon' node first described by Rouviere in 1932. This node is situated on the right, lateral to the para-aortic nodes between the level of the first and third lumbar vertebrae. This 'echelon' or sentinel node has been demonstrated at lymphography by cannulating the spermatic cord at the time of orchidectomy (Chiappa et al 1966). Although the technique has been useful for confirming the anatomy of the lymphatic vessels it has no place in routine clinical staging. There is also evidence that an 'echelon' node exists on the left (Macdonald & Paxton 1976).

The distribution of involved nodes in testicular tumours was studied by Wilkinson & Macdonald (1975). They found that in 71% of patients the involved nodes were on the ipsilateral side to the tumour, 9% had involvement of the contralateral side only and 20% showed bilateral involvement. Recently, Dixon et al (1986) reported an analysis of the pattern of lymph node involvement as demonstrated by CT. In this series contralateral involvement without ipsilateral disease was not seen. They suggest that the differences in their

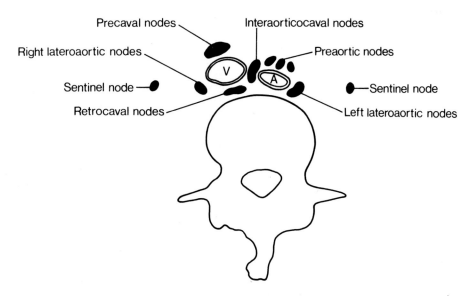

Fig. 10.1 Diagram to show the position of retroperitoneal nodes in cross-section at the level of the second lumbar vertebra. A = aorta; V = inferior vena cava.

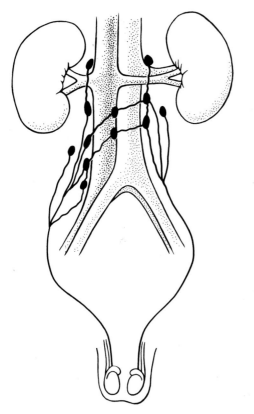

Fig. 10.2 Diagram to show the pattern of lymphatic spread of testicular tumours to the retroperitoneal nodes.

results compared with Wilkinson and Macdonald (1975), who analysed lymphographic findings, may be due to the demonstration of involved ipsilateral sentinel nodes with CT which are not opacified at lymphography.

Supradiaphragmatic spread from testicular cancer occurs by lymphatic and haematogenous pathways. Tumour spread via the thoracic duct may lead to involvement of the supraclavicular and superior mediastinal nodes Spread of tumour from the retroperitoneum may occur directly through the retrocrural space to involve the posterior mediastinal nodes and subcarinal nodes.

Haematogenous tumour spread is predominantly to the lungs but liver metastases are not infrequently seen in advanced disease. When widespread dissemination occurs metastases develop in other sites such as the bone and brain. The predominance of lung metastases is probably due to dissemination via the thoracic duct which drains directly into the venous circulation at the junction of the jugular and subclavian veins. The primary tumour may also directly invade the spermatic vein leading to pulmonary and other blood-borne metastases.

DIAGNOSIS

Imaging has only a limited rôle in detecting a testicular tumour and careful examination of the swollen testicle remains the best method of diagnosis. The differential diagnoses include epidydimitis, torsion, tuberculous and granulomatous orchitis. A simple hydrocoele is readily distinguished from tumour because it is transilluminable but occasionally a tumour may be associated with a hydrocoele.

Ultrasound has recently been employed for imaging the testes (Fig. 10.3). It is particularly valuable in those patients who are difficult to examine clinically and in patients who present with metastases in whom an 'occult' primary tumour of the testis is suspected (Hendry et al 1984). Ultrasound is also a useful technique for examining the contralateral testis as bilateral tumours occur in 2–3% (Sokal et al 1980) of patients although the second tumour usually presents at a later date. Following clinical diagnosis and serum marker estimations, orchidectomy is performed using an inguinal incision (Hendry 1981).

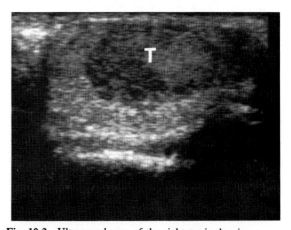

Fig. 10.3 Ultrasound scan of the right testis showing a primary testicular tumour (T). The tumour has a heterogeneous echo pattern. (By courtesy of Dr David O Cosgrove).

STAGING

Following orchidectomy the tumour is classified histologically and staging investigations are then undertaken to define the sites and volume of metastases as accurately as possible. The staging classification currently used at the Royal Marsden Hospital incorporates a statement on tumour volume as well as sites of disease (Table 10.2) (Peckham et al 1979). Staging investigations rely heavily on imaging and conventional radiology.

Over the past decade there have been major advances in imaging, in particular the introduction of whole body computed tomography (CT) and real-time ultrasound. CT is now established as a reliable staging investigation for various solid tumours. However, controversy regarding the relative rôles of CT and lymphography for examination of retroperitoneal nodes still exists and there is continuing debate with respect to the use of ultrasound and CT for evaluation of the liver. The way in which these techniques are deployed depends on many factors such as the availability of equipment, expertise of the radiologist, the tumour type being investigated and the impact of the results on therapeutic management.

In this discussion the detection of testicular tumour metastases will be considered according to the sites of disease and the advantages, limitations and pitfalls of the different techniques will be emphasized.

The retroperitoneum

Since testicular tumours spread in a logical manner first to the retroperitoneal nodes, the most important questions posed to the radiologist are firstly, is there evidence of retroperitoneal lymph node involvement and secondly, if disease is present what is its extent?

During the early 1960s bipedal lymphography became an established technique and for several years was the only method of assessing retroperitoneal lymph nodes. Considerable expertise was acquired not only in performing lymphography but also in interpretation of the results. Today, CT has completely replaced lymphography in many centres, particularly in the United States, but in the author's view there is still a well-defined place for lymphography in the assessment of testicular tumours.

Lymphography

Following injection of oily contrast medium into the lymphatic vessels, lymph nodes in the external iliac, common iliac and para-aortic chains are opacified. It is important to remember that contrast medium opacifies normal lymphoid tissue within the node and is not taken up by tumour. Thus, metastases appear as filling defects within involved nodes and contrast medium is compressed around the deposit (Fig. 10.4) (Wallace & Jing 1970). Filling defects within nodes may also be due to fibro-fatty replacement from old infection and, in addition, the normal lymph node hilum occasionally produces an identical appearance. These filling defects can usually be distinguished from metastases because they do not appear to expand the node, but it may be impossible to distinguish a small deposit from a benign filling defect on the 24-hour postlymphogram films. In this situation further follow-up films after two to three weeks will usually resolve the problem by demonstrating further expansion of the defect if it is due to tumour. With lymphography, lymph node deposits can be detected down to a

Table 10.2 Staging for testicular tumours used at the Royal Marsden Hospital. (In Stages III and IV abdominal status is defined as for Stage II).

I	No disease after orchidectomy
IM	Marker elevation after orchidectomy without detectable metastatic disease
II	Infradiaphragmatic node involvement
IIA	Metastases <2 cm diameter
IIB	Metastases from 2–5 cm diameter
IIC	Metastases >5 cm diameter
III	Supradiaphragmatic node involvement
M+	Mediastinal node involvement
N+	Neck node involvement
IV	Extranodal metastasis
L1	<3 metastases in number
L2	>3 metastases in number <2 cm diameter
L3	>3 metastases in number >2 cm diameter
H+	Hepatic involvement
	Other sites, e.g. bone, brain are specified

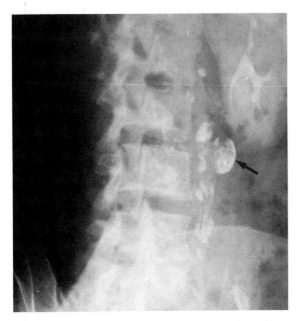

Fig. 10.4 Lymphogram film (oblique view) showing an involved node (arrowed) in the left para-aortic chain in a patient with a testicular teratoma.

size of about 1 cm but smaller filling defects should be observed over a period of a few weeks before a definitive diagnosis is made.

As a lymph node metastasis grows it compresses the nodal capsule and eventually breaks through it into the adjacent tissues. When this occurs the lymphogram demonstrates only that portion of the node which is not replaced by tumour. Characteristically, a crescent of compressed contrast medium is seen. Diagnosis of metastatic involvement is made on the basis of an abnormal pattern of contrast but the precise volume of the lymph node mass can only be assessed indirectly. Multiple involved nodes frequently coalesce to form a conglomerate tumour mass containing little, if any, contrast medium. Intravenous urography has been used as part of the lymphogram investigation to identify displacement of the kidneys by large retroperitoneal masses, hydronephrosis or deviation of the ureters (Fig. 10.5). Such information is helpful for defining tumour extent and, in addition, the intravenous urogram may demonstrate a congenital anomaly of the renal tract. This information is important as, for example, demonstration of a horseshoe kidney would significantly affect radiotherapy treatment plans.

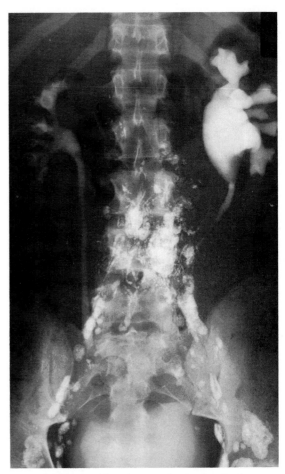

Fig. 10.5 Abnormal lymphogram showing involved retroperitoneal nodes from testicular teratoma. A large portion of the mass has not been opacified. There is left hydronephrosis and deviation of the left ureter. The volume of the mass is not precisely delineated.

The major limitations of lymphography are that it is an unpleasant procedure, may be technically difficult to perform and only opacifies certain lymph node chains. In testicular tumours the retroperitoneal nodes at the level of the renal hilar are most frequently involved and metastases may occur in those sites not opacified at lymphography. These include lymph nodes above the origin of the thoracic duct at about the level of the upper border of the second lumbar vertebra and more importantly the 'echelon' nodes lying lateral to the para-aortic chain.

The lymphogram appearances do not permit distinction between the various histological types of testicular tumour but in the majority of patients this is irrelevant because the histological diagnosis has been made prior to staging. In patients with an occult primary tumour who present with an abdominal mass, the lymphogram findings are usually sufficiently characteristic to distinguish metastatic disease from a lymphoma, although approximately 10% of patients with metastatic testicular tumours show a pseudolymphoma pattern on lymphography (Macdonald 1981).

Computed tomography

CT scanning elegantly shows the retroperitoneal structures and the high quality images obtained with current scanners allow normal lymph nodes to be appreciated in a high proportion of patients.

Techniques and pitfalls. When using CT as a staging investigation to survey the retroperitoneum for lymph node spread, it is appropriate to adopt a standard technique for all patients. Dilute oral contrast medium (e.g. 600 ml 2% Gastrografin – sodium meglumine diatrizoate) is given at least 45 minutes before the examination to outline the bowel. Patients should be fasted for four hours before the procedure because intravenous contrast medium may be required.

CT slice thickness varies with different scanners but, in general, sections 8–10 mm thick are used for most abdominal examinations. The inter-slice gap is optional but bearing in mind that the aim in testicular cancer is to detect lymph node deposits as early and therefore as small as possible, a slice interval no greater than 1.5 cm is recommended. Slice intervals of 2 cm are used in some centres but with this practice a node of 1 cm diameter may be completely missed.

The abdomen and upper pelvis are examined from the domes of the diaphragm to just above the acetabulae. Images through the pelvis are included because isolated involvement of an upper external iliac node has been documented and the time taken to include this area does not significantly prolong the examination. The initial scan is undertaken without the use of intravenous contrast medium. The reasons for this are firstly, that in most patients the examination is either definitely abnormal or definitely normal and the use of intravenous contrast material would not alter interpretation and is therefore unnecessary; secondly, it is preferable to use intravenous contrast medium to resolve specific problems because it can then be given with appropriate timing of the scans through the questionable areas.

The initial scan of the abdomen and pelvis should be reviewed by the radiologist while the patient is still on the table. Particular attention should be given to all soft tissue structures seen in the retroperitoneum, but especially to those just below the renal vessels. If these structures cannot be explained on an anatomical basis an involved node should be suspected and steps taken to confirm or refute this suspicion. Using this approach lymph node metastases down to the size of 8–10 mm can be diagnosed with CT.

The most common pitfall in diagnosing lymphadenopathy in the retroperitoneum is concerned with the distinction of vessels from suspected nodes but inadequately opacified small bowel may also have identical appearances to a soft tissue mass (David et al 1982). The crura of the diaphragm may stimulate lymphadenopathy but should not cause a real problem once experience in CT has been gained.

Vessels mistaken for enlarged nodes include the inferior mesenteric artery, lumbar veins, anomalies of the inferior vena cava and the inferior vena cava itself. Close examination of slices above and below the suspicious area may demonstrate the tubular nature of a vessel thus allowing correct interpretation without the need for intravenous contrast medium. However, if doubt persists a bolus injection of intravenous contrast material is required. Slices should be taken through the suspicious area using a bolus injection of 100 ml intravenous contrast material (300–370 mg iodine/ml). The first 50 ml is given prior to the commencement of the scan. Sequential dynamic scanning facilitates this type of study because several cms can be imaged while contrast medium remains in the vessel. An enlarged node lying anterior to the inferior vena cava may compress it and since there is frequently no significant difference between the attenuation values of the cava and the enlarged node, the mass may be missed (Fig. 10.6). Sudden change in shape of the apparent inferior vena cava should alert the radiologist to the presence of a mass. Once suspicion has been raised then it is easy to

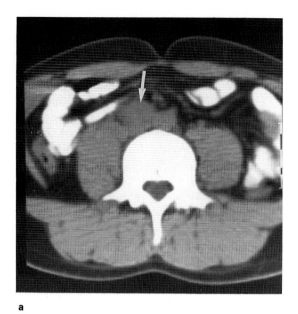
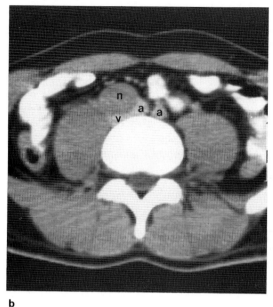

a

b

Fig. 10.6   (a) Precontrast scan showing an apparent large IVC (arrowed). (b) Following injection of contrast medium an enlarged node (n) is easily identified. The IVC is compressed (v). a = common iliac arteries.

confirm or exclude the presence of an enlarged node with dynamic scanning using intravenous contrast medium as described above.

Difficulties are not infrequently encountered in distinguishing small bowel from tumour. This is most often seen in thin patients in whom the bowel is closely related to the retroperitoneal structures. When this occurs several manoeuvres can be adopted to solve the problem but a successful manoeuvre in one patient will not necessarily prove helpful in another. The general rule is to give the patient a further dose of oral contrast medium and to rescan the area after a delay of approximately 15–20 minutes. When rescanning it is helpful to place the patient in the prone or lateral decubitus position because bowel frequently moves or changes shape when the patient is turned. Furthermore, air may be trapped within the apparent mass, thus confirming that it represents bowel. Intravenous contrast medium may occasionally be helpful because the small bowel wall opacifies but this technique is less reliable than those previously mentioned.

CT findings. With CT, normal lymph nodes appear as soft tissue density structures which are often only about 5 mm or less in diameter. A

lymph node containing a tumour deposit usually appears as a soft tissue density structure and distinction cannot be made between the normal and abnormal part of the node. The larger the node the easier it is to identify with CT and if several nodes are enlarged the diagnosis is simple.

Metastases from seminoma are of soft tissue density (Fig. 10.7) but in patients with testicular teratoma cystic deposits may also be seen. Small volume low density teratoma deposits are easier to distinguish from vessels than soft tissue opacities (Fig. 10.8). Large volume disease is often seen as a single mass with no obvious involvement of other retroperitoneal sites. In seminoma even the very large masses over 10 cm in diameter are predominantly of soft tissue density. Central areas of diminished density, presumably due to areas of necrosis, may be seen but this is unusual. The aorta and inferior vena cava may be obscured within the mass because tumour completely surrounds these structures which are of similar density to tumour. Displacement of the kidneys and/or hydronephrosis is associated with bulky disease and is readily demonstrated on CT.

In malignant teratoma approximately 50% of large volume retroperitoneal masses contain cystic

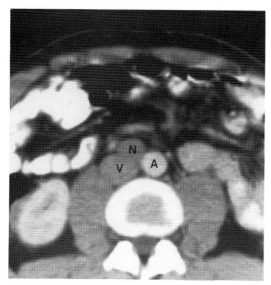

Fig. 10.7 Interaorto-caval lymph node metastasis (N) in a patient with a right-sided seminoma. A = opacified aorta; V = inferior vena cava.

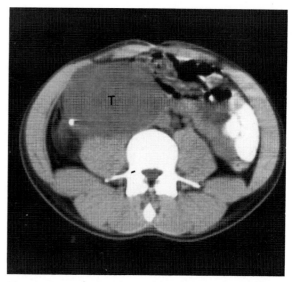

Fig. 10.9 Pretreatment low density teratomatous mass (T). The ureter is opacified and is closely related to the lateral aspect of the mass.

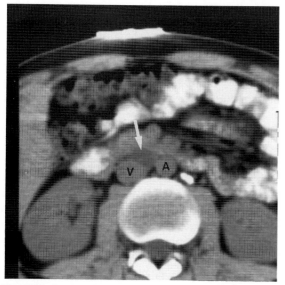

Fig. 10.8 Low density lymph node metastasis (arrowed) from a right-sided testicular teratoma. A = aorta; V = inferior vena cava.

areas (Husband et al 1980). The attenuation values of these cystic components are of the order of 5–15 Hounsfield units (Fig. 10.9). In those patients with solid soft tissue teratomatous masses distinction between seminoma and teratoma cannot be made.

One of the advantages of CT is its ability to detect enlarged nodes high in the retroperitoneal space, in the retrocrural space and lateral to the para-aortic chain. Demonstration of disease in these sites is clearly important, not only for staging purposes but also for identifying the extent of disease prior to surgery. These nodes, as in other areas, may be of soft tissue density or of low attenuation depending on the histology of the primary tumour.

Ultrasound

Advances in ultrasound during recent years have rendered the technique suitable for examination of the retroperitoneum. Its major limitations include interference by bowel gas and difficulty in visualizing the retroperitoneum in obese patients (Poskitt et al 1985). However, in thin patients ultrasound may on occasion be superior to CT. Enlarged nodes from testicular cancer appear as relatively echo-free soft tissue structures (Fig. 10.10). As with CT, in patients with testicular teratomas, cystic areas may be seen within the mass (Burney & Klatte 1979). Although ultrasound may demonstrate retroperitoneal lymphadenopathy, the precise extent of tumour is

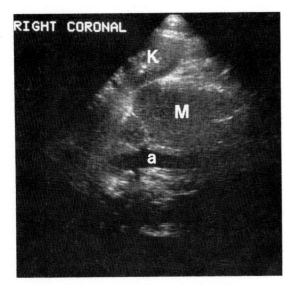

Fig. 10.10 Coronal ultrasound scan showing a large retroperitoneal mass on the left (M). The left kidney (K) is displaced laterally. a = aorta. (By courtesy of Dr David O Cosgrove.)

often difficult to visualize and for this reason ultrasound should be regarded as inferior to CT for staging even in patients with advanced disease.

The accuracy of CT, lymphography and ultrasound

Data obtained at staging laparotomy has shown that approximately 20–30% of patients considered to be stage I harbour occult microscopic deposits in retroperitoneal nodes (Kademian & Wirtanen 1977, Thomas et al 1981). These microscopic lesions cannot be identified by imaging techniques currently available and therefore, at best, we can only expect lymphography or CT to be accurate in about 80% of patients.

With CT, size is the key criterion for diagnosing lymph node deposits but in testicular teratomas the density of the suspected node is also significant. It has been widely accepted in the literature that a diameter of 1.5 cm should be considered as the upper limit of normal for a lymph node both in the pelvis and in the retroperitoneum (Best et al 1978, Husband 1985, Samuelsson et al 1986). This criterion worked well in practice during the early years of CT but today superior image quality and increasing expertise make it possible to diagnose abnormal retroperitoneal

nodes down to the size of 8–10 mm diameter. However, if nodes of 1 cm or less are taken as abnormal, specificity is reduced (Lien et al 1986). It is therefore important to seek other confirmatory evidence of metastatic disease, such as cytology or elevation of serum markers.

Criteria for diagnosing lymph node metastases with lymphography rely on the characteristics of the uptake of contrast medium as well as size of a filling defect. With this technique lymph node deposits can also be detected down to the size of just under 1 cm in diameter.

In the United Kingdom data comparing lymphography and CT with staging lymphadenectomy in testicular tumours is not available but several studies have been conducted to address this topic in other countries where retroperitoneal lymphadenectomy is undertaken. The accuracy of bipedal lymphography has been reported to range from approximately 60% to 90% giving an overall accuracy of 77% (Cook et al 1965, Storm et al 1977, Wallace & Jing 1977, Marincek et al 1983, Tesoro-Tess et al 1985). The overall sensitivity (ability to identify disease) is approximately 75% and the specificity (ability to exclude metastases) is of the order of 88%. Fewer studies have been conducted comparing the results of CT with those of lymphadenectomy but the reports which are available indicate that the accuracy of CT is similar to that of lymphography, with results for overall accuracy also ranging from about 60% to 90% (mean 76%). The mean reported sensitivity is 70% and the mean specificity is 86% (Dunnick & Javadpour 1981, Ehrlichman et al 1981, Thomas et al 1981, Marincek et al 1983, Tesoro-Tess et al 1985). The results of these studies imply that either lymphography or CT may be employed for staging testicular cancer with equal effectiveness. However, some of the studies with CT were undertaken in the early days with slow and relatively inferior image quality scanners. There is now a greater awareness of the ability of CT to detect small (approximately 1 cm) abnormal nodes and this should improve CT statistics in future studies. Furthermore, there is no doubt that CT defines tumour volume more accurately than lymphography as tumour is imaged directly (Marincek et al 1983). In a series reported from the Royal Marsden Hospital, CT was compared with lymphography in 225 patients (Husband % Grimer 1985). Involved nodes were identified with CT in 7 patients which were not opacified at lymphography, but in 3 patients the lymphogram showed small metatases in nodes which were only minimally enlarged and were not identified on CT. This series incorporated results from 1977 to 1984. The three patients in whom metastases were missed on CT were all scanned using a 20 second scanner. Since the installation of a fast scanner in 1981 we have not seen any patients with a negative CT scan but a positive lymphogram. In this series CT defined the extent of disease more accurately than lymphography and upgraded the stage from IIA or B to IIB or C when compared with lymphography in 16 patients.

The accuracy of ultrasonography has also been compared with CT and with lymphography in testicular cancer. The results for ultrasound indicate that it is equally as accurate as CT for identifying bulky retroperitoneal disease; in one study both techniques revealed accuracies of 90% (Poskitt et al 1985). In other studies both the sensitivity and specificity of CT have been higher than ultrasonography when all stages of disease are considered (Williams et al 1980, Rowland et al 1982). In a series reported by Poskitt et al (1985) CT was more accurate than ultrasound for identifying patients with small volume disease. Their data support our results from the Royal Marsden Hospital in which CT and ultrasound were compared in 89 patients (Husband et al 1981). With CT there were no false positive and 2 false negative examinations and with ultrasound there were 3 false positive and 15 false negative examinations. In addition, there were 15 technical failures with ultrasound compared with 1 technical failure with CT. Rowland et al (1982) also reported a high technical failure rate (17%) with ultrasound.

The chest

In patients with testicular teratoma lung metastases are often seen without mediastinal involvement and mediastinal disease is usually accompanied by pulmonary metastases, thus Stage III disease is relatively uncommon. Conversely, in seminoma, mediastinal disease is often seen in the absence of pulmonary metastases and pulmonary metastases are usually associated with mediastinal deposits.

Conventional radiology

Plain chest radiographs are mandatory for staging in all patients with testicular tumours and may reveal both pulmonary and mediastinal disease. If lymphography has been performed uptake of contrast medium into the mediastinum is occasionally observed and nodes may also be opacified in the supraclavicular fossa. Although these nodes are opacified they are not necessarily abnormal and the same criteria should be adopted for diagnosing deposits as in the retroperitoneum. Adequate penetration of the standard chest film is essential so that the mediastinal pleural reflections can be seen well. Particular attention should be given to the posterior mediastinum and subcarinal region as these are the most common sites of mediastinal disease.

Conventional or whole lung tomography was used for the detection of pulmonary metastases routinely in patients with negative plain chest films until the introduction of CT. Reports in the literature indicate that conventional whole lung tomography may detect pulmonary metastases in about 25% of patients who have negative chest films and, furthermore, tomography may reveal multiple metastases when only one lesion is visible on the plain film (Niefeld et al 1977, Bergaman et al 1980).

Computed tomography

Technique. CT scanning is carried out using 8 or 10 mm collimation contiguously from the lung apices to the lower borders of the costophrenic recesses. Scans are taken in full inspiration and it is important that the patient is instructed to withhold respiration at the same phase of the cycle for each scan so that areas of the lung are not missed due to erratic breathing. As in the abdomen, intravenous contrast medium is not routinely given but is reserved to resolve specific difficulties encountered when the complete examination is reviewed. In thin patients the mediastinal vessels may be difficult to separate from each other and minimally enlarged lymph nodes may be missed.

However, in the majority of patients the vascular anatomy is clearly displayed and even in those with anomalous vessels contrast medium is not always required.

The scans should be reviewed on lung window settings while the patient remains on the table as change in a patient's position may be helpful for distinguishing a pulmonary nodule from a vessel (see below).

Mediastinum. The most common site of mediastinal involvement in testicular tumours is the posterior mediastinum and disease in this area is well demonstrated with CT.

Posterior mediastinal lymphadenopathy appears as a soft tissue mass which produces a convex outline to the mediastinal contour. Extension of disease to the subcarinal nodes produces a characteristic appearance of a convex opacity in the azygo-oesophageal recess (Fig. 10.11).

Superior mediastinal lymphadenopathy is usually seen as a single enlarged node or as multiple discretely enlarged masses of soft tissue density. As in other sites, teratomatous metastases may appear cystic but this is less frequently seen in the chest than in the abdomen.

In the mediastinum, lymph nodes greater than 1 cm in diameter are considered abnormal but in

our experience patients in whom mediastinal spread is diagnosed on CT usually have relatively large obvious masses.

The lungs. It is widely accepted that CT is the most sensitive technique in radiology for identifying pulmonary metastases because nodules can be detected at the lung periphery down to the size of 3–4 mm in diameter (Muhm et al 1977, Schaner et al 1978).

Pulmonary metastases from testicular tumours are well circumscribed, round lesions, which are only distinguished from adjacent blood vessels seen in cross-section by virtue of their size compared to the size of the vessels in that region. There are two main problems in the interpretation of CT scans of the lungs when looking for metastatic disease. In the central areas of the lung where the vessels are relatively large, differentiation of pulmonary metastases from vessels is difficult and occasionally whole lung tomography may show a deposit which is missed on CT. Careful interrogation of these areas by following major vessels from slice to slice should therefore be carried out if whole lung tomography is not employed. When there is doubt as to whether an opacity represents a pulmonary metastasis or a vessel seen end-on, rescanning in the prone or lateral positions frequently solves the problem. The patient should be turned so that the area under review is situated uppermost in the scanner, thus making use of the gravitational effect of blood flow.

The second major difficulty is that pulmonary nodules may be due to granulomata, pleural lymph nodes or areas of inflammation (Chang et al 1979). These may have identical or similar appearances to deposits. Granulomatous disease is less common in the UK than in other countries such as the USA, and a patient with a known testicular tumour in whom multiple round pulmonary nodules are seen on CT can be presumed to have metastatic disease. However, if only one lesion is seen caution should be exercised. Our policy is to rescan the patient after a period of six weeks to demonstrate whether the lesion has significantly increased in size (Fig. 10.12). If the lesion has not changed, further follow-up is continued without treatment. If there is no change in the size of the lesion after six months then the nodule is presumed to be benign. This policy works well in practice and we have now

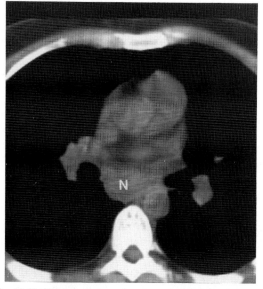

Fig. 10.11 Metastatic spread to the subcarinal nodes (N) in a patient with a pure seminoma.

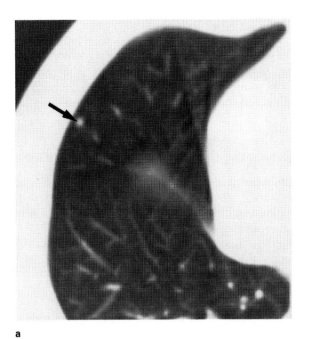 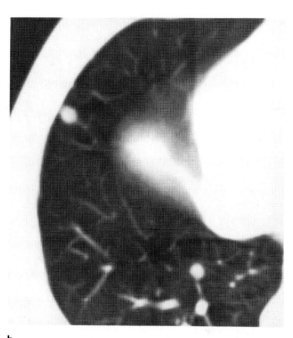

a   b

Fig. 10.12   (a) Initial CT of the chest showed a 4 mm nodule at the periphery of the right lung (arrowed). (b) A repeat CT six weeks later revealed obvious increase in size of the lesion indicating malignancy.

seen several patients in whom minute pulmonary nodules have persisted unchanged for periods of up to three or four years. In some patients lesions identified on the initial scan disappear on follow-up examinations. These opacities presumably represent areas of inflammation but it should be remembered that a small nodule may not be visualized on a follow-up scan because the patient's breath-holding is inconsistent.

Since testicular teratomas occur at an earlier age than seminomas, benign pulmonary nodules are likely to be seen less frequently in teratoma patients. In seminoma, pulmonary involvement is less common than in teratoma but if it does occur metastases tend to be larger at the time of diagnosis. In a group of 200 patients with seminoma in whom the chest manifestations were recently reviewed, benign pulmonary nodules were observed in 12 patients and in those with lung metastases at least one deposit was greater than 1 cm in diameter in each patient. Pleural metastases and pleural effusions are also seen more frequently in seminoma than teratoma (Williams et al 1987a).

Accuracy of CT. Computed tomography (CT) is the most sensitive technique for detecting mediastinal and pulmonary metastases but it is impossible to provide statistics for the accuracy of CT compared with histology because few patients with testicular tumours undergo surgery at presentation. The patient's clinical course during continued follow-up is the only way of determining accuracy and a mass which resolves on treatment is considered to be involved.

The detection of mediastinal lymph nodes in patients with lung cancer has received much attention because pathological correlation at surgery and mediastinoscopy is available. These studies have shown that CT is sensitive for detecting lymph nodes of 1 cm in diameter or greater, but specificity is low (Ekholm et al 1980). Since testicular tumour mediastinal metastases tend to be greater than 1 cm in diameter when diagnosed, false positive examinations are likely to be few. Two different series from the Royal Marsden Hospital have shown that CT has a yield over conventional radiography of approximately 15% in the detection of enlarged mediastinal nodes (Husband & Grimer 1985, Williams et al 1987a).

Provided strict criteria are observed CT is highly

accurate for diagnosing pulmonary metastases. The yield over conventional radiography including tomographs is as high as 20% (Chang et al 1979, Husband & Grimer 1985) and in addition to identifying metastases in patients with negative conventional films, CT may also show a greater number of deposits, thus upstaging patients from L1 or L2 disease to L2 or L3.

Other sites of disease

The liver

Hepatic involvement is seldom seen at presentation except in patients with advanced disseminated disease. It most frequently occurs in patients who fail to respond to first-line chemotherapy or in those who relapse after initial treatment.

Radionuclide scanning, ultrasound and CT may all be used for imaging the liver. CT is used for surveying retroperitoneal nodes. Examination of the liver is also included in the abdominal scans and it is therefore debatable whether further investigation of the liver by any other technique is required. Certainly, radionuclide scanning seems unnecessary but on occasion ultrasound may demonstrate a liver metastasis which is not visible on the CT scan (Husband et al 1981). For this reason we still employ liver ultrasound as part of the staging procedure.

With ultrasound liver metastases in testicular cancer usually appear as lesions of low echogeneity compared with normal liver parenchyma. With CT they are seen as areas of diminished density with ill-defined borders. In testicular teratoma hepatic metastases may appear cystic both on ultrasound and CT. If obvious liver metastases are demonstrated on the initial CT scan, enhanced scans are not taken. Intravenous contrast medium is only used if there is doubt regarding the presence of a metastasis or if an obvious solitary lesion is seen as this may represent an haemangioma.

The accuracy of ultrasound and CT in the detection of liver metastases in testicular tumours has not been evaluated in any large series but in our experience the techniques appear to be equally accurate.

Bone

Bone metastases are rare and are seldom seen at presentation. They occur in patients with progressive, uncontrolled disease or at the time of relapse. Symptoms usually indicate the site of involvement but occasionally unsuspected deposits are detected either on conventional radiographs or with CT.

Brain

Brain metastases occur in patients with progressive disseminated disease. They are more common in patients with trophoblastic teratomas than any other histological type. As in other tumours CT is the best method of demonstrating these deposits and radionuclide scanning is now rarely undertaken if CT is available.

Unusual sites of metastases

The widespread use of CT scanning has revealed disease in many different sites not previously recognized. In an analysis of 397 patients with testicular tumours who had metastatic disease (Husband & Bellamy 1985) unusual sites of thoraco-abdominal metastases were identified in 20 patients (23 sites). These sites included the kidneys, adrenal glands, the inferior vena cava, striated muscle, the spleen, the stomach, seminal vesicles, the prostate and the pericardium. Although such metastatic involvement may be seen at presentation it is more likely to occur later during the clinical course. This study emphasizes that any unusual finding on CT should be regarded with suspicion in a patient who has known metastases or has previously been treated for metastatic disease.

THE USE OF IMAGING FOR STAGING

A strategy for the use of imaging should be made in each department according to the availability of equipment, expertise and treatment protocols employed. Since these factors vary widely between different centres treating patients with testicular tumours, it is impossible to adopt a universal approach. Strong liaison between the clinician and the radiologist is essential so that the contribution of the radiology department is utilized as effectively as possible. The imaging strategy put forward in the following paragraphs refers to patients attending the Royal Marsden Hospital where chemotherapy is given to all patients with non-seminomatous germ cell tumours who have metastatic disease and to patients with advanced seminoma (Peckham et al 1983). Radiotherapy is only given to patients with seminomas who have small volume (IIA) disease. Patients with stage I malignant teratomas and seminomas are treated by orchidectomy alone and are entered into a surveillance policy (see below).

CT staging is undertaken in all patients with testicular tumours. If a plain chest radiograph has identified advanced lung or mediastinal disease then chest CT is not undertaken. However, if the patient has early lung disease (stages L1 or L2) or mediastinal lymphadenopathy only is identified then a chest CT scan is still required. All patients who do not fall into these groups have CT scans of the chest, abdomen and pelvis according to the techniques outlined above.

Although the accuracy of CT in the detection of retroperitoneal nodes in both seminoma and teratoma appears to be similar, the rarity of serum markers as an indicator of active tumour in seminoma makes radiology even more critical for the detection of small volume disease. For this reason these different histological types will be considered separately.

In patients with seminoma CT of abdomen and pelvis is undertaken as discussed above. If the abdominal CT examination is negative a lymphogram is performed with the objective of identifying disease in normal or only minimally enlarged nodes which may have been missed on CT. A lymphogram is also performed if the CT examination is inconclusive which is most frequently seen in very thin patients. If the CT study is definitely positive and only one enlarged node less than 2 cm diameter is seen (IIA disease) then fine needle aspiration is carried out under CT control to obtain cytology (Fig. 10.13). If the result of cytology confirms seminoma then therapy is instigated. If cytology is negative the node may be removed surgically to obtain histology. Progressive enlarge-

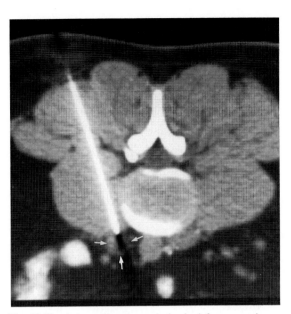

Fig. 10.13 A 1 cm diameter node in the left para-aortic chain (arrowed) in a patient with a left-sided seminoma. Cytology confirmed metastatic disease.

ment of the node demonstrated on a subsequent CT examination is also accepted as confirmatory evidence of metastatic disease.

Patients with non-seminomatous germ cell tumours are divided into those who are (a) serum marker negative at orchidectomy or have raised markers which return rapidly to normal following orchidectomy and (b) those who have rising serum markers at the time of staging.

(a) In those who are serum marker negative an identical approach to patients with seminoma is used. If the serum markers are elevated at orchidectomy but return to normal by the time of staging the presence of active tumour is less likely and CT alone is undertaken. However, it should be remembered that marker-producing primary tumours do not necessarily invoke marker-producing metastases and if a minimally enlarged node is seen on CT, then cytology is obtained. As in seminomas, lymphography may be used if the CT study is negative.

(b) If serum marker levels are rising following

orchidectomy and CT is definitely positive, treatment with chemotherapy is commenced without further confirmation. If the CT scan is negative a lymphogram may be employed but its use in this way is decreasing because such patients are treated with chemotherapy irrespective of identifying the site of disease.

A scheme for this approach for radiological staging of seminomas and malignant teratomas is shown in Figure 10.14.

MONITORING TREATMENT RESPONSE

Radiology is equally as important in patient follow-up as in initial staging. Timing and frequency

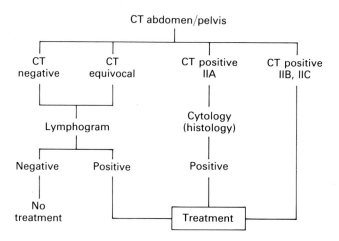

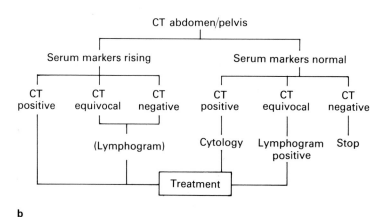

Fig. 10.14 Schematic approach to abdominal staging in testicular tumours. (a) Seminoma and serum marker negative teratoma. (b) Malignant teratoma — serum markers elevated at orchidectomy.

of follow-up investigations should be designed according to treatment protocols and clearly vary in different centres. In general, patients are re-evaluated fully following initial treatment whether this is with chemotherapy or radiotherapy. After this, continued radiological assessment is dependent on the stage of disease, the measured treatment response and future management strategy.

The abdomen

Before the days of ultrasound and CT postlymphangiogram films were the only method of assessing regression of retroperitoneal tumour. Since metastatic lymph node deposits do not take up lymphographic contrast medium, reduction in size is often difficult to assess accurately on follow-up radiographs. Another problem with postlymphogram films is that contrast medium is continually lost from opacified nodes making assessment increasingly difficult after the first few months.

If CT is undertaken for staging there is no doubt that it should be used for monitoring response to therapy. CT can accurately depict changes in tumour volume and may also show alteration in tumour composition (Husband et al 1982). In patients who undergo postchemotherapy lymphadenectomy CT is also highly accurate for localizing the site of residual disease, the size of the mass and its relationship to major vessels (Kennedy et al 1985). This information is required for surgical planning because residual masses above the renal hilar are approached using a thoraco-abdominal incision whereas disease confined below the renal vessels is approached using a midline abdominal incision.

Seminomatous masses shrink rapidly on chemotherapy and radiotherapy. In the majority of patients a soft tissue residuum is seen in the retroperitoneum (Fig. 10.15) (Stomper et al 1985). These masses usually persist but may show further minimal regression up to two years after therapy (Williams et al 1987c). Seminoma residua are rarely excised because previous lymphadenectomy data has shown that they usually represent areas of fibrosis (Stanton et al 1985).

Retroperitoneal teratoma masses show different patterns of tumour response. For instance, a soft

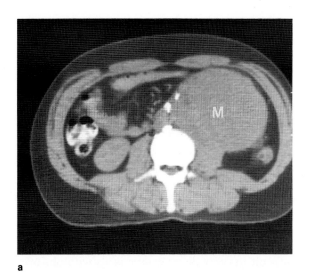

a

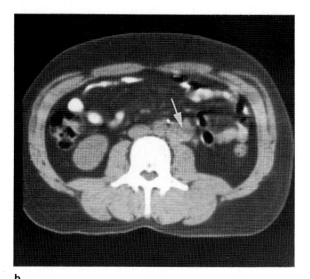

b

Fig. 10.15 Metastatic seminoma. (a) Pretreatment. (b) Postchemotherapy. The large soft tissue mass (M) has shown excellent regression leaving a small soft tissue residuum (arrowed).

tissue teratoma mass may respond in a similar way to a seminomatous mass leaving a small soft tissue residuum after treatment. Alternatively, cysts may appear within the mass during the treatment or cysts seen initially may become larger. We observed that cystic change during treatment was usually associated with a striking increase in tumour volume and an overall reduction in the mean attenuation values of the tumour (Husband et al 1982). We correlated the mean attenuation values of residual teratomatous masses with histology in 26 patients. The results showed that low attenuation values (less than 30 Hounsfield units) strongly indicated that the masses were cystic and consisted of differentiated teratoma with no evidence of active malignancy (Fig. 10.16). This topic was subsequently addressed by Scatarige et al (1983). They found low attenuation values in 10 patients (43.5%) but biopsy was only available in 3 patients who had received treatment. Two of these showed residual active tumour and these findings therefore disagree with ours. However, the series reported by Scatarige et al (1983) is a small and heterogenous group and it is therefore difficult to make direct comparisons with our own series. Stomper et al (1985) also reviewed CT density values in patients treated for non-seminomatous germ cell tumours. They found that uniform low attenuation values of residual

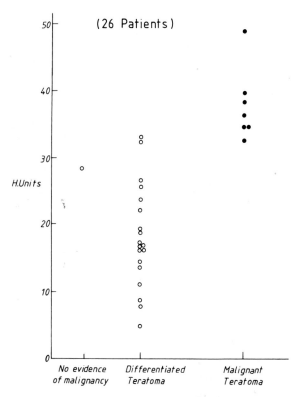

Fig. 10.16 Correlation of mean CT attenuation values of postchemotherapy residual masses with histology in 26 patients with testicular tumours. (Reprinted with permission from Husband 1982.)

masses (16 patients) were not associated with persistent malignancy and in this respect their results support our findings. Further investigation of this interesting phenomenon is warranted.

The chest

Chest radiographs are the mainstay of monitoring tumour regression provided metastases can be clearly identified on standard films. As in the abdomen, surgery may be indicated following treatment to remove residual lung and mediastinal disease (Goldstraw 1986). Immediately before surgery CT is helpful not only to confirm the number and position of obvious metastases but also to identify deposits not seen on the plain film. In addition, CT is helpful for defining the extent and position of abnormal mediastinal nodes.

Small pulmonary metastases, only identified initially on CT, usually disappear completely after treatment and only the larger deposits remain as residual lesions. Activity is impossible to assess in the lungs but treated lesions often have an irregular outline and sometimes cavitate.

Mediastinal regression is well shown with CT. Occasionally a teratoma lymph node deposit may become cystic and increase in size in the same way as in the retroperitoneum.

DETECTION OF RELAPSE

Patients with testicular tumours are followed clinically for several years but it is difficult to justify continued routine follow-up CT examinations after completion of successful treatment. In patients with teratomas who have undergone post-treatment lymphadenectomy further CT examinations are not undertaken at the Royal Marsden Hospital unless there is clinical suspicion of relapse or a rise in the serum markers. In seminoma patients we undertake CT immediately after treatment and then at twelve months following diagnosis. Further CT follow-up may show further regression of a small soft tissue residuum but is considered unnecessary unless new symptoms develop.

The objective of a surveillance policy for stage I disease is to avoid unnecessary treatment in those patients who are truly stage I, and to identify at the earliest opportunity the group of approximately 25% who will relapse. All patients considered to have stage I testicular teratoma who meet certain criteria are entered into this surveillance policy at the Royal Marsden Hospital. These criteria include histological confirmation of non-seminomatous germ cell tumours of the testis, no clinical or radiological evidence of spread, absence of tumour at the cut end of the spermatic cord and either negative serum marker levels or marker levels which rapidly return to normal (Peckham et al 1982).

We have recently analysed the role of radiology in a group of 147 patients with non-seminomatous germ cell tumours of the testis on surveillance (Williams et al 1987b). 37 patients relapsed, 86% of these during the first year. CT scanning identified relapse in the retroperitoneum in 18 out of 19 patients. In one patient the lymphogram follow-up abdominal film showed a growing deposit four weeks after a normal lymphogram and CT scan. This was the only patient in whom lymphogram follow-up films detected relapse. In eight patients serum markers only were elevated. Radiological investigations failed to demonstrate the site of disease which was presumably microscopic or very small. Relapse was diagnosed in the chest in 15 patients; 13 had pulmonary metastases and 2 had posterior mediastinal lymphadenopathy. In those with pulmonary metastases CT identified deposits in all patients and chest radiographs were diagnostic in 8. In the 2 patients with mediastinal involvement CT detected relapse which was visible on chest radiographs after review. The results of this analysis clearly indicate that CT is essential for identifying relapse in stage I testicular tumours if a surveillance policy is adopted. The need for lymphography is debatable. Certainly, in our series, postlymphogram films only identified disease in 1 out of 37 patients but this deposit would probably have been detected on CT at the subsequent examination. For this reason we no longer undertake lymphography except in patients with negative markers. CT is carried out at three-monthly intervals during the first year, then at 18 months and two years.

EFFECT OF TREATMENT ON NORMAL TISSUES

Radiotherapy to retroperitoneal nodes does not induce obvious fibrosis of the retroperitoneal structures on CT and interpretation is therefore not hampered. However, mediastinal irradiation, sometimes used for the treatment of seminoma, often induces intense fibrosis of the mediastinum and adjacent lung. In this situation it may be impossible to identify residual tumour or indeed early relapse.

A common complication of combination chemotherapy is bleomycin-induced lung damage. Pulmonary function tests are the most sensitive method of identifying early damage but these tests are not specific (Comis et al 1979). Plain chest radiographs demonstrate characteristic appearances in patients with moderate and severe damage but are insensitive for detecting early changes (Bonadonna et al 1971). CT is superior to chest radiographs for detecting early damage and shows characteristic pleurally-based peripheral lung opacities (Bellamy et al 1985). As damage increases the central areas of the lungs become progressively involved. Recognition of bleomycin damage on CT is important so that bleomycin can be discontinued if rapid progression occurs. Bleomycin damage should not be confused with developing metastases but occasionally distinction between these entities is difficult. Regression of a metastasis in an area of bleomycin damage is also difficult to assess.

Thymic hyperplasia is another effect of chemotherapy which may be seen in adults as well as children. We found an incidence of obvious thymic enlargement in 11.6% of patients treated with chemotherapy for non-seminomatous germ cell tumours of the testis (Fig. 10.17) (Kissin et al 1987). Thymic hyperplasia is thought to occur as a result of reduction in tumour burden in response to treatment but the phenomenon is not well understood. There is an increase in thymic volume and histology reveals true hyperplasia with increase in both lymphoid and epithelial components of the gland. It is important to recognize thymic hyperplasia as a cause of an enlarging anterior mediastinal mass in a patient who has recently received chemotherapy so that relapse is not erroneously diagnosed.

MAGNETIC RESONANCE IMAGING

So far, magnetic resonance imaging (MRI) of the

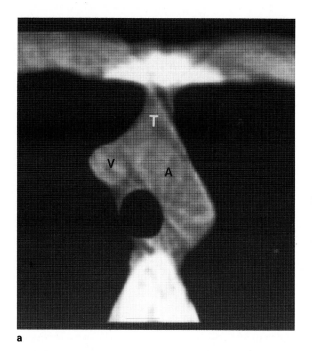
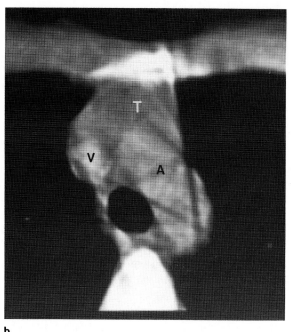

a

b

Fig. 10.17   A patient treated with chemotherapy over six months for metastatic testicular teratoma. (a) Pretreatment. (b) Thirteen months later. The scan shows an obvious increase in size of the thymus gland (T) following chemotherapy. V = superior vena cava; A = aorta.

chest and abdomen has not had the same dramatic impact on the management of cancer patients which CT enjoyed, but the technique is still at an early stage of development. It seems unlikely that MRI will replace CT for staging mediastinal and abdominal disease in testicular tumours because spatial resolution, at least on current scanners, is inferior to CT and the lungs cannot be assessed for the presence of pulmonary metastases. An early report in the literature has not shown any obvious benefit of MRI over CT for staging testicular tumours (Ellis et al 1984). The rôle of magnetic resonance imaging is more likely to be that of monitoring treatment response by demonstrating alteration in signal intensities related to changes in T_1 and T_2 values and possibly by obtaining information from spectroscopy. As yet no data is available on these aspects of magnetic resonance in testicular tumours and these comments are therefore purely speculative.

CONCLUSIONS

Present knowledge of tumour morphology before,

during and after treatment is partly the result of information derived from CT but is also firmly based on observations made by anatomists and radiologists for at least two decades before the advent of this new technology. As a result, we now understand tumour behaviour better and are in a position to use the information in a highly specific way for individual patient groups.

The crux of the value of any technique is its effect on patient management and there can be no doubt that radiology, and in particular CT, not only influences patient management but directly determines approach in a high proportion of patients. In 1981 we analysed results of management decisions based on CT findings in testicular tumours and showed that CT altered treatment choice in 30% of patients (Husband et al 1981). Today, such an analysis would show that CT, together with serum marker estimations, determines treatment policy in practically all our patients except those with plain film evidence of supradiaphragmatic disease. The technique is likely to remain the best imaging method for assessment of testicular tumours in the foreseeable future.

ACKNOWLEDGEMENTS

I wish to thank the Cancer Research Campaign for supporting work undertaken by the CRC Radiology Research Group at the Royal Marsden Hospital, Sutton.

I would like to acknowledge the close co-operation between the Testicular Tumour Unit and the Radiology Department and I would like to thank Professor Alan Horwich personally for reading this manuscript.

I would also like to thank Mrs Janice O'Donnell for typing this manuscript and Mrs Dorothy Mears and Mrs Jacqueline Seckel for their help in the preparation of the illustrations.

REFERENCES

Ball D, Barrett A, Peckham M J 1982 The management of metastatic seminoma testis. Cancer 50: 2289–2294

Bellamy E A, Husband J E, Blaquiere R M, Law M R 1985 Bleomycin-related lung damage: CT evidence. Radiology 156: 155–158

Bergaman S M, Lippert M, Javadpour N 1980 The value of whole lung tomography in the early detection of metastatic disease in patients with renal cell carcinoma and testicular tumors. Journal of Urology 124: 860–862

Best J K, Blackledge G, Forbes W St C et al 1978 Computed tomography of the abdomen in the staging and clinical management of lymphoma. British Medical Journal 2: 1675

Bonadonna G, DeLena M, Bartoli C et al 1971 Studio preliminare della fase I della bleomicina un nuovo farmaco antitumocale. Tumori 57: 21–53

Bradey N, Johnson R J, Read G 1987 Abdominal computed tomography in teratoma of the testis. British Journal of Radiology 60: 487–491

Burney B T, Klatte E C 1979 Ultrasound and computed tomography of the abdomen in the staging and management of testicular carcinoma. Radiology 132: 415–419

Calman F M B, Peckham M J, Hendry W F 1979 The pattern of spread and treatment of metastases in testicular seminoma. British Journal of Urology 51: 154–160

Chang A E, Schaner E G, Conkle D M, Flye M W, Doppman J L, Rosenberg S A 1979 Evaluation of computed tomography in the detection of pulmonary metastases. Cancer 43: 913–916

Chiappa S, Uslenghi C, Bonadonna G, Marano P, Ravasi G 1966 Combined testicular and foot lymphangiography in testicular carcinomas. Surgery, Gynecology and Obstetrics 123: 10–14

Comis R L, Kuppinger M S, Ginsberg S J et al 1979 Rôle of single-breath carbon monoxide-diffusing capacity in monitoring the pulmonary effects of bleomycin in germ cell tumor patients. Cancer Research 39: 5076–5080

Cook F E Jr, Lawrence D D, Smith J R, Gritti E J 1965 Testicular carcinoma and lymphangiography. Radiology 84: 420–427

David E, van Kaick G, Ikinger U, Gerhardt P, Prager P 1982 Detection of neoplastic lymph node involvement in the retroperitoneal space. European Journal of Radiology 2: 277–280

Dixon A K, Ellis M, Sikora K 1986 Computed tomography of testicular tumours: distribution of abdominal lymphadenopathy. Clinical Radiology 37: 519–523

Dunnick N R, Javadpour N 1981 Value of CT and lymphography. Distinguishing retroperitoneal metastases from non-seminomatous testicular tumors. American Journal of Roentgenology 136: 1093–1099

Ehrlichman R J, Kaufman S L, Siegelman S S, Trump D L, Walsh P C 1981 Computerized tomography and lymphangiography in staging testis tumors. Journal of Urology 126: 179–181

Einhorn L H, Donohue J P 1977 Cis-diaminedichloroplatinum, Vinblastine and Bleomycin in combination chemotherapy in disseminated testicular cancer. Annals of Internal Medicine 87: 293–298

Einhorn L H, Donohue J P, Peckham M J, Williams S D, Loehrer P J 1985 Cancer of the testes. In: DeVita V T, Hellman S, Rosenberg S A (eds) Cancer principles and practice of oncology, 2nd edn. Lippincott, Philadelphia, pp 979–1011

Ekholm S, Albrechtsson U, Kugelberg J, Tylen U 1980 Computed tomography in pre-operative staging of bronchogenic carcinoma. Journal of Computer Assisted Tomography 4: 763–765

Ellis J H, Bies J R, Kopecky K K, Klatte E C, Rowland R G, Donohue J P 1984 Comparison of NMR and CT imaging in the evaluation of metastatic retroperitoneal lymphadenopathy from testicular carcinoma. Journal of Computer Assisted Tomography 8: 709–719

Goldstraw P 1986 Thoracic surgery for germ cell tumours. In: Jones W G, Milford Ward A, Anderson C K (eds) Germ cell tumours II, Advances in the Biosciences vol 55. Pergamon Press, Oxford, pp 419–421

Hendry W F 1981 Diagnosis and management of the primary testicular tumour. In: Peckham M J (ed) The management of testicular tumours. Edward Arnold, London, pp 83–88

Hendry W F, Garvie W H H, Ah-See A K, Bayliss A P 1984 Ultrasonic detection of occult testicular neoplasms in patients with gynaecomastia. British Journal of Radiology 57: 571–572

Husband J E, Hawkes D J, Peckham M J 1982 CT estimations of mean attenuation values and volume in testicular tumours: a comparison with surgical and histologic findings. Radiology 144(3): 553–558

Husband J E 1985 Staging of bladder and prostate cancer. In: Walsh J W (ed) Computed tomography of the pelvis, in the series Contemporary issues in computed tomography vol 6. Churchill Livingstone, New York, pp 135–162

Husband J E, Bellamy E A 1985 Unusual thoracoabdominal sites of metastases in testicular tumors. American Journal of Roentgenology 145: 1165–1171

Husband J E, Grimer D P 1985 Staging testicular tumours: the rôle of CT scanning. Journal of the Royal Society of Medicine 78: 25–31

Husband J E, Peckham M J, Macdonald J S 1980 The rôle of abdominal computed tomography in the management of testicular tumours. Computerised Tomography 4: 1–16

Husband J E, Barrett A, Peckham M J 1981 Evaluation of computed tomography in the management of testicular teratoma. British Journal of Urology 53: 179–183

Husband J E, Hawkes D J, Peckham M J 1982 CT

estimations of mean attenuation values and tumour volume in testicular tumours: a comparison with operative findings and histology. Radiology 144: 553–558

Johnson D E, Bracken R B, Blight E M 1976 Prognosis for pathologic stage I non-seminomatous germ cell tumors of the testis managed by retroperitoneal lymphadenectomy. Journal of Urology 116: 63–65

Kademian M T, Wirtanen G 1977 Accuracy of bipedal lymphangiography in testicular tumors. Urology 9: 218–220

Kademian M T, Bosch A, Caldwell W L 1976 Seminoma: results of treatment with megavoltage irradiation. International Journal of Radiation Oncology Biology and Physics 1: 1075–1079

Kennedy C L, Husband J E, Bellamy E A, Peckham M J, Hendry W F 1985 The accuracy of CT scanning prior to para-aortic lymphadenectomy in patients with bulky metastases from testicular teratoma. British Journal of Urology 57: 755–758

Kissin C M, Husband J E, Nicholas D, Eversman W 1987 CT demonstration of benign thymic enlargement in adult patients after chemotherapy. Radiology 167: 67–70

Lien H H, Stenwig A E, Ous S, Fossa S D 1986 Influence of different criteria for abnormal lymph node size on reliability of computed tomography in patients with non-seminomatous testicular tumor. Acta Radiologica Diagnosis 27(2): 199–203

Macdonald J S 1981 Lymphography in testicular tumours. In: Peckham M J (ed) The management of testicular tumours. Edward Arnold, London, pp 102–118

Macdonald J S, Paxton R M 1976 Lymphography. In: Williams D I, Chisholm G D (eds) Scientific foundations of urology vol II. Heinemann Medical, London, p 226

Marincek B, Brutschin P, Tiller J, Fuchs W A 1983 Lymphography and computed tomography in staging non-seminomatous testicular cancer: limited detection of early stage metastatic disease. Urologic Radiology 5: 243–246

Mostofi F J, Price E B Jr 1973 Tumors of the male genital system. In Atlas of tumor pathology, Fascicle 8, Series 2. Armed Forces Institute of Pathology, Washington

MRC Working Party on testicular tumours 1985 Prognostic factors in advanced non-seminomatous germ cell testicular tumours. Results of a multicentre study. Lancet 1: 8–11

Muhm J R, Brown L R, Crowe J K 1977 Detection of pulmonary nodules by computed tomography. American Journal of Roentgenology 128: 267–270

Muir C S, Nectoux J 1979 Epidemiology of cancer of the testis and penis. National Cancer Institute Monographs 53: 157–164

Niefeld J P, Michaelis L L, Doppman J L 1977 Suspected pulmonary metastases: correlation of chest X-ray, whole lung tomograms and operative findings. Cancer 39: 383–387

Peckham M J 1981 Investigation and staging: general aspects and staging classification. In: Peckham M J (ed) The management of testicular tumours. Edward Arnold, London, pp 89–101

Peckham M J, Barrett A, McElwain T J, Hendry W F 1979 The combined treatment of malignant testicular teratoma: a preliminary report. Lancet 2: 267–270

Peckham M J, Barrett A, Husband J E, Hendry W F 1982 Orchidectomy alone in testicular stage I, non-seminomatous germ cell tumours. Lancet ii: 678–680

Peckham M J, Barrett A, Liew K H et al 1983 The treatment of metastatic germ cell testicular tumours with

bleomycin, etoposide and cis-platin (BEP). British Journal of Cancer 47: 613–619

Peckham M J, Horwich A, Hendry W F 1985 Advanced seminoma: treatment with cis-platin based chemotherapy or carboplatin (JM8). British Journal of Cancer 52: 7–14

Poskitt K J, Cooperberg P L, Sullivan L D 1985 Sonography and CT in staging non-seminomatous testicular tumors. American Journal of Roentgenology 144: 939–944

Pugh R C B 1976 Pathology of the Testes. Blackwell Scientific Publications, Oxford

Ray B, Hajdu S I, Whitmore W F 1974 Distribution of retroperitoneal lymph node metastases in testicular germinal tumors. Cancer 33: 340–348

Rouviere H 1932 Anatomie des lymphatiques de l'homme. Masson et Cie, Paris

Rowland R G, Weisman D, Williams S D, Einhorn L H, Klatte E C, Donohue J P 1982 Accuracy of preoperative staging in stages A and B non-seminomatous germ cell testis tumors. Journal of Urology 127: 718–720

Samuelsson L, Forsberg L, Olsson A M 1986 Accuracy of radiological staging procedures in non-seminomatous testis cancer compared with findings from surgical exploration and histopathological studies of extirpated tissue. British Journal of Radiology 59: 131–134

Scatarige J C, Fishman E K, Kuhajda F P, Taylor G A, Siegelman S S 1983 Low attenuation nodal metastases in testicular carcinoma. Journal of Computer Assisted Tomography 7: 682–687

Schaner E G, Chang A E, Doppman J L, Conkle D M, Flye M W, Rosenberg S A 1978 Comparison of computed and conventional whole lung tomography in detecting pulmonary nodules: A prospective radiologic–pathologic study. American Journal of Roentgenology 131: 51–54

Sokal M, Peckham M J, Hendry W F 1980 Bilateral germ cell tumours of the testis. British Journal of Urology 52: 158–162

Stanton G F, Bosl G J, Whitmore W F et al 1985 VAB-6 as initial treatment of patients with advanced seminoma. Journal of Clinical Oncology 3: 336–339

Stomper P C, Jochelson M S, Garnick M B, Richie J P 1985 Residual abdominal masses after chemotherapy for non-seminomatous testicular cancer: correlation of CT and histology. American Journal of Roentgenology 145: 743–746

Storm P B, Kern A, Loening S A, Brown R C, Culp D A 1977 Evaluation of pedal lymphangiography in staging non-seminomatous testicular carcinoma. Journal of Urology 118: 1001–1003

Tesoro-Tess J D, Pizzocaro G, Zanoni F, Musumeci R 1985 Lymphangiography and computerized tomography in testicular carcinoma: how accurate in early stage disease? Journal of Urology 133: 967–969

Thomas J L, Bernardino M E, Bracken R B 1981 Staging of testicular carcinoma: comparison of CT and lymphangiography. American Journal of Roentgenology 137: 991–996

Tyrrell C J, Peckham M J 1976 The response of lymph node metastases of testicular teratoma to radiation therapy. British Journal of Urology 48: 363–370

van Oosterom A T, Williams S D, Cortes Funes H, ten Bokkel Huinink W W, Vendrik C P, Einhorn L H 1986 The treatment of advanced seminoma with combination chemotherapy. In: Jones W G, Milford Ward A, Anderson C K (eds) Germ cell tumours II Advances in the Biosciences vol 55. Pergamon Press, Oxford, pp 229–233

Wallace S, Jing B-S 1970 Lymphangiography: diagnosis of nodal metastases from testicular malignancies. Journal of the American Medical Association 213: 94–96

Wilkinson D J, Macdonald J S 1975 A review of the rôle of lymphography in the management of testicular tumours. Clinical Radiology 26: 89–98

Williams M P, Husband J E, Heron C W 1987a Intrathoracic manifestations of testicular seminoma: radiologic appearances. American Journal of Roentgenology 149: 473–475

Williams M P, Husband J E, Heron C W 1987b Stage I nonseminomatous germ cell tumours of the testis: radiologic follow-up after orchidectomy. Radiology 164: 671–674

Williams M P, Naik G, Heron C W, Husband J E 1987c CT scanning of the abdomen in advanced seminoma: response to treatment. Clinical Radiology 38: 629–633

Williams R D, Feinberg S B, Knight L C, Fraley E E 1980 Abdominal staging of testicular tumors using ultrasonography and computed tomography. Journal of Urology 123: 872–875

11. The ovary

R. J. Johnson

INTRODUCTION

This chapter deals with malignant epithelial tumours of the ovary which are the commonest form of death from gynaecological malignancy in the UK and the USA. There are approximately 3800 deaths per annum in England and Wales and 11 000 deaths per annum in the USA (Office of Population Censuses and Surveys 1985, American Cancer Society 1975). It is estimated that 1 in 70 liveborn females will develop the disease, 40% at under 60 years of age. The overall 5-year survival of between 30% and 35% has not improved significantly in the past few decades (Doll et al 1966, Cutler et al 1975).

SCREENING

The stage of disease (Table 11.1) at diagnosis is important in determining survival with 5-year survival rates ranging from 65% for FIGO stage Ia to 3% for FIGO stage IV (Table 11.2) (Tobias & Griffiths 1976). Unfortunately, due to the insidious nature of the disease, the unreliability of clinical examination and the lack of an effective screening technique, the majority of patients (60–70%) present with stage III and IV disease. The patients may be asymptomatic at diagnosis and even those with advanced disease may only have vague symptoms of abdominal discomfort or distension. Earlier diagnosis, when surgery would be curative, may therefore have a major impact on survival and it has been calculated that by increasing the proportion of patients with stage I and II disease from 40% to 75%, the overall 5-year survival rate would increase from 28% to 45% (Crowther & Wagstaff 1986).

Table 11.1 FIGO* staging for ovarian carcinoma

FIGO stages	Extent of disease
I	Tumour limited to the ovaries.
Ia	Tumour limited to one ovary. No ascites.
Ib	Tumour limited to both ovaries. No ascites.
Ic	Tumour limited to one or both ovaries. Ascites containing malignant cells or with positive peritoneal washings.
II	Tumour involving one or both ovaries with pelvic extension.
IIa	Tumour with extension and/or metastases to the uterus and/or one or both tubes but with no involvement of visceral peritoneum. No ascites.
IIb	Tumour with extension to other pelvic tissues and/or with involvement of visceral peritoneum. No ascites.
IIc	Tumour with extension to uterus and/or one or both tubes and/or to other pelvic tissues. Ascites containing malignant cells or with positive peritoneal washings.
III	Tumour involving one or both ovaries with extension to small bowel or omentum limited to the true pelvis or intraperitoneal metastasis beyond the true pelvis or positive retroperitoneal nodes or both.
IV	Spread to distant organs.

*International Federation of Gynaecologists and Obstetricians

Attempts to improve early diagnosis by routine annual pelvic examination and cervical cytology or examination of peritoneal fluid by transvaginal aspiration have either failed, or been impractical for routine use (McGowan et al 1966, Julian & Woodruff 1969, Tobias & Griffiths 1976). As yet no circulating tumour associated antigen specific for ovarian carcinoma which will enable detection

Table 11.2 Relation of stage to prognosis

Stage	No. of patients	5-year survival (%)
I	751	61
IA	528	65
IB	130	52
IC	80	52
II	401	40
IIA	40	60
IIB	205	38
III	539	5
IV	101	3

of early disease has been identified. A number of polyclonal antibodies have been raised against soluble antigens extracted from ovarian tumours or cancer cell lines. At least three radio-immunoassays have been developed using the following:

(a) Ovarian carcinoma associated antigen (OCAA) (Bhattacharya & Barlow 1978)
(b) Ovarian carcinoma antigen (OCA) (Knauf & Urbach 1978)
(c) NB/7TK (Knauf & Urbach 1981).

Although these antigens are present in the sera of 70% of patients with ovarian cancer, they also occur in 10% of healthy individuals and in a substantial proportion of patients with other malignancies. Whilst they may be of value in monitoring patients during and after therapy, they are unlikely to be a useful screening technique.

A monoclonal antibody, CA125, has been raised against a cell surface glycoprotein (Bast et al 1981). Radio-immunoassays with the antibody have detected circulating antigen in 1% of normal individuals, 5% of patients with non-gynaecological malignancies and up to 80% of patients with epithelial ovarian carcinoma. A study is at present being undertaken in 1000 patients with benign gynaecological disease to ascertain the rôle of this antibody in detecting ovarian pathology (Bast & Knapp 1984). A prospective study in a large series of women will be necessary to determine the value of this monoclonal antibody as a screening technique.

Radiological techniques may provide reliable screening. The use of CT is prohibited for reasons of cost, availability and the use of ionizing radiation. Ultrasound is more available, is quicker and less expensive and does not use potentially harmful radiation. The ovaries can usually be identified, volume measurements made (Campbell et al 1982) and differences in ovarian size in individuals recorded. This applies equally in postmenopausal women in whom the ovaries decrease in size.

Early published data (Goswamy et al 1983) indicates that ultrasound screening will detect small ovarian neoplasms. However, the interval needed between repeat scans in order to detect the majority of Stage I disease is uncertain. It is also not known if the diagnosis and removal of asymptomatic benign neoplasms such as serous cyst adenomas, mucous cyst adenomas or endometriomas prevents uterine tumours undergoing malignant change and so reduces the incidence of invasive ovarian carcinoma. The important question of cost effectiveness has also to be answered.

DIAGNOSIS AND PREOPERATIVE ASSESSMENT

Limited disease

Approximately 30% of patients with ovarian carcinoma have tumour limited to the pelvis at the time of diagnosis. Detection is usually a chance occurrence, either on routine pelvic examination or at surgery for non-related disease (Fisher & Young 1977).

The management of a patient with an adnexal mass found on pelvic examination depends on the age of the patient, history, physical findings and the experience of the clinician (Schwartz & Weiner 1979). If malignancy cannot be excluded, surgery is usually undertaken and radiological investigations may be superfluous. However, satisfactory pelvic examination is not always possible, especially in obese patients, those who have had previous surgery or radiotherapy, those with pelvic inflammatory disease and in children. Experienced clinicians may find it difficult to determine the site of origin of a mass, e.g. whether it is uterine or ovarian. This can lead to difficulties in management and in these cases radiological investigation is justified. Even in those patients in whom the clinician is confident of his findings, radiological investigation may identify unsuspected pathology.

The radiological investigation of choice is pelvic ultrasound. When compared with surgery as a 'gold standard', ultrasound will detect and identify the site of origin of a pelvic mass in approximately 90% of patients (Levi & Delval 1976, Lawson & Albarelli 1977, Fleisher et al 1978, DeLand et al 1979, Walsh et al 1979). The size of the lesion can be measured and solid and cystic components identified. It is important to realise that ultrasound cannot characterize tissue and predict histology. It has been suggested that certain features allow for distinction between benign and malignant lesions (Morley & Barnett 1970, Kobayashi 1976, Meire et al 1978) but these are not reliable in practice (Goswamy et al 1983).

CT is less operator-dependent than ultrasound and will provide similar information as to the presence, site of origin and extent of a pelvic mass (Walsh et al 1978, Amendola et al 1981, Coulam et al 1982, Sanders et al 1983). It should be reserved for those patients who require further investigation following an equivocal ultrasound scan or when ultrasound has failed to identify a mass detected clinically.

Like ultrasound, CT cannot characterize tissue but both techniques can be combined with percutaneous needle aspiration biopsy to obtain a tissue diagnosis. This may be of value in patients with a primary tumour elsewhere who develop a pelvic mass. Distinction between a second primary tumour and a metastasis may be made and appropriate therapy given.

Radiolabelled monoclonal antibody imaging is not yet a reliable technique in distinguishing between uterine and ovarian masses or between benign and malignant lesions. Magnetic resonance imaging (MRI) is only available in a limited number of centres at present and its potential role is discussed later.

If surgery for suspected ovarian malignancy is indicated, then should radiological staging be undertaken prior to laparotomy? Surgery is indicated for confirmation and exclusion of malignancy. In the former case, surgery will provide tissue for histology, and if performed properly is the 'gold standard' for staging and the primary treatment. Ideally, all tumour should be removed and a bilateral salpingo-oopherectomy, hysterectomy and omentectomy performed. The abdomen should be explored, particularly the undersurface of the hemidiaphragms, and multiple peritoneal and lymph node biopsies should be taken. The only evidence of disease outside the pelvis may be found in these biopsies and may measure only a few millimetres in diameter. The inability of CT or ultrasound to characterize tissue and to detect lesions less than 1 cm in diameter excludes them from replacing surgery as a staging technique. It is therefore difficult to justify undertaking investigations which are time-consuming, and may be expensive, to identify disease which can only be detected at laparotomy. In those patients who do not have a malignancy, any preoperative staging investigations will have been unnecessary and wasteful of time and money.

In those patients referred for diagnostic ultrasound or CT in whom a mass with features of ovarian malignancy is identified, examination of the abdomen, with special attention being paid to the known sites of metastasis, can be justified. Some surgeons may require to know whether there is disease outside the pelvis in order to plan the optimal surgical approach, and whether there is any urinary tract obstruction or bowel involvement. Barium studies may be required to identify those patients who require bowel resection or diversion.

The role of preoperative lymphography is discussed in a later section.

Advanced disease

Invasion of other pelvic organs and extension into the abdomen of ovarian carcinoma can cause few if any symptoms and as a result the majority of patients present with advanced disease (Stage III and IV). Patients may notice increasing abdominal girth or have non-specific symptoms related to the gastrointestinal or genitourinary tracts. Physical examination often reveals an abdominopelvic mass and gynaecologists will proceed to laparotomy with minimal radiological investigations being undertaken. These can include a chest radiograph to identify cardiopulmonary disease, an intravenous urogram to demonstrate the anatomy of the urinary tract and occasionally barium studies to identify those patients who require bowel resection and/or diversion. An ultrasound scan may be performed to confirm an abdominopelvic mass of probable ovarian origin.

The arguments for and against preoperative staging are similar to those described in the previous section. Surgery is undertaken both as the staging procedure and as treatment. No radiological techniques can replace surgical staging although they may complement it. Identification of extent of disease prior to surgery is likely to be a local preference and is unlikely to alter immediate patient management.

Magnetic resonance imaging

The display of pelvic anatomy is well suited for study by MRI due to the absence of motion artefact. There is a high intrinsic contrast between pelvic fat, urine in the bladder, air and faeces in the rectum and the pelvic soft tissues which MRI, with its superior contrast resolution to ultrasound and CT, should be able to exploit thereby improving the staging of pelvic malignancy. The ability to image directly in the coronal and sagittal planes in addition to the transverse axial plane enables anatomical relationships to be better displayed and appreciated and should allow better identification and delineation of tumour spread from one site to adjacent structures, the pelvic floor and perineum.

As yet, MRI is unable to detect metastases in normal-sized lymph nodes or to distinguish between lymphadenopathy secondary to metastatic disease or other causes. However, it can readily distinguish between lymph node and pelvic side wall vasculature on T_1 or intermediate T_1-weighted sequences. This may improve the sensitivity of detection of lymphadenopathy, especially in the presence of ectatic vessels, a not uncommon problem in older patients (Fig. 11.1).

MRI has the potential to characterize tissue and to distinguish between benign and malignant lesions. This has implications in the diagnosis and staging of ovarian carcinoma. Tissue characterization can be approached in a variety of ways, viz. measurement of proton density, relaxation times, blood flow, chemical shift and/or the use of paramagnetic tracers. Using measurements of relaxation times, Johnson et al (1987) have demonstrated that by using a robust and reproducible method of T_1 and T_2 relaxation time measurement (Waterton et al 1984, Hickey et al 1986) distinction between recurrent rectal tumour and fibrosis can be made.

In the normal female pelvis, images obtained with T_2-weighted sequences demonstrate an intermediate signal intensity from the myometrium and a high signal intensity from the endometrium. Surrounding the endometrium is a low signal intensity band within the myometrium, the nature of which is uncertain (Fig. 11.2). It has been ascribed to the stratum basalis of the endometrium (Hricak et al 1983), a compacted muscle layer at the myometrial/endometrial junction (Worthington B S et al 1985) or as having a vascular basis (Worthington J L et al 1986). The zonal anatomy of the uterus is influenced by the hormonal environment and undergoes changes during the menstrual cycle. The normal ovary is more difficult to visualize, having a low to medium signal intensity on T_1-weighted images, and is best seen on heavily T_2-weighted sequences when the signal intensity approaches that of surrounding fat. The vessels surrounding the ovaries are identified as tubular structures at their periphery (Fig. 11.3).

In the assessment of adnexal mass lesions the characteristic zonal anatomy of the uterus facilitates assessment of the site of origin of the mass and for ovarian lesions, simple fluid-containing cysts can be separated from other types of lesions (Dooms et al 1986). The contents of cysts associated with endometriosis can be identified from the signal intensities obtained following the application of different pulse sequences (Worthington B S et al 1986). There have been anecdotal reports on the

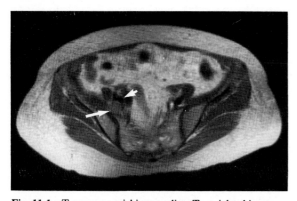

Fig. 11.1 Transverse axial intermediate T_1-weighted image (SE 1100/60) demonstrating lymphadenopathy (arrowed) lying posteriorly to the iliac vessels (arrowhead). Note the difference in signal intensity between the lymphadenopathy and the vessels.

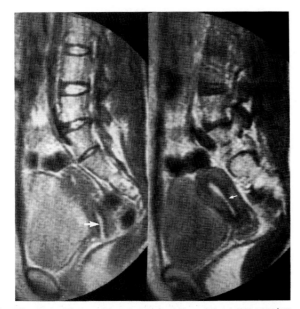

Fig. 11.2 Two multisection sagittal T_2-weighted (SE 3000/60) images demonstrating the normal uterus. There is a high signal intensity from the endometrium and the cervical mucous within the mucus-secreting glands and cervical plug (large arrow). The low intensity band between the endometrium and myometrium is well shown (small arrow). The low intensity band in the cervix probably represents stromal tissue with a high collagen content.

appearances of ovarian carcinoma on MRI but, as yet, no study comparing MRI with CT and surgery has been published.

Radiolabelled monoclonal antibody imaging (radio-immunoscintigraphy)

The aim of this technique is to detect tumour cells in vivo by using radio-isotopes attached to antibodies which bind to tumour-associated antigens on the cell surface. The use of radiolabelled antibodies to detect and visualize antibody/antigen interaction in vivo was first reported by Pressman & Keighley (1948) but clinical experience has only been gained more recently. Ward and Shepherd (1986) state that this technique can, theoretically, be used in three situations:

1. As a replacement for exploratory surgery, particularly second look laparotomy. The rôle of second look laparotomy is contentious and it is more likely to be informative than therapeutic. Radio-immunoscintigraphy is one method of restaging patients and determining end points of treatment.

2. As a means of improving the accuracy of preoperative staging, particularly to reduce the number of patients requiring bowel resection, which in their experience is approximately 25%.

3. It may have a rôle to play in association with screening programmes.

However, they admit that practical problems are preventing the translation from theoretical use. These problems are related to the antibody, the antigen, the isotope and the tumour itself. Initial studies using the antibody $HMFG_2$, conjugated to ^{123}I, correlating extent of tumour with surgery are encouraging and they report detection of lesions less than 1 cm^3 in size using subtraction techniques.

POSTOPERATIVE ASSESSMENT

Surgery is accepted as the primary treatment for ovarian carcinoma. Postoperative radiotherapy will improve the 5-year survival in patients with stage II disease and may be beneficial in stage III patients who have been optimally debulked, i.e. who have no residual disease greater than 2 cm in diameter (Bush & Dembo 1986, Spooner 1986).

Management of advanced epithelial ovarian carcinoma depends on maximum surgical effort to reduce tumour bulk to a minimum followed by the use of systemic chemotherapy. Although intensive combination chemotherapy will increase response rates and improve progression-free intervals, its use has not led to an improvement in overall survival. At present, only a small percentage of patients with advanced disease will be 'cured' and this may relate more to the tumour and patient characteristics than the chemotherapy regimen. The place of toxic combination chemotherapy has not been determined and it may well be that outside trial situations there is little place for its use and that single agents or less toxic regimens may be more appropriate (Lawton & Blackledge 1986). However, it is important that well planned, randomized clinical trials are conducted to evaluate the true rôle of chemotherapy. In these trials, stratification for the important prognostic factors must be made. Stage of disease at presentation or the amount of tumour remaining after surgery are two of these factors.

Accurate staging is important as the detection of

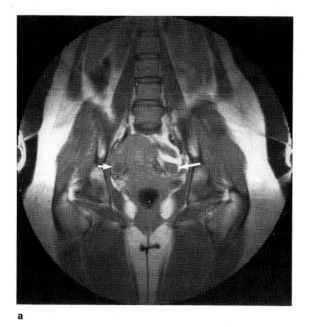

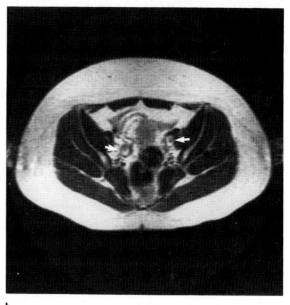

a   b

Fig. 11.3   (a) Coronal intermediate T_1-weighted image (SE 1100/60) demonstrating both ovaries (arrowed). (b) Transverse axial T_2-weighted image (SE 1500/80) demonstrating both ovaries (arrowed) of high signal intensity surrounded by a low intensity ring which represents the vessels.

unsuspected disease may alter the choice and efficacy of subsequent therapy. Surgery is the accepted 'gold standard' for staging techniques but is not 100% accurate. Between 20% and 50% of women who have had surgery, with or without additional radiotherapy for localized disease (stage I and II), will relapse and require further treatment (Munnel 1968, Bagley et al 1972). Some of these patients will have been initially understaged (Bagley et al 1973, Knapp & Friedman 1974, Rosenoff et al 1975). In patients with advanced disease it may not be possible either to adequately stage them or to remove all tumour. Only one third of patients referred to Manchester Ovarian Cancer Group Studies on combination chemotherapy in advanced disease have had adequate staging and surgical procedures. Between 15% and 20% have only had a biopsy.

There is, therefore, a case for additional staging procedures to be undertaken as follows:

1. To identify disease missed at surgery and assess its volume. This avoids the use of inappropriate additional therapy, for example, the use of postoperative radical megavoltage radiotherapy in patients thought to have only microscopic residual tumour.

2. To stage those patients in whom surgery has been incomplete, especially if toxic combination chemotherapy regimens are to be used. In these situations, clinicians require a more sophisticated staging technique than clinical examination to identify sites of disease and obtain baseline measurements prior to commencing treatment.

Imaging techniques must be able to identify tumour at the predicted sites of spread. The FIGO staging system is based on the concept that ovarian cancer spreads first within the pelvis, then within the peritoneum and does not metastasize outside the peritoneum until quite late in the course of the disease. Five pathways of metastatic spread have been described;

1. Local extension to contiguous structures.
2. Transcoelomic spread to involve the peritoneum, including the undersurface of the hemidiaphragms, liver capsule, omentum and visceral serosa.
3. Lymphatic spread to involve iliac, para-aortic and paracaval nodes.

4. Haematogenous spread to the liver parenchyma and rarely to lung or bone.

5. Transdiaphragmatic spread to involve mediastinal nodes.

The commonly used imaging techniques are CT, ultrasound and lymphography. MRI and radioimmunoscintigraphy have been discussed in previous sections.

CT as an adjunct to surgical staging

There have been several reports on CT in ovarian carcinoma and its rôle in the diagnosis and management of this disease (Schaner et al 1977, Amendola et al 1981, Mamtora & Isherwood 1982, Johnson et al 1983). In a series of 120 patients, Johnson et al (1983) demonstrated that CT compared favourably with surgical staging in the pelvis and abdomen and was superior to clinical examination of the pelvis and abdomen by experienced physicians. Disease at the predicted sites of metastasis could be demonstrated. Whilst surgical staging was the most important investigation, it did not identify all the sites of disease. Six patients who had had their liver inspected and palpated at surgery and were thought to be clear were shown to have metastases on CT. These metastases were usually situated posteriorly in the right lobe, a site difficult for the surgeon to assess (Fig. 11.4).

Uterine involvement, confirmed by repeat laparotomy, and retroperitoneal lymphadenopathy were other sites of disease missed at initial surgery but identified on CT. Blaquiere and Husband (1983) have also reported patients with liver metastases only identified by CT.

CT is therefore a non-invasive technique capable of identifying disease missed at surgery. The finding of unsuspected liver metastases has important implications for further treatment, especially if this is the only site of disease outside the pelvis. As it can image all metastatic sites, CT can be used as a single staging investigation when surgery has been inadequate. In both these situations it will provide objective baseline measurements so that response to additional treatment can be assessed.

Some of the disadvantages and limitations of the technique have been mentioned. These include cost and limited availability and an inability to characterize tissue and to detect lesions less than 1 cm in diameter. Difficulties can be experienced in interpreting the changes related to the vault of the vagina up to three months postoperatively and in distinguishing between unopacified bowel loops and residual tumour.

Ultrasound as an adjunct to surgical staging

Ultrasound findings in advanced ovarian carcinoma

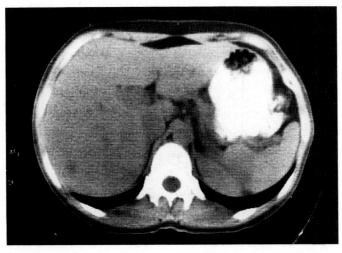

Fig. 11.4 CT scan through the liver demonstrating metastases posteriorly in the right lobe.

have been reported (Paling & Shawker 1981, Requard et al 1981) and there have been several comparisons of CT and ultrasound as staging techniques (Cosgrove et al 1980, Coulam et al 1982, Sanders et al 1983). Blackledge et al (1987) have recently completed a study comparing CT and ultrasound with surgical staging and clinical examination. The overall findings demonstrate that both CT and ultrasound compare favourably in identifying disease within the pelvis and liver but CT is superior in detecting disease in the peritoneal cavity and the retroperitoneum. Real-time ultrasound can often solve the dilemma on CT of distinguishing between unopacified bowel loops and a tumour mass.

If access to a CT scanner is limited, then ultrasound will provide a useful alternative staging investigation, especially for assessment of disease within the pelvis and liver.

If there is access to both CT and ultrasound then a rational policy should be adopted for the use of these techniques as adjuncts to surgical staging. For those patients who have had inadequate surgery, particularly when only a biopsy has been done, and who have a bulk tumour present, ultrasound is the appropriate technique for obtaining baseline measurements prior to chemotherapy. For those patients who have had adequate surgery, or who have minimal residual disease, CT is a more appropriate technique. For those patients who fall in between these two groups a flexible imaging policy should be adopted.

Lymphography as an adjunct to surgical staging

The lymphatics are a recognized pathway for the spread of ovarian carcinoma. The lymphatics of the ovary follow the ovarian veins and on the right ascend to lymph nodes in the paracaval region at the level of L2 and L3. On the left the lymphatics drain into nodes in the renal hilar and para-aortic areas at the level of L1. Accessory lymphatic channels may drain to the external iliac nodes. Extension of ovarian carcinoma to other pelvic organs provides additional pathways of lymphatic spread. Tumour cells within the peritoneum will flow preferentially into the lymphatics of the right hemidiaphragm and then to the mediastinum.

Detection of lymph node involvement is important, especially in patients with clinical stage I and II disease, as it may alter the choice of additional therapy. Knapp and Friedman (1974) performed aortic node biopsy in 26 patients with apparent stage I ovarian carcinoma and found metastases in 6. They did not think it feasible on the basis of palpation alone to determine if grossly enlarged nodes contained tumour or whether normal-sized nodes were free of tumour, and they therefore recommended routine biopsy of retroperitoneal nodes as part of surgical staging. This is now accepted practice.

Bipedal lymphography is used in many centres to detect lymph node involvement by primary and secondary malignancy. Its accuracy in detecting lymph node involvement in ovarian carcinoma has been reported, with an incidence of 8–22% in stage I, 5–20% in stage II, 29–41% in stage III and more than 50% in stage IV disease (Fuchs 1969, Hanks & Bagshaw 1969, Parker et al 1974, Musumeci et al 1980). In the series reported by Musumeci et al (1980), they were able to compare the lymphography findings with histology in 96 patients. Radiological accuracy was confirmed in 33 out of 33 positive and 55 out of 63 negative lymphograms; of the 8 false negative examinations, 5 were due to the presence of micrometastases.

The newer imaging modalities of CT and ultrasound will detect lymph node metastases. The criterion for tumour involvement is node size and metastases in normal-sized nodes cannot be detected. If a node is enlarged due to reactive hyperplasia or from an associated inflammatory process, then it will be falsely regarded as involved by tumour. Accuracy can be improved by the use of fine needle aspiration biopsy. Lymphography will estimate node size and internal architecture and is, therefore, capable of detecting metastases in normal-sized nodes, although the changes are often difficult to interpret. Equivocal lymph glands can be further evaluated by fluoroscopically guided percutaneous needle biopsy (Dunnick et al 1980). Follow-up radiographs are important as initially negative examinations may become positive (MacDonald 1982).

The disadvantages of bipedal lymphography compared with CT and ultrasound are that it is an invasive procedure associated with morbidity and rarely mortality. It is an uncomfortable procedure for the patient and requires expertise to perform and, more important, to interpret the radiographs, particularly when there are abnormalities in normal-sized nodes. Whilst lesions in normal-sized nodes can be identified, micrometastases are still missed. Certain lymph node areas which are the sites of metastases are not imaged. These include external and internal iliac, renal hilar, upper para-aortic/paracaval and retrocrural nodes. Lymphography does not give any information about disease at other sites within the abdomen.

Preoperative bipedal lymphography has been undertaken routinely in some centres (Musumeci et al 1980). In view of the limitations and morbidity associated with this procedure, it does not seem justified to use the technique on all patients with apparent stage I and II disease in whom the diagnosis of malignancy is not confirmed. In those patients subsequently shown to have malignancy, the identification of lymph node metastases would not preclude surgery as histology is required and the patient needs to be properly staged and treated. The preoperative identification of lymph node metastases in patients with advanced disease should not affect immediate management or preclude adequate surgical staging.

Lymphography would appear to be most valuable in identifying metastases in normal-sized nodes in those patients with stage I and II disease in whom surgery and non-invasive techniques have not identified disease outside the pelvis. In the absence of nodal metastases these patients may be treated by pelvic radiotherapy alone, or in certain categories of stage I disease by follow-up only.

ASSESSMENT OF TUMOUR RESPONSE

The assessment of the end point of treatment in ovarian cancer, particularly of combination chemotherapy, is difficult. A large number of studies have been designed to answer the question as to whether combination chemotherapy is better than a single agent and it is important when assessing these trials to define the end point criteria, particularly when and how response is assessed and when survival is documented; a marked difference in the survival curves for two regimens at

two years may be less obvious or non-existent at three or four years.

Invasive and non-invasive techniques can be used to assess response. The invasive techniques are either peritoneoscopy or second look laparotomy. The more commonly used non-invasive techniques are ultrasound and CT.

Peritoneoscopy or laparoscopy allows evaluation of the inferior diaphragmatic surfaces, liver, omentum and pelvis. Washings for cytology can be obtained. However, this technique has a high false negative rate and in patients who have had previous surgery or radiotherapy, the entire peritoneal cavity cannot be examined. The retroperitoneum cannot be visualized therefore lymph node status is not documented and tumour deep within the pelvis may be missed (Fisher & Young 1977, Berek et al 1981, Williams 1986).

Second look laparotomy, defined as 'an operation performed to assess disease status and to resect residual tumour whether or not its presence was suspected preoperatively' (Luesley & Chan 1986), has a number of benefits and advantages, some of which are theoretical. A second look laparotomy provides the most accurate definition of tumour response rate to chemotherapy. If the patient is found to be in a surgically documented complete remission, then unpleasant toxic chemotherapy can be stopped and trials of maintenance or consolidation therapy can be started from a defined point. It may provide the opportunity to resect residual tumour masses which have been rendered operable by chemotherapy and if minimal residual disease is detected by an early second look procedure, new treatments may be introduced in an attempt to convert a partial response to a complete one (Williams 1986).

A surgically documented complete remission confers a significant survival advantage (Cohen et al 1983) but does not imply a cure as patients can relapse (Schwartz & Smith 1980); also this survival advantage is not due to or influenced by the operation. There is currently little evidence that second look surgical debulking or second line therapy improve survival. The rôle of second look laparotomy is therefore controversial, but it is undoubtedly the most accurate method of defining tumour response to combination chemotherapy and its use should probably be confined to trials testing its usefulness and those assessing the usefulness of second line therapy in patients with minimal residual disease (Williams 1986).

The non-invasive techniques of ultrasound and CT can be used to restage patients at the end of a defined course of combination chemotherapy. CT, being able to visualize all metastatic sites, is preferable. Identification of residual or progressive disease can lead to modification or continuation of therapy. Those patients in whom further surgery is not warranted, for example those with bulk disease involving multiple bowel loops, can be identified. Previously inoperable disease may be assessed as operable or an isolated abnormality may be seen which can be an indication for further surgery, for example an abnormal uterus (Johnson et al 1983). If the ultrasound or CT scan is negative, the limitations of these techniques, particularly the inability to detect residual disease of small volume, do not preclude second look laparotomy at institutes where this is being performed (Amendola et al 1981, Brenner et al 1983, Calkins et al 1987). However, they may influence the timing of the second look laparotomy. In those centres where second look laparotomy is not performed and the scan data is relied upon for determining the end point of chemotherapy, a negative scan should not be equated with complete remission.

SUMMARY

1. Early diagnosis of ovarian carcinoma should improve overall survival and a reliable method of achieving this would be an important advance in the management of this disease; ultrasound may be such a method.

2. Ultrasound is the radiological investigation of choice in patients found to have a pelvic mass on clinical examination which warrants further assessment e.g. identification of site of origin or whether the lesion is cystic or solid, and in those patients in whom clinical examination is inadequate and disease is suspected.

3. Surgery is the most important treatment and staging technique in ovarian carcinoma. Some patients will have had inadequate staging and surgical procedures and if these patients are entered into randomized trials of combination chemotherapy then additional staging investigations are required. CT, despite its limitations, is the best single technique for this. Awareness of the postoperative appearances in the pelvis and the use of real time ultrasound when there are unopacified bowel loops present will reduce the number of interpretive errors. If access to a CT scanner is limited, then ultrasound is reliable in assessing disease within the pelvis and liver. It is less reliable than CT for detecting disease within the peritoneal cavity and retroperitoneum.

4. Newer imaging techniques have the potential to overcome some of the limitations of ultrasound and CT. Radio-immunoscintigraphy may enable the identification of small volume disease, even micrometastases. MRI has the potential to characterize tissue i.e. to distinguish between benign and malignant lesions. It is not likely to be able to provide histological diagnosis.

REFERENCES

Amendola M A, Walsh J W, Amendola B E, Tisnado J, Hall D J, Goplerud D R 1981 Computed tomography in the evaluation of carcinoma of the ovary. Journal of Computer Assisted Tomography 5: 179–186

American Cancer Society 1975 Cancer facts and figures. American Cancer Society, New York

Bagley C M Jr, Young R C, Canellos G P, DeVita V T 1972 Treatment of ovarian carcinoma: possibilities for progress. New England Journal of Medicine 287: 856–862

Bagley C M Jr, Young R C, Schein P S, Chabner B A, DeVita V T 1973 Ovarian carcinoma metastatic to the diaphragm: frequently undiagnosed at laparotomy. A preliminary report. American Journal of Obstetrics and Gynecology 116: 397–400

Bast R C Jr, Knapp R C 1984 Immunological approaches to the management of ovarian carcinoma. Seminars in Oncology 11: 264–274

Bast R C Jr, Feeney M, Lazarus H, Nadler L M, Colvin R B, Knapp R C 1981 Reactivity of a monoclonal antibody with human ovarian carcinoma. Journal of Clinical Investigations 68: 1331–1337

Berek J, Griffiths C T, Leventhall J 1981 Laparoscopy for second look evaluation in ovarian cancer. Obstetrics and Gynaecology 58: 192–198

Bhattacharya M, Barlow J J 1978 Ovarian tumour antigens. Cancer 42: 161–162

Blackledge G, Johnson R J, Kelly K Comparison with computed tomography, ultrasound, surgery and clinical examination in the assessment of ovarian cancer. Submitted for Publication

Blaquiere R M, Husband J E 1983 Conventional radiology and computed tomography in ovarian cancer: discussion paper. Journal of the Royal Society of Medicine 76(7): 574–579

Brenner D, Grosh W, Jones H 1983 An evaluation of the accuracy of computed tomography in patients with ovarian carcinoma prior to second look laparotomy. Proceedings of the American Society of Clinical Oncology 2: 149

Bush R S, Dembo A J 1986 Radiation therapy of ovarian cancer – the Toronto experience. In: Blackledge G, Chan K K (eds) The management of ovarian cancer. Butterworths, London, pp 119–127

Calkins A R, Stehman F B, Wass J L, Smirz L R, Ellis J H 1987 Pitfalls in interpretation of computed tomography prior to second look laparotomy in patients with ovarian carcinoma. British Journal of Radiology 60: 975–979

Campbell S, Goessens L, Goswamy R, Whitehead M 1982 Real time ultrasonography for determination of ovarian morphology and volume: a possible early screening test for ovarian cancer? Lancet 1: 425–426

Cohen C J, Brookner H W, Goldberg J D, Holland J F 1983 Improved therapy with cisplatin regimen for patients with ovarian carcinoma (FIGO III and IV) as measured by surgical end staging (second look surgery): The Mount Sinai experience. Clinics in Obstetrics and Gynaecology 10: 307–324

Cosgrove D O, Barker G H, Husband J E, McReady V R, Pussell S J, Wiltshaw E 1980 Carcinoma of the ovary: an evaluation of the rôle of ultrasound and CT scanning in its management. Ultrasound in Medicine and Biology. In: Wagai T, Omoto R, McCready V R (eds) Proceedings of the second meeting of the World Federation for Ultrasound in Medicine and Biology, Miyazaki, 22–27 July 1979. Excerpta Medica International Congress Series 505. Excerpta Medica, Amsterdam, Elsevier, New York, pp 25–29

Coulam C M, Julian C G, Fleisher A 1982 Clinical efficacy of CT and US in evaluating gynaecologic tumours. Applied Radiology Jan/Feb 1982: 79–87

Crowther D, Wagstaff J 1986 Future approaches. In: Blackledge G, Chan K K (eds) Management of ovarian cancer. Butterworths, London

Cutler S J, Myers M H, Green S B 1975 Trends in survival rates of patients with cancer. New England Journal of Medicine 293: 122–124

Deland M, Van-Nagell J R, Donaldson E S 1979 Ultrasonography in the diagnosis of tumours of the ovary. Surgery, Gynaecology and Obstetrics 148(3): 346–348

Doll R, Payne P, Waterhouse J 1966 Cancer incidence in 5 continents. International Union Against Cancer: Springer-Verlag, New York

Dooms G C, Hricak H, Tscholakoff D 1986 Adnexal structures: MR Imaging Radiology 158: 639–646

Dunnick N R, Fisher R I, Chu E W, Young R C 1980 Percutaneous aspiration of retroperitoneal lymph nodes in ovarian cancer. American Journal of Roentgenology 135: 109–113

Fisher R I, Young R C 1977 Advances in the staging and treatment of ovarian cancer. Cancer 39: 967–972

Fleisher A C, Everette James A Jr, Millis J B, Julian C 1978 Differential diagnosis of pelvic masses by gray scale sonography. American Journal of Roentgenology 131: 469–476

Fuchs W A 1969 Malignant tumours of the ovary. In: Fuchs W A, Davidson J W, Fischer H W (eds) Recent Results in Cancer Research – Lymphography in Cancer. Springer-Verlag, New York, pp 119–123

Goswamy R K, Campbell S, Whitehead M I 1983 Screening for ovarian cancer. Clinics in Obstetrics and Gynaecology 10: 621–643

Hanks G E, Bagshaw M A 1969 Megavoltage radiation and lymphangiography in ovarian cancer. Radiology 93: 649–654

Hickey D S, Checkley D R, Aspden R M, Naughton A, Jenkins J P R, Isherwood I 1986 A method for the clinical measurement of relaxation times in MRI. British Journal of Radiology 59: 565–576

Hricak H, Alpers C, Crooks L E, Sheldon P E 1983 Magnetic resonance imaging of the female pelvis. American Journal of Roentgenology 141: 1119–1128

Johnson R J, Blackledge G, Eddleston B, Crowther D 1983 Abdominopelvic computed tomography in the management of ovarian carcinoma. Radiology 146: 447–452

Johnson R J, Jenkins J P R, Isherwood I, James R D, Schofield P F 1987 Quantitative magnetic resonance imaging in rectal carcinoma. British Journal of Radiology 60: 761–764

Julian C G, Woodruff J D 1969 The rôle of chemotherapy in the treatment of primary ovarian malignancy. Obstetrical and Gynaecological Survey 24: 1037–1342

Knapp R C, Friedman E A 1974 Aortic lymph node metastases in early ovarian cancer. American Journal of Obstetrics and Gynaecology 119: 1013–1017

Knauf S, Urbach G I 1978 The development of durable antibody radio-immunoassay for detecting ovarian tumour associated antigen fraction OCA in plasma. American Journal of Obstetrics and Gynaecology 131: 780–787

Knauf S, Urbach G I 1981 Identification, purification and radio-immunoassay of NB/70K, a human ovarian associated antigen. Cancer Research 41: 1351–1357

Kobayashi M 1976 Use of diagnostic ultrasound in trophoblastic neoplasm and ovarian tumours. Cancer 38: 441–452

Lawson T L, Albarelli J N 1977 Diagnosis of gynaecologic pelvic masses by gray scale ultrasonography: Analysis of specificity and accuracy. American Journal of Roentgenology 128: 1003–1006

Lawton F G, Blackledge G 1986 Chemotherapy of ovarian cancer. In: Blackledge G, Chan K K (eds) The management of ovarian cancer. Butterworths, London, pp 97–108

Levi S, Delval R 1976 Value of ultrasonic diagnosis of gynaecologic tumours in 370 surgical cases. Acta Obstetrica et Gynecologica Scandinavica 55: 261–266

Luesley D M, Chan K K 1986 Second look laparotomy. In: Blackledge G, Chan K K (eds) The management of ovarian cancer. Butterworths, London, pp 79–96

MacDonald J S 1982 Lymphography in lymph node disease. In: Kinmouth J B (ed) The Lymphatics, 2nd edn. Edward Arnold, London, pp 237–371

McGowan L, Stein D B, Miller W 1966 Cul-de-sac aspiration for diagnostic cytology study. American Journal of Obstetrics and Gynaecology 96: 413–417

Mamtora H, Isherwood I 1982 Computed tomography in ovarian carcinoma: patterns of disease and limitations. Clinical Radiology 33: 165–171

Meire H B, Farrant P, Guha T 1978 Distinction of benign from malignant ovarian cysts by ultrasound. British Journal of Obstetrics and Gynaecology 85: 893–899

Morley P, Barnett E 1970 The use of ultrasound in the

diagnosis of pelvic masses. British Journal of Radiology 43: 602–616

Munnel E W 1968 The changing prognosis and treatment in cancer of the ovary. American Journal of Obstetrics and Gynaecology 100: 790–805

Musumeci R, De Palo G, Kenda R, Tesoro-Tess J D, Di Re F, Petrillo R, Rilke F 1980 Retroperitoneal metastases from ovarian carcinoma: reassessment of 365 patients studied with lymphography. American Journal of Roentgenology 134: 449–452

Office of Population Censuses and Surveys 1985 Mortality Statistics 1985 HMSO, London

Paling M R, Shawker T H 1981 Abdominal ultrasound in advanced ovarian carcinoma. Journal of Clinical Ultrasound 9: 435–441

Parker B R, Castellino R A, Fuks Z Y, Bagshaw M A 1974 The rôle of lymphography in patients with ovarian cancer. Cancer 34: 100–105

Pressman D, Keighley G 1948 The zone of activity of antibodies as determined by the use of radioactive tracers: the zone of activity of nephritoxic antikidney serum. Journal of Immunology 59: 141–146

Requard C K, Meitler F A, Wicks J D 1981 Preoperative sonography of malignant ovarian neoplasms. American Journal of Roentgenology 137: 79–82

Rosenoff S H, DeVita V T, Hubbard S, Young R C 1975 Peritoneoscopy in the staging and follow-up of ovarian cancer. Seminars in Oncology 2: 223–228

Sanders R C, McNeil B J, Finberg H J, Hessel S J, Siegelman S S, Adams D F, Alderson P O, Abrams H L 1983 A prospective study of computed tomography and ultrasound in the detection and staging of pelvic masses. Radiology 146(2): 439–442

Schaner E G, Head G L, Kalman M A, Dunnick N R, Doppman J L 1977 Whole body computed tomography in the diagnosis of abdominal and thoracic malignancy: review of 600 cases. Cancer Treatment Reports 61: 1537–1560

Schwartz P E, Smith J P 1980 Second look operations in ovarian cancer. American Journal of Obstetrics and Gynaecology 138: 1124–1130

Schwartz P E, Weiner M 1979 Ultrasound in gynaecology: a clinician's viewpoint. Clinics in Diagnostic Ultrasound 2 Genitourinary Ultrasonography: 183–190

Spooner D 1986 Radiation therapy in the management of ovarian malignancy. In: Blackledge G, Chan K K (eds) The management of ovarian cancer. Butterworths, London, pp 128–139

Tobias J S, Griffiths C T 1976 Management of ovarian carcinoma. New England Journal of Medicine 249: 818–823

Walsh J N, Rosenfield A T, Jaffe C C, Schwartz P E, Simeone J, Dembner A G, Taylor K J W 1978 Prospective comparison of ultrasound and computed tomography in the evaluation of gynaecologic pelvic cases. American Journal of Roentgenology 131: 955–960

Walsh J N, Taylor K J W, Wasson J F M, Schwartz P E, Rosenfield A T 1979 Grey-scale ultrasound in 204 proven gynaecologic masses: accuracy and specific diagnostic criteria. Radiology 130: 391–397

Ward B G, Shepherd J H 1986 The role of monoclonal antibodies in the diagnosis and investigation of ovarian cancer. In: Blackledge G, Chan K K (eds) The management of ovarian cancer. Butterworths, London, pp 46–55

Waterton J C, Checkley D R, Jenkins J P R, Naughton A, Zhu X P, Hicky D S, Isherwood I 1984 Use of the Total Saturation Recovery sequence in MRI: An improved approach to the measurement of T_1. Proceedings of the Third Annual Meeting of the Society of Magnetic Resonancing Medicine: New York. Society of Magnetic Resonance in Medicine, Berkeley, California, pp 736–737

Williams C J 1986 Second look laparotomy in epithelial ovarian carcinoma. In: Blackledge G, Chan K K (eds) The management of ovarian cancer. Butterworths, London, pp 76–82

Worthington B S, Powell M C, Buckley J H, Womack C, Symonds E M 1985 The low intensity band on spin echo images of the uterus: anatomic and clinicopathologic study. Radiology 157: 310

Worthington B S, Powell M, Symonds E M 1986 The rôle of MRI in the evaluation of endometriosis. Radiology 16(p) 306

Worthington J L, Balfe D M, Lee J K T et al 1986 Uterine neoplasms: MR imaging. Radiology 159: 725–730

12. The cervix

B. Eddleston

INTRODUCTION

In the United Kingdom approximately 4000 new cases of cervical cancer are recorded each year. The disease accounts for 2.9% of all deaths due to cancer in women (OPCS 1985). The commonest age groups affected used to be those between 45 and 55 years, but in the past decade more cases have been arising in younger women. There is evidence that the present generation of young women who have an exceptionally high incidence may continue to be at increased risk throughout their lives unless control measures are successful.

Considerable variation in geographic distribution of this disease has been recognized and it is normally the commonest cause of malignancy in women in developing countries. Classically there has been recognized to be a high incidence in women of lower socioeconomic status, the multiparous, those who begin sexual activity at an early age and those who have had more than one sexual partner. It is rare in virgins and some Jewish women. The reason for this latter finding is not completely clear, although there is some indication that ethnic patterns of sexual behaviour and/or genetic factors have a determining influence.

There has been very little change in the UK national incidence and mortality of the disease over the last two decades, but some Scandinavian countries and North American States have seen major falls in both incidence and mortality. Successful population screening may be responsible.

AETIOLOGY

Apart from the extreme rarity of cervical cancer in women who have never been known to be sexually active, and the greatly increased incidence in the lower socioeconomic groups of the population, many additional factors have been considered in relation to the cause of this disease including dietary habits, general hygiene and cigarette smoking. The strongest association by far is that of the age of first sexual intercourse and it is now generally considered to be a sexually related condition. The human papilloma virus (HPV) has been implicated as the aetiological agent, particularly types 16 and 18 where the viral DNA actually integrates into the nuclear DNA of the cell. Other papilloma virus types 6, 10, 11 and 32 have also been identified in cervical dysplasia and cervical intraepithelial neoplasia. The absolute relationship of HPV infection to the development of carcinoma of the cervix is still not firmly established; a recent critical review of the epidemiological evidence has been published by Munoz et al (1988). Herpes simplex virus (HSV) may be a cofactor, as may be tobacco metabolites and the immunosuppressive action of seminal fluid on an already damaged and infected cervix.

PROGNOSIS

Prognosis depends on the stage of the disease at presentation (Pettersson 1988). To date this has been dominated by the extent of the primary tumour, and patients with extension of disease beyond the pelvis have been shown to have a prognosis dependent on the degree of spread (Ward et al 1985). A survival rate of 50% for those patients with spread to one group of nodes unilaterally falls to virtually 0% for those who have microscopic spread to the para-aortic chains. A considerable number of the younger age group are diagnosed as having early clinical stage disease at presentation, but are shown surgically to have disseminated metastases (Hall & Monaghan 1983). Patients with primary tumours over 4 cm in diameter, with disease affecting more than two-thirds of the thickness of the cervix, poorly differentiated histology and vascular invasion have a worse prognosis.

PATHOLOGY

Cancer of the cervix was traditionally described as being 95% squamous cell carcinoma and 5% adenocarcinoma, with the rare occurrence of sarcoma, malignant melanoma and primary lymphoma. Recently Buckley et al (1988) have identified a changing pattern, with approximately 70% of the cases proving to be pure squamous cell carcinoma, 16% adenocarcinoma and 14% adenosquamous carcinoma. Furthermore, it would appear that it is the younger age group of women who are presenting with non-squamous and mixed cell tumours.

Cervical cancer spreads by local extension to the endometrium, the parametrium and thence to the pelvic side walls in direct continuity. Occasionally it can extend antero-posteriorly affecting the bladder, rectum and lower ureters. Very importantly it extends via the lymphatic vessels to the pelvic nodes, the para-aortic lymph nodes and even as high as the retrocrural, mediastinal and supraclavicular lymph nodes. The later the clinical stage the more likely lymphatic spread is to occur, but recently Buckley et al (1988) have identified lymph node metastases in 43.2% of surgical specimens removed for early stage cervical carcinoma. In younger patients blood-borne metastases give rise to distant metastatic involvement of lung, bone, liver and very rarely brain.

APPLIED ANATOMY

The relationship of the uterine cervix to other tissues and organs, together with the lymphatic vessels and blood supply, is extremely important in determining the spread of disease and the problems which may stem from lack of response or complications of treatment. Peritoneum, covering the uterus, extends as low as the posterior supravaginal cervix and then turns on to the anterior rectum a short distance from the posterior fornix of the vagina. Anteriorly this peritoneal sheet reflects on to the upper surface of the bladder via the vesicouterine recess. The result is that above and behind the cervix there are intestinal loops in close apposition. As the cervix projects into the vagina, forming the fornices, it is separated from the bladder by cellular connective tissue, the parametrium, which also envelops the sides of the cervix and extends laterally into the broad ligament. The bladder lies directly in front with the rectum and sigmoid colon positioned behind. As the ureters descend to the bladder they lie between 1 and 4 cm lateral to the supravaginal cervix before turning medially in front of the upper vagina. Lymphatic vessels from the cervix pass in three directions:

(i) Laterally in the parametrium to reach the external iliac nodes via the paracervical and obturator glands.
(ii) Postero-laterally to the internal iliac nodes.
(iii) Posteriorly to the presacral nodes.

These pathways link up with vessels from the vagina which drain into the inguinal and external iliac nodes. Ramifications pass out over the surface of the bladder and these can establish considerable collateral circulation when normal lymphatic drainage is obstructed. Blood supply is provided from two uterine branches of the internal iliac arteries, which anastamose superiorly with the ovarian and inferiorly with the vaginal vessels. At the level of the external opening of the cervix, two veins run with the arteries to the internal iliac veins and communicate with the vaginal vessels (Gray 1973).

DIAGNOSIS

Unfortunately cervical cancer may be symptomless, or symptoms unappreciated or ignored until late stage disease has developed. The identification of its presence rests on three possible lines of approach:

(i) Exfoliative cytology screening – the examination of a cellular smear taken by spatula or brush directly from the cervix;

(ii) Clinical examination of women presenting with conditions not related to the reproductive system;
(iii) Clinical assessment arising from gynaecological symptoms, particularly abnormal bleeding or discharge.

Clinical examination

Under this heading there are three categories of patients:

(i) Those who have abnormal smear findings.
(ii) Those who may be found to have cervical cancer when seen for unrelated medical conditions.
(iii) Those who present with definitive symptoms related to the reproductive tract.

Assessment involves a detailed history followed by clinical examination of the upper vagina and cervix. This leads to colposcopy or examination under anaesthesia, resulting in biopsy of overtly abnormal or suspicious sites, and evaluation of adjacent tissues, organs and lymph node areas. Only beyond these stages of the identification of disease can radiology have a place in the evaluation of carcinoma of the cervix.

STAGING

By tradition, staging of cervical cancer is a clinical exercise, using an agreed international system (FIGO 1985).

Stage 0 within the original classification has been replaced by the category cervical intra-epithelial neoplasia (CIN), which is subdivided into three groups, CIN3 corresponding to the previous stage 0. None of these stages represent invasive carcinoma. The FIGO classification for invasive carcinoma is as follows:

Stage I – Invasive tumour confined to the cervix.
IA – Microinvasive carcinoma (early stromal invasion).
IB – Clinically diagnosed cancer, remaining limited to the cervix or extending purely to the uterine body (cases of occult cancer are included).

Stage II – Tumour extending to:
IIA – The upper two-thirds of the vagina but not involving the parametrium.
IIB – Involvement of the parametrium but not reaching to the pelvic wall.

Stage III – Tumour involves either:
IIIA – The vagina in its lower third, or
IIIB – Through the parametrium as far as the pelvic side wall. (All cases associated with obstructive uropathy leading to hydronephrosis or non-functioning kidney).

Stage IV – Tumour involves either:
IVA – The mucosa of the bladder or rectum, or
IVB – Spread to tissues beyond the true pelvis.

The classification based on clinical assessment by vaginal and rectal examination, and then by the results of cystoscopy, histology and excretion urography, is primarily intended for use in relation to decisions about whether to use primary surgery. Kademian & Bosch (1977) cited the accuracy of clinical staging as between 60 and 70%, both in terms of understaging and over-staging patients treated surgically.

Averette et al (1975) compared surgical to clinical staging. 207 patients with invasive cervical cancer had been clinically staged from IB to IV prior to surgical exploration. Of 145 patients classed as stage IB, 26% were found to be more advanced and the majority of these (18%) were reclassified as stage IIIB or IV disease. Of 20 cases in clinical stage IIA, surgical exploration revealed more advanced disease in 9 (45%). Again, more than half of the restaged patients had stage IIIB or IV disease. 10 out of 20 patients with clinical stage IIB disease were reclassified as IIIB or IV. Two out of three patients with stage IIIA disease were reclassified as stage IV because of invasion of the bladder or rectum. In 16 patients with clinical IIIB disease the staging error was found to be 94%. 12 cases (75%) had surgical stage IV involvement (invasion of the bladder or rectum, or metastases to aortic lymph nodes) whilst 3 cases (18.5%) were restaged to category IIB disease.

In terms of prognosis, anomalies of the FIGO method have been commented upon by Bond (1985) and Benstead et al (1986). Bond's analysis revealed that stages IIB and IIIB each contained two subgroups with differing prognosis, depending on whether one or both parametria were involved. Similarly, in the report from Benstead et al it was noted that patients included in FIGO stage III with only one pelvic side wall involved showed a considerably improved survival rate over those in whom both pelvic walls were involved by extra-parametrial spread.

A major difficulty in clinical staging stems from the fact that the primary tumour is often associated with surrounding inflammatory disease, so that it may be impossible to determine how much of any parametrial thickening or fixation is due to growth extension.

RADIOLOGICAL ASSESSMENT

Staging by imaging methods has attracted much attention over the years. The procedures employed must, of course, concern themselves with identification of:

(i) The primary tumour.
(ii) The degree to which direct extension has occurred.
(iii) Demonstration of lymph node involvement, including the central abdominal lymph chains.
(iv) The identification of distant metastases other than in lymph nodes.

Prior to the availability of CT and refined ultrasound technology, radiological procedures which had any influence were the chest radiograph, excretion urography, pelvic and caval venography, bipedal lymphangiography and the barium enema. These were (and still may be) of value in revealing:

(i) Obstructed urinary pathways, with or without hydronephrosis.
(ii) The presence of poorly excreting or non-functioning kidneys.

(iii) 'Rat-tailing' of the distal ureters due to extravesical tumour extension (Fig.12.1).
(iv) Invasion of the bladder.
(v) Displacement of the kidneys and/or ureters by enlarged lymph nodes.
(vi) Pressure on the main pelvic and abdominal venous pathways from lymphadenopathy.
(vii) Replacement of lymph node architecture by metastases (Fig. 12.2).

The chest radiograph is of limited value except to demonstrate intercurrent disease (where clinically indicated), to examine a possible site of metastatic spread in late stage cancer, or to be a baseline for assessment on follow-up. Griffin et al (1976) reported that out of 227 patients suffering from cervical cancer who had pretreatment chest radiography, only 2 (0.88%) were discovered to have abnormal findings which were directly related to the primary disease.

Satisfactory excretion urography requires good ureteric demonstration, and to this end the large volume infusion technique gives good consistent results. Renoureteric displacement usually occurs only if lymph node enlargement is considerable, though it is sometimes possible to diagnose the presence of less gross disease by finding evidence of external pressure on well-filled ureters, as for

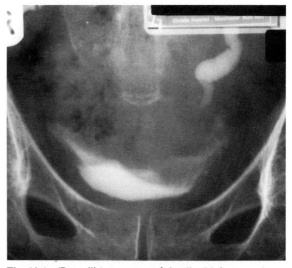

Fig. 12.1 'Rat-tail' appearance of the distal left ureter due to extracervical malignant infiltration.

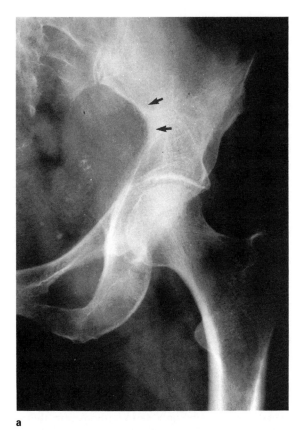 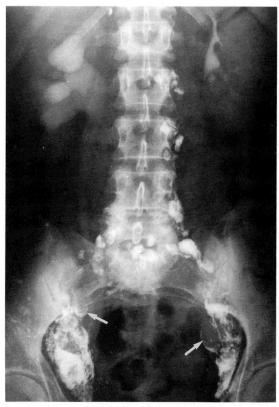

a   b

Fig. 12.2   (a) Large left soft tissue mass of metastatic lymph nodes showing direct invasion of the bony pelvic brim (arrows).
(b) Lymphadenogram and excretion urogram demonstrating lymph node metastases (arrows) together with lateral displacement
of the dilated right ureter, from para-aortic adenopathy. These lymph nodes have not taken up the contrast medium. ((b) is
reproduced by courtesy of Dr J Husband.)

example when they are dilated by incomplete
obstruction occurring from disease extension in the
pelvis. Bladder invasion is difficult to diagnose by
urography unless it is advanced or associated with
vesicovaginal fistula.

Lymphography

Bipedal lymphography (using iodinated poppy
seed oil) is not a particularly pleasant procedure
for the patient to undergo. It is capable of
demonstrating metastatic filling defects in lymph
nodes which are not enlarged, up to the level of
the kidneys. Problems arise with:

(i)   Difficulties in technique which result in
      underfilling from too little contrast.
(ii) Totally replaced nodes which do not take
      up the contrast.

(iii) Small metastases which do not produce
      significant distortion of lymph node
      architecture, to the point where there is
      diagnostic confidence of identification.
(iv) Interpretative errors due to difficulty in
      separating abnormal nodes affected by
      inflammatory as opposed to malignant
      disease.
(v)   Failure to opacify all of the lymph nodes
      in the upper pelvic and para-aortic chains.
(vi) The fact that the deep pelvic nodes, which
      are first involved in lymphatic spread, are
      not demonstrated by this technique.

Multiple reviews of the value of bipedal
lymphography for demonstrating lymph node disease in both lymphoma and metastatic carcinoma
from various sites have appeared over a period of
many years. In a critical evaluation of lymphangio-

graphy, Schaffer et al (1964) concluded that the procedure was of less value in patients with metastatic carcinoma than in those with lymphoma. A number of studies have been concerned with the particular application of the technique to cervical cancer (Piver et al 1971, Douglas et al 1972, Terry et al 1972, Smales et al 1986). There can be no doubt that this technique surpasses clinical evaluation of the pelvic and abdominal lymph nodes, both in demonstrating metastatic disease in normal-sized nodes and in revealing involvement missed by clinical examination in sites where the degree of nodal enlargement is only moderate.

In a study of the value of lymphography in stage IB cervical carcinoma, De Muylder et al (1984) examined 100 patients. 5 of these were diagnosed as positive, 15 as suspicious and 80 as negative. Subsequent histology showed 18 positive cases – all 5 of those with positive lymphograms, 3 of those with suspicious findings and 10 cases where the lymphograms had been regarded as entirely negative. Smales et al (1986) reported a 5-year survival rate for stage I patients with positive lymphograms of 55%, and for those with negative lymphograms 94%. This compared favourably to surgically staged IB patients, where the survival rates were 53% with identified lymph node metastases and 92% when no metastases were found (Martimbeau et al 1982). 80% of patients with positive lymphograms in the Smales series eventually died with disease outside the pelvis. Prognosis was especially poor in those patients who had para-aortic lymph node involvement, as had been previously quoted by Chism et al (1975) and Piver and Barlow (1981). However, 31% of patients with negative lymphograms at the outset eventually died of metastatic disease. Needless to say, the incidence of lymph node involvement rises as the clinical stage worsens. Douglas et al (1972) quoted 6% positivity in stages I and II and 10% in stage III, whereas Gerteis (1967) quoted the incidence of para-aortic lymph node disease as being 9% in stage I and 21% in stage III. In those patients who were subjected to Wertheim hysterectomy, 7% of the cases with negative lymphography showed positive nodes at surgery but 28% with reported positive lymphography did not have metastatic nodes identified. Fuchs et al (1969) expressed an overall diagnostic error rate of 15% in determining lymph node disease from lymphangiography.

For years it has been accepted that there is potential value to be gained in lymphography from a follow-up abdominal radiograph, which may demonstrate changes in lymph node patterns as unsuspected disease progresses. However, contrast retention in nodes is variable and may not be sufficient to assess changes after more than a short interval. Lee et al (1980) considered CT to be a more reliable modality for determining changing lymph node status after initial lymphography.

So-called false positive lymphangiograms, compared to histological identification of disease, may well be due to a failure to sample 'appropriate' nodes at laparotomy. This problem has been addressed by intraoperative lymphoscintigraphy (Gitsch et al 1984). Using technetium-99m labelled antimony sulphide and a gamma camera operating table, it was reported that the percentage of total lymphadenectomies in radical surgery for cervical cancer was raised from 53% to 88%.

Lymphography, therefore, shows significant deficiencies in its ability to identify the presence and extent of metastatic disease. Even though it has the advantage of being able to demonstrate abnormality in lymph nodes of less than 1.5 cm diameter, the precision with which it is capable of doing this is unreliable. Furthermore, it has distinctive limitations because of the failure to opacify nodes totally replaced by tumour.

Pelvic angiography as a staging procedure has been described by Lang (1980). Arteriographic diagnosis was based on identifying highly specific tumour neovascularity separate from that vascular change due to inflammatory disease. No understaging was said to occur, but some overstaging was reported in respect of failure to analyse the vascular appearances correctly. The technique, which does not identify lymph node metastases, is highly invasive, only applicable to direct tumour extension, and would appear to be of suspect value in recognizing infiltration of the parametrium.

Computerized tomography (CT)

The advent of CT has had a major impact on the assessment and management of cervical cancer, since this was the first time an imaging method could be deployed to examine directly the site of tumour origin and its soft tissue surroundings. The interrelationship between spatial resolution and density discrimination, related to transaxial sections, offered an entirely new concept in the appreciation of normal and pathological pelvic anatomy, coupled with the ability to view simultaneously the organ relationships, the pelvic side walls and the related lymph node areas (both pelvic and para-aortic) as well as to identify the effects on the urinary tracts and distant spread to bone, liver and brain with excellent accuracy.

CT is, however, a purely morphological tool in which the ability for boundary definition is extremely important. This is limited by the degree of spatial resolution obtained, and the influence of partial volume effect. Tissue characterization has not been possible. In all abdominopelvic studies there is a need to opacify the bowel, and the better this is achieved the less likelihood there is of misinterpreting intestinal loops as abnormal soft tissue masses. Unfortunately, there is no method of assuring that opacification occurs to the optimal degree in any individual patient. Gut motility may be inhibited by a suitable paralysant for the duration of the examination, and to this effect hyoscine-N-butylbromide (Buscopan) is a suitable agent in an intramuscular or intravenous dose of 20 mg. For the assessment of pelvic malignancy, renal excreted iodinated contrast medium should be given with the usual precautions. Unless there is evidence or suspicion of impaired renal function, 20 ml of iodinated contrast (iodine concentration approximately 300 mg/ml) is usually sufficient. As a cost saving exercise we do not use the newer low-osmolar agents unless the patient is identified as being in a 'risk category'. Each patient has a vaginal tampon and rectal balloon catheter inserted. Negative or positive contrast medium can be injected through the rectal catheter.

A standard programme of scanning is to produce 10 mm thick contiguous sections from the perineum to the iliac crest, 10 mm sections at 20 mm intervals to the level of the kidneys for assessment of pelvicalycine dilatation, and only to ascend to examine the areas above this if there is evidence of para-aortic adenopathy at renal levels, or a definite need on the part of the clinician to confirm liver metastases. However, since liver metastases occur infrequently, this problem is usually evaluated by ultrasound and/or radionuclide examination. In clinically staged early disease the programme ends at renal level.

The important question is 'Which, if not all, presenting cases of cervical cancer should be examined by CT?' CT criteria in the initial assessment of cancer of the cervix have been documented by a number of authors (Kilcheski et al 1981, Walsh et al 1981, Brenner et al 1982, Whitley et al 1982, Villasanta et al 1983, Vick et al 1984), where comparisons have been made with clinical or surgical staging or both.

Vick et al (1984) examined the question of parametrial invasion using CT and defined the difference between normal and abnormal appearances, the latter being:

(i) Poor definition or irregularity of the lateral cervical edges.
(ii) Prominent parametrial soft tissue strands extending into the surrounding fat.
(iii) Obliteration of the periureteral fat plane, with or without changes of urinary obstruction (Fig. 12.3).

The last two features were said to be always present in tumour infiltration; the first two could also be found in local inflammatory reaction.

King et al (1986) commented that CT evaluation of parametrial infiltration showed a true prediction rate of only 64%, and that the procedure added little to clinical assessment.

Out of 63 stage I patients examined, we found 13 with no demonstrable abnormality and 50 with abnormal features – usually related to distortion of the parametrium, about which it was not possible to predict whether malignant infiltration was occurring. The area of the parametrium is frequently the most difficult to evaluate, especially when there is no indication of disease elsewhere, because of the not uncommon association with inflammatory reaction.

In a series of 77 patients of average age 56 years, Walsh and Goplerud (1981) claimed that CT agreed with clinical staging in 65% of cases, advanced the stage in 19% and down-staged in 16%.

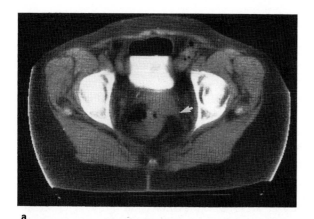

a

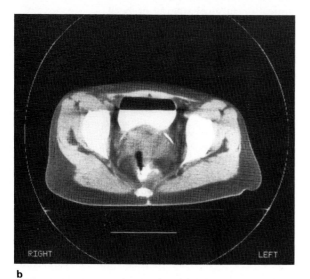

b

Fig. 12.3   CT scans demonstrating (a) left parametrial infiltration (arrow); (b) bilateral obliteration of the periureteral fat plane.

It was not accurate in differentiating stage IB from IIB lesions, but this was ascribed to the characteristics of the equipment being used. Endometrial extension was said to be diagnosable when the corpus uteri contained low density material – not a feature of our own experience of 83 patients in clinical stages I and II. Identification of the cervical tumour was claimed in 51 patients from the size of the mass (greater than 3 cm in AP diameter) and the presence of low density areas due to necrosis or ulceration. Smooth lateral cervical margins and preservation of the parametrial fat were regarded as indicators of stage I disease.

Stage IIA lesions could not be separated because of problems in demonstrating invasion of the upper vagina, and we have also found this to be a problem. IIB tumours showed irregular lateral cervical margins with parametrial extension but no involvement of the pelvic side wall, and the cervix itself was correspondingly bulkier. Identification of stage III and stage IV disease was made on finding pelvic side wall spread, invasion of the bladder (Fig. 12.4), loss of the posterior perivesical fat plane, nodular indentation of the bladder wall or intraluminal tumour and rectal involvement by obliteration of the fat plane over its anterior surface. Of itself, fat plane loss is not a reliable criterion for the extent of spread. Lymph node metastases were detected in 24% of patients examined using the standard criteria of size, but histological correlation was only available in 8 of these and 6 turned out to have only reactive hyperplasia in the nodes. A feature the authors stressed was that cervical tumour size appeared to be directly related to the likelihood of parametrial involvement and subsequent central recurrence.

Burghardt (1984) has stressed the relationship of tumour volume to the likelihood of presence of lymph node metastases, irrespective of the depth of penetration of the disease. Below 200 mm³ the risk of extension to lymph nodes is negligible. From 200 to 500 mm³ the risk is low unless vascular permeation has occurred, and above a volume of 500 mm³, when the tumour ceases to be of microinvasive type (Burghardt et al 1973), lymph node invasion is highly probable.

Whilst it is true that accuracy in identifying all sites of involvement by clinical assessment increases as the disease becomes more advanced, there is a major problem – to distinguish differences in clinical early stage disease where a therapeutic option, based on such information, would be possible. To this end, CT is capable of showing a worse situation in terms of identifying a large local mass, transpelvic spread, major involvement of bladder and rectum and enlargement of pelvic and para-aortic nodes. However, there remain distinctive problems of determining whether or not the bladder and rectum are truly invaded. Loss of fat planes (real or apparent) is by no means easy to diagnose with confidence in the individual case, and is not necessarily synonymous

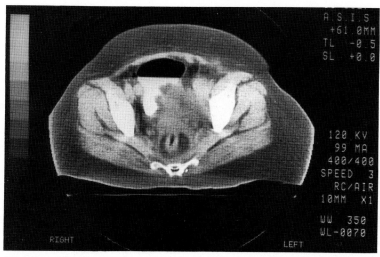

Fig. 12.4   CT scan demonstrating direct cervical tumour extension to the bladder.

with organ involvement. Furthermore, lymph node enlargement may be erroneously diagnosed because of ectatic vessels in close association (especially in the pelvis), or because they are affected by reactive hyperplasia or infection. Node size cannot be relied upon to exclude the presence of metastases.

Tindall (1987) quotes lymph node disease as now being recognized in 15–20% of clinical stage I tumours, 33% of those graded as stage II and 45% of those classified as stage III.

Ginaldi et al (1981) studied 24 patients with carcinoma of the cervix by both CT and lymphography, and confirmed that CT was better in detecting nodes completely replaced by neoplasm, those affected but not filled adequately by lymphography, and in determining extension of disease to other non-nodal sites. CT, as stated before, was incapable of demonstrating metastases in smaller nodes (less than 1.5 cm diameter), or of indicating the presence of reactive hyperplasia.

A survey (Dixon 1985) of current practice of lymphography where CT facilities exist covered a substantial area of the UK, and showed that there had been a major fall in the number of lymphograms performed. Radiologists prefer to forego any advantage of lymphography over CT for defining lymph node architecture against the ability of CT to look at more nodal sites, provide more information outside of the lymphatic system, and to be a more satisfactorily tolerated procedure (Fig. 12.5).

CT, whilst offering a wider comprehensive visualization of the regions of involvement in cervical cancer, also has distinctive limitations which may be summarized as follows:

(i)   Difficulty in evaluating the extent and volume of tumour confined to the cervix.

(ii) Problems in determining the presence of extension into the parametrium.

(iii) Identification of deep pelvic nodes until they are of a substantial size; 1–1.5 cm diameter, with greater than 2 cm likely to be malignant.

(iv) An inability to assess the likelihood of metastatic nodal disease in the common iliac, external iliac and para-aortic areas by size alone, with no ability to distinguish malignant infiltration from inflammatory disease or reactive hyperplasia.

(v)   Difficulty in assessing whether there is true invasion of the bladder and/or rectum unless there is major infiltration of either of these structures.

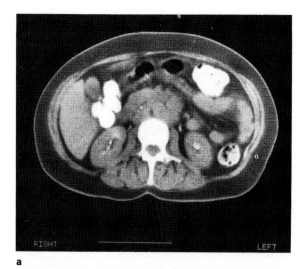

a

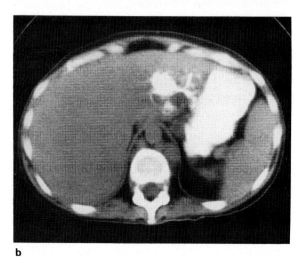

b

Fig. 12.5 (a) Substantial retroperitoneal lymphadenopathy in a patient clinically diagnosed as early stage disease. (b) Retrocrural lymphadenopathy. This could not have been diagnosed by clinical or surgical assessment and is too high to be shown by lymphography.

The advantages of CT over other methods of investigation described previously are:

(i) Demonstration of the extension of the malignant process beyond the parametria and the extent to which this is occurring on either side.

(ii) Demonstration of bone involvement before it is detectable by plain radiography, especially on the pelvic side wall and in the lumbosacral spine by direct infiltration from metastatic nodes.

(iii) The ability to recognize the presence of enlarged lymph nodes which have been totally replaced by tumour and would not be demonstrable by lymphography.

(iv) Identification of nodal disease above the levels which lymphography is capable of reaching.

Ultrasound

Application of ultrasound imaging to the female pelvis has demonstrated its capability to define abnormal morphological features in the region of the upper vagina, the cervix, the body of the uterus and the bladder. Additionally, it has been possible to gain information about the presence of bulky lymph node disease in the external and common iliac areas. Earlier applications of the technology embodied the use of abdominal surface probes of 3.5 MHz output, and examining the patient with fully distended bladder. The identification of a bulky cervix, the presence of ascites, the demonstration of a substantial mass spreading across the pelvis and lymphadenopathy, together with the revelation of the presence of obstructive uropathy, proved possible. However, inability to perform tissue characterization meant that there was considerable difficulty in separating malignant disease from inflammatory disease and fibrosis. Interference from gas in bowel loops proved to be a major factor affecting identification. Early local spread, especially into the parametrium and beyond, could not be adequately assessed. Sanders et al (1983) compared CT and abdominal surface ultrasound in the detection and staging of pelvic masses. Their results showed a slightly greater accuracy for CT (68%) than for ultrasound (56%). 28 of their cases with carcinoma of the cervix had surgical staging, and in 10 of these both ultrasound and CT underestimated the extent of disease because of micrometastatic spread or failure to appreciate non-bulky nodal disease.

Later developments of ultrasound have resulted in the application of transrectal, transurethral, transvesical and transvaginal techniques. Of these the transrectal (TRU) technique is the easiest and most consistently reproducible procedure. Di Candio et al (1984) in 10 patients demonstrated good correlation between TRU and the subsequent histopathological examination of parametrial infiltration. Zaritzky et al (1979) examined TRU specifically in the evaluation of cervical cancer. This report on 30 patients with documented evidence of tumour suggested that good imaging of the cervix and the parametrium could be obtained with a differential echo pattern at the site of tumour invasion, also that invasion of the bladder could be identified, but there was no indication as to the effectiveness of producing information on the pelvic lymph node status (Fig. 12.6). Magee & Pointon (1988) examined a group of 65 patients with cervical cancer before radiotherapy. Both transurethral and TRU procedures were carried out, but the latter was found to be more satisfactory using a 4 MHz transducer. Central pelvic disease could be visualized and any parametrial extension noted. Difficulties arose in distinguishing tumour from normal tissue in small growths localized to the cervix. Many such tumours were found to contain highly echogenic areas, but this was not a constant finding. The technique proved useful in identifying bulky (barrel-shaped) stage I tumours. However, assessment of pelvic lymphadenopathy proved unrewarding.

Yuhara et al (1987) used TRU to examine 108 patients with cervical cancer. In 29 cases parametrial infiltration was defined, and increases in parametrial dimension, internal echo intensity and shift of the cervix to the side of greater involvement were recorded. Greater parametrial bulk corresponded to wider malignant infiltration at surgery. A relationship was claimed between the width of the parametrial echo and the degree of induration as an index of parametrial infiltration.

As with CT, however, limitations still exist in being able to identify early local spread and lymph node involvement with an accuracy much greater than clinical assessment, and certainly less than surgical exploration. Nevertheless, the place of ultrasound, and the transrectal approach in particular, needs to be explored more fully with regard to its value in staging cervical cancer. The success of all ultrasound examination is greatly operator-dependent, and therefore greater application to technique, along with surgical correlation

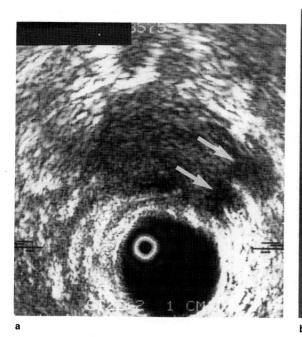

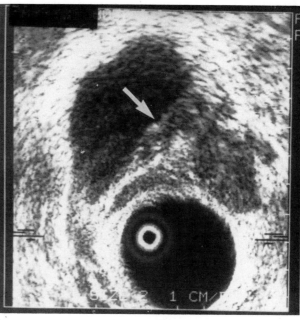

a　　　　　　　　　　　　　　　　　　　　b

Fig. 12.6 Transrectal ultrasound examination demonstrating (a) the presence of left parametrial infiltration (arrows); (b) early bladder invasion.

as far as possible, may hold out the promise of a relatively simple procedure which is much cheaper and less time-consuming than more elaborate methodology as an aid to staging.

Magnetic resonance imaging (MRI)

The use of magnetic resonance imaging (MRI) in cervical cancer is still in a relatively early phase of development. Its advantages are that it offers the facility of multiplanar imaging, avoids ionizing radiation and has, as yet, no proven biological hazard. The use of different radio frequency pulse sequences enables the production of images weighted for T_1 and T_2 relaxation times, and proton density, so as to effect the tissue contrast. The only adverse features of MRI imaging are:

(i) Cost of the technology.
(ii) Length of time for individual examination.
(iii) Patient intolerance of the procedure (under 2%).

The application of MRI to the problem of carcinoma of the cervix has recently been addressed by Powell et al (1986), assessing the potential for staging against clinical methods. Study of a group of 25 patients showed that 4 out of 7 clinical stage I patients had disease of a more advanced nature. This was also true in 3 out of 5 in clinical stage IIA, in 2 out of 6 in clinical stage IIB, in 1 out of 2 in clinical stage IIIA, and in 1 out of 4 in clinical stage IIIB. 9 of the patients were surgically staged and there was correlation with the MRI findings in 8 of these.

It has already been stated that tumour involvement of the parametrium proves to be the most difficult aspect to assess clinically, especially in the establishment of a tumour-free plane internal to the obturator internus muscle. This is of considerable importance in the question as to whether surgical resection should be undertaken, and it is by no means always possible for CT to evaluate this (Walsh & Goplerud 1981).

Hricak et al (1988) compared MRI and surgical findings in 57 patients with invasive cervical cancer. They claimed accurate staging in 46 cases (81%). However, confining comparison to those cases which were surgically staged as higher than IIA, the accuracy fell to 74%. Imaging was claimed to be more than satisfactory for demonstrating spread of tumour into the lower uterine segment, vaginal extension and parametrial invasion. Bladder and rectal involvement were assessed with a high accuracy. Baltzer (1979) and Dargent et al (1985) have stressed the relationship of primary tumour volume to the chances of cure, and MRI is capable of achieving quantitative assessment of volume (Fig. 12.7). In the series of Hricak et al (1988), MRI measurement of tumour size was in accord with that determined pathologically in 70% of patients.

In regard to the rôle of MRI in identifying lymphadenopathy, Lee et al (1984), using various pulse sequences, emphasized the similarity between demonstrating abdominal and pelvic lymphadenopathy by MRI and CT, but showed that the former was better in separating out nodes from adjacent vascular structures without the need for intravascular iodinated contrast injection, especially where problems of identification were related to variable position and tortuosity of vessels in the older patient. CT, on the other hand, offered better spatial resolution and shorter examination time. MRI, like CT, cannot yet offer reliable tissue characterization. The similarity between MRI and CT for detecting abdominopelvic lymphadenopathy has also been reported by Dooms et al (1984).

Dooms et al (1985) investigated the ability of MRI to characterize disease within lymph nodes. They concluded that it is unreliable in distinguishing benign from malignant conditions, but that useful information could be obtained to distinguish nodes enlarged from acute inflammatory lesions from enlargement due to other benign conditions or neoplastic infiltration. CT on the other hand, can only raise suspicion of inflammatory disease in nodes, related to patterns of postcontrast enhancement and/or associated features of tissue necrosis.

Whether the use of paramagnetic contrast agents such as gadolinium-DTPA will result in increased detection of early lymph node metastases remains to be seen.

Summary

In the problem of staging cervical cancer the ques-

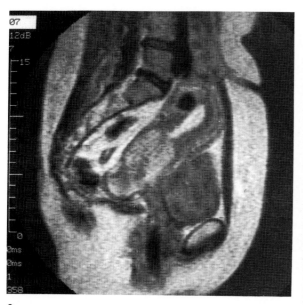
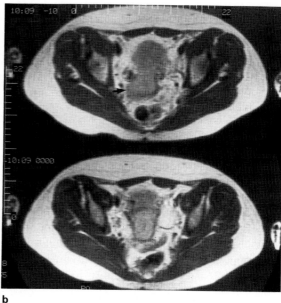

Fig. 12.7 (a) Sagittal MR images of a bulky cervical tumour extending into the corpus. The rounded low intensity lesion in the upper uterine body is a fibroid. The bladder is not invaded. Inferiorly the cervical tumour extends into the upper vagina. (b) Axial MR images of the same patient demonstrating right parametrial infiltration (arrow). The maximal orthogonal diameters can be measured and the volume calculated. (Reproduced by courtesy of Dr R J Johnson.)

tion arises as to whether any truly satisfactory policy can be evolved and implemented on a practical basis. Clinical assessment falls short of that which can be achieved by imaging methods, and both of these approaches have proven less accurate than surgical staging. However, even the latter is capable of failure because of the difficulties in producing adequate clearance of lymph nodes, together with the inability to attack all of the nodal areas which can be involved in this disease. Only positive findings are of value, and it seems likely at the present time that there will continue to be a significant number of patients in whom the presence of micrometastatic disease will not be demonstrated. Clinical, imaging and pathological features of the primary lesion have been shown to be of prognostic significance, and it has become increasingly easy to show unsuspected late stage disease. However, negative findings in even the most extended methods of staging (by utilizing all available approaches) will still mean that patients will continue to return with recurrent disease when the primary site of involvement remains clinically healed.

TREATMENT

The primary treatment of cervical cancer lies in the direction of either surgery or radiation therapy. Surgery for stages I and IIA takes the form of Wertheim's hysterectomy, involving removal of the Fallopian tubes, broad ligament, parametria and an upper vaginal cuff, together with resection of the pelvic lymph nodes. Some surgeons dissect above the common iliac node groups into the lower para-aortic areas. The effectiveness of lymph node removal is variable (see previous comments on operative lymphoscintigraphy) and the line of dissection does not always include the whole of the parametria. Residual central disease may therefore exist where the initial clinical staging was wrong, and the patient should have been categorized as stage IIIB. Furthermore, as we have already seen, the incidence of lymph node metastases having already occurred in early clinical stage disease is high. This is significantly greater in women below the age of 40. The figures of Buckley et al (1988) show differential incidence of 50% versus 24% in the two groups.

Treatment by radiation may be intracavity alone, intracavity plus external X-ray, or external X-ray alone. The stage of disease at presentation determines the method adopted. In the 5301 cases of cervical cancer treated at the Christie Hospital and Holt Radium Institute between 1969 and 1983 inclusively, 39.1% had intracavity therapy only, 50.6% had intracavity plus external radiation therapy and 9% had external X-ray treatment only. External X-ray fields are applied to the pelvis to include both the cavity itself and the pelvic node areas, but routine radiation of the bifurcation and para-aortic nodes is not undertaken.

Chemotherapy, using single or combined agents, is a palliative treatment reserved for those patients who have relapsed following radiation treatment. It is usually not given to patients over the age of 60 and the patients must have adequate renal function demonstrated by excretion urography and/or radionuclide renography.

The post-treated case

Significant 'relapse' rates occur in women with cervical cancer. Disease identified at the primary site up to six months after treatment is regarded as residual, whilst from that time onwards it is termed recurrent (Singleton & Orr 1983). The descriptions overlap as there are no means of identifying whether an individual tumour underwent complete remission without resource to impractical, repetitive follow-up examinations. Recurrence following what has been considered clinically adequate therapy usually occurs within two years, but may be delayed by up to ten years or more. The presence of recurrence may be clinically apparent.

The rôle of radiology in determining recurrence centres round the following problems:

(i)   Distinction of primary recurrence from pelvic fibrosis.
(ii) Detection of metastatic lymphadenopathy (Fig. 12.8).
(iii) Distinction of metastatic tumour from benign lesions (Fig. 12.9).
(iv) Demonstration of vascular occlusion by pelvic mass.
(v)   Invasion of other organs such as the bladder and rectum.

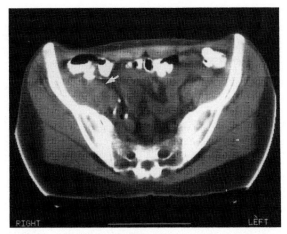

Fig. 12.8 Metastatic lymphadenopathy on the right pelvic side wall (arrow). The iliacus muscle is slightly swollen, indicating the probability of direct invasion.

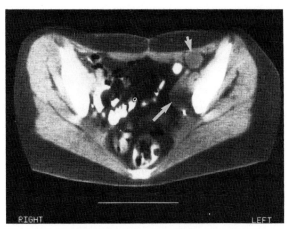

Fig. 12.9 Palpable left pelvic mass demonstrated on CT to be benign postoperative lymphocoeles (arrowed).

(vi) Definition of distant spread to bone, lung, liver or brain.

The choice of investigatory method is determined by the patient's symptoms and clinical condition on physical examination. Factors (i), (ii) and (v) above are best examined by CT or MRI, though excretion urography, contrast cystography and barium enema examination may be required to provide additional information for the surgeon contemplating radical resection. Factors (i), (ii) and (v) may also be assessed by ultrasound, though its accuracy at this stage of the disease process is less than that of CT The inability of CT to provide tissue characterization limits its value in assessing the distinction between fibrosis and residual/recurrent malignancy, and MRI may have considerably more promise in this direction.

Ebner et al (1988) report that at 1.5 T the distinction between recurrent tumour and fibrosis is facilitated with heavily T_2-weighted pulse sequences, i.e. TE greater than 60 ms. They report highly significant differences in the signal intensity of recurrent tumour and localized fibrotic masses one year after treatment. However, they are sceptical of the ability of MRI to make the distinction between tumour and changes consequent upon radiation treatment at an earlier stage. Furthermore, through its ability for improved boundary definition via multiplanar imaging and the use of T_1 and T_2-weighted sequences, MRI shows more likelihood of identifying adjacent organ involvement at an earlier stage. Demonstration of vascular occlusion can be undertaken by selective venography using direct catheterization in the absence of gross lower limb swelling, the intraosseous approach via the femoral trochanter, or by employing gamma camera, high resolution, radionuclide studies with ^{99m}Tc-labelled microspheres (Fig. 12.10). Distinction between metastatic tumour and benign lesions is most usually assessed today by CT or ultrasound.

Where there is doubt as to the nature of a soft tissue density, the procedure of percutaneous needle biopsy can be undertaken using ultrasound or CT-guided control, allowing calculation of depth from skin surface and angle of needle approach (Zornosa et al 1977, Jacques et al 1978, Husband & Golding 1983). For transperitoneal approaches, or in the case of masses closely related to blood vessels, a 22–23 gauge needle is employed, but larger diameter ones (e.g. 19 gauge) may be used for those procedures which do not involve peritoneal penetration. For biopsying through muscle, a Trucut needle may be employed. Good identification of tissue type can be obtained from cytological or histological examination of the specimen, though Jacques et al (1978) pointed out that cytology of cyst fluid can prove to be less satisfactory. Failure rates are low — especially in CT-guided procedures — and the method can be applied in patients with both

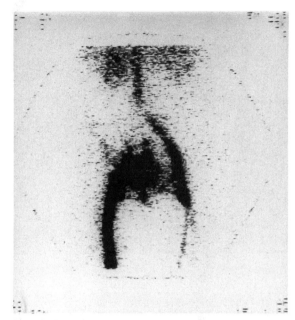

Fig. 12.10   Isotope venogram demonstrating complete occlusion of the right common iliac vein.

primary and recurrent tumours, including those in whom an imaging pattern of disease does not fit in with expected findings (Fig. 12.11). As a follow-on from the diagnostic procedure, the method may also be used to drain inflammatory collections in appropriately accessible sites.

The incidence of distant metastases from carcinoma of the cervix rises progressively with the clinical stage. Carlson et al (1967) examined the distribution of metastases in 2220 cases of cervical cancer. 341 of these showed positive identification, ranging from 0.74% in stage 1A to 100% in stage IV. Included in the survey were patients with lymph node involvement outside of the pelvis, even as high as the supraclavicular and cervical node areas. From this survey it is interesting to note that, in spite of an overall incidence of metastases of 15.4%, the number of patients developing spread to lung, bone, liver and brain was small in relation to the total number of patients surveyed. Clearly, the survey antedates the advent of more sophisticated investigatory technology, but provides a reasonable expression of the relative infrequency of metastases outside the lymphatic system.

Osseous metastases from carcinoma of the cervix

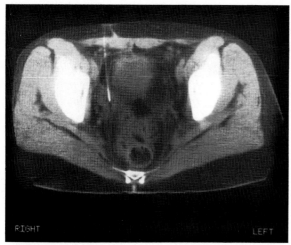

a

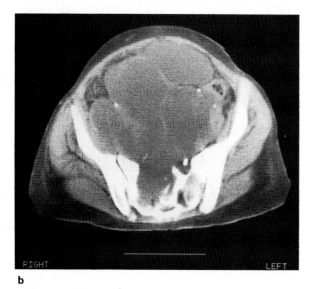

b

Fig. 12.11 (a) CT-guided biopsy of recurrent mass in the right pelvis. (b) Uncommon, bulky, locular, cystic type of recurrence of cervical cancer mimicking a disease pattern seen in carcinoma of the ovary.

were reviewed by Bassan & Glaser (1982). In all but one case of bony dissemination the histology of the primary tumour showed it to be poorly differentiated. Griffin et al (1976) predicted that follow-up examination of patients with cervical cancer having normal pretreatment chest radiography could be expected to reveal tumour-related abnormalities in approximately 6% over their period of survival.

In looking purely at recurrent pelvic cancer, Meanwell et al (1987) reported their experience of transrectal ultrasound, emphasizing the value of a simple, easy to perform and comfortable procedure for assessing presence of disease on both pelvic side walls, in the bladder, and in the central and presacral regions.

Walsh et al (1981) investigated the value of CT in patients thought to have recurrent cervical cancer. Of 29 biopsy confirmed recurrences, CT was correct in 82%, with the false negatives being due to the tumour volume being too small to be detected, and the false positives resulting from an inability to distinguish radiation change from active disease. CT is the method of choice for monitoring disease response to chemotherapy, which is usually reserved as a last option method of treatment following radiation and/or surgery.

In the pursuit of non-lymph node disease, the radiological approaches centre around:

(i) Conventional radiography of the chest and the skeletal system, including the use of tomography where indicated.
(ii) Radionuclide scanning for bone and liver metastases.
(iii) Ultrasound scanning for liver metastases and pelvic recurrence.
(iv) CT scanning for pelvic recurrence and distant metastases.

For the identification of distant metastatic spread to hilar or mediastinal nodes the method of choice is CT, but in our experience it is rarely indicated after full evaluation of a three film series, which includes the conventional PA radiograph, the penetrated AP and the lateral projection. Where conventional radiology has demonstrated metastatic destruction in the central skeletal axis, it is not our policy to proceed with further evaluation of the patient by CT examination, unless there is a need to identify that erosion is being caused by direct extension from metastatic lymph nodes in areas where radiation therapy may still be possible, or the patient is to receive chemotherapy.

The complications of therapy

These may be classified as immediate or delayed. Immediate reactions include radiation-induced cystitis and mild to moderate enterocolitis, and are usually amenable to treatment by conservative measures. Occasionally, during or immediately after a course of radiotherapy, a patient may develop an acute abdomen due to tubo-ovarian abscess, other pelvic inflammatory disease or obstruction of an irradiated bowel segment. Delayed reactions may supervene after a latent period of six months to 20 years following resolution of the initial problems. They may involve the urinary tract, the distal small bowel, the sigmoid colon and the rectum, and are increased by the combination of intracavity therapy with radical external beam radiation.

In a review of 831 patients with cervical cancer treated with both forms of radiation in doses ranging from 3000 to 7000 cGy, Strockbine et al (1970) documented the occurrence of severe persistent cystitis, ureteral strictures, bladder and rectal ulcers, small bowel necrosis, fistulae (vesico-vaginal and rectovaginal), and ulcerating sigmoiditis. In general, the more severe complications were related to high radiation doses, but the individual patient sensitivity was variable. Kline et al (1972) reported an increased risk of complications in treated patients, with more severe immediate bowel symptoms, but stressed that absence of symptoms was no assumption that later problems would not occur. Mason et al (1970) emphasized that radiation damage to bowel (at surgery or autopsy) can be present beyond the confines revealed by radiological study. Our own surgeons' experience is that changes are invariably more severe than radiology demonstrates. Changes in the small bowel ranged from nodular filling defects in the wall to established strictures and mechanical obstruction. In the distal large bowel, spasm, stricture, simulation of carcinoma, ulceration and perforation with abscess formation were various features identified.

In the series of Shibata et al (1982), 24 out of 52 irradiated patients (46%) developed mild enterocolitis, successfully managed by conservative measures, but 28 required surgical intervention which was mainly of resective type. They considered that a risk of radiation injury of 1–5% occurs to the small bowel with doses of 4500 cGy and to the colon and rectum with doses of 5500 cGy. At doses of 6000 and 8000 cGy respec-

tively, the risk was said to rise to 25–30%.

It is interesting to note that, 50 years ago, Corscaden et al (1938) reported 139 out of 350 cases of cervical cancer with changes related to the lower alimentary system following radiation therapy, and that these ranged from congestion of the mucosa to ulceration and stricture formation. They referred to the fact that susceptibility of intestinal mucosa to radiation had long been known — since the 1920s — and was originally reviewed by Desjardins (1931).

67 patients with evidence of radiation damage, proven surgically and/or histologically, have been reviewed by Taylor et al (1989). Patients with known recurrent or metastatic disease were not included, and all those analysed had had combined external beam and intracavitary radiotherapy. 16 patients had small bowel damage. Patients with severe injuries often had more than one site involved. 31 patients showed large bowel damage, mainly as strictures in the rectosigmoid colon. 36 patients were shown to have abnormalities in the urinary tract, usually lower ureteric strictures and hydronephrosis. Reduction in bladder size and mucosal irregularities were associated findings.

Radiation bowel damage

In the series of Taylor et al (1989) features in the small bowel were as follows:

(i) Plain radiograph evidence of incomplete ileal obstruction.
(ii) On small bowel enema examination, fixed intestinal loops, associated thickening of bowel wall or strictures (Fig. 12.12).
(iii) Mucosal irregularities embracing spiky distortion and nodular filling defects (Fig. 12.13).
(iv) Fistulae to the skin surface after previous small bowel resection.

These findings accord with those of Mason et al (1970).

In the large bowel the findings on double contrast barium enema were:

(i) Stricture — the commonest abnormality, involving the rectosigmoid area in 27 patients, and measuring between 3 and 30 cm in length (Fig. 12.14).

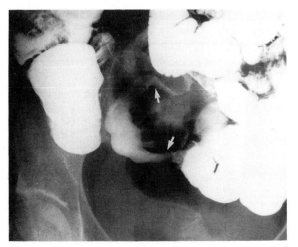

Fig. 12.12 Late stage radiation small bowel damage with established stricture formation (arrows).

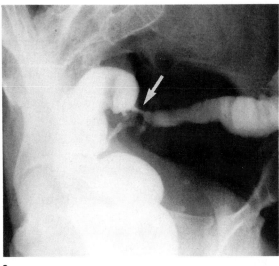

a

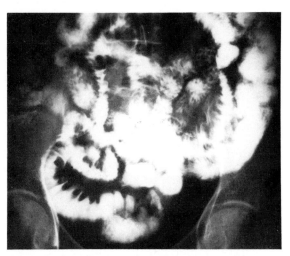

Fig. 12.13 Small bowel barium enema demonstrating mucosal abnormality and separation of pelvic bowel loops but no identifiable stricture.

(ii) Mucosal irregularity embracing fine ulceration, deeper focal ulcers and generalized mucosal thickening, not dissimilar to the findings in Crohn's disease.

(iii) Widening of the presacral space.

(iv) Fistulae which were either rectovaginal, rectouterine, rectovesicovaginal, from colon to jejunum or into abscess cavities (Fig. 12.15).

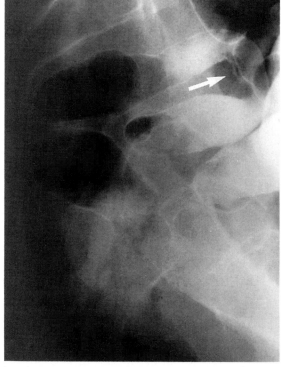

b

Fig. 12.14 (a) Very tight pelvirectal stricture in a classic area after cervical cancer irradiation. (b) Double contrast study illustrating radiation bowel disease in the sigmoid. Changes are by no means as dramatic as in the other case, but were proven at surgery. This illustrates the need for great care in looking for radiation bowel damage by radiological examination.

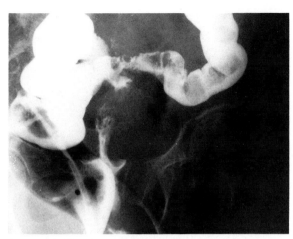

Fig. 12.15 Fistulous connection between the distal large bowel and the utenus.

(v) Hypertrophy of circular muscle without stricture or diverticular disease.
(vi) Distortion of the outline of sigmoid diverticulae.

Damage to bowel is due to the induction of an endarteritis obliterans. The rate of onset of the injury and its type — perforation of fistula or stricture — is a manifestation of the degree of vascular damage.

Ludgate & Merrick (1985) reported the investigation of absorption of vitamin B12 (^{58}Co B12), and a synthetic bile analogue 75 SeHCAT, measured simultaneously in 26 patients with diarrhoea following pelvic irradiation for cervical cancer. They identified four separate groups in which the therapeutic implications were different. All patients had received external beam radiotherapy plus intracavity radiation with Caesium-137.

In considering the surgical treatment of radiation bowel disease, the question arises as to whether the diseased segment should be bypassed or resected, and whether the blood supply may be jeopardized further by assiduous attention to freeing adhesions. It is certainly possible that the identification of a segment of bowel which has been injured by radiation treatment may not be the end of the story, and the condition may well be progressive, so that each case needs to be individually assessed on the basis of the radiological findings and the symptoms which are being en-

countered. The sensitivity to radiation of different structures which lie in apposition to the radiated cervix is known to vary (Maruyama et al 1974, Goldstein 1979).

Factors which predispose to the development of radiation bowel injury are:

(i) Pre-existing ischaemic bowel disease, especially in hypertension and diabetes (Van Nagel et al 1974).
(ii) Pelvic inflammatory reaction inhibiting bowel movement (Stockbrine et al 1970).
(iii) Adhesions from previous surgery.
(iv) Closeness or otherwise of a bowel loop to the radiation source.
(v) Individual patient/organ sensitivity.

The incidence of radiation damage to bowel has been variously assessed. Corscaden et al (1938) described only 12 out of 190 patients with postradiation lower bowel symptoms developing late complications in the form of ulcers and strictures. Woon Sang Yu et al (1982) used CT to demonstrate anatomical relationships in intracavity radiation therapy so as to illustrate the relative positions of the adjacent bladder, small bowel and rectosigmoid, and to calculate the likely dose received by each of these structures. Sherrah-Davies (1985) compared the incidence of morbidity in patients treated by the standard Manchester radium technique, with that of patients treated by Selectron after-loading therapy. He concluded that the general use of low dose rate after-loading machines represented progress in that radiation dose to staff is reduced, but that the morbidity, in terms of radiation damage to adjacent organs, might be higher than with the old radium method.

In the search for evidence of radiation injury to the bowel, there are several points which need to be borne in mind:

(i) The likelihood of its occurrence in the knowledge that the patient has had X-ray therapy of a type and to a dose level at which the risk is finite.
(ii) Only subtle changes may be present in the symptomatic patient, and great care should be taken to examine the rectosigmoid in as many different positions as necessary and

to produce delineation of the whole segment.

(iii) Changes in the distal large bowel may mimic other disease, e.g. pseudocarcinoma (Todd 1938).

(iv) Distorted diverticular may be due to radiation effect and not a result of simple inflammatory reaction.

(v) Abscess formation from perforation, in the presence of diverticula, may be very difficult to differentiate as being radiation induced, and careful attention to other associated features is necessary.

(vi) The small bowel enema should be pursued with considerable diligence through the ileal segment, and caution taken not to overfill with too-concentrated contrast. Insufflated air can often be of major assistance in evaluating overlapping of adherent bowel segments.

(vii) Small bowel changes may simulate other disease, e.g. lymphoma, carcinoid.

Genitourinary

In the series of Taylor et al (1989), 31 patients with urinary tract abnormality had 48 ureteral strictures, leading to hydronephrosis, usually at or immediately above the union with the bladder (Fig. 12.16). Evaluation of the cause of tract dilatation necessitated the extension of investigation from infusion excretory urography to ultrasound, CT, retrograde pyelography and antegrade pyelography — with or without nephrostomy — in 27 patients. Postradiation ureteric strictures may appear similar to those due to early involvement of the distal ureter by extracervical extension of the primary malignant process. They may be of considerable length. Abnormality of the bladder following radiation presents as mucosal distortion, ranging from granular irregularity, through a coarse globular pattern, to deep fissuring due to marked ulceration. Changes in bladder volume and shape, at the time of maximum filling, may be noted when comparing post-treatment with pretreatment excretory urography. Fistulae involving the bladder are almost invariably vesicovaginal in nature, but may be associated with a rectovaginal communication.

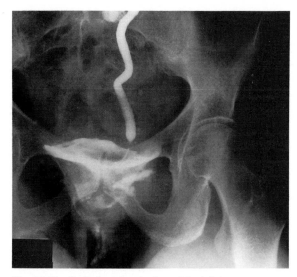

Fig. 12.16 Radiation cicatrisation of the left lower ureter with an associated vesicovaginal fistula.

Ultrasound examination proved to be of value in assessing urinary tract dilatation where renal function had ceased, as assessed by excretory urography, and in guidance for antegrade pyelo-ureterography. The latter is always performed during the course of percutaneous nephrostomy in order to demonstrate the extent to which the ureter is compromised and at what level. Nephrostomy itself is carried out in order to gain time in the further assessment of the uraemic patient for corrective (diversion) surgery. CT has been useful in 11 patients in revealing presacral fibrosis, para-aortic lymphadenopathy causing ureteric compression, the demonstration of vesicovaginal fistula and in coincidentally diagnosing pyometrium (Fig. 12.17). Radioactive renography is of value in showing differential renal function in the patient with distorted biochemistry from urinary tract damage, and especially in relation to deciding on which, if not both kidneys, to perform nephrostomy drainage.

Other late complications

An increased incidence of second cancers developing in patients who have previously received radiation therapy has been reported by a number of authors (Smith 1962, Dickson 1972, El Castro et al 1973, Lee et al 1982, Quilty & Kerr 1987).

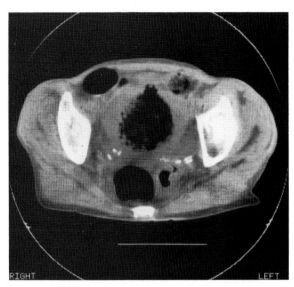

Fig. 12.17 Pyometrium due to gas-forming organisms following radiation therapy with stenosis of the cervical canal.

In the series of El Castro et al (1973), 26 patients were identified and analysed. The time interval between irradiation and new disease was between 5 and 30 years, but the expected rate in an untreated population was not discussed, and two-thirds of the cases were more than 60 years old at the time of identification of the second tumour. However, nearly 50% of patients showed evidence of bowel radiation at the site of a new cancer. Dickson (1972), from an analysis of 913 women surviving more than five years after treatment for cervical cancer, found a higher than expected death rate from cancer of the rectum, colon, bladder and lung. Quilty and Kerr (1987) identified 27 patients with bladder cancer treated years previously for menorrhagia. Tumours were high grade and advanced, and only 32% of these patients survived more than one year. Patients who had had high dose therapy had a shorter time interval to the appearance of the vesical cancer than those whose treatment involved low dosage.

The WHO international radiation study group has indicated an increased incidence of rectal, ovarian and bladder cancer in patients surviving for long periods after radiation therapy for carcinoma of the cervix, and who had had high doses of radiation. Lower doses may also be implicated in the late incidence of bladder cancer (Day & Boice 1983). The radiological input to this problem of very delayed further malignant disease is simply that of identification and delineation of the second tumour through whatever methods are appropriate to the individual case, and consideration of the treatment options available.

Radiation induced bone damage, leading to necrosis, is not a complication which arises from radiotherapy employing intracavity radiation alone: it may be seen with treatments which combine external beam radiation with intracavity radiation. The incidence in the presence of megavoltage therapy is less than with the old kilovoltage techniques. Typical appearances are of irregular bony sclerosis, with distortion of trebecular pattern and the development of pathological fractures. The number of cases in the Christie Hospital and Holt Radium Institute identified as having this complication from treatment for cervical cancer has been no more than a handful in the past 20 years.

Radiology and treatment planning

This subject is treated elsewhere in this volume (Ch. 18). Suffice it to say that there are three approaches of relevance:

(i) Verification of source placement for intracavity radiation and/or field application for external irradiation, through conventional radiography.
(ii) CT radiation planning for intracavity therapy.
(iii) The still to be evaluated applications of MRI.

SUMMARY

The traditional hope that earlier diagnosis leads to earlier treatment and better survival rates remains difficult to apply across the spectrum of cervical cancer. The natural fall in incidence of the disease is unfortunately being offset by a higher mortality rate in younger age groups. Problems relating to the accuracy of clinical staging are well known, particularly the identification of tumour volume, the extent of disease of the cervix and lymph node metastases. Imaging methods allow distinctive improvement in the staging process, but only for certain groups in whom management can be affected, and they are not sufficient for the identification of total disease. Whilst both investigatory and surgical staging may be more accurate, the emphasis in such methods is usually to reveal a worse than suspected state. Neither radiology nor surgery is capable of revealing fully the true extent of spread to pelvic and para-aortic lymph nodes. Micrometastatic disease and skip lesions remain a considerable problem.

Earlier identification of cervical cellular dysplasia through exfoliative cytology may go some way to reducing the numbers of women presenting with invasive cancer, but the success of this is dependent on screening intervals which presently look to be too widely spaced. Improved application of histological methods has been shown to lead to a better predictability regarding those patients who might have a worse prognosis for the clinically assessed disease stage with which they present.

The value of radiological methods in the staging process, the assessment of the patient in the period after treatment and in the identification of complications due to therapy has been reviewed. The interplay between histopathological identification of the high risk case and the investigative techniques of radiology needs to be more clearly defined if improved methods of treatment are to develop.

Within the field of diagnostic radiology, the highest yield of information is likely to lie with:

(i) Ultrasound, using improved transrectal techniques.

(ii) Increased facility of CT and its application to earlier clinically staged disease, especially in identifying those patients who have unsuspected spread beyond the local environs of the cervix and the parametrium.

(iii) Greater availability and application of MRI for assessment of primary tumour volume, local extension and the subsequent distinction of fibrosis from recurrent malignancy. The promise of improved staging in relation to available treatment options already exists.

With the advent of more sophisticated imaging techniques, it is doubtful whether there still remains a rôle for lymphography. Any small benefit which it may be thought to confer might now be considered offset by its distinctive limitations in determining therapy. At the same time it has to be said that ultrasound, CT and MRI have nothing to offer in the identification of micrometastatic disease, and this is a very real problem in all cases of cervical cancer which are considered to have been picked up at an early point in the disease process.

REFERENCES

Averette H E, Ford J H Jr, Dudan R C, Girtanner R E, Hoskins W J, Lutz M H 1975 The staging of cervical cancer. Clinical Obstetrics and Gynaecology 18 (3): 215–232

Baltzer J 1979 Tumour size and lymph node metastases in squamous cell carcinoma of the uterine cervix. Archives of Gynecology 227: 271–278

Bassan J S, Glaser M G 1982 Bony metastases in carcinoma of the uterine cervix. Clinical Radiology 33(6): 623–625

Benstead K, Cowie V J, Blair V, Hunter R D 1986 Stage III carcinoma of the cervix. The importance of increasing age and extent of parametrial infiltration. Radiotherapy and Oncology 5: 271–276

Bond W H 1985 Carcinoma of the cervix: the staging anomaly. Clinical Radiology 36: 625–628

Brenner D E, Whitley N O, Prempree T, Villasanta U 1982 An evaluation of the computed tomographic scanner for the staging of carcinoma of the cervix. Cancer 50: 2323–2328

Buckley C H, Beards C S, Fox H 1988 Pathological

prognostic indicators in cervical cancer with particular reference to patients under the age of 40 years. Journal of Obstetrics and Gynaecology 95: 47–56

Burghardt E 1984 Micro-invasive carcinoma in gynaecological pathology. Clinics in Obstetrics and Gynaecology 22(1): 239–257

Burghardt E et al 1973 Der unterchied zwischen der zervixkrebs def ftadiums 1A under dem begriff microkarzinoma. Geburtshilfe und Fraunheilkunde 33(3): 168–172

Carlson V, Declos L, Fletcher G H 1967 Distant metastases in squamous cell carcinoma of the uterine cervix. Radiology 88: 961–966

Chism S E, Park R C, Keys H M 1975 Prospects for para-aortic irradiation in treatment for carcinoma of the cervix. Cancer 35: 1505–1509

Corscaden J A, Kasabach H H, Lenz M 1938 Intestinal injuries after radium and roentgen treatment of carcinoma of the cervix. American Journal of Roentgenology 2 (6): 871–887

Dargent D, Frobert J L, Bean G 1985 V factor (tumour volume) and T factor (FIGO classification) in the assessment of cervix cancer prognosis: the risk of lymph node spread. Gynaecological Oncology 22: 15–22

Day N E, Boice J D Jr 1983 Second cancer in relation to radiation treatment for cervical cancer. International Agency for Research on Cancer, Lyon

De Muylder X, Belanger R, Vauclair R, Audett-Lapointe P, Cormier A, Methot Y 1984 Value of lymphography in stage IB cancer of the uterine cervix. American Journal of Obstetrics and Gynaecology 148: 610–613

Desjardins E U 1931 Action of roentgen rays and radium on gastro-intestinal tract: experimental data and clinical radiotherapy. American Journal of Roentgenology and Radiation Therapy 26: 145, 335, 493

Di Candio G, Campatelli A, Mosca F, Gadducci A, Nuzzi F M, Facchina V 1984 Transrectal ultrasonography and cervical neoplasia. European Journal of Gynaecological Oncology 3: 124–202

Dickson R J 1972 Late results of radium treatment of carcinoma of the cervix. Clinical Radiology 23: 528–535

Dixon A K 1985 The current practice of lymphography: A survey in the age of computed tomography. Clinical Radiology 36: 287–290

Dooms G C, Hricak H, Crooks L E, Higgins C B 1984 Magnetic resonance images of the lymph nodes: comparison with CT. Radiology 153: 719–728

Dooms G C, Hricak M, Moseley M E, Bottles K, Fisher M, Higgins C B 1985 Characterisation of lymphadenopathy by magnetic resonance relaxation times: Preliminary results. Radiology 155: 691–697

Douglas B, MacDonald J S, Baker J W 1972 Lymphography in carcinoma of the uterus. Clinical Radiology 23: 286–294

Ebner, F, Kressel H Y, Mintz M C et al 1988 Tumour recurrence versus fibrosis in the female pelvis: differentiation with MR imaging at 1.5 T. Radiology 166: 333–340

El Castro B, Rosen P P, Quan S H H 1973 Carcinoma of large intestine in patients irradiated for carcinoma of the cervix and uterus. Cancer 31: 45–52

Fuchs W A, Davidson J W, Fischer H W 1969 Diagnosis of cancer metastases in lymph nodes. Lymphography in cancer (Recent results in cancer research) Heinemann, London; Springer-Verlag, Berlin, pp 107–119

Gerteis 1967 Progress in lymphology. Ruttiman W, Thieme G (eds). Verlag, Stuttgart, p 209

Ginaldi S, Wallace S, Jing B-S, Bernardino M E 1981 Carcinoma of the cervix. Lymphangiography and computed tomography. American Journal of Radiology 136: 1087–1091

Gitsch E, Phillipp K, Pateisky N 1984 Intra-operative lymph scintigraphy during radical surgery for cervical cancer. Journal of Nuclear Medicine 25: 486–489

Goldstein H M 1979 Small bowel and colon. In: Libshitz H I (ed) Diagnostic roentgenology of radiotherapy change. Williams & Wilkins, Baltimore, pp 85–100

Gray's Anatomy (35th Edn) 1973 Warwick R, Williams P L (eds) Longman, London

Griffin T W, Parker R G, Taylor W J 1976 An evaluation of procedures used in staging carcinoma of the cervix. American Journal of Roentgenology 127: 825–827

Hall S W, Monaghan J M 1983 Invasive carcinoma of the cervix in younger women. Lancet 1: 731

Hricak H, Lacey C G, Sandles L G, Chang Y C F, Winkler M L, Stern J L 1988 Invasive cervical carcinoma: comparison of M R imaging and surgical findings. Radiology 166: 623–631

Husband J E, Golding S J 1983 The rôle of computed tomography-guided needle biopsy in an oncology service. Clinical Radiology 34: 255–260

Jacques P F, Staab E, Richey W, Photopulos G, Santon M 1978 CT-assisted pelvic and abdominal aspiration biopsies in gynaecological malignancy. Radiology 128: 651–655

Kademian M T, Bosch A 1977 Staging laparotomy and survival in carcinoma of the uterine cervix. Acta Radiologica (Stockholm) 16: 314–323

Kilcheski T S, Arger P H, Mulhern C B, Coleman B J, Kressel H Y, Mikuta J I 1981 Rôle of computed tomography in the pre-surgical evaluation of carcinoma of the cervix. Journal of Computed Assisted Tomography 5 (3): 378–383

King L A, Talledo O E, Gallup D G, El Gammal T A M 1986 Computed tomography in evaluation of gynaecologic malignancies: A retrospective analysis. American Journal of Obstetrics and Gynaecology 155: 909–964

Kline J C, Buckler D A, Boone M L, Peckham B M, Carr W F 1972 The relationships of reactions to complications in the radiation therapy of cancer of the cervix. Radiology 105: 413–416

Lang E K 1980 Angiography in the diagnosis and staging of pelvic neoplasms. Radiology 134: 353–358

Lee J K T, Stanley R J, Sagel S S, Merson G L, Koehler R E 1980 Limitations of the post-lymphangiogram plain abdominal radiograph as an indicator of recurrent lymphoma. Comparison of computed tomography. Radiology 134: 155–158

Lee J K T, Heiken J P, Ling D et al 1984 Magnetic resonance imaging of abdominal and pelvic lymphadenopathy. Radiology 153: 181–188

Lee J Y, Perez C A, Ettinger N, Fineber B B 1982 The risk of second primaries subsequent to irradiation for carcinoma of the cervix. International Journal of Radiation Oncology, Biology, Physics 8(2): 207–211

Ludgate S M, Merrick M V 1985 The pathogenesis of post-irradiation chronic diarrhoea: Measurement of SeHCAT and B12 absorption for differential diagnosis determines treatment. Clinical Radiology 36: 275–278

Magee B J, Pointon R S 1988 Assessment of cervical carcinoma with transrectal and transurethral ultrasound. Clinical Radiology 39: 350

Martimbeau P W, Kjorstad K E, Iveren T 1982 Stage IB carcinoma of the cervix. The Norwegian Radium Hospital: II Results when pelvic nodes are involved. Obstetrics and Gynaecology 60: 215–218

Maruyama Y, Van-Nagell J R, Utley J, Vider M L, Parker J C 1974 Radiation and small bowel complications in cervical carcinoma therapy. Radiology 112: 699–703

Mason G R, Dietrich P, Friedland G W, Hanks G E 1970 The radiological findings in radiation-induced enteritis and colitis. Clinical Radiology 21: 232–247

Meanwell C W, Rolfe E B, Blackledge G, Docker M F, Lawton F G, Mould J J 1987 Recurrent female pelvic cancer. Assessment with transrectal ultrasound. Radiology 162: 278–281

Munoz N, Bosch X, Kaldor J M 1988 Does human papilloma virus cause cervical cancer? The state of epidemiological evidence. British Journal of Cancer 57: 1–5

Pettersson F (ed) 1988 Annual report on the results of treatment in gynaecological cancer. International

Federation of Gynaecology and Obstetrics, Stockholm

Piver M S, Barlow J J 1981 Five-year survival (with no evidence of disease) in patients with biopsy-confirmed aortic node metastases from cervical carcinoma. American Journal of Obstetrics and Gynaecology 139: 575–578

Piver M S, Wallace S, Castro J R 1971 The accuracy of lymphangiography in carcinoma of the uterine cervix. American Journal of Roentgenology 111: 278–283

Powell M C, Worthington B, Sokal S, Wastie M, Buckley J, Symmonds E M 1986 Magnetic resonance imaging — its application to cervical carcinoma. British Journal of Obstetrics and Gynaecology 93: 1276–1285

Quilty P M, Kerr G R 1987 Bladder cancer following low or high dose pelvic irradiation. Clinical Radiology 38: 583–585

Office of Population Censuses and Surveys 1985 Cancer Statistics: Registrations and Mortality Statistics (1983 & 1985). HMSO, London

Sanders R C, McNeil B J, Finberg H J et al 1983 A prospective study of computed tomography and ultrasound in the detection and staging of pelvic masses. Radiology 146: 439–442

Schaffer B, Koehler P R, Daniel C R et al 1964 A critical evaluation of lymphangiography. Radiology 80: 917–930

Sherrah-Davies E 1985 Morbidity following low-dose-rate selectron. Therapy for cervical cancer. Clinical Radiology 36: 131–139

Shibata H R, Freeman C R, Roman R D 1982 Gastro-intestinal complications after radiotherapy for carcinoma of the uterine cervix. Canadian Journal of Surgery 25(1): 63–66

Singleton H M, Orr W O Jr 1983 Cancer of the cervix. Current Reviews in Obstetrics and Gynaecology. Churchill Livingstone, Edinburgh

Smales E, Perry C M, MacDonald J E, Baker J W 1986 The value of lymphography in the management of carcinoma of the cervix. Clinical Radiology 37: 19–22

Smith J C 1962 Carcinoma of the rectum following irradiation of carcinoma of the cervix. Proceedings of the Royal Society of Medicine 55: 701–702

Strockbine M R, Hancock J E, Fletcher G E 1970 Complications in 831 patients with squamous cell carcinoma of the intact uterine cervix treated with 3000 rad or more whole pelvis irradiation. American Journal of Roentgenology 108(2): 293–304

Taylor P M, Johnson R J, Eddleston B 1989 Radiology of radiation injury. In: Schofield P F, Lupton E (eds) The causation and clinical management of pelvic radiation disease. Springer-Verlag, London, pp 37–57

Terry L N Jr, Piver S S, Franks J E 1972 The value of lymphangiography in malignant disease of the uterine cervix. Radiology 103: 175–177

Tindall V 1987 Tumours of the cervix uteri. In: Jeffcoate's principles of gynaecology, 5th edn. Butterworths, London, pp 395–416

Todd T F 1938 Rectal ulceration following irradiation treatment of carcinoma of the cervix uteri. Pseudocarcinoma of the rectum. Surgery, Gynaecology and Obstetrics 67: 617–631

Van Nagel J R, Maruyama Y, Parker J C, Dalton W L 1974 Small bowel injury following radiation therapy for cervical carcinoma. American Journal of Obstetrics and Gynaecology 118: 164–167

Vick C W, Walsh J W, Wheelock J B, Brewer W H 1984 CT of the normal and abnormal parametria in cervical cancer. American Journal of Radiology 143: 597–603

Villasanta U, Whitley N O, Haney P J, Brenner D 1983 Computed tomography in invasive carcinoma of the cervix: an appraisal. Obstetrics and Gynaecology 62: 218–224

Walsh J W, Goplerud D R 1981 Prospective comparison between clinical and CT staging in primary cervical cancer. American Journal of Radiology 137: 997–1003

Walsh J W, Amendola M A, Hall D J, Tishnado J, Goplerud D R 1981 Recurrent carcinoma of the cervix: CT diagnosis. American Journal of Radiology 136: 117–122

Ward B G, Shepherd J E, Monaghan J W 1985 Occult advanced cervical cancer. British Medical Journal 290: 1301–1302

Whitley N O, Brenner D E, Francis A et al 1982 Computed tomographic evaluation of carcinoma of the cervix. Radiology 142: 439–446

Woon Sang Yu, Sagerman R H, Chung T C et al 1982 Anatomical relationships in intra-cavity irradiation demonstrated by computed tomography. Radiology 143: 537–541

Yuhara A, Akamatsu N, Sekiba K 1987 Use of transrectal radial scan ultrasonography in evaluating the extent of uterine cervical cancer. Journal of Clinical Ultrasound 15: 507–517

Zaritzky D, Blake D, Willard B S, Resnick M 1979 Transrectal ultrasonography in the evaluation of cervical carcinoma. Obstetrics and Gynaecology 53(1): 105–108

Zornosa J, Wallace S, Goldstein H M, Lukeman M, Jing Bao-shan 1977 Transperitoneal percutaneous retroperitoneal lymph node aspiration biopsy. Radiology 122: 111–115

13. The lymphatic system

J. J. K. Best   R. Jones

Hodgkin's disease (HD) and the non-Hodgkin's lymphomas (NHL) form an important group of malignancies. They are uncommon compared with the major cancers, but are amongst the most treatable at the present time. In the UK, lymphoma accounts for 5–6% of malignancies (Callender et al 1987). Crude incidence in the United States for whites is 3.3 per 100 000 per year for HD and 9.4 per 100 000 per year for NHL (Young et al 1981).

Survival rates for lymphoma have dramatically improved over the past 20 years. The reasons for this are multiple and include improved understanding of the natural history of these diseases, more accurate staging methods and the emergence of improved therapeutic regimes, especially multi-agent chemotherapy. HD has a bimodal age distribution, with peaks around 30 and 70 years (Young et al 1981). NHL tends to affect the elderly, incidence increasing with age beyond 40 years and being commonest between 75 and 79 years. Both appear to be more prevalent in males than females, the difference being more apparent in HD. Both incidence and mortality rates are lower in non-whites (Young et al 1981).

Imaging procedures permitting accurate assessment of extent of disease have played a major part in the development of current lymphoma management. Lymphography was introduced in 1952 (Kinmonth 1952), and was the first imaging method for delineating extent of abdominal disease. The routine use of splenectomy and laparotomy for staging of HD helped to demonstrate the orderly progression through lymph node groups, as well as giving accurate staging of disease extent. Laparatomy is less important in NHL but has provided a useful tool for investigation of tumour behaviour. Computed tomography (CT) now plays a large part in lymphoma staging, and has come to replace many of the older imaging techniques.

Imaging procedures in lymphomas can be helpful in three main ways: in diagnosis, in staging and in follow-up/remission status assessment. Diagnosis is essentially clinicopathological in most cases, but radiology may provide much valuable information in some patients, especially those whose disease is more cryptic, e.g. isolated mediastinal disease or extranodal involvement. Radiology is also increasingly able to provide methods of cytological and pathological diagnosis by guided biopsy and aspiration cytology techniques using fluoroscopy, ultrasound or CT.

Investigation of patients, however, should always be considered in the light of possible treatment options and assessment of progress of disease and overall patient prognosis. It is unnecessary to carry out examinations which will not alter the clinical management of the patient. Close liaison between clinicians and radiologists is important, and the radiologist should be cognisant of current treatment methods and the indications for changing them.

PATHOLOGY AND CLASSIFICATION

Hodgkin's disease is still staged according to the Ann Arbor classification (Carbone et al 1971). Pathologically, the Rye classification of lymphocyte predominant/depleted, mixed cellularity or nodular sclerosing types is still the mainstay of diagnosis (Table 13.1) (Lukes & Butler 1966). More recently, tumour behaviour and patterns of spread of the different types of HD have become

Table 13.1 Rye classification of Hodgkin's disease (Lukes & Butler 1966)

Histology	Distinctive features	Relative Frequency (adults) %
Lymphocytic	Abundant stroma of mature lymphocytes and/or histiocytes; no necrosis, Reed–Sternberg cells may be sparse.	10–15
Nodular sclerosis	Nodules of lymphoid tissue separated by bands of doubly refractile collagen; atypical 'lacunar' Hodgkin's cells in clear spaces within the lymphoid nodules.	20–50
Mixed cellularity	Usually numerous Reed–Sternberg cells and mononuclear Hodgkin's cells in a pleomorphic stroma of eosinophils, plasma cells, fibroblasts and necrotic foci.	20–40
Lymphocytic depletion	Reed–Sternberg cells usually, although not always, abundant; marked paucity of lymphocytes; diffuse non-refractile fibrosis and necrosis may be present.	5–15

better understood. Hodgkin's disease tends to spread along contiguous node groups but rarely affects some lymph node groups such as the mesenteric, hepatic hilar, presacral or popliteal groups (Bonnadonna & Santoro 1985a). Patterns of disease presentation before treatment are largely determined by pathological subgroups. Thus, most patients with lymphocyte predominant histology present with local disease in upper cervical nodes, those with lymphocyte depleted histology present with abdominal nodes and extranodal disease, and those with nodular sclerosing histology present with supradiaphragmatic disease and in particular mediastinal node involvement. Patients with mixed cellularity histology present with either cervicothoracic disease or lymphoma on both sides of the diaphragm with no particular lymph node group predilection. These observations form the

basis of prophylactic irradiation techniques in patients with apparent localized disease (Kaplan 1980).

NHL is a much more heterogeneous group of diseases. The old classification of lymphosarcoma, reticulum cell sarcoma and giant follicular lymphoma has been largely replaced by the Rappaport classification (Rappaport 1966), and later modifications (Garvin & Berard 1980). This classifies NHL into two broad groupings of (a) diffuse and (b) nodular pattern of lymph node involvement, and further categorizes according to predominant cell type – small cells (lymphocytes), large cells (histiocytes), mixed or undifferentiated.

Lately there have been multiple attempts at reclassification largely based on the origin of the cell type of the lymphomas: T or B lymphocytes, or monocyte/macrophage lineage. 60% of all lymphomas in the UK/Europe are of B-cell origin, 10% T-cell, 5% monocyte/macrophage type and 14% Hodgkin's disease. In the remainder there is no distinct cell origin type (Callender et al 1987). Subgroups of all these types have been further described and classified, with high, intermediate and low grade variants. A Working Group in lymphoma produced a full classification in 1982 (Rosenberg et al 1982), and together with the Kiel/Lennert system (Lennert et al 1975) these are the main classifications used today (Table 13.2).

NHL is more likely to be widespread at presentation and does not spread in the same orderly manner as HD. It also accounts for the majority of the 25% of lymphoma cases presenting with extranodal disease.

Treatment varies according to the grade of tumour as well as degree of spread. Low grade tumours, 70% of NHL, including CLL (Callender et al 1987) may receive no treatment at all for many years, whereas high grade tumours behave like poor histological grade Hodgkin's disease and require aggressive multi-agent chemotherapy.

Lymphomas in children have a different spectrum pathologically. Mixed cellularity HD is more common than in adults, and the lymphocyte depleted type is almost never seen in the younger child. NHL are typically high grade: lymphoblastic type, behaving more like acute lymphoblastic leukaemia than adult non-Hodgkin's lymphoma; Burkitt's/undifferentiated lymphomas;

Table 13.2 Classification of non-Hodgkin's lymphoma: Rosenberg et al 1982 (columns 1 + 4), Lennert et al 1975 (column 2), Rappaport 1966 (column 3), Kim et al 1982 (column 5)

Working formulation	Kiel	Rappaport	Median survival (yrs)	% Total NHL
Malignant lymphoma (ML)				
Low grade				
A. ML: Small Lymphocytic Plasmacytoid	ML: Lymphocytic, cell (B or T cell) Lymphoplasmacytic Hairy cell leukaemia	Well differentiated lymphocytic	5.8	3.6
B. ML: Follicular Predominantly small cleaved cells	ML: Centroblastic — centrocytic — follicular	Nodular poorly differentiated lymphocytic	7.2	22.5
C. ML: Follicular Mixed small cleaved and large cells		Nodular mixed cell type	5.1	7.7
Intermediate grade				
D. ML: Follicular Predominantly large cells	ML: Centroblastic — centrocytic/centroblastic — follicular	Nodular histiocytic	3.0	3.8
E. ML: Diffuse Small cleaved cells	ML: Centrocytic	Diffuse, poorly differentiated lymphocytic	3.4	6.9
F. ML: Diffuse Mixed small and large cells	ML: Centroblastic — centrocytic — diffuse	Diffuse, mixed cell type	2.7	6.7
G. ML: Diffuse Large cell Large cleaved cell Large non-cleaved cell	ML: Centrocytic (large) ML: Centroblastic	Diffuse, histiocytic	1.5	19.7
High grade				
H. ML: Large cell immunoblastic Plasmacytoid Clear cell Polymorphous	ML: Immunoblastic (B or T) Pleomorphic T cell lymphoma	Diffuse, histiocytic	1.3	7.9
I. ML: Lymphoblastic Convoluted cell Non-convoluted cell	ML: Lymphoblastic (T)	Lymphoblastic	2.0	4.2
J. ML: Small non-cleaved cell Burkitt's	ML: Lymphoblastic (B) Burkitt's Non-Burkitt's	Diffuse, undifferentiated Burkitt's Non-Burkitt's	0.7	5.0
Miscellaneous				12.0

and histiocytic/large cell types. The latter behave similarly to adult types of NHL (Murphy 1980).

Patterns of relapse are interesting and should help to guide the use of follow-up investigations and indicate likely anatomical areas of recurrence. In HD, 80–90% of those who relapse do so within two to three years of the initial course of treatment (Bonnadonna & Santoro 1985a). In patients treated with radiotherapy, new disease is frequently seen in the next adjacent lymph node chain outside the treated field, or less commonly in non-contiguous areas, usually because of limitations of diagnostic methods in initial staging (Kaplan 1980). Patients treated with chemotherapy initially tend to recur in sites the same as or contiguous to the original disease (Bonnadonna & Santoro 1985a).

Lymphomas of the non-Hodgkin's type are seen in a significant proportion of AIDS patients, and are usually of intermediate or high grade histological type (Ciobanu et al 1983). Early studies suggest that at least 10% of AIDS patients develop lymphomas (Portlock 1985). Primary involvement of the brain occurs more commonly than in other cases of non-Hodgkin's lymphoma (Snider et al 1983). Prognosis is poor since the lymphomas tend not to respond to treatment (Portlock 1985).

STAGING AND IMAGING METHODS

The initial diagnosis of lymphoma occurs in many ways. The typical clinical presentation of lymphadenopathy, with or without constitutional symptoms such as malaise or fever, accounts for most cases. Incidental lymph node enlargement may be seen on a routine chest radiograph. There may be local symptoms referrable to an extranodal site, such as bone pain or gastrointestinal bleeding, leading to plain radiographs, isotope examinations or contrast studies revealing the diagnosis. A full account of possible diagnostic pathways and appearance of lymphoma in all its guises is not within the remit of this chapter.

Since 1971 the Ann Arbor classification for staging Hodgkin's disease has gained widespread acceptance and use (Table 13.3) (Carbone et al 1971). It is frequently used to stage NHL; childhood NHL has its own staging schemes. The Ann Arbor classification distinguishes between clinical and pathological staging. Clinical staging is based on initial biopsy results, history, examination, laboratory results and imaging investigations. Pathological staging uses the results of gross and microscopic histology, splenectomy, liver, bone marrow and lymph node biopsy with findings at laparotomy. Suffix letters further determine involvement of spleen (S), liver (H), marrow (M), lung (L), pleura (P), bones (O), or lymph nodes (N). A and B indicate the absence or presence of certain constitutional symptoms (fever, night sweats, weight loss of greater than 10% in six month). The letter E is used to denote extranodal

Table 13.3 Ann Arbor staging classification (Carbone et al 1971)

Stage	Classification
I	Involvement of a single lymph node region (I) or of a single extralymphatic organ or site (I_E).
II	Involvement of two or more lymph node regions on the same side of the diaphragm or localized involvement of an extralymphatic organ or site and one or more lymph node regions on one side of the diaphragm.
III	Involvement of lymph node regions on both sides of the diaphragm (III), which may also be accompanied by involvement of the spleen (III_S) or by localized involvement of an extralymphatic organ or site (III_E) or both (III_{SE}).
IV	Diffuse or disseminated involvement or one or more extralymphatic organs or tissues, with or without associated lymph node involvement.

The absence or presence of fever >38°C, night sweats or unexplained weight loss of 10% or more of body weight in the six months preceding admission are to be denoted in all cases by the suffix letters A or B respectively.

sites affected by direct spread of disease from local node involvement.

In many centres, and in cases of widespread lymphoma, pathological staging is limited and may be restricted to a single node or tissue biopsy. This places the onus on clinical staging to be as accurate and complete as possible.

Routine screening methods are of value if the method used has a high level of accuracy in assessing areas of disease, e.g. CT or lymphography in retroperitoneal nodes. Sites infrequently affected should not be routinely screened, e.g. the gastrointestinal tract and the renal tract. If the disease occurs frequently, but in organs where no satisfactory imaging method exists, inaccurate methods should not be used, e.g. isotope scans in splenic disease. If symptoms indicate specific local sites appropriate imaging should be carried out, e.g. barium studies with gastrointestinal symptoms.

Imaging techniques should be assessed against pathological data for assessment of their sensitivity (ability to detect disease without false negatives), specificity (ability to confirm lack of disease without false positives) and overall accuracy (sum of sensitivity and specificity).

The main imaging techniques will be considered, together with an assessment of the rôle of staging laparotomy.

Plain radiographs and conventional tomography

Chest radiographs remain the mainstay of evaluation of thoracic involvement by lymphoma, being quick, sensitive, cheap and easy to repeat for evaluation of treatment and relapse. Although not all affected areas may be shown, the method is often sufficient to stage disease in the chest, and CT or other imaging techniques are unnecessary as the findings will not affect management.

Limitations of plain chest films include the inability to image many lymph node groups well, especially the subcarinal, peri-oesophageal and tracheobronchial nodes and nodes situated in the cardiophrenic angles. They are also poor at detecting pericardial or chest wall involvement, and cannot distinguish between nodes and other mass lesions.

Whole lung tomography is often able to demonstrate additional sites of disease to those shown by plain chest radiography. In a study of 243 patients additional involvement was seen in 21.3% of cases, although this changed staging in only 1.2% of patients (Castellino et al 1976). In most centres thoracic CT has replaced plain tomography.

A major study of 300 untreated patients with HD and NHL was carried out in 1976 to assess distribution of disease in the thorax using plain radiographs and tomography (Filly et al 1976). In Hodgkin's disease, two-thirds of patients have intrathoracic node disease on presentation. The superior mediastinal nodes are almost always affected in this group. 22% of patients have hilar node involvement. Thoracic involvement is less common in young children and predominantly affects the anterior mediastinum. 25% to 30% of newly diagnosed NHL cases have intrathoracic node disease (see also Fig. 13.1 and Table 13.4).

Parenchymal lung disease is seen in 11.6% of patients with Hodgkin's disease, often with ipsilateral hilar and mediastinal nodes, and in 3.7%

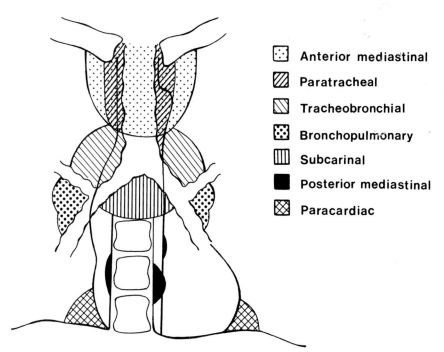

Anterior mediastinal
Paratracheal
Tracheobronchial
Bronchopulmonary
Subcarinal
Posterior mediastinal
Paracardiac

Fig. 13.1 Schematic representation of the locations of the various lymph node groups analysed in patients presenting with lymphomas (Filly et al 1976).

Table 13.4 Incidence of various intrathoracic abnormalities noted radiographically in patients with previously untreated lymphomas (modified from Filly et al 1976)

	Hodgkin's disease (%)	Non-Hodgkin's lymphoma (%)
Intrathoracic disease	67	43
Anterior mediastinal	46	13
Tracheobronchial	45	13
Paratracheal	40	13
Bronchopulmonary	20	9
Subcarinal	10	4
Internal mammary	7	1
Posterior mediastinal	5	10
Paracardial	2	4
Lung	12	4
Pleura	8	10
Bone	4	1

of patients with NHL at presentation (Filly et al 1976).

Pleural effusions are seen in 7% of patients with HD and 10% with NHL. The presence of pleural effusions and similarly lymphatic oedema on chest radiographs does not necessarily signify local infiltration, as shown by the resolution of these findings following mediastinal radiotherapy alone. Pleural effusions are almost never seen in children with Hodgkin's disease (Parker et al 1976), but are relatively common in NHL, particularly with Burkitt's lymphoma (Dunnick et al 1979).

The presence of bulky mediastinal disease in HD, defined as a mass whose transverse diameter is greater than one-third of the chest at the level of T5–T6 on a standing PA chest radiograph, is an adverse prognostic factor and is usually treated with chemotherapy or combination treatment even in the absence of more widespread disease (Mauch et al 1982).

Plain radiograph skeletal surveys to detect occult bone lesions are not carried out routinely in view of the very low incidence of bone lesions on presentation, although they are performed if local symptoms indicate possible bony involvement.

Radio-isotopes

Various radio-isotopes have been used to stage lymphoma. Bone scintigraphy using technetium-labelled diphosphonates is an accurate and effective method of assessing skeletal involvement, but its value as a staging procedure is limited because of the low incidence of bone lesions at presentation. Children have a higher incidence of bone lymphoma than adults (18%) but rarely, if ever, have asymptomatic disease (Castellino et al 1975).

Gallium scanning (using gallium-67 citrate) has been used to localize tumours for the past 20 years. Lymphomas take up the isotope and the use of gallium scanning in staging lymphoma, particularly HD, was first reported in 1971 (Pinsky et al 1971). The exact mechanism of gallium uptake into tumours and inflammatory disease is still unknown. Gallium is taken up by leucocytes which migrate to areas of inflammation and into some tumours (Larson 1978). Gallium scanning in lymphomas has had varying degrees of reported success. It appears to be more effective at demonstrating disease above the diaphragm than below (Johnston et al 1977). Sensitivities for detection of disease below the diaphragm are only about 0.5 (0.5 for nodes, 0.38 for liver, 0.49 for spleen) (Turner et al 1978). It also appears to be better at imaging some forms of lymphoma than others, notably HD and high grade NHL (Anderson et al 1983). Gallium scanning is also not specific for lymphoma, as gallium is taken up by other tumours including lung, liver and testicular neoplasms, as well as in assorted inflammatory conditions such as infection and sarcoidosis.

Optimal gallium localization of lymphoma requires high doses, 400 MBq compared with the more usual 100–150 MBq, together with gamma cameras equipped with triple window pulse height analysers. Under these conditions, sensitivity and specificity of greater than 0.90 have been reported (Anderson et al 1983). The use of CT scanning of the chest has reduced the use and need for gallium scanning, and in our centre it is only used to differentiate between active disease and post-treatment fibrosis above the diaphragm where CT shows a residual mass. Some centres, however, still advocate the use of gallium as a routine staging procedure (Joshua et al 1984).

The use of technetium-labelled sulphur colloid in assessing liver and spleen involvement is uncommon. This technique shows the extent of relative uptake between liver, spleen and other reticuloendothelial tissues (notably bone marrow), but is poor at detecting focal disease deposits of less than 1.5 cm in diameter. Most deposits are smaller than this in the liver and spleen on presentation and we do not recommend this examination routinely in staging.

Ultrasound

Ultrasound examination may be used both in the detection of disease and as an aid to obtaining histological specimens. Compared with other imaging modalities, ultrasound is the most operator dependent. It can visualize the retroperitoneum well and enlarged lymph nodes can be clearly shown, but has the disadvantage of not being able to penetrate bowel gas or bone, and examinations of obese patients are often difficult. Node size determines abnormality in ultrasound examinations, and no useful information regarding the cause of enlargement or internal architectural detail can be obtained. Studies suggest that the retroperitoneum can be examined as well as in CT scanning in only 30–50% of cases, and the extent of disease is often underestimated (Neumann et al 1983). Evaluation of the liver and spleen by ultrasound is widely used for many clinical applications. It is a cheap and often effective examination. In lymphoma patients, however, only large focal lesions (over 1.5 cm) can be detected, and often the only possible indicator of involvement of these organs is by size estimation. It must be remembered, however, that organ size correlates poorly with organ involvement. Enlarged liver and spleen may not contain lymphoma, and disease may be present in normal-sized organs. Sometimes the overall echo pattern of organs, particularly the liver, may appear coarse, indicating possible diffuse involvement without clear focal lesions. This assessment is difficult to quantify and the majority of diffuse or small nodular involvement by lymphoma is not seen by ultrasound. Ultrasound is useful in guiding aspiration or biopsy of lesions in order to obtain histology. Size and type of sample vary according to the depth and position of the material biopsied and the expertise and experience of the operator. Good pathological and cytological expertise is needed to maximize benefit from samples obtained. Ultrasound is not used at our centre for the routine staging of lymphomas.

Lymphography

Bipedal lymphography has been used for many years in the evaluation of lymphoma. The technique demonstrates the position and size of lymph nodes of the external and common iliac groups, and those of the para-aortic nodes up to the level of the hila of the kidneys. Above this, opacification is much less reliable and attempts to overfill the abdominal nodes may result in significant respiratory impairment by contrast microemboli in the pulmonary capillary bed. The examination involves cannulation of lymphatics in the dorsum of the foot following opacification with methylene blue dye injected into the first and second web spaces. Oily contrast media are used, the volume used varying according to the height of the patient. As well as the size and shape of lymph nodes, lymphography is able to demonstrate disturbances of nodal architecture and therefore can distinguish disease in normal-sized lymph nodes. It can also distinguish between nodes enlarged by tumour or reactive hyperplasia. The latter is relatively common, especially in children (Castellino et al 1977).

Lymphography does not demonstrate all the nodes in any nodal group, and cannot opacify mesenteric nodes, the nodes at the hila of the spleen, liver or kidneys, or any node group above the diaphragm apart from occasional nodal filling along the line of drainage from para-aortic nodes to the thoracic duct. It also does not demonstrate nodes completely replaced by lymphoma. In centres which do not carry out lymphography regularly the techniques may become difficult, and the examination can be uncomfortable for the patient.

In areas of nodal opacification, lymphography has high specificity, sensitivity and overall accuracy in studies with pathological correlation based on laparotomy data (Marglin & Castellino 1981, Castellino et al 1984). Most large studies show higher accuracy in detection of disease in the retroperitoneal nodes with lymphography compared with CT scanning (Castellino & Marglin 1982, Castellino et al 1984). Patterns of nodal opacification and size vary between histologically different lymphomas. HD tends to give only moderate nodal enlargement and the nodes themselves are often affected focally rather than in a diffuse manner, particularly with the nodular sclerosing type. NHL tends to produce larger, more diffusely diseased nodes, especially the nodular types.

Interpretation of lymphography is dependent on the expertise and experience of the radiologists involved. Where lymphography is not routinely carried out, the small (7%) advantage in accuracy of staging lymphography over CT may be lost (Castellino et al 1984). There is little doubt that lymphography is less often performed with the increasing availability of CT. In our centre, lymphography is only performed if abdominal CT is regarded as negative on initial presentation and in types of lymphoma known to show only minor nodal enlargement, e.g. nodular sclerosing HD.

Computed tomography

CT is now widely accepted as a valuable technique in the assessment of neoplasms, and the lymphomas are one of the disease groups where the examination is most useful. As far as routine staging of lymphoma is concerned, examination of the thorax, abdomen and pelvis only need be considered.

CT of the thorax delineates anatomy more clearly and completely than plain radiographs or tomograms, particularly in the mediastinum (Heitzmann et al 1977). It is able to give more information as to the type of tissue of origin of mediastinal masses than plain films, especially if scanning is carried out following intravenous contrast. It gives excellent visualization of lymph node groups not easily seen on plain radiographs (see previous section), and accurate information about pericardial, pleural, lung and chest wall disease often not seen on chest radiographs.

A recent study showed abnormal findings on CT in 28% of NHL patients with no definite chest radiograph abnormalities. The same paper showed that 6 out of 11 abnormal chest radiographs were not due to lymphoma (Khoury et al 1986).

Experience with mediastinal node spread from bronchogenic carcinoma as assessed by CT compared with pathological confirmation found at operation in a study of 46 patients demonstrates the overall sensitivity of the technique as high with an accuracy of 89%, but overall the specificity was low, only 57%, because of small lymph nodes involved by metastatic disease and large lymph nodes showing reactive hyperplasia (Reid 1988).

The use of thoracic CT in staging is not universal, and the change in staging grade and prognosis produced by the extra information given compared to plain radiographs may be small compared with cost and examination time. We perform thoracic CT on all cases of lymphoma. It provides a base line for follow-up studies and is the most accurate method of staging disease at the present time. Even when treatment options would not be influenced, as with bulk mediastinal disease, CT still provides information about other sites in the chest not seen on plain radiographs which may be the only site of lymphoma in post-treatment studies, and it therefore helps to make important management changes.

Abdominal CT has been advocated for 10 years for staging lymphomas (Best et al 1978) and is increasingly used. In detection of lymph nodes only size can be used as a criterion of involvement as nodal architecture cannot be seen. A diameter of 1.5 cm is generally accepted as the upper limit of normal size. Nodes smaller than this in certain anatomical locations, e.g. the retrocrural space, may be interpreted accurately as being abnormal because of the uniformity of normal findings in these areas. Nodes are best seen where there is a reasonable amount of fat between them, and for this reason CT is often less helpful in children. Adequate opacification of the bowel by oral and/or rectally administered contrast is also important to avoid false positive results given by loops of bowel in the posterior peritoneum.

The inability of CT to detect disease in normal-sized lymph nodes or to distinguish between moderately enlarged nodes due to disease or reactive changes has been well described. Although lymphography may be superior to CT in these respects, possible abnormality on lymphography alone may not be sufficient to convince clinicians of the true extent of disease and further investigations, such as biopsy, might be needed regardless of the lymphogram result.

CT is more accurate in assessing para-aortic/retroperitoneal nodes than mesenteric nodes, especially in HD, where affected nodes in the mesentery are often of normal size (Best & Black-ledge 1980, Castellino 1983). In NHL, mesenteric nodes are often quite large and may be much more obviously involved by disease than para-aortic nodes, thereby making CT a better indicator of disease extent than 'ymphography.

CT has been shown to be capable of revealing disease in nodes when lymphography has been reported as normal (Best & Blackledge 1980). It also may show greater extent of disease in the para-aortic region compared with lymphography (Kreel 1976, Schaner et al 1977). In the high para-aortic nodes, CT is the only commonly available modality capable of showing nodal enlargement. The prognosis and treatment of stage III HD patients has been shown to be altered by the extent of nodal and/or organ involvement in the ab-domen, more particularly whether disease is confined to above the renal hila or otherwise (Stein et al 1982). CT is better able to answer this ques-tion than other imaging techniques. Even advocates of lymphography in the staging of lym-phomas agree to the use of CT in the abdomen in NHL patients because of the reasons previously outlined. We would use CT in HD also, accepting its limitations, and would argue that any difference in the detection of disease does not alter the even-tual outcome, especially with improvement in treatment regimes.

Assessment of the liver and spleen by CT has been disappointing. Much of the published litera-ture on the subject has shown that CT (with and without contrast enhancement) often fails to detect disease in these organs (Best & Blackledge 1980, Castellino 1983, Castellino et al 1984). If the lym-phoma nodules are over 1 cm in diameter the ability to detect disease increases but at presen-tation liver and spleen are rarely affected by large bulky disease. Assessment of organ involvement by estimation of size alone is inaccurate, except when organs are massively enlarged. One-third of patients with normal splenic size in HD have been shown at laparotomy to have involved organs. Liver involvement is relatively uncommon in lym-phomas at presentation, being 6–9% in HD (Kaplan 1980) and 14% in NHL (Goffinet et al 1977), but splenic involvement is common, especially in HD. It is this fact plus evidence that disease cannot be accurately detected by any imaging method, which has led to the persistent need for staging laparotomy. Splenic involve-ment in NHL is usually seen in association with widespread disease and there is often clear evidence of disease elsewhere in the abdomen or in the bone marrow. Documentation of splenic disease in NHL is therefore less likely to be im-portant regarding treatment planning for these patients than for those with HD.

Emulsified oily contrast agents have been developed which show more parenchymal detail within the liver and spleen, and which allow the detection of more and smaller lesions within these organs (Vermess et al 1980). Again, the method is not specific for lymphoma and will not distinguish lymphoma from benign lesions like granulomata.

CT is useful in assessing other sites of lym-phoma such as intracranial involvement or skeletal disease. This is carried out only if there are specific indications of disease in these areas.

Magnetic resonance imaging

Magnetic resonance imaging (MRI) is being evaluated as a diagnostic tool in many clinical fields. It can detect nodal and organ enlargement, but it does not appear to have any advantage in this respect over CT, and one study suggests that CT may be better able to detect nodes, especially in the neck and abdomen (Dooms et al 1984). MRI image quality is still in a phase of rapid im-provement and any deficit in spatial resolution compared with CT may only be a temporary phenomenon. MRI may also be able to demon-strate disease in the bone marrow not able to be imaged by other means (Olson et al 1986). Quan-titative MRI measuring T_1 relaxation times has been demonstrated to be a sensitive method for detecting liver involvement by malignant lym-phoma (Richards et al 1986). MRI is also able to give an excellent demonstration of the meninges, brain stem and spinal cord and is now the imaging method of choice for disease in these areas. The equipment is expensive, examination times are long and the number of MRI scanners is still ex-tremely small compared with the number of CT scanners. We do not envisage routine MRI scan-ning for the staging of lymphomas in the forseeable future.

Staging laparotomy

Staging laparotomy has been the keystone of the progress in assessing the accuracy of imaging staging techniques. Although not within the remit of a chapter on radiology, evaluation of the need for this procedure as a routine investigation is of relevance since its performance alters the need for other imaging procedures.

Staging laparotomy is rarely carried out in patients with NHL. CT and bone marrow examination are often able to stage fully the disease, which is often widespread in these patients at presentation. Isolated splenic involvement is also uncommon in patients on presentation, unlike those with HD.

In HD, the role of staging laparotomy is under critical re-evaluation. Some centres still perform this routinely in clinical stage I/II due to supradiaphragmatic node disease, and about 20% of these patients have occult abdominal disease (liver 1–6%, spleen 15–20%, nodes 5–10%) (Bonnadonna & Santoro 1985b). Some clinicians believe that early splenic involvement presents a high risk for concomitant or subsequent hepatic and marrow disease and use this as an argument for laparotomy (Kaplan 1980, Proceedings 1982). Others would dispute this. Laparotomy should only be carried out if the detection of splenic disease will alter management.

Modern combined radiotherapy and chemotherapy regimes are being increasingly used in the initial treatment of HD, thus making laparotomy and the assessment of splenic disease less critical. Also, the prognosis following salvage chemotherapy given to patients who relapse after having had radiotherapy alone is no worse than for those given combination treatment initially (Kaplan 1981, Hoppe et al 1982). The risks of fulminant septicaemia following splenectomy should also be considered, and it is rarely performed in young children for this reason. In children, because of the significant risk of splenectomy and also because of the important risk of growth retardation when radiotherapy alone is used in treatment, the modern therapy usually comprises combination chemotherapy and low dose involved field radiotherapy, thus obviating the need for accurate anatomical staging.

Staging laparotomy is now hardly ever carried out in our centre.

REMISSION STATUS/FOLLOW-UP

The growing effectiveness of treatment for lymphoma, especially HD, makes the assessment of treatment response an important part of the function of imaging in these patients. It is important to identify areas affected by lymphoma which are not responding to first line therapy, especially as alternative chemotherapy regimes are still able to provide long term remissions. The choice of imaging techniques and their frequency depends on the individual clinician caring for the patient. The site of disease may also be important. If disease is clearly seen on simple investigations such as chest radiographs, serial examinations help to monitor progress. If disease is only present in areas detected by CT scanning, then serial CT examinations are required. Investigations are usually performed at the end of induction of clinical remission and then at routine intervals dictated by the anticipated relapse interval. Accurate documentation of remission involves full clinical and laboratory tests, and may also include bone marrow or liver biopsies, CSF examination or other procedures depending on the original extent of disease. Plain radiography and follow-up lymphography films may also be taken. Experience shows that these tests may well underestimate the extent of residual disease.

CT is used to assess as fully as possible the true remission status. CT of the thorax and abdomen is carried out to optimize assessment of any areas of possible persistent disease activity. It has been shown that many patients who are clinically in remission are shown by CT to have disease, and that the presence of this disease has an adverse effect on prognosis (Blackledge et al 1981). It also provides a useful baseline for comparison with later examination in assessment of treatment required. We feel that CT is better able to give an overall assessment of remission status than other imaging methods.

The radiologist needs to be aware of change that may occur as a result of the therapy used. If treatment is by radiotherapy, there may be pneumonitis within the radiation field as early as 1–3 months later. The incidence of this varies from 5–20% (Mauch 1985). Perihilar and perimediastinal pulmonary fibrosis may be seen from six months after treatment. These latter changes are usually asymptomatic but must not be confused with recurrent disease or intercurrent infection. Comparison with previous films tends to show the progressive shrinkage of lung typical of post-treatment fibrosis, but this may sometimes be a very difficult problem to resolve, and biopsy may be required. Radiotherapy may also affect the heart, most commonly producing asymptomatic pericardial effusions but sometimes leading to tamponade and constrictive pericarditis.

When chemotherapy has been used, there may be changes on the chest radiograph for several reasons. Firstly, there may be idiosyncratic or allergic phenomena, with pulmonary infiltrates. The possibility of direct fibrotic damage caused by the drugs used should also be considered, especially with bleomycin (Morrison & Goldman 1979). Adriamycin may cause cardiac failure by direct toxicity leading to cardiomyopathy. The changes of any opportunistic infection must always be considered. Induced thrombocytopenia may cause pulmonary haemorrhage.

Follow-up of patients involves clinical and laboratory assessment, as well as imaging techniques. We consider routine use of CT to be the most useful imaging technique. Relapse in lymphoma following treatment tends to occur within five years of initial treatment (87% within three years in HD) (Weller et al 1976). Lymphographic contrast has been shown to remain within the lymph nodes for varying times, with only about half of the patients retaining diagnostic amounts of contrast at 15 months (Fabian et al 1966). This gives the plain radiograph follow-up film limited value. Repeated lymphography is often difficult practically, and uncomfortable for patients. We feel that follow-up lymphography is probably less helpful than follow-up CT, and other studies support our view (Lee et al 1980). In cases of clinically suspected relapse, CT will often show unsuspected disease below the diaphragm, or more extensive abdominal disease than expected. In patients with no abnormal physical findings but symptoms of possible relapse, CT often demonstrates active disease (Blackledge et al 1981).

Second malignancies following treatment for lymphomas should be borne in mind. These are more commonly seen after treatment for HD, probably because of the better prognosis for these patients. The most common malignancy is non-lymphoblastic leukaemia, seen particularly in patients who have received chemotherapy, especially with alkylating agents (Coleman 1982). NHL may develop in patients following treatment for HD (Krikorian et al 1979, Coleman et al 1982). These tend to be of aggressive histological subtypes. In cases followed up for ten years or longer, the risk of developing NHL is of the order of 5–15%, the interval between diagnosis of HD and NHL being 44 to 124 months (Portlock 1985). Development of NHL appears greatest in those receiving both radiation and chemotherapy (Krikorian et al 1979, Coleman 1982).

SUMMARY AND CONCLUSIONS

Diagnosis, staging and follow-up of patients with lymphoma requires close co-operation between oncologist and radiologist for optimal management. Knowledge of the latest advances in therapy and imaging methods is important to maximize survival in this group of patients where prognosis is continually improving.

Accurate histological diagnosis may be made using needle aspiration cytology with ultrasound or CT guidance (Zornoza et al 1981). This is already the case for large cell lymphomas, but by using stains for T and B cell markers, monoclonal antibodies, looking for light chain restriction in cells and other immunocytochemical techniques, further improvements in diagnostic accuracy may become possible (Mason & Gatter 1987). At present, however, most pathologists still prefer large pathological specimens for histological architecture analysis of lymphomas. In the case of aspiration cytology for follow-up when the original lymphoma cell-line is known, cytological diagnosis may be easier.

For staging of lymphoma we feel that CT is the single most important investigation. We accept that in HD, lymphography in good hands has some advantage in assessment of retroperitoneal nodes, but for practical purposes CT gives better overall assessment of the whole extent of disease.

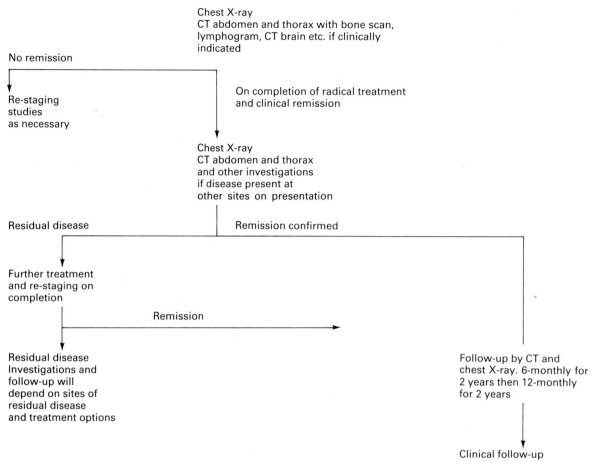

Fig. 13.2   Investigation of Hodgkin's disease.

Thoracic CT, in addition to plain radiography, can give a better estimate of mediastinal extent, and is able to be performed at the same time as abdominal and pelvic examinations. Lymphography can be difficult both practically and in interpretation, and outside centres of high expertise becomes less useful as a diagnostic tool. We would therefore advocate its use only in certain well-defined circumstances, such as in nodular sclerosing HD stage I–II where CT has proved negative. Figures 13.2 and 13.3 give suggested protocols for investigation and follow-up for patients with HD and NHL.

As treatment improves, the overall aim of staging appears to have been simplified. The treatment options, especially in HD, are now less complicated and less reliant on anatomical extent than in the past. Practically, there may be only two groups of HD patients: those who may be cured by radiotherapy alone (clinical stage I and II without B symptoms or mediastinal bulk disease), and those who need combination treatment or chemotherapy (Wiernik & Slawson 1982). It may be that disease bulk rather than anatomical extent determines prognosis, and more quantitative or structured methods of reporting with accurate assessment of tumour volume may become important. CT, again, would appear to be best able to carry out this form of assessment.

Liver and spleen assessment is difficult using any form of imaging. Newer contrast media may help to improve this in CT, but disease is still likely to be missed in a proportion of cases. Change in treatment regimes, however, has made accurate

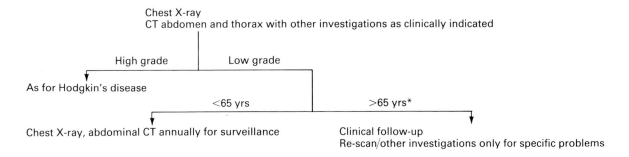

*Age limits are arbitrary and act only as a guideline

Fig. 13.3 Investigation of non-Hodgkin's lymphoma.

detection of disease in the spleen less important, and salvage chemotherapy following relapse after radiotherapy is now so good that overall prognosis would not seem to be affected in these cases. We therefore feel that staging laparotomy may no longer be routinely indicated. Isotope examinations using gallium citrate, technetium colloid examinations of liver and spleen and technetium diphosphonate examinations of bone are not used as routine staging procedures. Gallium may well still have a place in the assessment of active disease in the chest, especially in difficult cases with post-treatment changes.

Ultrasound and MRI have little practical use in staging except in specific situations, e.g. assessment of ureteric obstruction using ultrasound, or assessment of meninges/brain stem with suspected lymphoma involvement by MRI.

In remission assessment and follow-up, simple investigations such as plain radiographs where applicable should be carried out. CT may be the only modality showing disease and serial examinations are then needed. Lymphography shows response to initial treatment well, but contrast loss over as short a period as one year often precludes accurate further assessment. Second or third lymphograms

may be difficult and uncomfortable procedures.

CT is perceived as an expensive technique but has become much more available as an imaging method, and all lymphoma patients in this and many other countries should have access to a scanner for staging and follow-up purposes.

Clinicians and radiologists should be aware of, and fully acquainted with, changes due to therapy and complications of treatment. The possibility of second malignancies developing should be borne in mind, particularly where lymphoma 'recurs' late and appears resistant to treatment.

Acquired immune deficiency syndrome (AIDS) is well described, and is becoming increasingly common. These patients are at risk of developing NHL of intermediate and high grade types. These lymphomas tend to present atypically and the possibility of AIDS should be considered, e.g. with cases of localized intracerebral disease.

The aim of imaging should always be to provide accurate and useful information where this information will alter management or prognostic outlook. As treatment methods and patient prognosis improves, methods for staging with imaging techniques should become less invasive and less unpleasant for the patient.

REFERENCES

Anderson K C, Leonard R C F, Canellos G P, Skarin A T, Kaplan W D 1983 High dose gallium scanning in lymphoma. American Journal of Medicine 75: 327–331
Best J J K, Blackledge G 1980 The use of computed tomography of the abdomen in the initial assessment and

monitoring of patients with lymphoma. In: Symington T, Williams A E, McVie J G (eds) Cancer assessment and monitoring (10th Pfizer International Symposium). Churchill Livingstone, Edinburgh, pp 188–203
Best J J K, Blackledge G, Forbes W St C et al 1978

Computed tomography of abdomen in staging and clinical management of lymphoma. British Medical Journal 2: 1675–1677

Blackledge G, Mamtora H, Crowther D, Isherwood I, Best J J K 1981 The role of abdominal computed tomography in lymphoma following treatment. British Journal of Radiology 54: 955–960

Bonnadonna G, Santoro A 1985a Clinical evolution and treatment of Hodgkin's disease. In: Wiernik P H, Canellos G P, Kyle R A, Schiffer C A (eds) Neoplastic diseases of the blood, vol II. Churchill Livingstone, New York, pp 789–790

Bonnadonna G, Santoro A 1985b Clinical evolution and treatment of Hodgkin's disease. In: Wiernik P H, Canellos G P, Kyle R A, Schiffer C A (eds) Neoplastic diseases of the blood, vol II. Churchill Livingstone, New York, pp 794–795

Callender S T, Burch C, Vanhegan R I 1987 The lymphomas. In: Weatherall D J, Leadingham J G, Warrell D A (eds) Oxford textbook of medicine, 2nd edn. Oxford University Press, Oxford

Carbone P P, Kaplan H S, Musshoff K, Smithers E W, Tubiana M 1971 Report of the committee on Hodgkin's disease staging. Cancer Research 31: 1860–1861

Castellino R A 1983 Newer imaging techniques for extent determination of Hodgkin's disease and non-Hodgkin's lymphoma. In: Miraud E L, Hutchinson W B, Milich E (eds) 13th International Cancer Congress part D: Research and treatment. Liss, New York, pp 365–372

Castellino R A, Marglin S I 1982 Imaging of abdominal and pelvic lymph nodes. Lymphography or computed tomography? Investigative Radiology 17: 433–443

Castellino R A, Bellani F F, Gasparini M, Musumeci R 1975 Radiographic findings in previously untreated children with non-Hodgkin's lymphoma. Radiology 117: 657–663

Castellino R A, Filly R, Blank N 1976 Routine full lung tomography in the initial staging of patients with Hodgkin's disease and non-Hodgkin's lymphoma. Cancer 38: 1130–1136

Castellino R A, Musumeci R, Markovits P 1977 Lymphography. In: Parker B R, Castellino R A (eds) Paediatric, oncologic radiology. C V Mosby, St Louis, pp 183–208

Castellino R A, Hoppe R, Blank N, Young S W, Neumann C, Rosenburg S A, Kaplan H S 1984 Computed tomography, lymphography, and staging laparotomy: correlations in initial staging of Hodgkin's disease. American Journal of Roentgenology 143: 37–41

Ciobanu N, Andreef M, Safai B, Koziner B, Mertelsmann R 1983 Lymphatic metaplasia in a homosexual patient with Kaposi's sarcoma. Annals of Internal Medicine 98: 151–155

Coleman C N 1982 Secondary neoplasms in patients treated for cancer: etiology and perspective. Radiation Research 92: 188–200

Coleman C N, Burke J S, Varghese A 1982 Secondary leukaemia and non-Hodgkin's lymphoma in patients treated for Hodgkin's disease. In: Rosenburg S A, Kaplan H S (eds) Malignant lymphomas: etiology, immunology, pathology, treatment. Bristol Myers Cancer Symposia vol 3. Academic Press, New York

Dooms G C, Hricak H, Crooks L E, Higgins C B 1984 Magnetic resonance imaging of the lymph nodes: comparison with CT. Radiology 153: 719–728

Dunnick N R, Reaman G H, Head G L, Shawker T H, Ziegler J L 1979 Radiographic manifestations of Burkitt's lymphoma in American patients. American Journal of Roentgenology 132: 1–6

Fabian C E, Nudelman E J, Abrams H L 1966 Postlymphogram film as an indicator of tumour activity in lymphoma. Investigative Radiology 1: 386–393

Filly R, Blank N, Castellino R A 1976 Radiographic distribution of intrathoracic disease in previously untreated patients with Hodgkin's disease and non-Hodgkin's lymphoma. Radiology 120: 277–281

Garvin A J, Berard C 1980 Comparative analysis of pathological classifications: current recommendations regarding new technical considerations. Seminars in Oncology 7: 234–244

Goffinet D R, Warnke R, Dunnock N R et al 1977 Clinical and surgical (laparotomy) evaluation of patients with non-Hodgkin's lymphoma. Cancer Treatment Reports 61: 981–992

Heitzmann E T, Goldwin R L, Proto A V 1977 Radiological analysis of the mediastinum using computed tomography. Radiological Clinics of North America 15: 309–329

Hoppe R T, Coleman C N, Cox R S, Rosenburg S A, Kaplan H S 1982 The management of stage I–II Hodgkin's disease with irradiation alone or combined modality therapy: the Standford experience. Blood 59: 455–465

Johnston G S, Go M F, Benua R S, Larson S M, Andrew G A, Hubner K F 1977 Gallium-67 citrate imaging in Hodgkin's disease. Final report of co-operative group. Journal of Nuclear Medicine 18: 692–698

Joshua D E, Dalgleish A, Kronenburg M 1984 Is staging laparotomy necessary in patients with supradiaphragmatic I and IIA Hodgkin's disease? Lancet 1: 847–848

Kaplan H S 1980 Hodgkin's disease, 2nd edn. Harvard University Press, Cambridge, MA

Kaplan H S 1981 Hodgkin's disease: biology, treatment, prognosis. Blood 57: 813–822

Khoury M B, Godwin J D, Halversen R, Hanun Y, Putman C E 1986 Rôle of chest CT in non-Hodgkin's lymphoma. Radiology 158: 659–662

Kim H, Zelman R J, Fox M A et al 1982 Pathology panel for lymphoma clinical studies: a comprehensive analysis of cases accumulated since its inception. Journal of the National Cancer Institute 68: 43–67

Kinmonth J B 1952 Lymphography in man: A method of outlining lymphatic trunks at operation. Clinical Science 11: 13–20

Kreel L, 1976 The EMI whole body scanner in the demonstration of lymph node enlargement. Clinical Radiology 27: 421–429

Krikorian J G, Burke J S, Rosenburg S A, Kaplan H S 1979 Occurrence of non-Hodgkin's lymphoma after therapy for Hodgkin's disease. New England Journal of Medicine 300: 452–458

Larson S M 1978 Mechanisms of localisation of gallium-67 in tumours. Seminars in Nuclear Medicine 8: 193–203

Lee J K, Stanley R J, Sagel S S, Melson G L, Koehler R E 1980 Limitations of the post-lymphangiogram radiograph as an indicator of recurrent lymphoma: comparison to computed tomography. Radiology 134: 155–158

Lennert K, Mohri N, Stein N, Kaiserling E 1975 The histopathology of malignant lymphoma. British Journal of Haematology (suppl) 31: 193–203

Lukes R J, Butler J J 1966 The pathology and nomenclature of Hodgkin's disease. Cancer Research 26: 1063–1081

Marglin S, Castellino R A 1981 Lymphographic accuracy in 623 consecutive previously untreated cases of Hodgkin's disease and non-Hodgkin's lymphoma. Radiology 140: 351–353

Mason D Y, Gatter K C 1987 The rôle of immunocytochemistry in diagnostic pathology. Journal of Clinical Pathology 40: 1042–1054

Mauch P 1985 Radiotherapeutic aspects of Hodgkin's disease. In: Wiernik P H, Canellos G P, Kyle R A, Schiffer C A (eds) Neoplastic diseases of the blood, vol II. Churchill Livingstone, New York, pp 827–839

Mauch P, Gorshein D, Cunningham J, Hellman S 1982 Influence of mediastinal adenopathy on site and frequency of relapse in patients with Hodgkin's disease. Cancer Treatment Reports 66: 809–817

Morrison D A, Goldman A L 1979 Radiographic patterns of drug induced lung disease. Radiology 131: 299–304

Murphy S B 1980 Classification, staging and end results of treatment of non-Hodgkin's lymphoma: dissimilarities from lymphomas in adults. Seminars in Oncology 7: 332–339

Neumann C H, Robert N J, Rosenthal D, Canellos G 1983 Clinical value of ultrasonography for the management of non-Hodgkin's lymphoma patients as compared with abdominal computed tomography. Journal of Computer Assisted Tomography 7: 666–669

Olson D O, Shields A F, Scheurich C J, Porter B A, Moss A M 1986 Magnetic resonance imaging of the bone marrow in patients with leukaemia, aplastic anaemia and lymphoma. Journal of Investigative Radiology 21: 540–546

Parker B R, Castellino R A, Kaplan H S 1976 Paediatric Hodgkin's disease. 1: Radiographic evaluation. Cancer 35: 2430–2435

Pinsky S M, Hoffer P B, Turner D A, Harper P V, Gottschack A 1971 Place of gallium-67 in staging of Hodgkin's disease. Journal of Nuclear Medicine 12: 385

Portlock C S 1985 Lymphomas occurring in association with other diseases. In: Wiernik P H, Canellos G P, Kyle R A, Schiffer C A (eds) Neoplastic diseases of the blood, vol II. Churchill Livingstone, New York, p 906

Proceedings of the symposium on contemporary issues in Hodgkin's disease: biology, staging and treatment (San Francisco, California, September 9–12, 1981) 1982 Cancer Treatment Reports 66: 601

Rappaport H 1966 Tumours of the haemopoietic system. In: Atlas of tumour pathology. Armed Forces Institute of Pathology, Washington DC

Reid W 1988 Personal communication

Richards M A, Wells J A, Reznek R H et al 1986 Detection of spread of malignant lymphoma to the liver by low field strength magnetic resonance imaging. British Medical Journal 293: 1126–1128

Rosenberg S A, Berard C W, Brown B W et al 1982 National Cancer Institute sponsored study of classification of non-Hodgkin's lymphomas: summary and description of a working formulation for clinical usage. Cancer 49: 2112–2135

Schaner E G, Head G L, Kalman M A, Dunnick N R, Doppman J L 1977 Whole body computed tomography in the diagnosis of abdominal and thoracic malignancy: review of 600 cases. Cancer Treatment Reports 61: 1537–1560

Snider W D, Simpson D M, Aronyk K E, Nielsen S L 1983 Primary lymphoma of the brain associated with acquired immune deficiency syndrome. New England Journal of Medicine 308: 45

Stein R S, Golomb H M, Wiernik P H et al 1982 Anatomical substages of stage IIIA Hodgkin's disease: follow up of a collaborative study. Cancer Treatment Reports 66: 733–741

Turner D A, Fordham E W, Ali A, Slayton R E 1978 Gallium-67 imaging in the management of Hodgkin's disease and other malignant lymphomas. Seminars in Nuclear Medicine 8: 205–218

Vermess M, Doppmann J L, Sugarbaker P H et al 1980 Clinical trials with a new liposoluble contrast material for computed tomography of the liver and spleen. Radiology 137: 217–222

Weller S A, Glatstein E, Kaplan H S, Rosenburg S A 1976 Initial relapses in previously treated Hodgkin's disease. I: Results of second treatment. Cancer 37: 2840–2846

Wiernik P H, Slawson R G 1982 Hodgkin's disease with direct extension into pulmonary parenchyma from a mediastinal mass: a presentation requiring special therapeutic considerations. Cancer Treatment Reports 66: 711–716

Young J L, Percy C L, Asire A J (eds) 1981 Surveillance, epidemiology and end results: incidence and mortality data, 1973–1977. National Cancer Institute Monographs no 57. US Government Printing Office, Washington

Zornoza J, Cabillas F F, Altoff T, Ordonez N, Cohen M A 1981 Percutaneous needle biopsy in abdominal lymphoma. American Journal of Roentgenology 136: 97–103

14. Bone and soft tissue

F. G. Adams

INTRODUCTION

A detailed description of the diagnostic features of bone and connective tissue tumours may be found in any standard radiological textbook. The main aims of this chapter are to explore the relationship between radiology and pathology with special emphasis on staging procedures, to examine the impact of new radiological techniques, and lastly to consider the economic aspects of radiological practice.

The subject is vast and may be approached in many ways. However, the tumours will be classified into primary connective tissue, marrow or haemopoetic and metastases because the incidence and management of these three groups is so disparate.

PRIMARY CONNECTIVE TISSUE TUMOURS

Malignant primary connective tissue tumours are rare. The incidence of such lesions in the west of Scotland from 1980 to 1984 is given by the standardized rate for males of 0.837 per 100 000. By comparison, the standardized rate for males suffering lung cancer is 100.98 per 100 000. Corresponding values for females are 1.8 and 32 per 100 000 respectively.

Clinical presentation

Pain associated with malignant bone tumours soon becomes constant and severe. Local tenderness is usually present before swelling. In advanced cases with highly vascular tumours, distended vessels are present in conjunction with increased skin temperature. Systemic symptoms such as fever, malaise, anaemia and pallor suggest a poor prognosis. Pathological fracture is uncommon in rapidly growing tumours as they usually present before the bone has been sufficiently weakened.

Routine haematology may reveal anaemia which is associated with a poor prognosis. Biochemical examination may reveal elevations of the serum calcium or alkaline phosphatase which are nonspecific, and are of little value in assessing the extent of the disease.

It is not intended to deal in depth with benign connective tissue lesions. Suffice it to say that the clinical presentation of benign lesions may be similar to that of the less aggressive malignant tumours. Such patients may present with vague discomfort or swelling. Complications due to pressure on adjacent nerves, vessels or joints, overlying bursitis or fracture through the stalk of an exostosis may simulate more sinister disease. Sudden onset of severe pain and loss of function may imply a pathological fracture.

Staging of malignant connective tissue tumours

It is crucial that the radiologist clearly understands the staging systems of any tumour before commencing investigations because such staging systems are usually designed to rationalize patient management. The staging systems become a common language shared by all members of the team involved in treating malignant disease. The staging system outlined in this chapter is that of Enneking (1983) and is based on the following assumptions:

1. Given a specific histology, the tissue of origin does not influence the prognosis, e.g. a high grade

fibrosarcoma of bone behaves like a high grade fibrosarcoma of soft tissues.

2. The purpose of staging is primarily for surgical management.

3. Marrow cell lesions behave differently and so require different staging and treatment.

4. Biological aggressiveness may be more accurately predicted by clinical presentation and radiological findings than by histological appearances.

5. The location of a lesion in relation to the anatomical barriers is more important than size.

6. Metastases to regional lymph nodes or lungs carry an equally bad prognosis.

7. The different categories of the staging system reflect a progressively poorer prognosis.

Surgical grading

This grading is based on a combination of histological, clinical and imaging information. Lesions which carry a better prognosis are graded G1 whilst those with a poorer prognosis are graded G2.

G1 or low grade lesions histologically exhibit few mitotic figures, are well differentiated, exhibit few atypical cells, have a more mature matrix and show no evidence of vascular invasion. Clinically the patient would complain only of discomfort and any swelling would have appeared slowly. Radiologically the lesion will be relatively well defined, show only slightly increased uptake on an isotope scan and little or no vascularity on an angiogram. Conversely, G2 or high grade lesions exhibit many mitotic figures, are poorly differentiated, exhibit many atypical cells, have an immature matrix and show vascular invasion. Clinically the patient will often complain of severe pain and/or a rapid increase in size of the swelling. Isotope scans show markedly increased uptake, usually more extensive than is suggested by the radiograph, which usually shows an ill-defined lesion. Increased vascularity is usually marked on an angiogram.

The term surgical grading is used in preference to histological grade because in some instances the biological aggressiveness of the tumour is more accurately predicted by clinical and radiological factors. Thus a tumour may be categorized as G2

on the basis of either histological appearances or a combination of clinical and radiological features. It is not the function of the radiologist to predict the exact histological origin of the tumour because such predictions are too inaccurate to form a basis for surgical management. It should be remembered that each tumour is managed uniquely and although some tumours such as parosteal osteosarcoma, Kaposi's sarcoma and chordoma present as G1 lesions and osteosarcoma, and Paget's sarcoma classically presents as G2 lesions, many tumours such as fibrosarcoma, giant cell tumour, haemangiopericytoma and alveolar cell sarcoma are variously graded as G1 or G2 lesions.

Surgical site

The site of the lesion is of paramount importance in surgical management. Lesions are categorized as compartmental (T1) if they are completely confined within a compartment such as a bone or a muscle, and extracompartmental (T2) if they have broken through these anatomical barriers or have actually arisen within fascial planes. Once tumours become extracompartmental, there is no anatomical barrier to further spread.

Metastases

Patients without metastases are categorized as M0 and those with metastases as M1. With sarcomas as opposed to carcinomas, the prognosis for metastases to regional lymph nodes is as bad as that for pulmonary metastases. However, patients tend to die of pulmonary metastases so that their recognition is generally more important (Enneking 1983).

Although it has been clearly stated that radiologists should not predict the histological origin of such tumours, this is not to deny that the histology is central to the overall management of the patient. Indeed, once the tumour has been staged locally, the results of the biopsy will guide the radiologist in the search for metastases. Connective tissue sarcomas normally metastasize to lungs or liver. Alveolar soft part sarcoma, rhabdomyosarcoma, epithelioid sarcoma, clear sarcoma, clear cell sarcoma and synovial sarcoma tend to spread to regional lymph nodes. Chordomas, giant cell tumours and aneurysmal bone cysts rarely metastasize.

Relationship between pathology and the staging system

Before reviewing the surgical implications of the staging system, some fundamental pathological features must be discussed.

In bone and soft tissue surgery, the term tumour includes the pseudocapsule and the surrounding reactive zone. Thus both the tumour and the reactive zone must be completely within the compartment if the lesion is to be classified as G1. The reason for this is that the reactive zone is a mechanism by which the tumour may spread due to new vessels being drawn into the tumour. Tumour may then escape through small spaces or invade the new vessels resulting in satellite tumours in the reactive zone. Thus a bone tumour becomes a G2 lesion if there is radiological evidence of periosteal reaction, the isotope bone scan shows reactive bone at the periosteum or an angiogram reveals new vessels around the periosteum. Similarly, soft tissue tumours become G2 lesions when radiographs, isotope scans or angiograms show similar features.

There are a number of spurious associations between prognosis and lesion size, lesion depth and proximity of lesions to vital structures. Enneking (1983) clearly showed that the poor prognosis associated with larger lesions is due to the fact that the majority of large lesions are T2. Curiously, very large lesions (> 20 cm) tended to have a better prognosis. Similarly, the truism that superficial lesions have a better prognosis is not because they are detected earlier but because the majority are G1 lesions. Lastly, the correlation between prognosis and proximity to vital structures is explained by the fact that involvement of neurovascular bundles by definition categorizes a lesion as T2.

In addition to the occurrence of small satellite tumours, approximately 25% of osteosarcomas exhibit skip lesions. These are defined as second tumours occurring in the same bone or on the opposite side of the joint with normal intervening tissue. According to Enneking & Kagan (1975) they are not multicentric tumours and most likely result from invasion of marrow sinusoids. This mechanism does not explain the transarticular skips or the occasional extra-osseous skip. Over 80% of the skip metastases occur in the lower limb.

Surgical implications of the staging system

Once the staging procedures have been completed, the patient will fall into one of the following six categories:

Stage 1A   G1 T1 M0
Stage 1B   G1 T2 M0
Stage 2A   G2 T1 M0
Stage 2B   G2 T2 M0
Stage 3A   G1 or G2 T1 M1
Stage 3B   G1 or G2 T2 M1

For stage 3 lesions, the therapeutic attention tends to shift to control of metastatic disease and so will not be considered further at this point. Patients with stage 1 and 2 lesions will generally fall into the surgical categories shown in Table 14.1. The term wide means that a large margin of approximately 10 cm of normal tissue surrounding the tumour should be removed. Radical means that the entire bone or muscle compartment must be removed. Thus a G2 T1 lesion will cause an entire bone or muscle group to be removed whilst a G1 T2 lesion will result in an amputation approximately 10 cm proximal to the nearest evidence of active tumour.

The key point which must be grasped by the radiologist is that he or she plays a crucial part in the GTM classification. The actual histology is determined by the pathologist whilst the radiologist must concentrate on defining the extent of the disease.

Biopsy

Although biopsy generally provides the essential

Table 14.1 Treatment related to the surgical grading and site of primary connective tissue tumours.

	T1	T2
G1	Wide excision	Wide amputation
G2	Radical excision	Radical amputation

information with which to grade the tumour, it has been shown by Mankin et al (1983) that it is neither as reliable nor as safe as many radiologists assume. These workers showed that with regard to diagnostic accuracy, differences in diagnosis between biopsy and final outcome occurred in 82 out of 329 patients (25%). These differences were categorized as major if they were likely to mislead the surgeon or alter treatment. Of the 82 differences, 60 (73%) were major and of those 43 (71%) were made at the referral centre. Complications of biopsy included fracture, wound breakdown, haemorrhage and infection and occurred in 57 patients (17.3%). In 30 of the 57 patients, complications adversely affected treatment or outcome. The complication rate was higher for those biopsied initially at the referring centre (44 out of 57).

As a result of these findings the following points should be considered in the approach to staging: the surgeon who is going to manage the patient should perform the biopsy, which should be so placed that it can be excised with the definitive operation and not interfere with skin flaps; for the general radiologist working in a District General Hospital the implication is that referral to the treatment centre should be advised instead of biopsy; and the enthusiastic interventional radiologist should not meddle with biopsies of connective tissue sarcomas. Staging procedures such as radionuclide scans and angiograms should be performed prior to biopsy to avoid false positive studies. Haematoma and swelling caused by the trauma of the biopsy will overestimate the size and site of the lesion whilst any increase in vascularity caused by repair will overestimate the aggressiveness of the lesion. Anatomical planes should not be violated, the smallest incision should be made and the most direct route taken through muscle rather than through fascial planes as it has been shown that tumour recurrences are nearly always extracompartmental, suggesting that previous biopsy has converted a T1 into a T2 lesion. Wherever possible biopsy of actual bone should be avoided; the soft tissue at the leading edge of the tumour should be sampled. In general needle biopsies, although attended by reduced complications, are not recommended, particularly in suspected cartilagenous tumours which tend to have polymorphous histology, or in soft tissue tumours in which large areas of necrosis may be present.

Therapeutic options

Surgery

Until a few years ago, the only choice was whether or not to operate. However, improvements in survival due to advances in radiation treatment and chemotherapy have forced the surgeon to consider limb salvage operations to maintain limb function. These limb salvage operations are generally carried out in patients with G1 tumours who are fully grown or nearly so in order to avoid problems of limb shortening. Predicted limb length discrepancy should not exceed 8 cm. The radiologist can offer the surgeon accurate staging of disease, and accurate measurements of the length of the limb and the width of the medullary canal of the relevant bone. Postoperatively these patients have a high complication rate, particularly when given adjuvant chemotherapy. They are a difficult group of patients because the allografts are frequently osteoporotic and obscured by the fixing devices so it is more difficult to obtain high quality radiographs.

Radiation therapy

Histology is essential for rational therapy. As a general working rule, if the surgical resection is considered successful then radiation therapy is not indicated although chemotherapy may be given to attempt to deal with micrometastases. If surgical removal is incomplete or in doubt then radiation therapy and/or chemotherapy are given. Within this general approach the radioresponsiveness of the tumour is important. Although many connective tissue sarcomas are not particularly radiosensitive, the response is variable and a trial of radiation therapy is often given. If the response is poor chemotherapy may be tried.

Thus although radiation is usually an adjuvant therapy, it may be the primary mode of treatment as in orbital rhabdomyosarcoma in children; it may be used to shrink the tumour mass as an aid to surgery or chemotherapy, and it is frequently used to relieve pain and to prevent pathological fracture. An important advantage of radiation therapy is that it is limb sparing.

The radiologist has an invaluable rôle in the management of connective tissue tumours. It has been clearly shown by Rothwell et al (1983) and Hobday et al (1979) that even the bladder carcinomas which are relatively well demonstrated by conventional imaging techniques are incompletely covered by radiation fields in up to 37% of cases. CT permits accurate determination of the site and hence the volume of the lesion. It may help spare damage to vital structures such as the eye, spinal cord, kidneys, and for cosmetic reasons, the skin.

Attenuation measurements enable calculation of correction factors to allow for decreased absorption by lung tissue. Thus CT scanning is important in planning for modern radiation therapy of connective tissue tumours and is particularly valuable when the CT scanner and radiotherapy planning computers are compatible.

Circumferential irradiation of a limb leads to extensive painful fibrosis and lymphoedema. These complications can be minimized by leaving a strip of unirradiated tissue. Similarly if uninvolved bones are not completely irradiated, the incidence of post-irradiation fractures is reduce (D'Angio 1985, Tepper & Suit 1985). If possible the radiotherapist would also try to avoid irradiating more than one epiphysis in a growing child to prevent problems of limb shortening. Tissue damage may also be lessened by employing a shrinking field technique, which necessitates replanning of radiation fields. Clearly all of these measures are designed to minimize the complications of radiation therapy and are much more easily carried out using CT.

When obtaining CT images, the radiographer should remember to incorporate an external marker, usually a wire on the patient's skin, to be used as a reference. If the CT room and the treatment planning room have identical laser lights increased precision will be obtained.

Chemotherapy

The generally poor results of the treatment of bone tumours either by surgery alone or combined with radiation therapy have led to the search for effective chemotherapeutic agents. In turn, improving prognosis has stimulated limb salvage procedures. Chemotherapy may be used to eradicate micrometastases or to control local disease while a custom-made prosthesis is being constructed. Biological allografts suitable in benign lesions are not appropriate for malignant tumours as the chemotherapy interferes with host acceptability.

Most of the studies on bone tumours have related to osteosarcoma and the trend is to reject single agent regimes. Currently the best results are reported by Rosen et al (1982) who based postoperative chemotherapy on the response to the preoperative chemotherapy. As osteosarcoma is a rare tumour, historical studies have been bedevilled by a lack of randomization and controls. It is important that the radiologist, as part of the oncology team, obtains copies of the appropriate staging protocols of patients entered into trials.

The rôle of chemotherapy in soft tissue sarcomas is less clear because they form an even rarer heterogeneous group of patients with a variable response to treatment. With the exception of the commonest tumour, rhabdomyosarcoma of childhood, randomized trials have proven impossible. The treatment of soft tissue sarcoma is also primarily surgical and the general approach is similar to that for bone tumours. Adjuvant chemotherapy is based on experience gained with the Intergroup Rhabdomyosarcoma Study (IRS).

The IRS clinical grouping classification is as follows:

Group I: Localized disease, completely excised (regional nodes not involved).

(a) Confined to muscle or organ of origin.
(b) Contiguous involvement with infiltration outside the muscle or organ of origin, as through fascial planes.

Group II: Grossly excised tumour with microscopic residual disease.

(a) No evidence of gross residual tumour. No evidence of regional node involvement.
(b) Regional disease, completely excised (regional nodes involved and/or extension of tumour into an adjacent organ). All

tumour completely excised with no microscopic residual tumour.

(c) Regional disease with involved nodes, grossly resected, but with evidence of microscopic residual disease.

Group III: Incomplete resection or biopsy with gross residual disease.

Group IV: Distant metastatic disease present at onset (lung, liver, bones, bone marrow, brain and distant muscle and nodes).

Soft tissue sarcomas are routinely treated by chemotherapy as a multiagent cocktail. Less intensive regimes are given to groups I and II. Additionally, with tumours adjacent to the skull base, the basal meninges are irradiated unless the CT scan shows basal involvement in which case the entire meninges are treated. Extremity lesions are associated with an unusually poor prognosis and are always given intensive regimes (Maurer & Mc-Williams 1985).

Radiological management

Logically it follows from the calculus of the staging system that the rôle of the radiologist in the primary management of connective tissue tumours is early detection of the lesion, assessment of the aggressiveness and local extent of the lesion and the detection of metastases.

Plain radiographs

To confirm as soon as possible that the patient's symptoms are due to malignancy requires meticulous radiographic technique. The key to bone radiology is trabecular detail, thus fine grain rare earth screens should be used for extremity work. It is advisable to match film and screen combinations from the same manufacturer. Exposures are usually in the 75 kV range for the pelvis, 60 kV range for extremities and 50 kV range for soft tissues. Coning is an essential part of good radiographic technique.

Early radiological signs of a tumour are loss of definition of trabecular detail accompanied by an area of either increased or reduced radiodensity and irregularity of the cortical margin. Early tumours are illustrated in Figures 14.1 and 14.2.

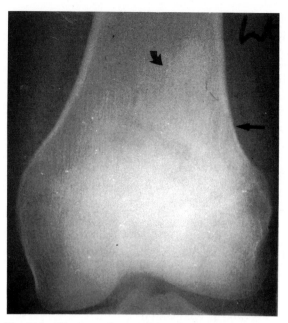

Fig. 14.1 The key to bone radiology is observation of trabecular detail. This radiograph, originally passed as normal, was of a young girl complaining of persistent pain for about three weeks. There is a diffuse increase in bone density extending upwards from the lateral femoral condyle towards the curved arrow and involving two thirds of the diameter of the femoral shaft. The horizontal arrow reveals thinning and early cortical destruction as compared with the other side. There is no periosteal reaction.

The aggressiveness of the lesion is assessed by examining the growing edge of the tumour. If the lesion is surrounded by a sclerotic margin then a slow-growing benign condition can be confidently diagnosed. If the lesion has a well-defined geographical area of bone destruction then the lesion is either benign or G1 (Lodwick 1965). If the lesion exhibits moth-eaten or permeative bone patterns of bone destruction then it is a G2 lesion. If the patient is in a District General Hospital, the radiologist should now advise referral to a specialist orthopaedic surgeon so that appropriate staging investigations can be carried out prior to biopsy.

The local extent of the lesion is assessed by the detection of periosteal reaction. If the bone is expanded and yet the cortex is intact and any periosteal reaction which is present is solid, then a benign condition may be diagnosed. If the periosteal reaction is interrupted and the pathology is that of malignancy, the tumour is graded as T2 or extracompartmental. By corollary, if the lesion is arising in the soft tissues then periosteal reaction also indicates a T2 lesion. Examples of the value of radiology in staging connective tissue tumours are given in Figures 14.3 and 14.4.

Although regional lymph node metastases carry the same ominous prognosis as pulmonary metastases, patients tend to die because of the latter and chest radiographs are mandatory. If these are normal then further investigation is required, ideally by CT scanning.

With regard to soft tissue tumours, plain radiographs may reveal periosteal reaction suggesting spread to adjacent bone; otherwise they are of little value in assessing the extent of the disease.

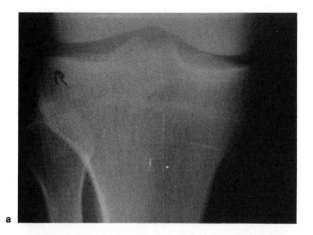

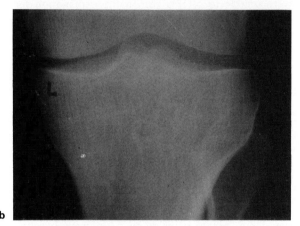

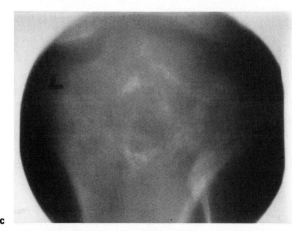

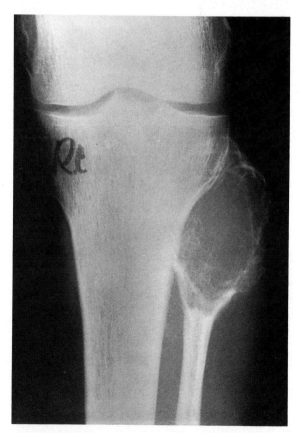

Fig. 14.2 Radiographs of a middle-aged man complaining of persistent pain in the left knee for several months. The right tibia for comparison reveals a normal trabecular pattern (a). On the left side there is irregularity of the trabeculae and loss of definition of the residual epiphyseal line (b). The changes are more clearly demonstrated by the tomogram (c).

Fig. 14.3 Radiograph of a G1 T1 tumour. Although the bone is expanded there was no evidence of cortical break or periosteal reaction. The tumour is well-defined and the boundary between abnormal and normal bone is easily seen.

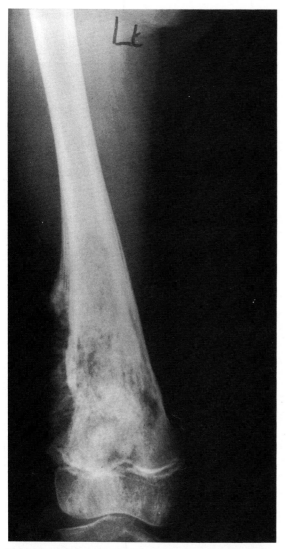

Fig. 14.4 Radiograph of a G2 T2 tumour. This tumour is aggressive and the boundary between normal and abnormal bone is not clearly defined. Extensive periosteal reaction indicates that the tumour has breached the bony compartment and extends into the soft tissues.

Isotope bone scans

A full discussion of the value of isotope bone scans will be given in the section on metastatic disease of bone and soft tissue. Aggressive G2 lesions exhibit markedly increased uptake whilst G1 lesions tend to show slightly or moderately increased uptake. (It should be accepted that a normal isotope scan virtually excludes a malignant bone lesion.)

Some G1 lesions have a surrounding ring of increased uptake whilst the centre of the lesion may show normal or reduced uptake. A positive scan with a normal radiograph should not be ignored. As malignant primary tumours tend to occur in young adults, the differential diagnosis is usually trauma and rarely infection. Paget's disease and, generally speaking, arthritis are excluded. Either a biopsy or a further period of observation is indicated.

If isotope accumulation is seen outside the confines of the bone then the tumour is graded as T2. However, Chew & Hudson (1982) describe falsely extended uptake patterns in osteosarcoma. They were unable to offer a reasonable explanation for this phenomenon and their observations have led to a loss of confidence in isotope scanning in local staging of bone tumours. However, they failed to consider the likely explanation of extended uptake not being histological but simply technical. When images are obtained using the present count technique, which is usual to allow for variations in decay of radio-isotope, then a very active lesion in the field of view will quickly saturate the film, particularly if the intensity settings are too high. The result is a large concentration of uptake whilst the rest of the image is poorly defined. Similar appearances are also found in the pelvis if the bladder is full of urine or in patients with active Paget's disease of a limb.

The intensity of uptake in an isotope scan cannot be used to predict the aggressiveness of a tumour. Benign lesions are generally 'cooler' than malignant lesions but there is a large overlap between the two groups. An example is illustrated in Figure 14.5. Similarly, isotope scanning cannot be used to confirm malignant transformation in a benign tumour: even a change in serial scans might simply relate to a growth spurt or associated trauma. Once a pathological fracture occurs, the only value of an isotope scan in such conditions is documentation of the presence of multiple lesions.

Meticulous technique is required by the radiographer. Skip lesions may be missed by poor technique or mimicked by urine contamination on clothing and this possibility must be rigorously excluded as the vast majority of skip lesions occur in the lower limb.

In patients with primary connective tissue

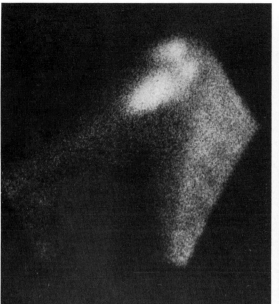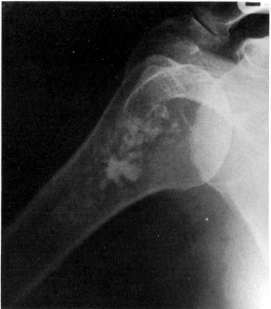

Fig. 14.5 Discordance between isotope scan and radiograph. The isotope scan shows moderate increase in uptake which in the absence of any clinical information might suggest a malignant process. The radiograph reveals a benign condition.

tumours, careful correlation with radiographs is advised, not only preoperatively but also post-operatively in the assessment of complications or allografts and prostheses. The examinations should be monitored to obtain the best projections free from metal components.

Computed tomography

The main value of CT in bone tumours is the demonstration of a soft tissue extension and its relationship to the neurovascular bundles and key organs. This is particularly useful in difficult areas such as the pelvis and paravertebral regions where surgery could be precluded because of the risk of nerve palsies or haemorrhage. When the surgeon is planning conservative or reconstructive surgery in a limb, he needs to know how many muscle groups have to be resected so that he can estimate if the postoperative limb is likely to be stable.

Although the axial anatomy is usually well demonstrated, it is often difficult to be sure about the lower or more importantly the upper limits of the tumour.

Scanning should be performed to maximize the chance of detecting marrow skip lesions. If necessary, the neurovascular bundles or the tumour can be enhanced using i.v. contrast. Ideally the opposite limb should be scanned for comparison, but in patients with a large tumour, severe pain or muscle spasm this may not be possible. Patients with severe pain or muscle spasm should have adequate sedation and analgesia.

The use of raw data reconstructed enlargements of areas of particular interest can result in easier interpretation of abnormal findings, and facilitate measurements within the medullary cavity. Errors in measurement are likely to occur due to varying window levels and window widths, and if possible the scan should be calibrated using known phantoms. Detailed measurements of the size of the femoral head are also useful in limb salvage operations.

As might be anticipated, CT scanning is of even more value in soft tissue tumours. With the exception of phleboliths, which indicate an arteriovenous malformation, or very low attenuation values (in the order of −90 to −150 HU) indicating a fatty tumour, CT does not give histological information (Golding & Husband 1982).

Blurring of planes, presumably due to oedema,

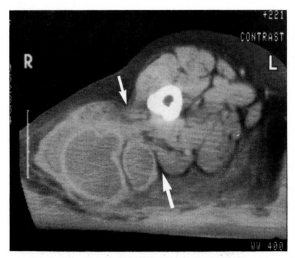

Fig. 14.6 The advantage of CT. This patient with neurofibromatosis presented with a huge tumour in the thigh. CT clearly reveals the size of the tumour and its relationship to the femur and thigh muscles and neurovascular bundles. The clear plane of cleavage is demonstrated between the normal tissue and the tumour (arrows).

and poorly defined margins are highly suggestive of malignancy. However, histological predictions should not be offered as substitutes for histology as some benign tumours, most notably desmoid tumours, are locally invasive and are associated

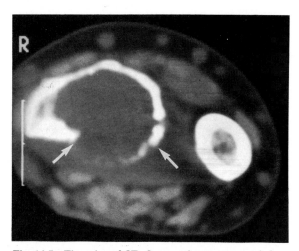

Fig. 14.7 The value of CT. Conservative surgery was being planned for this tumour which although histologically benign had broken through the cortex (arrows) and extended into the soft tissues. The surgeon can predict which muscles may have to be sacrificed and whether a stable functional result is likely.

with high recurrence rates. When the tumour encircles bone and is in contact with a significant though undefined portion of the circumference, some surgeons regard these as T2 lesions (Weis et al 1978). Bone involvement is uncommon (Weekes et al 1985) and is best demonstrated by radiographs when the tumour is in an extremity but by CT when the tumour is in an awkward region such as the pelvis (Egund et al 1981). There is a negative correlation between the amount of tissue necrosis and a favourable outcome (Costa et al 1984, Weekes et al 1985). Some illustrative examples of the value of CT are given in Figures 14.6–14.9. As with bone lesions, the search for lung metastases is mandatory unless already present on the chest radiograph.

Angiography

The use of angiography in connective tissue tumours was popularized in America before the advent of CT. If CT shows that the tumour is avascular then there is little point in proceeding to angiography. The upper limit of a vascular tumour is better demonstrated by angiography (Egund et al 1981). In vascular tumour, knowledge of the site of the main draining veins may assist the surgeon in placing tourniquets and in subsequent dissection particularly if conservative surgery is being contemplated. When a muscle compartment is ex-

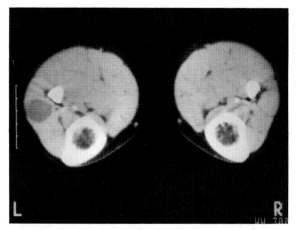

Fig. 14.8 The value of CT. This patient presented with ill-defined discomfort in the left leg and a CT scan reveals a well-defined hypodense lesion confined to one muscle compartment. Amputation is likely to be avoided.

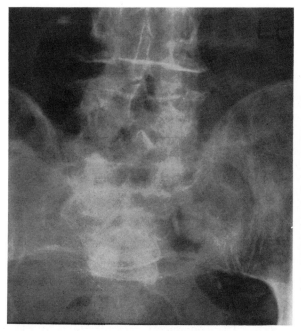
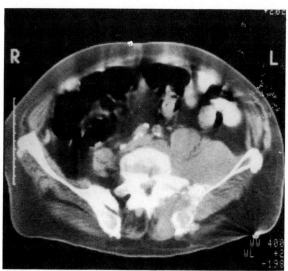

Fig. 14.9 The value of CT. Although the radiograph reveals destruction of part of the left ala of the sacrum, the true extent of the tumour mass is better delineated on the CT scan. Massive extension anterior to the iliac blade is well demonstrated. This information is of benefit to the surgeon planning a more accessible route for biopsy or to the radiotherapist for treatment planning.

panded by tumour the angiogram will necessarily overestimate the size of the tumour. The resolution of detail on digital vascular imaging with intravenous injections is too poor for the technique to be of value in the extremities, and the problem of multiple overlapping gut vessels virtually precludes its use in abdominal tumours.

However, digital vascular imaging with arterial injections will provide high resolution angiograms and will permit lower doses of contrast. The value of digital vascular imaging in retroperitoneal and mediastinal tumours is likely to be limited because these tumours take their blood supply from many sources and there are multiple overlapping vessels. However, if the technique is performed bowel paralysis is essential. Embolization of vascular tumours is a useful technique for symptomatic relief when surgery is not considered feasible for very vascular tumours such as haemangiomas.

Magnetic resonance imaging and ultrasound

As magnetic resonance imaging (MRI) does not produce signals from cortical bone, its rôle may be limited. It can be particularly useful for assessing soft tissue extension, satellite lesions and marrow skip lesions. Theroretically it could be of value in detailed analysis of the soft tissue mass and in differentiating tumour from haematoma or necrosis, with obvious impact on treatment.

The facility of high quality coronal scans is particularly useful for seeing the upper and lower limits of the tumour but the anterior and posterior limits can be poorly defined unless axial scans are also obtained.

The resolution of MRI does not match the current generation of CT scanners but developments in the use of surface coils in conjunction with high field systems may overcome this. Although MRI is more expensive and not as widely available, a fuller investigation might show it to be cost effective in this small group of patients. A comparison of MRI and CT scans is given in Figure 14.10.

The cost and spatial resolution of modern equipment makes ultrasound the modality of choice for detecting liver metastases. Beyond this

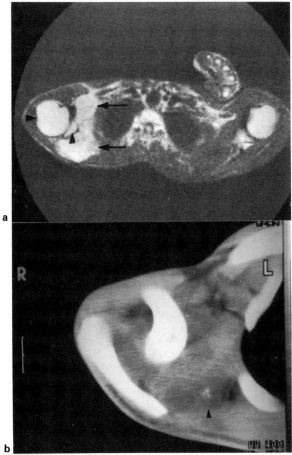

Fig. 14.10 Comparison of (a) MRI and (b) CT. This patient has had a partial scapulectomy for chondrosarcoma and the black arrowhead in the CT scan reveals a hypodense area containing a cluster of calcifications. This represents recurrence of cartilagenous tumour. In the T_2-weighted MR image, the arrowheads indicate the humeral head and the glenoid fossa. A large area of increased signal is noted medial to this which represents recurrence of tumour. The MRI findings correlated more accurately with the clinical situation. Note that as the CT scan was obtained with the patient lying supine and the MRI scan with the patient lying prone, it is impossible to obtain absolutely comparable images.

ultrasound has little to offer in connective tissue tumours.

MARROW TUMOURS

This section will be brief because most of these tumours are in the realm of the paediatric radiologist. Additionally, although the radiologist

plays a crucial rôle in the staging of these tumours, procedures tend to be the same regardless of the tumour histology.

Clinical presentation and laboratory findings

Ewing's sarcoma occurs in children and young adults and usually presents as a rapidly enlarging painful mass with systemic manifestations of weight loss, fever and malaise. Involvement of the small bones of the hand is rare. Pathological fracture is a more common presentation than with malignant connective tissue tumours. Lymphomatous bone involvement is a disease of late adolescence and early middle age and it is an uncommon presentation. Gradual onset over two or three months is the rule and pain is the commonest presenting symptom. Constitutional symptoms of fever, malaise and weight loss are less marked. Myeloma is a disease of late middle age and the elderly. The commonest presentation is diffuse skeletal pain and anaemia.

With Ewing's tumours, a markedly raised ESR is usually present. A raised white cell count with a shift to the left and anaemia may mimic infection. In lymphoma the blood count is usually normal but an absolute lymphopenia suggests advanced or aggressive disease. A blood smear may demonstrate lymphoma cells. Immunological markers are frequently specific. With myeloma, characteristic bands are classically seen on serum protein electrophoresis. In light chain disease, Bence-Jones protein may be present in the urine. A raised serum calcium sometimes fortuitously raises suspicion of the diagnosis.

Staging/pathology/biopsy

These diseases are systemic and frequently have multiple sites of origin or metastases. Thus irrespective of the staging system, the local tumour, the thorax and abdomen and any symptomatic site have to be examined.

Histology is absolutely essential. In Ewing's sarcoma the lesion is biopsied to exclude infection and to differentiate from osteosarcoma. In lymphoma a palpable lymph node should be excised if possible rather than risk bone biopsy. In myeloma biopsy is generally unnecessary.

All Ewing's sarcomas are high grade, extremely vascular lesions and frequently exhibit satellite and skip lesions. Lymphoma is not so vascular and does not show these features.

Therapeutic options

Increasingly, chemotherapy is becoming the mainstay of treatment. Local control in apparently localized disease is complemented by radiotherapy although there is an increasing trend to limb-sparing surgery in Ewing's sarcoma. The combination of alkylating chemotherapy and radiotherapy is avoided in young children because of complications of malignancy and limb deformity. The intensity of the chemotherapeutic regime corresponds to the aggressiveness and extent of the underlying disease.

Radiology

Radiographs

It is unusual for Ewing's tumour to be confined to bone. Exhuberant periosteal reaction and soft tissue mass are the rule, as is a permeative pattern of bone destruction. The main problem in Ewing's sarcoma is to demonstrate the extent of the soft tissue mass. Conventional tomograms are generally unhelpful. The appearances of lymphoma are not usually as aggressive as Ewing's sarcoma and slow-growing lesions are often sclerotic: chest radiographs are mandatory in both conditions. The punched-out lesions of myeloma are well known. Skeletal survey is the most sensitive method of staging the extent of the disease; 91% of lesions are detected as opposed to 46% by radio-isotope studies (Ludwig et al 1982). Occasionally myeloma exhibits diffuse osteoporosis but in the absence of lytic lesions there is no reason to suspect malignancy as the cause unless the patient is unusually young.

Isotope bone scans

This is the simplest and most accurate method of assessing the extent of skeletal involvement in Ewing's sarcoma and lymphoma. It is less useful in evaluating soft tissue extension. All imaging methods tend to underestimate the extent of bony involvement in Ewing's sarcoma. In lymphoma, multiple bone involvement at presentation is extremely rare and tends to occur late in the stage of the disease. As these patients tend to be older, arthritis and trauma enter the differential diagnosis, and correlation with radiographs is essential. Isotope scanning is not advised in myeloma unless the patient has unexplained bone pain. In general the positive areas in myeloma scans tend to occur in the spine and usually reflect pathological fracture rather than simple lytic deposits.

Computed tomography

In Ewing's sarcoma the advantages of CT for radiotherapy planning or limb-sparing surgery are as outlined previously for connective tissue tumours. The majority of Ewing's sarcomas have pulmonary metastases and a few have extra-osseous disease so CT of the lungs and abdomen is advised.

In lymphoma surgical treatment is not an option. However, examination of the abdomen and, in the presence of a normal chest radiograph, the mediastinum is carried out. Lung involvement in the absence of mediastinal disease is uncommon and occurs late in the disease. CT is not generally required for myeloma. It is required in the follow-up of lymphoma and the real therapeutic dilemma is not how to treat but when to stop treating; to continue increases the risks of iatrogenic disease and to stop risks a relapse which is generally not as responsive.

Angiography and lymphography

Angiography is seldom employed in marrow tumours. Lymphography has been replaced as the investigation of choice by CT. Some centres still perform lymphograms in lymphoma if the CT scans are normal.

METASTATIC BONE DISEASE

Economic approach

The moral and economic problems posed by metastatic bone disease are completely different from those of primary malignant connective tissue tumours. In the latter group, the frequency of disease is low and so the costs of diagnosis and treatment are less likely ever to become a major drain on resources. Furthermore, although the cost of the individual patient management may be high the benefits in terms of prolonged life expectancy or mobility, particularly in the event of a cure, are correspondingly greater. By contrast metastatic bone disease is common, frequently terminal and the patient outcome may not be significantly altered by expending scarce radiological resources. Thus the value of performing any radiological test should be critically evaluated, for example the value of routine scanning of asymptomatic patients for bone metastases, which is carried out in the vast majority of major departments.

Most doctors appreciate that high sensitivity (the proportion of positive tests in diseased patients) and high specificity (the proportion of negative tests in normal patients) confer increased value on a test and are constantly trying to refine and improve these parameters. However, very few are aware of the fact that the prevalence of disease (proportion of diseased patients in the population being studied) has a profound influence on the value of a test.

Let us examine the value of a very accurate test with 95% sensitivity and 95% specificity in staging 1000 patients in whom the prevalence of disease is 2%. This is not an unrealistically low figure because the incidence of bone metastases in early breast cancer, which is the commonest cancer in females to spread to the skeleton, is only of

the order of 4% (Gray et al 1980). From Table 14.2 we can see that as 1000 patients have been studied and the prevalence is 2% it follows mathematically that 980 are normal and 20 are diseased. As the test is 95% sensitive and specific, of the 20 abnormal patients 19 will be correctly detected and of the 980 normal patients 931 will be correctly identified. However, what is of more value than sensitivity or specificity to the clinician managing the individual patient is knowing the predictive value of a test. In other words, given that a test is positive what is the probability that the patient actually has the disease? In this case we can see that the test was positive in 68 instances but in only 19 cases was the patient actually diseased. Put formally, the predictive value of a positive test is only 19/68 or 27.9%. Thus the radiologist operating at these low levels of prevalence must accept that the majority of the positive tests will be false. Unless they are critical, clinicians can create complex problems by generating multiple false positive results to a battery of poorly thought-out investigations.

Contrast these results with those for a test with the same sensitivity and specificity, but where the prevalence of disease is increased to 50%. The predictive value of a positive test is now dramatically increased to 95% (see Table 14.3).

Radiologists must remember that when many tests are originally constructed with random control groups, the incidence of disease may be 50% and therefore the results of the tests will be very impressive. However, when the same tests are applied to the general population with a lower prevalence of disease, it will be impossible to

Table 14.2 Predictive values for a test which is 95% sensitive and 95% specific performed on 1000 patients with a disease prevalence of 2%.

	Test positive	Test negative	No. of patients
Disease positive	19	1	20
Disease negative	49	931	980
Total	68	932	1000
Predictive values	27.9%	99.8%	

Table 14.3 Predictive values for a test which is 95% sensitive and 95% specific performed on 1000 patients with a disease prevalence of 50%.

	Test positive	Test negative	No. of patients
Disease positive	475	25	500
Disease negative	25	475	500
Total	500	500	1000
Predictive values	95%	95%	

reproduce the same excellent results. The situation is even worse if the same test is used in a screening situation in which the prevalence of disease is only 4 or 5 cases per 1000. The predictive value of a test will then be approximately 5%, in other words 19 out of every 20 patients will be false positive.

Consider also the problems of sequential imaging where a clinician who is keen to exclude a certain pathology might 'reasonably' request a second test should the first test be normal. Let us assume that 1000 patients are again scanned with a prevalence of disease of 5%, that isotope scanning is 95% sensitive and 90% specific and that the second test is a plain radiograph with a sensitivity of 90% and a specificity of 95%. The results of performing the isotope scan first are detailed in Table 14.4. This test has correctly detected 47.5 out of 50 diseased patients. To detect the remaining 2.5 patients, 857.5 patients will have to be radiographed giving a prevalence of 0.29% and this will lead to the results detailed in Table 14.5. The predictive value of a positive test for plain radiographs will only be 5% because the first test, having filtered out the majority of positive tests, has dramatically lowered the prevalence of disease in the second test.

What then is the cost of these tests, having assessed their clinical value? In the sequential imaging example, assuming the average cost of an isotope scan to be £50, the average cost per case detected is $1000 \times 50/47.5 = £1052.63$. The marginal or extra cost of detecting the last 2.5 cases by plain radiography assuming that radiographs cost £25 per case is $857.5 \times 25/2.25 = £9527.77$. These are simply the costs to the radiology or nuclear medicine departments. Further consideration should also be given to the costs of investigation of the false positive studies, the cost to the patient of transport, anxiety and discomfort, and the additional cost in terms of administration.

In day-to-day radiological management of individual patients it is easy to agree to an additional apparently helpful test. However, unless radiologists adopt a critical economic approach they will simply continue to waste scarce resources which could be put to better use. Policies and priorities have to be developed: for example, if it has been shown that the incidence of metastatic bone disease in early breast cancer is only 4% should the policy be to desist from scanning asymptomatic patients except in a tightly controlled research situation?

Logistics of radiological management

The value of radiology in the management of malignant tumours is a function not only of the quality of the imaging modality but also of the communication processes between the clinician and the radiologist. Ideally, the radiological management of a patient should be decided after full consultation with the referring clinician. However, the usual mode of communication is the X-ray request form; clinicians and radiologists should learn to make full use of this important mode of communication. It is by no means an uncommon experience within departments of radiology to find that deficiencies of interpretation of imaging are related to the absence of relevant clinical detail. The clinical information section is the most abused part of the request form. Despite

Table 14.5 Predictive values for performing a plain radiograph which is 90% sensitive and 95% specific on 857.5 patients with a disease prevalence of 0.29%.

	Test positive	Test negative	No. of patients
Disease positive	2.25	0.25	2.5
Disease negative	42.75	812.25	855
Total	45.0	812.5	857.5
Predictive values	5%	99.9%	

Table 14.4 Predictive values for an isotope scan which is 95% sensitive and 90% specific performed on 1000 patients with a disease prevalence of 5%.

	Test positive	Test negative	No. of patients
Disease positive	47.5	2.5	50
Disease negative	95	855	950
Total	142.5	857.5	1000
Predictive values	33.3%	99.7%	

having immense potential for medical education and research, clinicians piously hope that radiologists will enlighten them on the subject of radiological management by producing a few simple algorithms. Algorithms as a guide to radiological investigation are useless because circumstances are so variable. What is appropriate in one hospital may be unobtainable in another; a technique may not be available within reasonable time due to absence of key personnel, equipment failure or maintenance.

Unfortunately, the assessment of the value of a test must include its impact on clinical management and the patient's health status. This can be achieved by ensuring that the X-ray request card poses a question related to clinical management which the radiologist may answer by whatever technique he thinks is most appropriate. A typical request card should read 'carcinoma breast, ?mets' or 'painful swelling right pubis ?mets'. In the first instance the radiologist might organize a bone scan whilst in the second he would advise a radiograph of the pelvis. Having forced the clinician to ask a question which must be answered then either the clinician or the radiologist may review the value of the test in answering the question. They can find out if the answers were accurate, whether the test influenced the clinical management, whether the radiologist issued vague reports, whether the test is capable of answering the question, and lastly how the test compared with clinical acumen. These are all topics which can be used as a basis for self-education or research by either the clinician or the radiologist.

If the clinician does not commit himself, possibly exposing his lack of expertise, he can never be shown to be right or wrong but then neither can the radiologist and so the value of a test in clinical management will never be established.

Clinical features

Metastatic bone disease is the commonest malignant tumour of bone. Metastases occur in the marrow-bearing areas with the vertebral column being the most frequently involved site (Meissner & Warren 1971). Clinical symptoms are usually due to:

1. An enlarging mass
2. A pathological fracture
3. A pathological fracture with instability
4. Cord compression.

The symptoms of cord compression may be due to an extradural deposit, pathological fracture with dislocation, spinal angulation secondary to vertebral collapse and rarely to intradural metastases (Boland et al 1982). Localized back pain and pressure is a common symptom most marked at night and aggravated by movement. Muscle weakness occurs and may progress to paraplegia. The rapidity of onset influences prognosis; if symptoms appear rapidly, i.e. in less than 24 hours, then the prognosis is poor even with treatment. Sensory levels are not a reliable guide to the site of a lesion except with conus medullaris lesions. In the early stages cord damage may be poorly developed both from a sensory and motor point of view. Bowel and bladder symptoms occur late and should be regarded as medical emergencies.

In metastatic bone disease pain is the usual symptom. It may initially be intermittent and multifocal in onset but soon becomes constant and poorly relieved by rest. Rarely the presentation may be breathlessness or fatigue due to extensive marrow replacement and associated marrow failure. Pathological fracture, nerve and vessel entrapment are less common presentations.

Leucoerythroblastic anaemia is characteristic. Elevated levels of serum calcium and alkaline phosphatase are frequently present. Elevated serum acid phosphatase is pathognomonic of prostatic metastases. As metastatic bone disease and Paget's disease both occur in elderly patients, isolated elevations of alkaline phosphatase generally reflect the latter condition.

Staging/biopsy

The detection of bone metastases invariably represents advanced disease and, except in some elderly patients whose lesions are hormonally dependent, carries a grave prognosis. As few patients survive beyond 18 months the diagnosis should not be made lightly. Localized bone pain in the presence of known malignancy which typically spreads to bone can be assumed to be a metastasis particularly if there is collaborative isotope scan or radiographic evidence. Biopsy is unnecessary, particularly in frail patients, and should not be performed unless it is essential for management and histology has not been obtained whilst assessing the primary tumour.

Therapeutic options

As a general rule asymptomatic metastases may be given no immediate treatment although radiation therapy may be given for certain strategic lesions such as metastases in the upper cervical spine if there is concern about stability.

Surgery

In spinal metastases the aim of treatment is to avert cord compression and paraplegia. Recently the use of high dose dexamethasone has enabled doctors to buy time and has allowed more accurate investigation. Cervical spine lesions with fracture dislocation are treated with a firm collar, radiation therapy and dexamethasone. Traction is reserved for those patients with marked subluxation. Upper dorsal fracture dislocations are naturally supported by the ribs and thoracic muscles; lower dorsal and upper lumbar fractures usually require a brace and surgical stabilization. Decompressive laminectomy with a posterior approach often yields poor results because of unsatisfactory access to the tumour which usually arises from the anteriorly placed vertebral body, and secondly removal of the posterior elements may aggravate any spinal instability. Anterior decompression is preferred and is relatively easy in the cervical spine. The transthoracic approach is difficult and requires a multidisciplinary approach. Morbidity is high and complete removal of tumour is impossible. In general the prognosis is very poor in the presence of complete paraplegia particularly if it has developed within 24 hours. Similarly, loss of sphincter control also carries a poor prognosis.

In non-spinal metastatic disease the general principles are that if surgery is to be employed, it should be aggressive as subsequent intervention is much less effective. As much of the malignant tissue as possible should be removed and replaced with methylmethacrylate and then some form of

internal fixation is inserted. Prophylactic fixation of long bone metastases should be considered if:

1. A femoral lesion is greater than 2.5 cm in diameter
2. There is lytic destruction of more than 50% of the cortex
3. There is persistent pain on weight-bearing despite radiation therapy (Harrington 1982).

Fracture healing is generally good following prophylactic fixation as bone union requires rigid fixation. Pelvic metastases are difficult to treat because of problems in predicting the exact degree of involvement; stability of acetabular fractures crucially depends on the degree of cortical involvement of the medial and superior walls.

Radiation therapy

Radiation therapy is indicated primarily for the relief of pain and to promote bone healing. Such treatments are usually palliative and therefore have wide margins. Detailed evaluation of tumour margins by expensive imaging modalities such as CT is not necessary. When there is a solitary lesion, long term control to avoid the necessity to repeat treatment justifies more intensive therapy and therefore more accurate radiotherapy planning.

Radiation therapy is employed after fixation of pathological fractures as continued tumour growth will lead to loosening of the fixing devices (Sherry et al 1982). Radiation therapy is also employed following prophylactic fixation of metastases. Surgery is performed prior to radiation therapy because the latter causes hyperaemia, usually maximal in the second week. This in turn causes bone softening and predisposes to pathological fracture because the bone is particularly sensitive to torsion stress when part of the cortex is destroyed. Surgery in a hyperaemic pathological fracture is clearly undesirable. In the spine, treatment usually includes two levels above and below the lesion and is combined with steroid therapy.

Chemotherapy

Although chemotherapy is occasionally employed in skeletal metastases with gratifying results in the short term, the patient's survival is generally not influenced unless the primary tumour is hormone dependent.

Radiology plays an important part in the assessment of the response to treatment. Although isotope scanning has been used, there are no generally agreed and defined criteria of response. Frequently the scan shows a marked increase in the number of metastases shortly after commencing treatment and this may represent a good response to occult metastases rather than the development of new metastases. Radiographs often underestimate the response to chemotherapy as new bone formation which represents bone healing clearly lags behind the antitumour effect (Bhardwaj & Holland 1982).

Criteria of response on radiographs could be:

1. Complete response – complete regression of all disease with recalcification of osteolytic lesions.

2. Partial response – 50–99% reduction in the products of two perpendicular diameters, one of which must represent the greatest diameter of the tumour.

3. Improvement – 25–49% reduction in the product of two perpendicular diameters, one of which must represent the greatest diameter of the tumour.

4. Stable disease – less than 25% reduction in the product of two perpendicular diameters, one of which must represent the greatest diameter of the tumour.

5. Progression – the appearance of a new lesion or an increase of more than 25% in the product of the perpendicular diameters, one of which must represent the greatest diameter of the tumour.

Radiology

Plain radiographs

Pathological fracture. The diagnosis is usually obvious with a large lytic lesion surrounding the fracture line. In the absence of an associated lytic lesion, the fracture is generally deemed to be simple.

Skeletal survey. As has already been conclusively shown by almost every comparative study in the literature, isotope scanning is more sensitive than radiology in the detection of bone metastases. This is because bone metastases occur in the marrow which contributes little to overall bone density on a plain radiograph. Secondly, approximately 50% of bone cortex has to be destroyed before the lesion becomes radiologically visible. Thirdly, even when visible, the lesion is often obscured by overlying composite shadows such as bowel gas. However, using the retrospectoscope metastases demonstrated by radio-isotopes do in fact show radiological abnormalities in the vast majority of cases, and it may therefore be worthwhile to carry out a skeletal survey, particularly if nuclear medicine facilities are not available. The extent of the skeletal survey is a trade-off between quality and throughput. Stewart-Scott & Adams (1974) showed that radiographs confined to the torso and proximal long bones would cover 90% of metastatic sites. In addition radiographs of symptomatic areas outside these sites would cover 50% of the remaining metastatic sites. The additional radiographs required to cover the last remaining 5% of metastatic sites would double the examination time and cost.

Difficult metastases

Pancoast tumour. Symptoms of Pancoast tumour are secondary to brachial plexus involvement. Bone involvement may be absent or minimal. Radiographs and isotope scans are relatively insensitive, and CT is the examination of choice.

Pelvic metastases. Difficulties in detecting pelvic metastases occur due to overlying bowel and soft tissue shadows and failure to examine the entire bone systematically. Special attention should be paid to:

1. The tear drop in the medial aspect of the hip joints.
2. Symmetry of sacral foramina.
3. The upper sacral margin.
4. The medial extent of the ilium as it extends behind the ala of the sacrum.
5. Symmetry of cortical thickness of the pelvic brim.
6. Trabecular symmetry, particularly in the lateral portions of the ilium, supra-acetabular region and pubic and ischial bones.

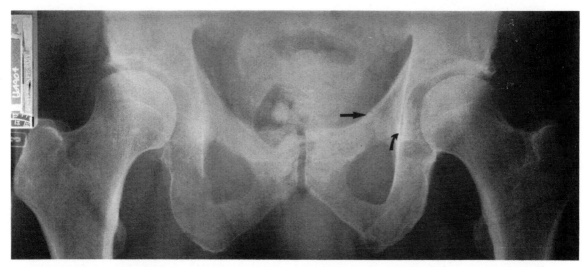

Fig. 14.11 Pelvic metastasis. On the normal side, the curved arrow indicates the tear drop sign whilst the horizontal arrow reveals a normal thickness of cortex of the superior ischial ramus. Absence of these signs on the right indicates a metastasis.

Spinal metastases. Like pelvic metastases, these are difficult to detect. A thorough appreciation of the anatomy will reduce errors of perception. The spine is composed of two parts: anteriorly there is a box in which the lateral margins are represented by two curved lines. The top and bottom of the end plates are seen as ellipses except at the level where the X-ray beam is centred, in which case the end plate is seen as a straight line. The posterior elements can be thought of as representing a starfish with the spinous process forming the body, and the laminae and pars interarticaularis and pedicles forming the four tentacles.

Paravertebral metastases. Involvement of the paravertebral and parapelvic soft tissues by metastases is generally not detected on radiographs or isotope scans and either CT or MRI is required.

Some of these aspects of detection of difficult metastases are illustrated in Figures 14.11–14.14.

Isotope scanning

It is generally agreed that isotope scanning is highly sensitive and, with less justification, that it is non-specific. The high false positive rate for metastatic disease in most studies is simply due to poor diagnostic criteria. Defining metastatic disease as 'multiple hot spots' without any qualification will lead to a high false positive rate.

Metastases, osteoarthritis, unrecognized or indeed recognized trauma and Paget's disease are all common in late middle aged and elderly populations. As all are associated with hot spots, it is hardly surprising that they may coexist and cause

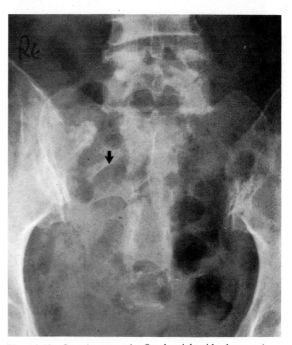

Fig. 14.12 Sacral metastasis. On the right side the sacral foramina are well outlined. The vertical arrow indicates the most cranial foramen. On the left side this foramen is destroyed by tumour.

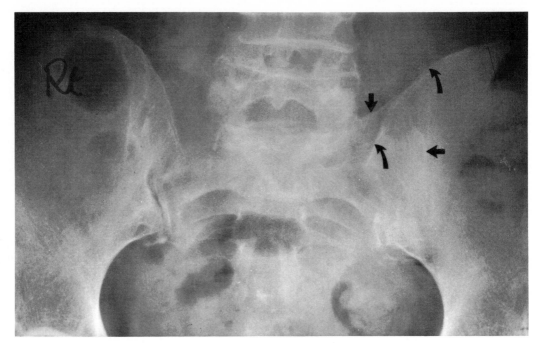

Fig. 14.13 Pelvic metastasis. On the left side the vertical arrow and the horizontal arrow indicate the superior and lateral margins of the ala of the sacrum. The curved arrows indicate the superior margin of the ilium which extends down behind the ala of the sacrum. On the right side there is loss of the superior and lateral margins of the ala of the sacrum.

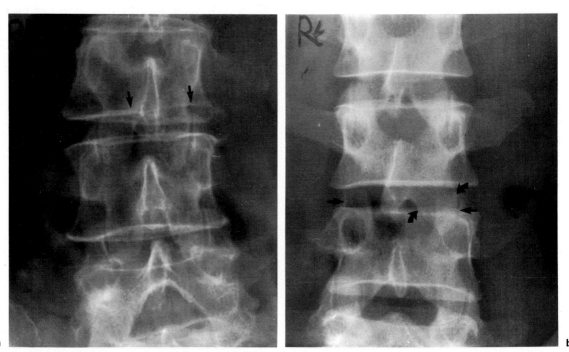

a   b

Fig. 14.14 In radiograph (a) the vertical arrows reveal partial collapse of the vertebral body. The inferior end plate is no longer represented as an ellipse as the anterior and posterior aspects of the ellipse diverge towards the left side of the body. Compare this with the inferior end plate of the vertebral body below. In radiograph (b) the laminae and the inferior articular facet on the left side of L3 are well seen (curved arrows) and the facet joint is indicated by the horizontal arrow. On the right side the inferior articular facet and the lamina are destroyed. The star fish has only three tentacles.

confusion with malignancy. However, once it is appreciated that these conditions have characteristic patterns of abnormality then the specificity of isotope scanning will improve.

Characteristically metastases present as multiple small discrete hot spots randomly distributed throughout the marrow bearing area. Total skeletal involvement is most likely to occur in cancer of the prostate or breast and sometimes scans may superficially appear normal but such 'super scans' can be identified by the lack of renal and soft tissue uptake. Furthermore, the intertrochanteric areas are usually hotter than the femoral heads and careful inspection of the ribs often reveals slight unevenness of uptake. Very rarely purely lytic metastases, usually from the lung, may exhibit reduced uptake or a cold spot. Clearly as one moves up the spectrum from increased uptake to decreased uptake some metastases must exhibit an identical degree of uptake to normal bone. This proportion is approximately 5% (Adams & Horton 1978).

It should be appreciated that the vast majority of osteoarthritic joints produce no abnormality on a bone scan and it is only the more advanced cases which produce hot spots, therefore unless radiographs show obvious sclerosis or osteophyte formation then caution should be exercised before attributing hot spots to arthritis. Other forms of arthritis such as rheumatoid disease or ankylosing spondylitis have much hotter foci, occur in different age groups and have their own characteristic distribution.

Unrecognized trauma is the commonest cause of false positive diagnosis. Isotope scanning detects not only fractures but haematomas and myositis ossificans. Thus the traumatic episode may be quite minor and go unnoticed by the patient even if mentally alert. Secondly, the changes of healing trauma, particularly fractures, persist for up to nine months and increased accumulation at the fracture site may occur for the rest of the patient's life, particularly if there has been marked displacement and callus formation. Vertical or oblique long bone fractures are characteristically elongated in appearance. In contrast, rib fractures tend to be very localized as opposed to metastases which tend to involve a length of rib. Solitary hot spots are common at the anterior ends of ribs and may represent fractures or stress at the costochondral junction. Simultaneous uptake in a vertebral body and the anterior of a rib is analogous to bony rings being fractured in more than one place. Multiple rib fractures do not show a random pattern but reflect the method of trauma.

Arthritis generally presents as areas of increased uptake on both sides of the joint or in the lateral third of the spinal column. The lower cervical and lower lumbar spines are most frequently involved.

Paget's disease characteristically arises at the end of long bones. Extensive or total bone involvement occurs whilst this pattern is very rarely seen in metastases with one notable exception, namely cancer of the prostate.

With regard to the intensity of hot spots, early or treated metastases, arthritis, trauma older than six months and mature Paget's disease tend not to exhibit marked uptake. A solitary hot spot does not represent a pattern and is truly non-specific. Such scans should always be viewed in the light of clinical findings and radiographs. The occurrence of persistent bone pain in a patient with a malignancy known to spread to bone is ominously suggestive of metastases unless the radiograph demonstrates a non-malignant cause.

The question of whether radiographs or isotope scans should be performed first is frequently asked. If one believes that isotope scanning is truly non-specific then the scans are going to have to be accompanied by radiographs in every instance. However, as outlined above, in many instances the combination of the history and characteristic scan appearances will enable a diagnosis to be made with a high degree of accuracy. In the small proportion of cases in which there is doubt then radiographs can be obtained, but this should not be necessary in more than 10%. Whether one wishes to perform a scan or radiographs depends on the precise nature of the clinical problem; if it is simply to exclude skeletal metastases then a bone scan is the test of choice as it is the more sensitive. If the scan is negative then the problem is solved. If the scan is positive then the pattern of abnormality may be diagnostic and as previously indicated only a minority require radiography. However, if the clinical problem is to determine the cause of pain at a specific site then radiographs should be obtained as they are more specific. Only if the radiographs are normal, meaning absence of disease and not simply absence of metastases, should a bone scan be considered. Although positive scans often precede radiographic abnormalities, and indeed clinical symptoms, caution should be advised in treating or equally importantly withholding treatment simply on the basis of scan findings, without giving due consideration to the clinical problem. Illustrative scans are shown in Figures 14.15–14.18.

Computed tomography

It is economically unsound to consider CT scanning as a substitute for radionuclide studies. Its use should be reserved for those situations when the isotope studies have not provided adequate information for treatment, or when there is impending paraplegia or severe focal pain without

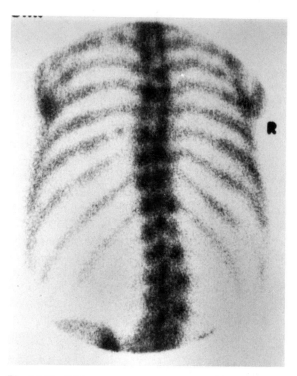

Fig. 14.16 Diffuse metastases — superscan. The bony skeleton is extremely well demonstrated and there is absence of renal uptake. Careful inspection of the ribs reveals non-uniformity of uptake which is also sometimes a clue to a 'superscan'.

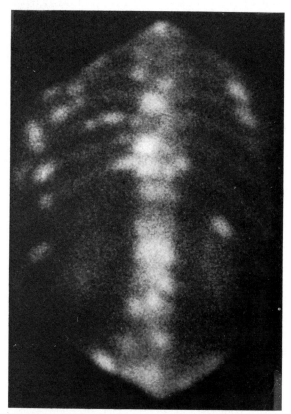

Fig. 14.15 Isotope scan — metastases. Note that metastatic bone disease characteristically presents as a random distribution of hot spots in the marrow bearing areas.

a demonstrable cause. In patients with abnormal neurological findings the question of performing unenhanced CT scans or CT myelography must be considered in relation to treatment options.

IATROGENIC COMPLICATIONS

This subject alone could occupy a chapter and in the interest of brevity the discussion will be confined to complications of radiation therapy.

The effect of radiation therapy on bone is governed by many factors such as the dose, beam hardness, methods of fractionation, specificity of bone irradiated, amount of bone irradiated, the presence of associated infection or trauma and lastly the age of the patient (Rubin & Casarett 1968). The spectrum of effect varies from a temporary cessation of bone metabolism to frank necrosis.

Whole bone irradiation in the growing skeleton leads to an overall decrease in bone size and bone

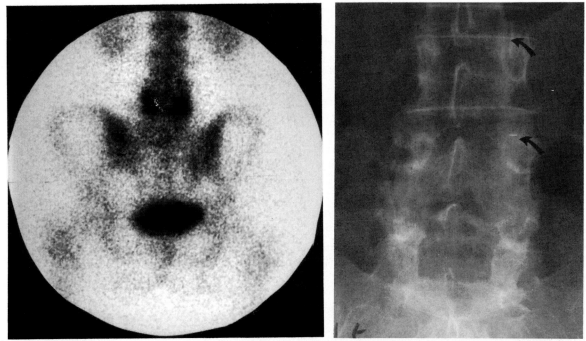

Fig. 14.17 Isotope scan — osteoarthritis. Increased uptake is noted in the lateral third of the spine bilaterally at L4/5 level. On the radiograph the normal facet joints in the upper vertebrae are well seen (curved arrows). The facet joints at the L4/5 level are not seen and there is diffuse sclerosis. These findings reflect osteoarthritis.

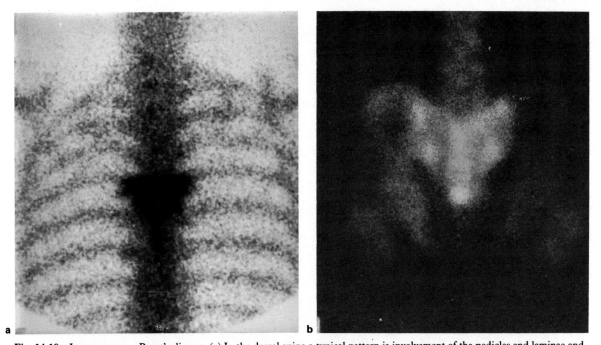

Fig. 14.18 Isotope scan — Paget's disease. (a) In the dorsal spine a typical pattern is involvement of the pedicles and laminae and this extends inferiorly into the spinous process which can be seen projected over the vertebra below. (b) In the sacrum there is complete involvement of the bone by Paget's disease. Complete bone involvement is extremely uncommon in malignant bone disease, except in prostatic cancer.

atrophy simulating osteogenesis imperfecta. Radiation of an epiphysis may result in premature arthritis, whilst damage to the epiphyseal plates will cause marked stunting of growth.

Metaphyseal irradiation leads to bowing whilst diasphyseal irradiation leads to undertubulation. Howard et al (1975) believe that radiation therapy causes bone atrophy but that bone necrosis requires associated trauma or infection. The healing bone may simply exhibit sclerosis or may additionally show areas of cortical thinning and sharply demarcated small spindle-shaped translucencies and a disorganized trabecular pattern.

Radiation effects in bone are most frequently found in radiographs of the rib and pelvis and to a lesser extent the spine and long bones, and are well described in standard texts. In departments which provide a full range of imaging facilities the effects of radiation therapy are also likely to be seen on isotope or CT images. Whilst these changes are unlikely to influence clinical management, their recognition helps to prevent misleading radiological reports. As isotope imaging tends to be functional as well as anatomical, evidence of radiation portals is often seen on bone scans, usually as areas of diminished isotope accumulation and poor anatomical detail. The spine is most frequently involved secondary to the treatment of lung and marrow tumours whilst asymmetry of ribs or pelvis may be seen in females.

Although radiation fibrosis is well recognized on chest radiographs it can increasingly be identified on CT scans in the mediastinal and retroperitoneal sections by noting obliteration of the fat compart-

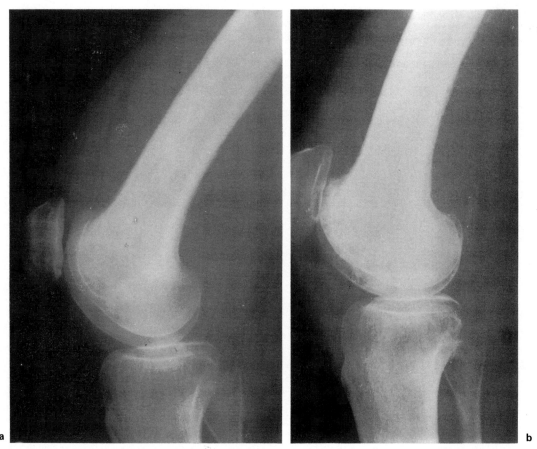

a b

Fig. 14.19 Radiation sclerosis. Following treatment of the soft tissue tumour anterior to the femur (a) diffuse increase in bone density developed (b).

ments of the fascial planes and thickening of fibrous tissue septa.

Differentiation between recurrence of tumour and radiation change can be a difficult and crucial problem as anatomically regions are rarely irradiated more than once: comparison of the radiographs with radiation simulator films can be valuable. Radiation changes tend to follow symmetrical patterns. The appearance of a soft tissue mass either on clinical examination or on ultrasound is highly suggestive of recurrence.

Some of these features are illustrated in Figures 14.19 and 14.20.

CONCLUSIONS

1. Don't waste time trying to predict the histology – it cannot be done reliably.

2. Concentrate on assessing the aggressiveness of tumours and their relationship to tissue compartments.

3. Adopt a critical attitude to the rôle of radiology in malignancy and only employ it if there is a reasonable probability that it will significantly alter the patient's management and health status.

4. Remember the effect of imaging patients when the prevalence of disease is low.

ACKNOWLEDGEMENT

I would like to acknowledge the valuable advice of Professor D. Hamblen in the preparation of this chapter.

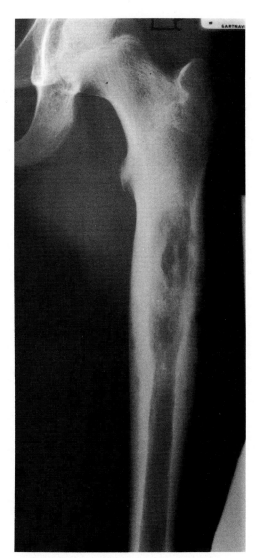

Fig. 14.20 Radiation necrosis. Following successful radiation treatment for a Ewing's tumour, multiple spindle-shaped lucencies developed. These findings are characteristic of radiation necrosis.

REFERENCES

Adams F G, Horton P W 1978 Rectilinear bone scanning: Differentiation between metastases and degenerative spinal disease. British Journal of Radiology 51: 281–285

Bhardwaj S, Holland J F 1982 Chemotherapy of metastatic bone cancer. Clinical Orthopaedics 169: 28–37

Boland P J, Lane J M, Sundaresa N 1982 Metastatic disease of the spine. Clinical Orthopaedics 169: 95–102

Chew F S, Hudson T M 1982 Radionuclide bone scanning of osteosarcoma: falsely extended uptake patterns. American Journal of Roentgenology 139: 49–54

Costa J, Wesley R A, Glatsein E, Rosenberg S A 1984 Grading of soft tissue tumours; results of a clinicopathologic correlation in a series of 163 cases. Cancer 53: 530–541

D'Angio G J 1985 Soft tissue sarcoma, radiation therapy. In: D'Angio G J, Evans A E (eds) Bone tumours and soft tissue sarcomas. Edward Arnold, London, pp 72–83

Egund N, Ekelund L, Sako M, Persson B 1981 CT of soft tissue tumours. American Journal of Roentgenology 137: 725–729

Enneking W F 1983 Musculo-skeletal tumour survey vol 1. Churchill Livingstone, New York, pp 69–88

Enneking W F, Kagan A 1975 The implication of 'skip' metastases in osteosarcoma. Clinical Orthopaedics 111: 33–42

Golding S J, Husband J E 1982 The rôle of computed tomography in the management of soft tissue sarcomas. British Journal of Radiology 55: 740–747

Gray I, Adams F G, Hogg R G, McCardle C S 1980 Detection of occult metastases. British Journal of Surgery 67: 380

Harrington K D 1982 New trends in the management of lower extremity metastases. Clinical Orthopaedics 169: 53–61

Hobday P, Hodson N J, Husband J, Parker R P, MacDonald J S 1979 Computed tomography applied to radiotherapy treatment planning: techniques and results. Radiology 133: 477–482

Howard W J, Loeffler R I C, Starchman D E, Johnson R G 1975 Post-irradiation atrophic changes of bone and related complications. Radiology 117: 677–684

Lodwick G S 1965 Tumours of bone and soft tissue. University of Texas M. D. Anderson Hospital and Tumour Institute. Year Book Medical Publisher, pp 49–68

Ludwig H, Kumpan W, Sinzinger H 1982 Radiography and bone scintigraphy in multiple myeloma: a comparative analysis. British Journal of Radiology 55: 173–181

Mankin J H J, Lange T A, Spanier S S 1983 The hazards of biopsy in patient with malignant primary bone and soft tissue tumours. Journal of Bone and Joint Surgery 64(A): 1121–1127

Maurer H M, McWilliams N B 1985 The chemotherapy of soft tissue sarcomas. In: D'Angio G J, Evans A E (eds)

Bone tumours and soft tissue sarcomas. Edward Arnold, London, pp 84–93

Meissner W, Warren S 1971 Distribution of metastases in 4012 cancer patients. In: Anderson W A D (ed) Pathology vol 1 edn 6. C V Mosby, St Louis, p 538

Rosen G, Caparros B, Huvos A G et al 1982 Preoperative chemotherapy for osteogenic sarcoma. Selection of postoperative adjuvant chemotherapy based on the response of the primary tumour to preoperative chemotherapy. Cancer 49: 1221–1230

Rothwell R I, Ash D V, Jones W G 1983 Radiation treatment planning for bladder cancer: A comparison of cystogram localisation with computed tomography. Clinical Radiology 34: 103–111

Rubin P, Casarett G W 1968 Clinical radiation pathology vol 2. W B Saunders, Philadelphia, p 518

Sherry H J, Levy R N, Siffert R S 1982 Metastatic disease of bone in orthopaedic surgery. Clinical Orthopaedics 169: 44–52

Stewart-Scott J, Adams F G 1974 The place of scintiscanning using Sr in the detection of osseous metastases. Clinical Radiology 25: 497–505

Tepper J E, Suit H D 1985 Radiation therapy of soft tissue sarcomas. Cancer 55: 2273–2277

Weekes R G, McLeod R A, Reiman H M, Pritchard D J 1985 CT of soft tissue neoplasms. American Journal of Roentgenology 144: 355–367

Weis L, Heelan R T, Caird-Watson R 1978 Computed tomography of orthopaedic tumours of the pelvis and lower limb. Clinical Orthopaedics 130: 254–259

15. The central nervous system

W. St Clair Forbes

METHODS OF INVESTIGATION

Conventional radiological examination of the skull has a very limited rôle in the diagnosis and follow-up of primary intracranial malignancy, being limited essentially to the detection of intracranial calcification and signs of raised intracranial pressure. Since its introduction into clinical practice in 1972, computed tomography (CT) has become the primary imaging modality for the diagnosis and follow-up of cerebral mass lesions. Its importance is unrivalled by other conventional imaging modalities such as selective angiography of the intracerebral vessels, air encephalography and isotope brain scanning. CT has largely replaced these methods of examination and has become the primary diagnostic method in the investigation of raised intracranial pressure and in patients who present with symptoms and signs of an intracranial space occupying lesion. Tumours are diagnosed earlier, resulting in more effective treatment. Important therapeutic management decisions are assisted by CT and in many instances biopsy and/or excision are deferred by the characteristic CT appearances. Despite its high cost, CT is very cost effective because it reduces in-patient stay and the need for expensive and invasive examination techniques which in many cases carry a lower sensitivity for demonstrating the abnormalities. Magnetic resonance imaging (MRI) has a similar capability and promises improved tissue characterization..

In the management of patients with primary and secondary malignancy of the spinal column including the paravertebral region and the intraspinal contents including the spinal cord and nerve roots, however, the conventional radiological methods of examination of plain radiographs, myelography using water soluble contrast and spinal angiography (rarely) have an important rôle to play in demonstrating the effects of malignant disease. CT in these cases has a complementary rôle and may be combined with myelography to examine accurately the contents of the spinal canal following localization of the abnormality demonstrated on the conventional radiological studies. MRI by imaging in the sagittal plane has distinct advantages over CT and accurately demonstrates the site and multiplicity of intraspinal lesions; it also does not use ionizing radiation. The supplementary rôle of conventional radiological investigation in the diagnosis of malignant disease of other organ systems which may metastasize to the central nervous system cannot be overemphasized.

TECHNICAL ASPECTS

The routine CT examination of the cranium comprises transaxial sections parallel to the orbito-meatal line. Thin sections (4, 5 or 6 mm slice thickness) of the posterior fossa are usually obtained while the supratentorial compartment is examined using thicker sections (8, 9 or 10 mm slice thickness). The examination is supplemented by an intravenous injection of contrast medium to show enhancement, either of the tumour or of the adjacent normal brain or vascular structures. The administration of intravenous contrast medium by infusion methods or bolus injection greatly improves CT sensitivity and specificity in tumour diagnosis. Some infiltrating tumours may be isodense with normal brain tissue, causing little or no mass effect, and may therefore be missed without contrast enhancement. Contrast enhancement occurs as a consequence of the breakdown of the blood–brain barrier and is usually demonstrated in those cases showing intracerebral oedema, which is itself another manifestation of a damaged blood–brain barrier. Steroid administration, used to decrease the mass effect from the associated oedema, may modify the contrast enhancement by causing a decrease in the intensity of enhancement without any reduction in the size of the tumour mass. Delayed scanning to detect enhancement occurring about one hour post-injection is sometimes useful to detect tumours with a slightly impaired blood–brain barrier.

Specialized CT techniques employing the use of thin sections (1.5, 2.0 or 3.0 mm), high doses of contrast medium (42 g or more) and the use of direct or reconstructed coronal and sagittal sections are required in the diagnosis of mass lesions of the pituitary gland, skull base, orbits and posterior fossa (particularly the cerebello-pontine angle). The specialized CT examinations which provide very accurate pretreatment information are time consuming and must be meticulously performed to take full advantage of the increased resolution obtained. Standard examination protocols are employed to monitor accurately the changes during and following therapy.

Thin section CT in the transaxial plane with or without intrathecal contrast (myelo-CT), is required in the investigation of spinal malignancies. Reconstructed images provide additional information regarding the extent and effects of the intraspinal or vertebral disease. For technical and logistical reasons, CT cannot cover the entire neural axis and the examination is therefore limited to a short segment(s). Intravenous contrast has a very limited rôle in CT examination of the spinal cord.

Cerebral angiography has a limited diagnostic rôle and is used primarily to identify the vascular structures preoperatively. This is particularly important in the suprasellar and pineal regions. Angiography may be indicated in those cases where CT is non-specific and can provide specific diagnostic information e.g. demonstrating extracranial supply in the meningiomas and the characteristic nodule in cerebellar haemangioblastoma, in which condition lesions unsuspected on CT may be demonstrated angiographically.

Interventional angiography has a limited rôle in the preoperative embolization of the extracranial supply of meningiomas (Hieshima et al 1980). Cerebral angiography should only be used to supplement the CT examination and should be performed in specialized units.

LIMITATIONS OF CT

Tissue characterization

Despite its ability to detect normal and abnormal soft tissue and specific tissue density such as calcification and fat, simple analysis of attenuation values does not permit precise tissue characterization. Dynamic CT scanning using a bolus injection of contrast medium followed by rapid sequence scanning at the same level provides temporal graphic displays of contrast enhancement and clearance from tissue, providing information about the vascularity of the tumour or brain parenchyma. Absorption coefficient measurements cannot accurately differentiate neoplasms from non-neoplastic processes, or benign from malignant or cystic neoplasm from solid lesions.

Common sources of error are:

1. A non-specific low density abnormality with mass effect, which could be
   (a) infarct
   (b) infection
   (c) tumour
   (d) trauma
   (e) gliosis
   (f) demyelination
2. A non-specific low density abnormality with absent or minimal mass effect, which could be
   (a) infarct
   (b) resolving haematoma
   (c) tumour
   (d) postoperative
   (e) infection
   (f) postradiotherapy
3. An area of ring enhancement with oedema and mass effect, which could be
   (a) glioma
   (b) abscess
   (c) resolving haematoma/infarct
   (d) early postoperative resection of tumour

4. A non-homogeneously enhancing mass, which could be
   (a) tumour
   (b) infection
   (c) demyelination
5. A midline hyperdense mass in the suprasellar region, which could be
   (a) pituitary adenoma
   (b) aneurysm
   (c) ependymoma
6. A midline hyperdense mass in the pineal region, which could be
   (a) pineal tumour
   (b) an aneurysm of the vein of Galen
7. Atypical appearances; cystic cerebello-pontine angle mass, which could be
   (a) acoustic neuroma
   (b) cystic meningioma
   (c) haemangioblastoma

CT also cannot differentiate a solitary metastasis from an intrinsic tumour.

In the diagnosis of tumours of the posterior fossa in children accurate differentiation between medulloblastoma, astrocytoma and ependymoma is not always possible.

Tumour margins

The margins of all tumours cannot be identified with accuracy for the following reasons:

1. Partial volume effect — the linear attenuation coefficient of a 'voxel' is related to the averaging of the tissue contained in the 'voxel'. No matter how small the volume of tissue, it is unlikely to contain entirely homogeneous material. High and low density substances may contribute disproportionately to the derived Hounsfield (H) number. This 'partial volume effect' becomes especially important when normal structures and disease processes interface within a section. Structural margins may be difficult to identify with precision and the accuracy of attenuation coefficient measurements is reduced.

2. Noise — this is the degree of random statistical variation in the CT image. Many factors contribute to the 'noise' of a system. These include kV, pixel width, slice thickness, size of subject, patient dosage and the efficiency of the detector system. Noise is related to the contrast resolution of the scanner and is a very important measure of performance since the naturally occurring contrast between normal tissue and tumour is low. Increased noise levels, therefore, have the effect of lowering the contrast difference between soft tissue structures leading to poorer resolution of the tumour margin.

3. Cerebral oedema — peritumoural oedema cannot be differentiated from low density tumour.

Patient movement

Movement of the patient's head results in some points appearing in different positions during the scanning cycle. These degrade the image quality. These streak artefacts are exaggerated by the presence of metallic density surgical or dental artefacts and by air.

Differential absorption artefacts

Streaks are produced where two tissues of greatly differing absorption are adjacent e.g. brain and air, brain and surgical clip.

Reproducibility

Precise positioning and accurate reproducibility of a thin section presents significant problems despite the use of a digital reconstructed radiograph ('Scannogram'). This limitation has important consequences for accurate follow-up. Stereotactic CT using a special frame overcomes this problem, but its use is time consuming.

Radiation dose

The radiation dose is variable, depending on the selection of radiographic factors. A maximum skin dose of 1 rad per section may be obtained on some systems. However, the maximum entry dose at the centre section is higher since radiation to one section results in scatter to the adjacent section. Any consideration of radiation dose must relate to the benefit to the patient.

Use of axial sections

The use of axial sections only is standard practice

in the diagnosis of brain tumours. This may lead to difficulties in the overall assessment of tumour size. Multiplanar and three-dimensional reconstructions are impractical in all cases with regard to time, radiation dose and clinical usefulness, particularly in those cases demonstrating clear cut evidence of aggressive parenchymal tumours. Lesions of the sellar region, skull base and posterior fossa should be examined using thin sections and multiplanar reconstructions. MR scanning has a dominant rôle in the diagnosis and management of these lesions.

False negative results

The detection of tumours is higher in cases presenting with signs of raised intracranial pressure or specific signs. False negative CT is more likely in patients presenting with epilepsy and transient ischaemic attacks. False negative CT may constitute 4% of the total number of patients with malignant glioma (Walker et al 1983). The first evidence of the tumour in such patients may be a slow wave abnormality on the EEG. False negative CT examinations may also be seen in patients with small isodense gliomas and intracerebral metastases who have strong clinical evidence of a tumour. Grades I and II astrocytoma, glioblastoma multiforme and metastases may not be visualized on the initial scan (Bolender et al 1983). Serial examinations may have to be performed in those patients suspected of having a brain tumour.

CT underestimates or misses diffuse leptomeningeal spread of tumour. Hydrocephalus in these cases may be absent and not all these lesions show contrast enhancement. Definitive diagnosis can only be made by CSF cytology.

Brain stem tumours may be obscured by petrous ridge artefacts, or a tumour near the skull base may be missed because of the 'partial volume effect'.

Small tumours may be missed if the scan is technically inadequate due to patient movement or suboptimal technique, including interrogation.

Non-specific CT findings

A significant minority of patients being investigated for intractable epilepsy have a non-specific calcified or low-density abnormality without mass effect on CT. Gliomas compromise the majority of these lesions which should be explored surgically.

Postoperative and post-therapy changes

In the early postoperative period, an area of brain swelling with rim enhancement is commonly present and cannot be reliably differentiated from tumour residue until approximately three months following surgery. The late radiotherapy effect of a mass which enhances cannot be differentiated from tumour.

THE ROLE OF CT IN INTRACEREBRAL TUMOURS

CT is extremely sensitive, detecting 98% of all intracranial masses (Davis 1977, Baker et al 1980). It has a lower specificity for individual tumours; histological confirmation, if possible, is therefore required in the assessment of all patients. In addition to detecting and localizing an intracranial mass, CT will identify invasion of adjacent structures including the dura and skull vault and may detect metastases through the cerebrospinal fluid which can occur with certain types of tumour. The associated mass effect can be assessed from the CT image and the ventricular size evaluated.

The prognosis of some intracerebral tumours, notably tumours of the posterior fossa, has improved because of earlier diagnosis and the detection of recurrence and complications.

DIAGNOSIS

Supratentorial tumours — the gliomata

Gliomas

Astrocytoma and glioblastoma multiforme account for 50% of all primary tumours and 75% of all gliomas. These tumours, which originate from astrocytes or their primitive precursors, usually arise from the central white matter of the cerebrum in adults and cerebellar hemispheres and brain stem in children. Gliomas have been classified by Kernohan as grades I to IV: the least malignant astrocytomas are grades I and II with glioblastoma multiforme representing grades III and IV. The CT appearances vary according to the grade (Williams 1985). The grade I astrocytoma is typically shown as a well-defined area of low attenuation with no surrounding peritumoural oedema and minimal mass effect (Fig. 15.1). The diagnosis is confidently predicted if calcification, which is seen in 50% of cases, is present (Leeds et al 1984). However, difficulties in diagnosis are presented by an uncalcified low grade astrocytoma which may resemble an acute infarct or area of demyelination.

The attenuation characteristics of a grade II astrocytoma are more heterogeneous. Central cysts may usually be differentiated from areas of necrosis. The tumour margin shows variable enhancement which may vary with time, and moderate peritumoural oedema and mass effect are present (Fig. 15.2). Calcification is unusual and these tumours must be differentiated from areas of infarction, cerebritis (abscess), resolving haematoma and other low grade neoplasms.

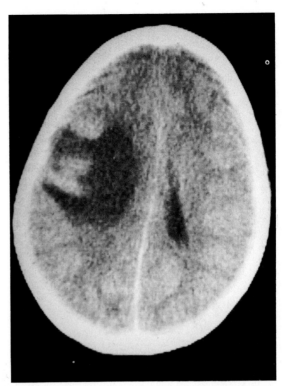

Fig. 15.2 Grade II astrocytoma. Enhanced scan shows a large mass of heterogeneous enhancement with a large cystic component on its medial aspect. Compression of the left lateral ventricle indicates a significant accompanying mass effect.

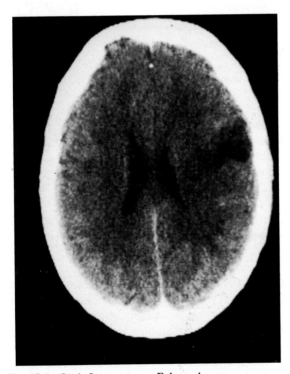

Fig. 15.1 Grade I astrocytoma. Enhanced scan demonstrates a well-defined low attenuation abnormality with no surrounding oedema and minimal mass effect in the right parietal region.

Glioblastoma multiforme shows more characteristic appearances indicative of the increased degree of malignancy. These rapidly growing, highly malignant tumours are characterized on the unenhanced CT scan as large mass lesions of heterogeneous attenuation. The tumour margins are irregular and poorly defined, and central hypodense zones are frequent. Calcification is uncommon. Intense, heterogeneous enhancement is usual and multiloculation with complete and incomplete thick-walled rings and nodules is frequently demonstrated. The associated mass effect due to the presence of peritumoural oedema is extensive. Severe ventricular compression and midline displacement is demonstrated (Fig. 15.3). The tumour may extend to the meninges. Differentiation from a large necrotic solitary or multiple confluent metastases may be difficult but the appearances are characteristic of malignancy.

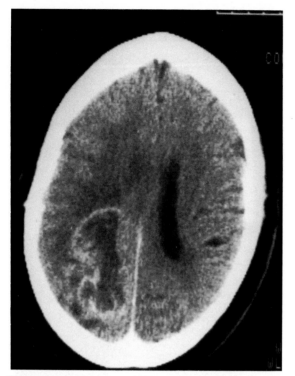

Fig. 15.3 Glioblastoma multiforme. Heterogeneously enhancing multiloculated mass with incomplete ring enhancement, surrounding oedema and mass effect.

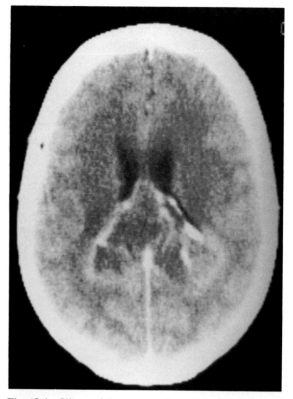

Fig. 15.4 Glioma of the corpus callosum. Irregularly enhancing tumour infiltrating the splenium of the corpus callosum, obliterating the posterior aspects of the lateral ventricles and demonstrating periventricular extension.

Angiography typically shows abundant neo-vascularity with arterio-venous shunting and abnormal deep veins. Infiltration of the corpus callosum resulting in compression and deformity or obliteration of the lateral ventricle may produce difficulty in diagnosis on the unenhanced scan as these tumours are often isodense. If the ventricles are symmetrically deformed they may appear small and slit-like on the unenhanced CT scan and, unless intravenous contrast is administered, the cause of the small ventricles may be overlooked. Bilateral enhancement is typical of callosal involvement (Fig. 15.4). Large areas of hae-morrhage within a glioma are uncommon: haemorrhage large enough to produce symptoms will obliterate evidence of the underlying neoplasm and will appear as a large haematoma. Haemor-rhagic gliomas and resolving haematomas may show similar appearances on serial CT. In ap-proximately 20% of haemorrhagic gliomas, a portion of the glioma may be spared.

Multicentric gliomas cannot be differentiated from metastases on CT and are usually diagnosed at autopsy.

Oligodendroglioma

These slow growing tumours which originate from oligodendrocytes in the central white matter ac-count for about 5% of intracranial gliomas. Characteristically, the tumours are very large at diagnosis and are located in the anterior half of the cerebrum (Vonfakos et al 1979). The abnormality is identified as a large, irregular mass of heterogeneous attenuation containing calcification and hypodense zones. Nodular or shell-like cal-cification is seen in 90% of tumours. The tumour margin may be discrete or poorly defined. Peritumoural oedema and enhancement is variable (Fig. 15.5). An oligodendroglioma without cal-

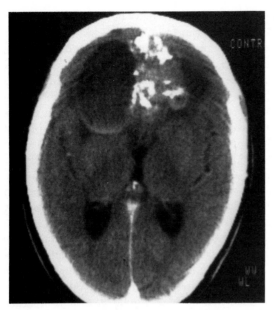

Fig. 15.5 Oligodendroglioma. Large predominantly well-defined hypodense mass in the frontal region, crossing the midline, with large calcified foci and minimal heterogeneous enhancement.

Primary intracerebral lymphoma carries a worse prognosis than lymphoma of corresponding cell types outside the central nervous system. Secondary CNS involvement is seen in 5–9% of patients with systemic lymphoma (Levitt et al 1980).

Hodgkin's disease rarely affects the central nervous system. Involvement of the brain parenchyma, leptomeninges, dura and epidural tissues may be seen in cases with advanced systemic disease and carries a poor prognosis.

The CT appearances of primary and secondary parenchymal lymphoma are similar. A parenchymal mass is reliably diagnosed but detection of leptomeningeal spread is unreliable. A mass may be isodense or slightly hyperdense, with moderate homogeneous and well circumscribed enhancement. Central necrosis is rare and there is variable peritumoural oedema. The parenchymal lesions may show transient spontaneous regression. Subependymal spread of lymphoma on CT cannot be differentiated from ependymoma or medulloblastoma (Fig. 15.6). Angiography shows an avascular

cification is difficult to differentiate from other large gliomas.

Ganglioglioma and ganglioneuroma

These are rare, relatively benign slow growing tumours containing mature ganglion cells and stromal elements derived from glial tissues. Malignant change is rare. The CT features are non-specific and include low attenuation or isodense mass lesions with frequent calcification and cysts. Homogeneous enhancement is seen in the majority of cases. The lesions cannot be differentiated on CT from astrocytomas or metastases.

Lymphoma

Primary lymphoma is rare, accounting for only 1.5% of all primary brain tumours. Immunosuppressed patients carry a higher risk of developing the tumour which is more common in males. The tumour may be solitary or multiple and shows a predilection for the basal ganglia, corpus callosum, thalami, periventricular regions, cerebellum and brain stem (Tadmor et al 1978, Holtas et al 1984).

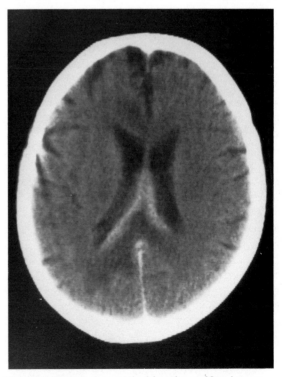

Fig. 15.6 Primary intracerebral lymphoma. Note intense ventricular ependymal enhancement indicating subarachnoid spread of tumour.

mass without tumour blush which may be helpful in differentiating lymphoma from glioma.

Spinal lymphoma cannot be readily differentiated radiologically from other masses.

Meningioma

This benign tumour of the meninges accounts for 16% of primary intracranial tumours. They are slow growing, well-encapsulated tumours and are normally treated surgically. These tumours have a dural attachment and their frequent invasion of the adjacent calvarium produces changes on the skull radiograph which may be the first indication of their presence. More importantly, compression of the adjacent brain parenchyma and dural sinuses can be detected on CT. Infiltration of the brain is rare; it is seen in cases undergoing malignant transformation. The commonest sites of origin in decreasing order of frequency are the vertex, sphenoid ridge, olfactory groove, supra/parasellar region and posterior fossa.

Meningiomas produce very characteristic CT appearances. The unenhanced scan shows an isodense or hyperdense mass with smooth margins.

Calcification, which may be either punctate or globular, is seen in 20% of cases. Hypodense lesions are rare. Intense, homogeneous enhancement of a well-defined mass is usual (Fig. 15.7) and areas of inhomogeneity resulting from cysts, necrosis or old haemorrhage may be seen in some cases. Intratumoural haemorrhage is rare. The tumours are usually round or globular but en-plaque lesions may be seen.

The location of a meningioma determines the degree of surrounding oedema. Extensive oedema is seen with lesions near the vertex. Oedema is absent or minimal with suprasellar, cerebello-pontine angle or intraventricular lesions. The degree of mass displacement, bowing of the falx, and ventricular compression may be less than expected in view of the long history.

Malignant transformation is suggested on CT by the presence of poorly-defined tumour margins and inhomogeneous enhancement, indicating parenchymal invasion, and central necrosis. Peritumoural oedema is variable in these cases, which must be differentiated from metastases, gliomas and lymphomas. The presence of hyperostosis virtually excludes a glioma, metastasis or lymphoma.

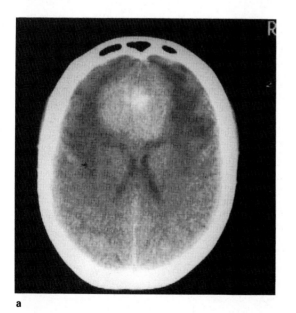

a

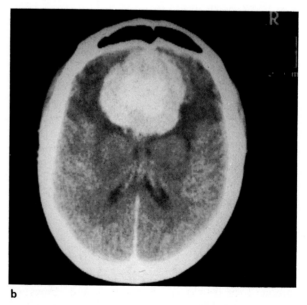

b

Fig. 15.7 Meningioma. (a) Precontrast, and (b) postcontrast scans. Well-defined hyperdense mass containing central calcification arising from the anterior falx. Homogeneous enhancement and extensive peritumoural white matter oedema and severe ventricular compression shown.

Angiography, by demonstrating a prolonged tumour blush, no arterio-venous shunting and meningeal supply may assist diagnosis.

The prognosis of meningiomas is related to their location, size, extent of resection and histological features. Recurrence is uncommon after total removal (less than 10%), but frequent after subtotal excision. The extent of resection and histological changes of pleomorphism are the only factors which correlate significantly with the recurrence rate.

Intra- and suprasellar tumours

Pituitary adenomas

Staging of aggressive tumours is influenced by the effects of the tumour on normal anatomical structures. Thin transaxial and direct coronal sections with contrast enhancement are necessary to appreciate fully the relationship between the sphenoid sinus, sella turcica, pituitary gland, suprasellar cisterns, cavernous sinuses and internal carotid arteries. Dynamic scanning may be required for differentiating the intracavernous carotid arteries, cavernous sinuses and pituitary gland and detecting vascular encasement. The pituitary gland does not have a blood–brain barrier and therefore opacifies in parallel with the blood iodine level. Time–density curves can be used to differentiate vascular structures from tumour. The optic chiasm and tracts have a characteristic shape on both axial and coronal images. The infundibulum and tuber cinereum are clearly visualized on thin section CT.

Enlargement of the pituitary gland is best determined by assessing the height of the gland because the border between it and the cavernous sinus is poorly defined. A gland height in excess of 9 mm is abnormal (Cusick et al 1980). The superior surface of the normal gland can be of any configuration i.e. concave, flat or convex.

Adenomas are classified as microadenomas (less than 10 mm) or macroadenomas. Microadenomas may be asymptomatic or symptomatic and may secrete prolactin, adrenocortical trophic hormone (ACTH) or human growth hormone. Microadenomas appear on CT as a hypodense area on unenhanced coronal CT sections. The gland has a convex upper surface and the infundibulum is displaced from the midline. The sella floor slopes to the affected side. CT can be used to gauge the response to therapy (Chernow et al 1982). Macroadenomas, on the other hand, usually produce symptoms by compressing the adjacent normal gland or optic chiasm. Macroadenomas are isodense and show intense homogeneous enhancement, and appear only slightly less dense than the cavernous sinuses postcontrast. Calcification and bone destruction are uncommon but may be seen in the more aggressive tumours. Tumour extension can be superior (most common), lateral, anterior, posterior or inferior. Areas of low attenuation indicating necrosis or fluid may be seen within a giant tumour (Fig. 15.8a). Lateral extension will be seen on coronal CT (Fig. 15.8b); the internal carotid arteries may be encased by enhancing tumour. Extension anteriorly into the orbit may be seen in the more aggressive tumours. A large enhancing mass in the pituitary or parasellar region must be differentiated from a giant aneurysm, meningioma of the tuberculum sella or nasopharyngeal carcinoma.

Craniopharyngioma

This tumour is derived from remnants of Rathke's Pouch and is the second most common suprasellar tumour. The peak incidence is in childhood (rare before 2 years of age), but it may also be seen in adults, usually in the fifth decade. Tumours are characteristically well-encapsulated and cystic and are intra- or suprasellar in location. Densely globular or peripheral curvilinear calcification occurs in 80% of cases in children but in only 40% or less of adult cases. Characteristically the tumour is demonstrated as a midline cyst with or without calcification and hydrocephalus (Fig. 15.9). A non-calcified cystic craniopharyngioma is difficult to differentiate from an epidermoid or arachnoid cyst. A craniopharyngioma may occasionally arise within the third ventricle, usually presenting with ventricular obstruction.

Colloid cyst

This occurs at the foramen of Monroe in the antero-superior portion of the third ventricle. Hydrocephalus may be intermittent due to a ball-valve effect of the tumour. It is a rounded tumour of increased attenuation which may show minimal enhancement due to choroid plexus wrapped around the tumour. The third ventricle is often collapsed.

Chiasmal gliomas

Visual abnormalities and optic atrophy are the clinical manifestations of these tumours which are associated with neurofibromatosis. They present on CT as well-defined masses with smooth margins and are isodense or show slightly increased attenuation values without focal calcification. The tumours show variable contrast enhancement. One or both optic nerves may be affected (Miller et al 1980).

Hypothalamic gliomas

These are tumours of infancy producing failure to thrive, unusual alertness and hyperactivity. The tumour is usually a benign astrocytoma. The CT appearances are of a large, well-defined tumour

with irregular or smooth outline. The tumours are predominantly low density showing multifocal areas of marked enhancement and calcification may be present (*see* Ch. 3).

Pineal region tumours

The two main types of neoplasm are pineal cell tumours (pineocytomas, pineoblastomas), and germ cell tumours. Radiological detection is less difficult than distinguishing between the two types. CT has an important rôle in identifying invasion of adjacent structures and in detecting metastases. Pineal tumours, especially those that seed via the CSF spaces or ventricles, have a poor survival rate. Pineal cell tumours occur with equal frequency in either sex, are less common than germ cell tumours and have a greater tendency to calcify. The pineocytoma may be found at any age and is a slow growing tumour confined to the posterior third ventricle. CT shows a slightly hyperdense mass which may enhance and frequently contains dense focal calcifications. The pineoblas-

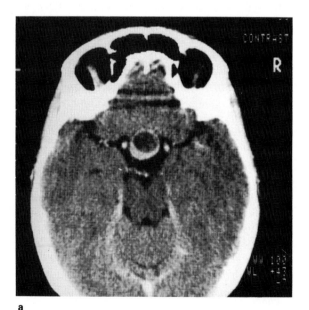

a

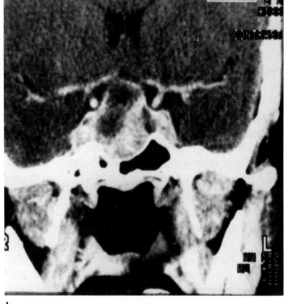

b

Fig. 15.8 Pituitary macroadenoma. Postcontrast scans (a) transaxial, and (b) direct coronal sections. Enhancing mass eroding the floor of the pituitary fossa with dome-shaped cystic extension superiorly into the suprasellar cistern. Note displacement of the terminal portions of both internal carotid arteries.

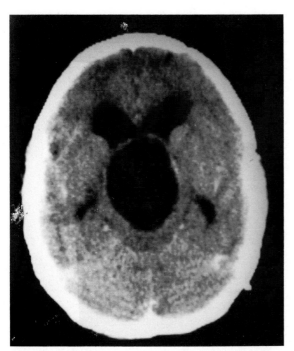

Fig. 15.9 Craniopharyngioma in a child. Well-defined low attenuation midline cyst obliterating the third ventricle and producing internal hydrocephalus.

toma is a highly malignant tumour of primitive pineal parenchymal cells occurring in both children and adults. The mass has poorly-defined margins on CT, shows dense, homogeneous enhancement and often contains calcification. Invasion of adjacent structures and CSF seeding may be seen with both tumours. Germ cell tumours of the pineal include germinoma, teratoma and teratocarcinoma. These tumours occasionally involve the suprasellar region. Both germinomas and teratocarcinomas may spread via the CSF pathways. Germinoma, a malignant germ cell neoplasm occurring almost exclusively in males, may occur either as an isolated posterior third ventricle mass or in association with a suprasellar germinoma. CT shows a hypodense, isodense or hyperdense mass with infrequent calcification (Fig. 15.10a). The tumour margins are frequently indistinct and irregular and the mass shows intense enhancement. Hydrocephalus is frequent because of the proximity of these tumours to the aqueduct. Ependymal or cisternal seeding appears as focal areas of contrast enhancement

(Fig. 15.10b). Teratoma is a rare benign tumour shown on CT as a mass of heterogeneous density containing areas of calcification and fat (Fig. 15.10c). The mass has irregular margins and shows only minimal enhancement. Intense enhancement in a teratoma would suggest malignant degeneration (Zimmerman et al 1980). Teratocarcinomas are malignant tumours which include embryonal cell and yolk sac carcinoma and choriocarcinoma. These tumours are characterized by intratumoural haemorrhage, invasion of adjacent structures and seeding via the CSF pathways. CT shows a hypodense, isodense or slightly hyperdense mass which enhances intensely. Calcification is absent.

Despite the characteristic CT appearances when present, differentiation of the varied types of tumour of the pineal region or differentiation from astrocytomas is not possible (Weisberg 1984).

Tumours of the optic nerve and sheath

Optic nerve glioma

Optic nerve glioma is the commonest tumour of the optic nerve. The optic nerves are involved bilaterally in some cases of neurofibromatosis. In older patients, unlike children, optic nerve gliomas follow a progressive malignant course. The CT shows a fusiform enlargement of the optic nerve. The tumour is isodense and enhancement is variable: tumour calcification and cystic changes are unusual (*see* Ch. 3, pp 67–69).

Optic nerve sheath meningioma

These tumours are similar to meningiomas elsewhere. Tumours involving the anterior part of the optic nerve sheath have a better prognosis than those at the orbital apex. The precontrast CT scan shows a smooth fusiform enlargement of the optic nerve which enhances homogeneously. There may be associated sphenoid bone hyperostosis and calcification.

Posterior fossa tumours

The detection of tumours of the posterior fossa by CT is very reliable. The CT criteria for predicting

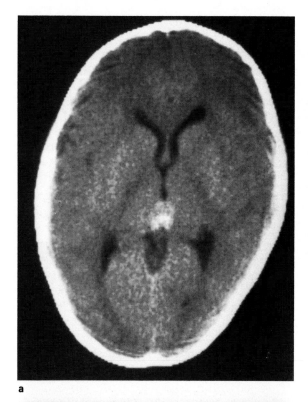

a

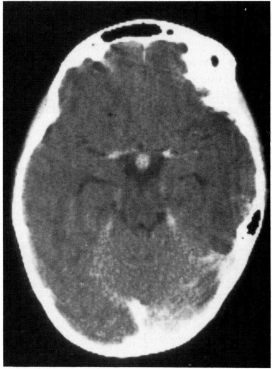

b

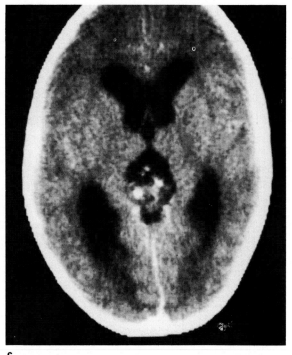

c

Fig. 15.10 Pineal region tumours. (a) and (b) germinoma. (a) Hyperdense mass with calcification in the region of the pineal with (b) an associated hyperdense metastatic suprasellar mass. (c) Teratoma: minimally enhancing heterogeneous mass containing fat and calcific densities compressing the posterior third ventricle producing obstructive hydrocephalus.

the histology of a posterior fossa tumour are about 80% reliable (Naidich et al 1977).

Posterior fossa gliomata

These tumours are among the few benign gliomas encountered: children and young adults are usually affected. Adults affected have the same tumour as that observed in the paediatric age group; cystic astrocytoma and ependymoma. Calcification is seen in 20% of cases. Cystic (50%) and solid (50%) tumours are the two main morphological types. The cystic type is more often found in the cerebellar hemispheres (80%) than in the vermis (20%). CT may show either a well-defined low density mass with rim enhancement in 50% of cases, where the tumour completely surrounds the cyst, or a small solid mass in the cyst wall seen as an area of focal nodular enhancement. Peritumoural oedema may be seen. Recurrence of the cystic glioma is rare after surgical excision. Solid tumours are more often seen in young adults. Unenhanced CT shows a mass lesion of ill-defined areas of mixed attenuation with zones of low attenuation predominating. A variable pattern of enhancement is demonstrated and a non-enhancing low density mass on CT may prove to be a solid astrocytoma. These solid tumours have a tendency to infiltrate through the close confines of the posterior fossa, extending into the cerebellar peduncles to involve the brain stem. Complete removal is often impossible because of infiltration into adjacent structures, and local recurrence is therefore more common. These solid tumours must be differentiated from medulloblastoma and ependymoma.

Brain stem gliomata

The main incidence of these tumours, which cause progressive cranial nerve palsies, is in older children and young adults. Accurate confirmation by high resolution, multiplanar CT is important because biopsy of the brain stem is hazardous. CT shows asymmetrical expansion of the brain stem which may show reduced attenuation (Fig. 15.11). Contrast enhancement is variable. Compression of the mesencephalic and pontine cisterns anteriorly and of the fourth ventricle posteriorly is usual. Hydrocephalus, however, is rare. A glioma must be differentiated from other causes of brain stem expansion which include infarction, vascular malformation and multiple sclerosis.

Medulloblastoma

This is a embryonal tumour and is the most common tumour of the posterior fossa in childhood. It arises in the roof of the fourth ventricle and tends to fill the fourth ventricle as it grows. It is characteristically located centrally in the posterior fossa. Tumours of the hemispheres are more often seen in older patients. CT characteristically shows a uniformly hyperdense mass which enhances intensely. The mass is usually well defined and cysts and necrotic areas may be present (Fig. 15.12a). Calcification is unusual, only being seen in 10%

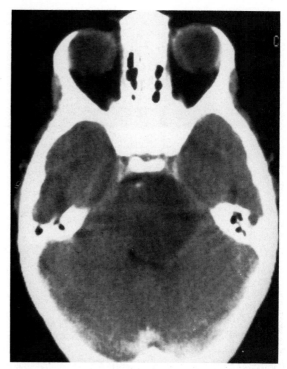

Fig 15.11 Brain stem glioma. The brain stem is expanded by a mass of low attenuation. Note posterior displacement of the fourth ventricle and obliteration of the mesencephalic cisterns.

of cases. Hydrocephalus is common and is seen in 85%. The tumour characteristically metastasizes along CSF pathways and this is seen in 10% at diagnosis. The seedings are recognized as irregular thickening of the ependyma and meninges (Fig. 15.12b) and may occur through ventricular shunts resulting in haematogenous spread and peritoneal seeding. CT is highly accurate, correlating with the histological findings in 90% of cases.

Ependymoma

Ependymomas of the fourth ventricle are more common in childhood than adulthood where the tumours are supratentorial and periventricular in location. CT characteristically shows a thin, well-defined low attenuation halo surrounding an isodense or hyperdense mass. The halo represents the distended and nearly effaced fourth ventricle surrounding the tumour. Fine, punctate calcification is seen in 50% of cases. The tumour shows

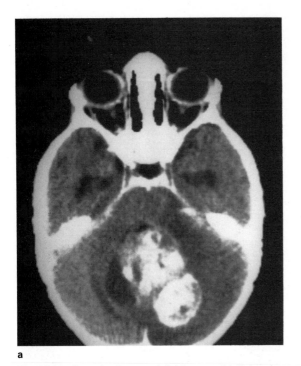

a

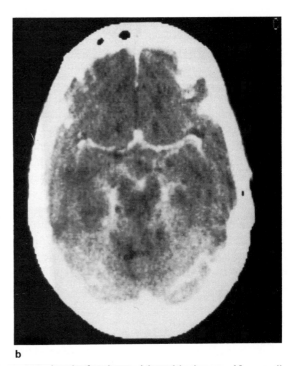

b

Fig. 15.12 Posterior fossa medulloblastoma. (a) Enhancing mass compressing the fourth ventricle and brain stem. Note small intratumoural cysts and surrounding oedema. (b) Meningeal enhancement, particularly in the cisterns around the midbrain, due to tumour infiltration.

heterogeneous enhancement with little or no oedema (Fig. 15.13). Cysts are uncommon but necrotic areas are seen frequently. Hydrocephalus is common. 60% of tumours extend through the foramina Luschka into the cerebello-pontine angles.

Haemangioblastoma

This tumour is the commonest primary cerebellar hemispheric tumour in adults, usually presenting in middle age. The association of haemangioblastoma with angioma of the retina is referred to as Lindau's syndrome. The von Hippel–Lindau syndrome, a phakomatosis, is characterized by lesions in the eye, brain and spinal cord. Cystic lesions with mural nodules are seen in 50%, the remainder being solid tumour masses with or without a central necrotic area. The CT scan appearances correlate with the pathological findings. The unenhanced scan shows a well-defined low attenuation cystic mass without peritumoural oedema and calcification. The postcontrast scan

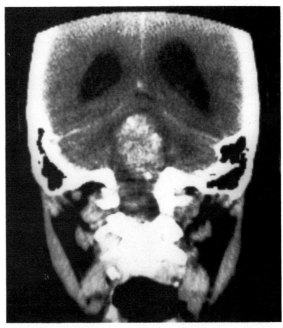

Fig. 15.13 Ependymoma of the fourth ventricle. A direct coronal section showing enhancing mass containing punctate areas of calcification and surrounding low attenuation halo.

characteristically shows an enhanced mural nodule. The solid tumour shows non-specific CT appearances which cannot be differentiated from those of an astrocytoma or metastasis. These tumours are usually smaller than 5 cm. Angiography is required and has an increased sensitivity and specificity for demonstrating the multiple small tumours which are characteristic of this condition.

Cerebello-pontine angle masses

Acoustic neuromas and meningiomas are the commonest tumours of the cerebello-pontine angle (CPA). These are usually readily distinguished by CT from an epidermoid which is an uncommon CPA lesion. CT is very accurate for diagnosing the presence of an acoustic neuroma in the CPA. Thin section, high resolution CT in the axial and coronal planes is required to show the enlargement of the internal auditory meatus which is commonly seen. The characteristic appearances are of an isodense mass extending into the CPA cistern. Calcification and cystic change are rare and the mass shows homogeneous enhancement (Fig. 15.14). Large tumours will displace the brain stem and fourth ventricle. Low attenuation changes indicating necrosis are uncommon. The presence of cystic changes with an acoustic neuroma will lead

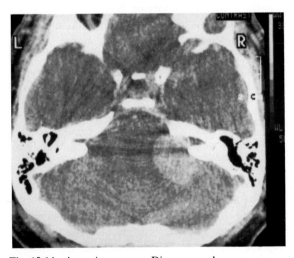

Fig. 15.14 Acoustic neuroma. Direct coronal section: well-defined enhancing mass in the right cerebello-pontine angle cistern compressing the brain stem. Note expanded internal auditory meatus.

to difficulty in differentiating it from an epidermoid. CT may miss tumours of 5 mm or less in diameter. These small, often intracanalicular tumours may require negative contrast (air or carbon dioxide meatography) combined with high resolution CT for diagnosis (Kricheff et al 1980). An intracanalicular tumour prevents filling of the internal auditory meatus with gas. Adhesions at the internal auditory meatus may, however, cause false positive appearances and the anatomical features of the area must be fully understood to assist interpretation.

MRI is more helpful for characterization of neuromas, epidermoid cysts and gliomas of the CPA, while CT is more informative for meningiomas, metastases and tympanomastoid cholesteatomas. MRI is more helpful in the diagnosis of CPA lesions in defining the full extent of the lesions and their relationships to contiguous structures (Gentry et al 1987).

Meningioma is the important differential diagnosis of an acoustic neuroma and may be difficult to differentiate on CT appearances alone. Meningiomas rarely cause bone erosion. Extension is towards the tentorium. CT usually shows a mass of increased attenuation with intense enhancement, often with cystic change. Unlike acoustic neuroma, calcification is frequent and the tumours are often larger. Angiography may be required in difficult cases to demonstrate the blood supply from the external carotid.

Epidermoid tumours enlarge the CPA cistern, do not distort the brain stem and are fat-containing, appearing as low density masses on CT. These tumours do not enhance and are large at diagnosis.

Glomus jugulare tumour (paraganglioma, chemodectoma)

This tumour causes destruction and irregularity of the cortical margins of the jugular fossa which may be detected on plain radiographs of the skull base. 50% of jugular foramina are asymmetrical with the right usually larger than the left. CT demonstrates a lobulated, uniformly dense and enhancing mass which shows hypervascularity on angiography. Jugular venography shows expansion of the jugular bulb.

Leukaemic infiltration of the meninges

The CNS is affected in about 10% of patients with acute leukaemia, usually in the form of meningeal infiltration (Pagani et al 1981). Intrathecal methotrexate and whole brain irradiation effectively eradicates leukaemic cells in the central nervous system. CT shows enhancement of the meninges in the sulci, fissures and basal cisterns (Fig. 15.12b). Less frequently, there is an isodense or slightly hyperdense parenchymal mass with a zone of surrounding oedema and homogeneous contrast enhancement.

PRETREATMENT ASSESSMENT (AND STAGING)

The TNM classification is of limited value because the tumour margins often cannot be accurately defined, the tumours do not spread to lymph nodes and rarely metastasize. CT in the axial and coronal planes will display the location of intracerebral tumours. Direct infiltration into vital areas and compression of adjacent normal tissue may be readily appreciated. The degree of malignancy of a primary intracerebral tumour can only be determined from the histological appearances following biopsy. Accurate biopsy is required but may be difficult in view of the location of the tumour, difficulties with defining tumour margin, the presence of surrounding oedema and the complications occurring within the tumour such as necrosis and haemorrhage. Stereotactic-guided CT biopsy offers a very precise and safe method of obtaining adequate specimens and holds promise for improving the surgical resection of some tumours. In many instances, however, biopsy may not be possible, e.g. in the case of nuclear and intra-axial tumours and infiltrating tumours in the dominant hemisphere.

CT criteria in pretreatment assessment

Tumour morphology

CT allows the precise localization of the mass and provides information regarding the size, shape, volume, enhancement characteristics, presence of calcification and cysts and haemorrhage within the tumour mass as well as the presence of surrounding oedema, displacement and compression of adjacent normal structures and the presence of obstructive hydrocephalus. However, the complex shape of most tumours is difficult to assess accurately from a series of transaxial sections. Coronal and reconstructed sagittal images are frequently required to supplement the information obtained from the conventional transaxial sections. A three-dimensional surface reconstruction algorithm has been developed using information obtained from a series of conventional thin CT sections. The algorithm accurately reconstructs the surfaces between contours of both supra- and infratentorial anatomical sites (Gillespie et al 1987). Volume and surface area of lateral ventricles and tumour site can be calculated and displayed as a three-dimensional image. The actual size and three-dimensional shape of the lesion and its topographical relationship to surrounding structures can be utilized to plan the surgical approach. The incorporation of this technique may greatly assist neurosurgeons and neuro-oncologists in planning multimodality therapy and also in the localization of small and relatively inaccessible lesions which may not be adequately assessed by conventional methods. Furthermore, the efficacy of radiotherapy and/or chemotherapy in brain tumours may be more accurately assessed.

Intraoperative CT scanning with a dedicated CT scanner provides accurate tumour localization, superior contrast and spatial resolution and cross-sectional anatomy of the entire brain. Further development of intraoperative CT guidance will allow safer and even complete removal of some previously unresectable tumours (Lunsford et al 1984).

Peritumoural oedema

Peritumoural oedema is caused by a breakdown in the blood–brain barrier and is frequently seen in both benign and malignant tumours; it may contribute quite significantly to the mass effect of these lesions. The degree of oedema can be graded by CT and the effects of steroid therapy monitored. Steroid therapy causes a progressive increase in the attenuation values of the white matter corresponding to a decrease in the oedema.

Staging of posterior fossa tumours

These tumours are often unresectable and respond to regimes of combined radiation and chemotherapy. Accurate pretreatment assessment of these tumours is paramount, prior to biopsy and definitive treatment. The use of direct coronal CT is advocated in the preoperative assessment of posterior fossa tumours. CT performed in this plane displays all the significant anatomical relationships in the exact orientation found during surgical dissection (Naidich et al 1985). Complete excision of posterior fossa tumours is the aim of most surgical approaches. Where infiltration is present, part of the cerebellar hemisphere and vermis can frequently be sacrificed to obtain a complete clearance but involvement of the brain stem and cerebellar peduncles prevents complete excision. Tumours completely filling the fourth ventricle can be accurately demonstrated on CT (Kingsley & Harwood-Nash 1984). CT is, however, less reliable in differentiating tumour from surrounding oedema where the fourth ventricle is completely obliterated, either by complete filling by tumour or extrinsic compression. MRI provides a more accurate means of assessing the posterior fossa and brain stem in children by readily imaging in the sagittal plane, thereby showing the extent of a tumour more accurately.

Intraoperative sonography

Both CT and ultrasound will define tumour masses but sonography is more effective than CT in determining whether a lesion is cystic, with or without septations or solid. CT, however, excels in defining the associated features of an intracranial neoplasm, such as surrounding oedema and details of enhancement. Sonography as an intraoperative localizing tool requires a surgically created cranial defect (Gooding et al 1984) and can be used for drainage of cysts and to resolve equivocal CT findings such as low density, non-enhancing masses in which low grade tumour cannot be reliably differentiated from necrosis or fluid.

Assessment of lesions unsuited to biopsy

Infiltrative tumours of the brain stem may be difficult to diagnose despite clinical evidence of their presence. These tumours may present as low density mass lesions only, without contrast enhancement or hydrocephalus. In this group much reliance is placed on the tumour morphology demonstrated on CT. Biopsy using routinely available techniques is difficult and hazardous. Tumours smaller than 5 cm in diameter and those with cysts or calcification may carry a better prognosis (Albright & James 1985).

Radiotherapy planning

Although CT has markedly improved the ability to detect tumours, the precise localization of tumour on projection radiographs remains difficult. Frequently, bony landmarks are used and fields are sized generously to assure that all tumour is included in the radiation portal. The difficulties are increased when oblique portals are used since the relationship between structures, as defined by the 'beam's view' of them, changes with gantry angle, and the recognition of bony landmarks in oblique projections may be difficult. A newly developed system (Haynor et al 1986) uses radio-opaque markers attached to the head as reference points. These markers are identified on both CT scans and simulation films and their locations entered into the treatment planning computer. The tumour and any desired normal structures are then outlined manually on each CT section. Transparent overlays produced by the computer show the position of the reference markers and tumour outlines for any combination of gantry angles and source–film distance. Because the overlays are scaled to the simulation films, the reference points enable precise alignment of overlay and films. The tumour outline thus appears on the simulation or verification films exactly as it is 'seen' by the therapy beam, making field verifications straightforward and accurate, even on oblique films.

Favourable prognostic signs

Certain CT features, either singly or in combination, may indicate a more favourable outcome following treatment. Well-defined cystic or enhancing lesions with smooth margins, well demarcated from the surrounding brain, with minimal or no surrounding oedema and minimal mass effect are often seen in low grade malignancies or benign tumours. Surgical resectability is improved where the tumour is located superficially in the cerebral or cerebellar hemispheres and in tumours of the non-dominant hemisphere.

Unfavourable prognostic signs

The prognosis of intracerebral tumours depends in part on the completeness or otherwise of the tumour excision. Large tumour size and heterogeneous enhancement are associated with poor resectability. Poorly-defined tumour margins and the presence of oedema are important criteria adversely affecting the prognosis. A large tumour with extensive oedema will produce a very significant degree of midline displacement and herniation which may have a serious adverse effect on the outcome unless treatment is instituted urgently. CT plays a very significant role in assessing the mass effect of such tumours. In cases of primary lymphoma treated by radiotherapy, the size of the lesion is the most important prognostic factor and is probably related to the location of the tumour (Cellerier et al 1984). The presence of contralateral extension, e.g. in callosal gliomas, and extension through the tentorial hiatus to the middle cranial or posterior fossae are poor prognostic signs. The CT appearances may provide some information about the margin of a tumour. A plane of cleavage may be present around the cystic component at the periphery of an astrocytoma, without surrounding oedema, and there may be sharp demarcation of a densely enhancing medulloblastoma or the centrally necrotic astrocytoma and its surrounding oedema from the normal brain. Infiltration is assumed to be present where the enhancing tumour margin is less well-defined, however. It is rare that the whole margin of a tumour is of sufficient density after contrast to suggest a well-encapsulated lesion. It is far more common for the edge of a tumour to enhance to a variable degree, and it is just this feature which has been shown to be an unreliable guide to infiltration (Kingsley & Harwood-Nash 1984). Stereotactic biopsy techniques in the supratentorial compartment have indicated a correlation between the pattern of CT changes with and without contrast and the microscopy findings (Boethuis et al 1978).

Seeding via CSF

Certain tumours e.g. medulloblastomas and ependymomas seed via the CSF spaces resulting in ependymal or meningeal spread. Intracranial subarachnoid metastases of medulloblastoma may be detected at the time of diagnosis. The introduction of thin section high resolution CT scanning has improved the detection rate. This may have an impact on the treatment of these patients, since the frequent appearance of metastases may indicate the need for more vigorous chemotherapeutic regimes (North et al 1985).

Cerebral metastases from lung carcinoma

CT plays an important role in those cases with vague neurological signs and in neurologically asymptomatic patients. Treatment decisions are based on accurate preoperative staging and the findings may obviate the need for lung resection (Tarver et al 1984).

INTERVENTIONAL CT

Stereotaxis

Stereotactic CT is used to obtain biopsy material of CT-proven lesions and thereby provide important therapeutic information. It is also used for therapeutic purposes combined with CO_2 laser and intracavitary and interstitial irradiation.

Biopsy

Two methods are commonly used:

(a) The simpler and less accurate method is to relate the CT abnormality from axial and longitudinal images to identifiable bony landmarks. The digitalized data are entered into a three-dimensional computer matrix which corresponds to the coordinate system of a standard stereotactic frame located in the operating theatre. A site for biopsy is selected by the cursor from the CT display screen. The computer calculates and gives out the mechanical adjustments of the stereotactic frame necessary to place the target point into the focal point of the frame.

(b) The second method uses a modified stereotactic device in the CT system; this is the preferred and more accurate method. Modified Riechert–Mundinger (Bullard et al 1983), Brown–Robert–Wells (Asakura et al 1985) or Gouda (Gouda et al 1983) stereotactic frames interface with the scanner. The patient, with the frame in position, is scanned and then transferred to the operating theatre for biopsy. The apparatus is equipped with a measuring phantom constructed of material such as carbon fibre allowing CT scanning without artefacts. The stereotactic co-ordinates (*xyz*) of any target can be taken directly from the transverse and longitudinal CT image with a high degree of accuracy. These target co-ordinates and the trajectory approach angles are calculated using a computer system in the operating room (Kelly et al 1985).

Tumours in various sites, including the brain stem, have been successfully biopsied. CT scans may be performed immediately afterwards with the frame in situ to assess post-biopsy complications. No mortality or permanent morbidity has been reported. The anatomical accuracy using both methods can be improved by performing limited CT arteriography (Nauta et al 1984) using a small volume bolus (4 cm) injected during scanning. The vessels are seen in the same CT image as that used for stereotactic localization and this greatly improves the assessment of the arterial and venous anatomy of the lesion, enabling the operator to avoid injury to vessels.

CT-guided stereotactic interstitial brachytherapy

Stereotactic CT techniques have extended the application of the implantation of radioactive sources into malignant, unresectable intra-axial brain tumours. Optimal application of this method of treatment requires careful preoperative planning, computer assisted dosimetry, and CT-guided stereotactic implantation of the isotope-bearing catheters. The technique can be used combining available CT software with a standard radiotherapy treatment planning computer and the Brown–Roberts–Wells stereotactic system. The method

combines preoperative imaging of tumour position and volume, dosimetry planning and brachytherapy catheter insertion (Maruyama et al 1984, Coffey & Friedman 1987). The dosimetry of radioactive phosphorus (^{32}P) for intracavitary treatment of cystic brain tumours is dependent on the accurate determination of the cyst volume which can be obtained by high resolution CT using standard software. Advances in imaging and the use of stereotactic techniques in interstitial brachytherapy or in combination with teletherapy may improve survival. Current use of these techniques should be limited to centres with both stereotactic and radiotherapeutic expertise where the risks and benefits can be investigated.

CT-guided stereotactic surgery

This method permits precise resection of certain deep-seated intracerebral neoplasms. After the tumour volume has been reconstructed from either CT or MR data, a computer-monitored, stereotactically directed CO_2 laser is used to vaporize the intracerebral tumour. The system provides safe surgical control in three dimensions for the resection of substantial amounts (as assessed by postoperative (CT) of intra-axial neoplasms (Kelly et al 1986). This is a promising new approach to intracranial lesions.

POSTOPERATIVE CHANGES

Early changes

CT scans performed in the early postoperative period following excision of an intra-axial tumour show enhancement at the margins of the tumour bed. This enhancement may occur as early as one week postoperative and may be seen at three months, gradually diminishing in intensity on serial CT scans. It is due to the disruption of the blood–brain barrier by the surgical excision and is difficult to differentiate from residual tumour, abscess, resolving haematoma or infarct. It may be seen at the surgical site after removal of a non-enhancing tumour. Early postoperative scans are an unreliable indicator of residual tumour volume but are useful for demonstrating the beneficial effects of surgery on hydrocephalus and midline displacement and for detecting complications of surgery. Surgical intervention may also cause oedema which will diminish over the ensuing few weeks. On the other hand, tumoural enhancement and peritumoural oedema associated with residual tumour will tend to increase over a period of weeks.

Late changes

The CT appearances depend on the completeness of the surgical excision and may be modified by changes induced by radiotherapy or chemotherapy. Serial examinations are required for accurate assessment and a baseline examination can be performed 1–3 months after treatment to serve as a guide for monitoring further changes. Serial CT over a period of 6–18 months will allow assessment of success of the surgical resection of a tumour. Tumour mass, associated oedema and intensity of enhancement are prognostic CT indicators after surgery for malignant glioma, the length of survival being inversely related to the amount of residual tumour, degree of postoperative oedema and intensity of enhancement (Andreou et al 1983).

POSTRADIOTHERAPY CHANGES

Early and late effects are recognized (Sheline 1980). CT performed during the course of therapy may show cerebral oedema which will respond to corticosteroids. A few weeks to months after therapy, CT may show dilated ventricles, fissures and sulci and a slight decrease in the attenuation of the white matter. These latter changes probably result from demyelination, and may be transient and reversible.

Abnormal CT scans are seen in a high proportion of long term survivors (2–10 years) following therapeutic or prophylactic cranial irradiation. CT shows progressive dilatation of the ventricles and subarachnoid spaces up to eight years after cessation of therapy. The CT abnormalities do not correlate with neurological or neuropsychological testing, and may be reversible; a normal cortex has been demonstrated at autopsy (Wang et al 1983).

White matter low density changes may be seen in normal brains postradiotherapy but may also be due to multifocal necrosis and progressive multifocal leukoencephalopathy.

Radiation necrosis, which may occur as a late complication, is sometimes progressive, often irreversible and dose-related. This is due to vascular changes and is more severe in the white matter. The CT scan shows deep, focal, low attenuation mass lesions in or near the irradiated tumour bed, but still within the radiation field. These lesions may show ring enhancement and cannot be differentiated from recurrent tumour, which may or may not be present within the zone of radiation necrosis. Rarely, surgery may be required to substantiate the nature of an enhancing lesion.

Mineralizing microangiopathy occurs following cranial irradiation and methotrexate chemotherapy and is seen in 25–30% of children with acute lymphoblastic leukaemia who have received either therapeutic or prophylactic cranial irradiation and methotrexate. CT characteristically shows bilateral, frequently symmetrical cortico-medullary

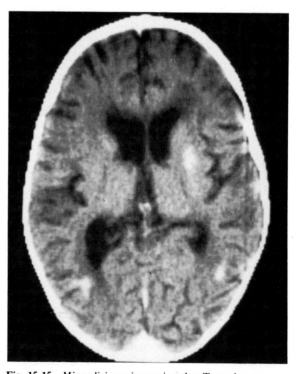

Fig. 15.15 Mineralizing microangiopathy. Treated acute lymphoblastic leukaemia: note enlarged sulci and ventricles with multifocal areas of calcification in the basal ganglia and at the cortico-medullary junction.

junction calcification and basal ganglia calcification. Mild dilatation of the ventricles and extracerebral CSF spaces accompanies these changes (Fig. 15.15). Although the three factors radiotherapy, chemotherapy and raised intracranial pressure probably have a synergistic rôle in the pathogenesis, it is believed that the methotrexate triggers the changes which are induced by the radiotherapy.

Necrotizing leukoencephalopathy is a less common but more serious complication seen in less than 10% of children with acute lymphoblastic leukaemia. This is characterized by demyelination, necrosis and gliosis. CT appearances are of bilateral diffuse or focal low attenuation changes in the periventricular white matter. A significant mass effect is uncommon and enhancement, which may be patchy or ring-like, is variable and may be confused with tumour recurrence. A combination of areas of decreased attenuation and severe atrophy carries a poor prognosis in these cases.

CT findings in long term survivors

Favourable CT signs in a patient with low grade astrocytoma surviving for ten years or more are loss of tumour bulk, the presence of a smooth-walled, non-enhancing porencephalic cavity replacing the original tumour, white matter low attenuation changes with no enhancement and signs of focal atrophy. Calcification may be present either within or adjacent to the irradiated tumour.

Residual tumour of less than 45 mm diameter on postoperative CT scan is associated with a 70% probability of long term survival, therefore radical surgical management of glioma should be undertaken where possible. Younger patients are more likely than older patients to attain long term survival.

COMPLICATIONS OF TREATMENT

CT has a major rôle to play in detecting important complications of treatment. Subdural hygromas occur frequently following excision of tumours of the posterior fossa and may be seen in the supratentorial compartment following tumour resection. These hygromas have a characteristic configuration and are of CSF density. Hygromas occurring in the supratentorial compartment may be associated with supra- and infratentorial tumours whilst hygromas occurring in the posterior fossa are not associated with supratentorial lesions. CT scanning will detect infected subdural hygromas (empyemas) by demonstrating enhancement of the rim and an associated mass effect. Intracranial haemorrhage, both parenchymal and subarachnoid, complicating treatment and cerebral infarction occurring secondary to malignancy and radiotherapy will be detected by CT. Furthermore, changes induced by radiotherapy will also be detected.

CRITERIA FOR TUMOUR RECURRENCE

The presence of areas of abnormal attenuation with or without enhancement, associated mass effect and oedema constitutes positive evidence of tumour recurrence in an appropriate clinical situation (Fig. 15.16). The demonstration of intraventricular or meningeal metastases is further evidence of tumour recurrence. Hydrocephalus and focal sulcal obliteration are secondary signs produced by the mass effect but may be present without an attenuation or enhancing abnormality. In the cases of tumours of the posterior fossa, CT has a high specificity for detecting recurrent medulloblastomas and astrocytomas in childhood.

It has been suggested that CT may be used to estimate the doubling time of recurrent tumours by analysing the volume of enhanced and unenhanced areas using the standard CT software and serial CT scans. In the author's view this is of limited value.

THE RÔLE OF SERIAL CT

Serial CT has a rôle to play in the following situations:

1. In the differentiation of a low attenuation tumour from an area of recent infarction or of cerebritis/abscess and tumour from oedema. In the latter, serial CT following corticosteroid administration may demonstrate a progressive increase in the attenuation values of the white matter corresponding to a decrease in the oedema and allowing earlier visualization of the mass lesion.

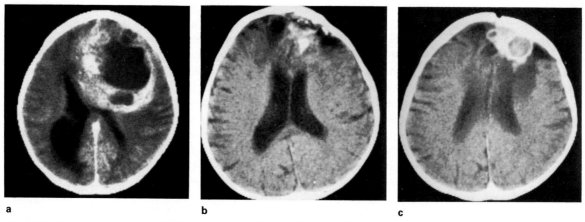

Fig. 15.16 Juvenile astrocytoma. (a) Pretreatment examination. Very large heterogeneously enhancing mass with severe ventricular compression and displacement. (b) Nine months following subtotal removal and radiotherapy. Unenhanced scan shows focal atrophy in the right frontal region with calcification at the site of the tumour. (c) The same patient: recurrent tumour. Enhanced scan shows irregular ring enhancement and mass effect.

2. In the identification of a biopsy site when the initial CT appearances were equivocal or where the age and clinical condition of the patient was a relative contraindication to biopsy at presentation.

3. In early diagnosis, where there is
   (a) a high clinical suspicion of a tumour or EEG abnormality and a normal CT scan. Serial scanning at three or six-monthly intervals is required. The optimum period for rescanning is not known and will depend on the clinical condition and the suspected histology.
   (b) an equivocal CT. Successful diagnosis depends on early investigation with CT and repeat CT where there is a high clinical suspicion of tumour. Successful early diagnosis may be limited by the small size of a tumour, an isodense tumour showing minimal mass effect and no enhancement and by the appearance of non-specific changes which may be confused with demyelination and infarction.

In both instances, MR scanning may provide more specific information and should be performed before the follow-up CT scan.

4. In the preoperative assessment to evaluate the secondary effects of the tumour on the ventricular system or on the adjacent normal tissues. A clinically 'silent' lesion in the dominant hemisphere may be kept under observation on serial CT to detect complications such as hydrocephalus or compression, providing the indication for operative/radiotherapeutic intervention.

5. In the detection of early and late post-treatment changes and complications.

6. In the detection of recurrent tumour.

7. To monitor suspected but unconfirmed tumours e.g. grade I astrocytoma in the dominant hemisphere. Surgery may be deferred if the CT signs are static. Changes may lead to earlier treatment.

8. To monitor known tumours. This includes inoperable tumours, tumours previously treated with radiotherapy, treatment of the oedema accompanying tumours, partially operated tumours and following shunt procedures.

TUMOURS OF THE SPINAL CORD, NERVE ROOTS AND MENINGES

Tumours of the spinal cord and its membranes are similar in type to those found in the cranial cavity. 50% of the neoplasms affecting the spinal cord arise from its enveloping structures and are about equally divided between meningiomas and neurinomas: gliomas only account for about 10%

(Taveras & Wood 1976). Involvement of the spinal cord by metastatic tumours occurs more frequently than cerebral metastases. Metastases to the spinal cord are usually epidural and rarely extend to the meninges to invade the spinal cord itself whereas intracranial metastases are invariably intracerebral. Two-thirds of all spinal metastases originate either in the lung or breasts.

Plain radiographic examinations have a more important rôle than that of CT in the initial diagnosis of primary and secondary tumours of the spinal column, meninges and contained neural tissue.

CT has a complementary rôle in defining the tumour morphology and local effects of the tumour and is usually combined with myelography (myelo-CT) to study more precisely the features of the tumour at the level of the myelographic block.

Primary spinal tumours produce characteristic changes in approximately 15% of cases. The three cardinal radiographic features are:

1. Enlargement of the vertebral canal as manifested by flattening or concavity of the pedicles, increased interpeduncular distance and scalloping of the posterior margins of the vertebral body and thinning of the laminae.
2. Enlargement of the intervertebral foramen in the case of dumb-bell shaped tumours.
3. Calcification within the tumour.

Intraspinal metastases produce either osteolytic or osteoblastic changes in the adjacent vertebrae. A paraspinal shadow may result from retropleural tumour.

Myelography using non-ionic water soluble contrast media is the definitive technique for localizing the site of a compressive lesion. Combined ascending and descending techniques may be required for assessing the upper and lower limits of a myelographic block and for determining the number of lesions present.

Intramedullary tumours e.g. glioma and ependymoma characteristically expand the spinal cord and produce partial or complete obstruction to the flow of contrast medium. Ependymomas comprise 70% of gliomas and originate most frequently in the conus medullaris. The tumour may extend along the filum terminale and in some cases may fill the lumbar canal throughout its entire length. Intradural, extramedullary tumours e.g. neurofibroma and meningioma produce typical findings of a sharply defined filling defect produced by the tumour which displaces and compresses the spinal cord. An extradural mass e.g. metastasis is characterized by narrowing of the contrast column as it reaches the widest portion of the tumour.

The rôle of CT

CT provides additional information regarding the soft tissue component of tumours. In bony spinal metastatic disease CT has an important rôle in showing the extension of the soft tissue mass into the spinal canal and the extent of involvement of the posterior elements. Myelo-CT may be required in cases of myelographic block to show the degree of cord compression.

CT may show specific tissue components of a tumour, e.g. fat in dermoids and calcification in meningiomas, which may not be apparent from plain radiographs or conventional myelography. Lack of tissue characterization is a serious disadvantage of CT in the evaluation of intraspinal neoplastic disease unless fat (e.g. dermoids) or calcification is present. Enhancement of the CSF using water soluble contrast medium is therefore frequently required to differentiate abnormal tissue from normal compressed tissue. The use of CT is further restricted by its inability to demonstrate the length of a long segment block unless an extensive examination is performed. CT is, therefore, confined to the level of the block and the use of high resolution thin sections and reconstructed images in additional planes will provide additional information regarding the morphology of the tumour, the extent of the soft tissue component and the localized effects on the adjacent axial skeleton (Tadmor et al 1983). Plain CT is valuable for identifying the presence and extent of vertebral metastases, as well as the presence of benign disease in cancer patients by examining isotope bone scan positive lesions (Redmond et al 1984).

MRI has a definite advantage over CT in its non-invasiveness and significantly in its ability to examine the spine in multiple planes, particularly in the sagittal plane permitting accurate visualization of the longitudinal extent of intra/extradural tumours and their effects on adjacent structures, paraspinal soft tissue extension and vascular involvement. CT without contrast medium is superior to MRI in showing cortical bone destruction and calcified tumour matrix (Beltran et al 1987).

REFERENCES

Albright A L, James H E 1985 Neurosurgical staging of midline intra-axial (nuclear) tumours. Cancer 56 (suppl 7): 1786–1788

Andreou J, George A E, Wise A, deLeon M, Kricheff I I, Ransohoff J, Foosh T 1983 CT prognostic criteria of survival after malignant glioma surgery. American Journal of Neuroradiology 4(3): 488–490

Asakura T, Uetsuhara K, Kanemaru R, Hirahara K 1985 An applicability study on a CT-guided stereotactic technique for functional neurosurgery. Applied Neurophysiology 48(1–6): 73–76

Baker H L, Houser O W, Campbell J K 1980 National Cancer Institute Study: evaluation of computed tomography in the diagnosis of intracranial neoplasms. I. Overall results. Radiology 136: 91–96

Beltran J, Noto A M, Chakeres D W, Christoforidis A J 1987 Tumours of the osseous spine: staging with MR imaging versus CT. Radiology 162(2): 565–569

Boethuis J, Collins V P, Edner G, Lewander R, Zajicek J 1978 Stereotactic biopsies and computer tomography in gliomas. Acta Neurochirurgica 40: 223–232

Bolender N F, Cromwell L D, Graves V, Margolis M T, Kerber C W, Wendling L 1983 Interval appearance of glioblastomas not evident in previous CT examinations. Journal of Computer Assisted Tomography 7(4): 599–603

Bullard D E, Nashold B S, Osborne D et al 1983 Experience using two CT-guided stereotactic biopsy methods. Applied Neurophysiology 46(1–4): 188–192

Cellerier P, Chiras J, Gray F, Metzger J, Bories J 1984 Computed tomography in primary lymphoma of the brain. Neuroradiology 26(6): 485–92

Chernow B, Buck D R, Early C B, Ray J, O'Brian J T 1982 Rapid shrinkage of a prolactin-secreting pituitary tumour with bromocriptine: CT documentation. American Journal of Neuroradiology 3: 442–443

Coffey R J, Friedman W A 1987 Interstitial brachytherapy of malignant brain tumours using computed tomography-guided stereotaxis and available imaging software: technical report. Neurosurgery 20(1): 4–7

Cusick J F, Haughton V M, Hagen T C 1980 Radiological assessment of intrasellar prolactin-secreting tumours. Neurosurgery 6: 376–379

Davis D O 1977 CT in the diagnosis of supratentorial neoplasms. Seminars in Roentgenology 12: 97–108

Gentry L R, Jacoby C G, Turski P A, Houston L W, Strother C M, Sackett J F 1987 Cerebello-pontine angle-petromastoid mass lesions; comparative study of diagnosis with MR imaging and CT. Radiology 162(2): 513–520

Gillespie J E, Adams J E, Isherwood I 1987 Three dimensional computed tomographic reformations of sellar and parasellar lesions. Neuroradiology 29: 30–35

Gooding G A, Boggan J E, Weinstein P R 1984 Characterisation of intracranial neoplasms by CT and intra-operative sonography. American Journal of Neuroradiology 5(5): 517–520

Gouda K I, Freidberg S R, Larsen C R, Baker R A, Silverman M L 1983 Modification of the Gouda frame to allow stereotactic biopsy of the brain using the GE8800 computed tomographic scanner. Neurosurgery 13(2): 176–181

Haynor D R, Borning A W, Griffin B A, Jacky J P, Kalet I J, Shuman W P 1986 Radiotherapy planning: direct tumour location on simulation and portfilms using CT. Part I: Principles. Radiology 158(2): 537–540

Hieshima G B, Everhart F R, Mehringer C M et al 1980 Pre-operative embolisation of meningiomas. Surgical Neurology 14: 119–127

Holtas S, Nyman U, Cronqvist S 1984 Computed tomography of malignant lymphoma of the brain. Neuroradiology 26(1): 33–38

Kelly P J, Earnest F, Kall B A, Goerss S J, Scheithauer B 1985 Surgical options for patients with deep-seated brain tumours: computer assisted stereotactic biopsy. Mayo Clinic Proceedings 60(4): 223–229

Kelly P J, Kall B A, Goerss S, Cascino T L 1986 Results of computer assisted stereotactic laser resection of deep-seated intracranial lesions. Mayo Clinic Proceedings 61(1): 20–27

Kingsley D P, Harwood-Nash D C 1984 Parameters of infiltration in posterior fossa tumours of childhood using a high resolution CT scanner. Neuroradiology 26(5): 347–350

Kricheff I I, Pinto R S, Bergeron R T, Cohen N 1980 Air-CT cisternography and canalography for small acoustic neuromas. American Journal of Neuroradiology 1: 57–63

Leeds N E, Elkin C M, Zimmerman R D 1984 Gliomas of the brain. Seminars in Roentgenology 19(1): 27–43

Levitt L J, Dawson D M, Rosenthal D S, Moloney W C 1980 CNS involvement in the non-Hodgkin's lymphomas. Cancer 45: 545–552

Lunsford L D, Parrish R, Albright L 1984 Intra-operative imaging with a therapeutic computed tomographic scanner. Neurosurgery 15(4): 559–561

Maruyama Y, Chin H W, Young A B et al 1984 CT and MR for brain tumour implant therapy using CF–252 neutrons. Journal of Neuro-oncology 2(4): 349–360

Miller J H, Pena A M, Segall H D 1980 Radiological investigation of sellar region masses in children. Radiology 134: 81–87

Naidich T P, Lin J P, Leeds N E, Pudlowski R M, Naidich J B 1977 Primary tumours and other masses of the cerebellum and fourth ventricle: differential diagnosis by computed tomography. Neuroradiology 14: 153–174

Naidich T P, Tomita T, Pech P, Haughton V 1985 Direct coronal computed tomography for presurgical evaluation of posterior fossa tumours. Journal of Computer Assisted Tomography 9(6): 1065–1072

Nauta H J, Guinto F C Jr, Pisharodi M 1984 Arterial bolus contrast medium enhancement for computed tomographically guided stereotactic biopsy. Surgical Neurology 22(6): 559–564

North C, Segall H D, Stanley P, Zee C S, Ahmadi J, McComb J G 1985 Early CT detection of intracranial seeding from medulloblastoma. American Journal of Neuroradiology 6(1): 11–13

Pagani J J, Libshitz H I, Wallace S, Hayman L A 1981 Central nervous system leukaemia and lymphoma: computed tomographic manifestations. American Journal of Radiology 137(6): 1195–1201

Redmond J, Spring D B, Munderloh S H, George C B, Mansour R P, Volk S A 1984 Spinal computed tomographic scanning in the evaluation of metastatic disease. Cancer 54(2): 253–258

Sheline G E 1980 Irradiation injury of the human brain: a review of clinical experience. In: Gilbert H A, Kagan A R (eds) Radiation damage to the nervous system. Raven Press, New York

Tadmor R, Davis K, Roberson G H, Kleinman G M 1978 Computed tomography in primary malignant lymphoma of the brain. Journal of Computer Assisted Tomography 2: 135–140

Tadmor R, Cacayorin E D, Kieffer S A 1983 Advantages of supplementary CT in myelography of intraspinal masses. American Journal of Neuroradiology 4(3): 618–621

Tarver R D, Richmond B D, Klatte E C 1984 Cerebral metastases from lung carcinoma: neurological and CT correlation. Work in progress. Radiology 153(3): 689–692

Taveras J M, Wood E H 1976 Part VII Diseases of the spinal cord. In: Diagnostic radiology, 2nd edn, vol 2, Williams & Wilkins, Baltimore, pp 1091–1251

Vonfakos D, Marcus H, Hacker H 1979 Oligodendrogliomas: CT patterns with emphasis on features indicating malignancy. Journal of Computer Assisted Tomography 3: 783–788

Walker R, Lieberman A N, Pinto R et al 1983 Transient neurologic disturbances, brain tumours and normal computed tomography scans. Cancer 52(8): 1502–1506

Wang A M, Skias D D, Rumbaugh C L, Schoene W C, Zamani A 1983 Central nervous system changes after radiation therapy and/or chemotherapy: correlation of CT and autopsy findings. American Journal of Neuroradiology 4(3): 466–471

Weisberg L A 1984 Clinical and computed tomographic correlations of pineal neoplasms. Computerized Radiology 8(5): 285–92

Williams A L 1985 Chapter 5: Tumours. In: Williams A L, Haughton V M (eds) Cranial computed tomography: a comprehensive text. C V Mosby, St Louis

Zimmerman R A, Bilaniuk L T, Wood J H, Bruce D A, Schut L 1980 Computed tomography of pineal, parapineal and histologically related tumours. Radiology 137: 669–677

16. The head and neck

W. D. Jeans

INTRODUCTION

The extracranial tissues of the head and neck considered here are the paranasal sinuses, nose, mouth, nasopharynx, larynx and pharynx, together with the base of the skull, salivary glands, cervical soft tissues, eye and ear. Radiological investigation of these tissues is generally by plain film radiography, followed when necessary by CT scanning or by conventional tomography if CT is not available. CT has been almost as useful in the extracranial region as within the head and has increased diagnostic accuracy significantly (Gatenby et al 1985). Magnetic resonance imaging (MRI) is more useful than CT scans if soft tissues alone are being examined, as in the soft tissues of the neck, but does not show early bone lesions in the detail required in lesions of the sinuses (Glazer et al 1986). Isotope imaging is of use in suspected bone lesions not visible on plain radiographs in this area, and angiography is useful only for benign lesions not considered here, and for the exclusion of vascular lesions in proptosis. Ultrasound has little part to play, apart from investigation of the eye. Interventional procedures are used to obtain fine needle aspiration biopsy specimens. Arterial infusions of cytotoxic agents have been used with limited success, although methotrexate given intravenously appears to act synchronously with irradiation to give improved survival rates (Pointon et al 1983).

Radiology is of help in the management of lesions in this area at three points in the progression of disease. Initially, the diagnosis is made, and possible differential diagnoses are considered. Secondly, the extent of the lesion is estimated since this influences the method of treatment, and lastly changes seen after treatment or during recurrence may be shown. The use of a standardized approach to initial investigation is commended (Eddleston 1980) and this allows later comparative assessment of patients. Radiography, normal anatomy and variations are not specifically discussed here, and can be found in textbooks covering the area (Bergeron et al 1984, Jeans 1984, Samuel & Lloyd 1978).

THE PARANASAL SINUSES

Incidence and presentation

Tumours of the sinuses are relatively rare in the UK, with about 370 new cases being registered annually in England and Wales under the International Classification of Diseases Code 160, which includes the nose as well as the sinuses. The incidence in males and females is almost the same at 0.8 and 0.7 cases/100 000 of the population, and there is no particular regional variation. Two aetiological factors have been described: nickel refining workers were found to have an increased incidence of carcinoma of the sinuses and of the bronchus which disappeared when the manufacturing process was changed (Doll 1967), and hard wood workers have also been found to have an increased incidence of sinus cancer (Acheson et al 1967). The tumours occur mainly in those aged 65 and over.

Symptoms depend on the primary site of the tumour, and the direction in which it has spread. The majority of tumours occur in the antra, followed in frequency by the antro-ethmoid angle, ethmoids, frontal sinus and sphenoid. Spread of tumour to the nose will cause nasal obstruction with a blood stained discharge: extension to the orbit may produce proptosis or displacement of the eye. Downwards extension from the antrum may produce dental symptoms or a mass in the roof of the mouth, whilst forward extension will cause swelling over the face. Frontal sinus tumours present with swelling over the forehead or with orbital symptoms. Sphenoid sinus tumours are very rare in the UK and because of their central situation present late, with pituitary or nasopharyngeal symptoms.

Pathology, site and spread

The majority of tumours of the sinuses are malignant and 80% of these are carcinomas, mostly squamous cell, with transitional cell, anaplastic and adenocarcinomas also occurring (Friedmann & Osborn 1976). A second form of adenocarcinoma is also seen in the antrum, and is sometimes known as a cylindroma. Lymphosarcomas, other sarcomas, plasmacytomas, melanomas and metastases may occur, and direct spread may occur from tumours in adjacent areas. Other destructive lesions which may cause radiological, clinical and sometimes pathological difficulty in diagnosis are osteomyelitis secondary to sinus infection, infection with aspergillosis being particularly destructive, muco- and pyo-coeles, and granulomata. These include those of unknown cause as with the Wegener's and necrotizing type, the infective granulomas which occur after surgery, and sarcoid.

Spread is by local invasion, and late in the disease by lymphatic spread to cervical glands and by haematogenous spread to the lung parenchyma.

Staging

The size of lesions within the sinuses and the extent of spread through the walls can only be determined by radiological methods prior to operation (Harrison 1978). No standard International Union against Cancer TNM classification is yet available (Harmer 1978) and a variety of methods are used. These can be standardized and compared using a computerized input, and this approach may give more information concerning the critical difference in prognosis related to stage

and treatment (Morton et al 1985). The essential points are that the prognosis for tumours of the antrum is worse when they are situated in the upper and in the posterior part of the cavity, presumably because spread may be greater before symptoms occur, and that retrospective staging is inaccurate and results in a greater number of 'unstaged' tumours.

80% of tumours of the sinuses are in the antrum and the following discussion refers to these. It is generally agreed that T1 tumours are those confined to the antrum – it is unusual to find tumours at this stage. T2 tumours are those which have spread through the wall medially, laterally or inferiorly: spread in other directions may cause an increase in stage in some classifications and not others. T3 and T4 lesions involve spread into the ethmoids, the orbit, the skin of the cheek, the pterygoid plates, pterygo-palatine fossa, base of the skull, nasopharynx and up into the cribriform plate, sphenoid sinus and cranial fossa. Extension into glands of the neck (N1–3) is late in the disease, and distant metastasis (M1+) is also rare and occurs late.

Radiology

Primary investigation is by plain radiography using occipito-mental, occipito-frontal, lateral and submento-vertical views (Bryan 1987). If the radiographs are normal no further investigation is usually needed, but if an abnormality is present in a patient with a history suggestive of a tumour (Fig. 16.1), further investigation will be required. Some radiologists prefer stereoscopic films of the occipito-mental and submento-vertical projections to demonstrate bone erosion and destruction (Eddleston & Johnson 1983). Linear or pluri-directional tomography will demonstrate bone lesions in more detail and reveal lesions hidden by overlying bone. If CT is available it should be performed using transverse axial sections (Fig. 16.2), initially without contrast medium since this does not help in T1 or 2 tumours (Forbes et al 1978). Its great advantage is that it shows soft tissues well (Hasso 1984) and there is little point in doing conventional tomography as well, since CT usually demonstrates the lesion better, occasionally resulting in staging being advanced (Jeans et al 1982),

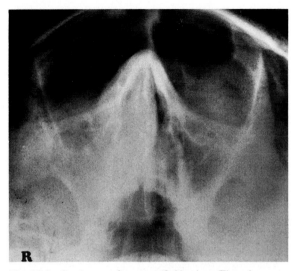

Fig. 16.1 Carcinoma of antrum, O.M. view. There is irregular opacification of the right antrum and the adjacent nasal cavity, in a patient with a bloodstained nasal discharge.

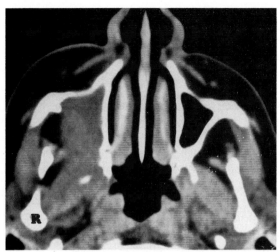

Fig. 16.2 Carcinoma of antrum, axial CT section. A soft tissue density extends postero-laterally on the right to become continuous with the lateral pterygoid muscle. There is loss of the postero-lateral antral wall and the lateral pterygoid plate.

and gives a better estimate of possible resectability (Lund et al 1983). In a small proportion of cases coronal CT sections will be needed to assess bone lying in the plane of the horizontal sections and high lesions close to the frontal fossa or involving the orbits. In the latter case contrast medium will

be needed to show possible intracranial spread (Fig. 16.3). It is preferable to do coronal sections directly rather than by reconstruction whenever possible.

In early lesions the antrum may show irregular opacification, but this is unusual. More often there

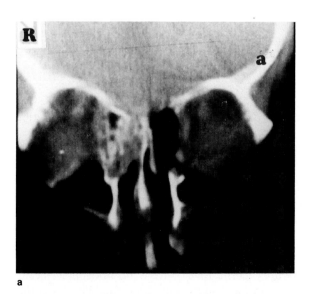

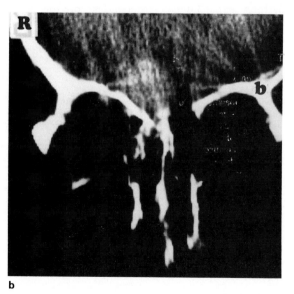

Fig. 16.3 Ethmoidal carcinoma, coronal sections before (a) and after (b) contrast medium. A soft tissue mass is shown in the right ethmoid. After contrast medium, enhancement is seen in the anterior cranial fossa adjacent to the mass, indicating a breach of the blood–brain barrier.

is irregular destruction of bone with a soft tissue mass extending into the nasal cavity or laterally (Table 16.1). One side of the atlas may be abnormally clearly seen on an occipito-frontal view when there is destruction of the alveolar bone (Kolbenstvedt et al 1985), and this observation makes the point that a mass causing bone thinning and destruction may result in other structures in the line of the primary beam being seen more clearly than usual. In both conventional and computerized tomography there may be apparent loss of bone radiologically which is not confirmed at surgery, when soft tissue is seen on both sides of a thin bony plate. This may be due to loss of contrast or to bone resorption and is seen both in tumours and in inflammatory disease.

The association of an opaque sinus, bone destruction and an adjacent soft tissue mass means that the patient has almost certainly got a carcinoma of the antrum, and a biopsy should be performed. The same appearances may also be caused by other malignant lesions listed in the section on pathology, and by granulomata. Changes seen in bone on CT should be treated with caution, since demineralization from chronic infection may cause apparent radiological bone loss in an area which appears normal at operation. MRI scans show a soft tissue mass and may show areas of high signal intensity (dependent on the pulse

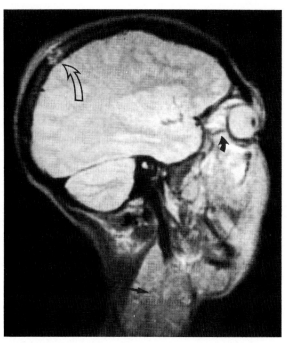

Fig. 16.4 Carcinoma of antrum and metastases, sagittal MRI section through right antrum. High signal intensity is shown from a tumour in the right antrum, extending posteriorly into the pterygoid region and upwards into the orbit (curved black arrow). Enlarged lymph nodes are seen in the neck (arrow), and a metastasis is seen in the vault (hollow arrow). (Spin echo SE 2000/80, reproduced by courtesy of Dr A. Leung of Mount Vernon Hospital.)

Table 16.1 Radiological signs in carcinoma of the antrum

Radiographs
Irregular soft tissue mass in antrum
Complete opacification of antrum (present in two-thirds)
Increase in size of inferior turbinate, together with antral mass
Soft tissue mass in nose or cheek
Partial loss of normal bony outline, adjacent to soft tissue mass
Irregular translucencies in bone, adjacent to soft tissue mass
Sclerosis of bone — rare and may only follow Caldwell–Luc
  operation

CT
Above signs together with:
Loss of low density area next to postero-lateral wall of antrum
Soft tissue mass extending out from antrum
Proptosis
Mass in orbit or cranial fossa continuous with mass in sinus
Enhancement of mass if blood–brain barrier breached

MRI
Soft tissue mass
Increase in signal intensity at site of tumour and metastases,
  depending on pulse sequences

sequences) both from the primary tumour and from metastases (Fig. 16.4).

The same signs are seen in tumours affecting the other sinuses. Those starting in the antro-ethmoidal angle have a soft tissue mass extending downwards into the antrum, so that the inferior part of the antrum may appear normal. There is bone destruction in the ethmoidal region and in the adjacent orbital margins, and it is in these tumours that coronal sections are needed to assess upwards spread. Contrast medium must be given to assess intracranial extension since this may not be visible on the plain scans, as shown in Figure 16.3. In the frontal sinus, extension into bone is seen as loss of the normal lamina dura of the sinus, with a permeative pattern of ill-defined lucent areas in the frontal bone. Radiologically this is the same appearance as that of osteomyelitis of the frontal bone.

Treatment

Treatment may be by surgery only in T1 lesions, by radiotherapy only in T3 lesions, or by a combination of the two in most patients (Hordijk & Brons 1985). The overall 5-year survival rate is 51%, with none of those patients having cervical nodes at presentation surviving. Occasionally T1 tumours may be removed at an initial excision biopsy, and the only signs then are of the lateral rhinotomy. Following radiotherapy, oedema or granuloma formation of the mucosa may be seen, and there is no radiological method of distinguishing this from recurrence. In patients with recurrence there may be a soft tissue density within the remaining antrum (Fig. 16.5), and later this increases and there is progressive bone destruction. It is useful to be able to recognize that a Caldwell–Luc procedure has been carried out, as it has in this patient, by the increase in thickness of the postero-lateral antral wall, partially absent medial wall and reduced antral volume, sometimes with inward bowing of the antero-lateral wall (Cable et al 1981).

THE NOSE

Tumours are most often squamous carcinomas, with malignant melanomas occurring second in order of frequency. These present with epistaxis, nasal obstruction, pain and swelling (Freedman et al 1973). They may recur an unexpectedly long time after removal of the primary lesions and may invade the adjacent sinus, when it is impossible to say on radiological grounds where the site of origin has been (Fig. 16.6). Lymphoma and plasmacytoma (Castro et al 1973) may also occur in the nasal cavity (Fig. 16.7), and chondrosarcomas may develop in the nasal cartilages (Zizmor & Noyek 1978).

Inverted papillomas of the nose are uncommon benign tumours which may recur after surgery, and have a spectrum of appearances ranging from the simple polyp to definitely neoplastic epithelium. Radiologically, in inverted papillomas the plain films may be normal or in one-third of patients show mucosal thickening only. There may be opacification of the antra, and less often of the ethmoids or frontal sinuses, together with a mass in the nasal cavity. In some cases the mass may show calcification on CT, and may extend into the antrum showing bone destruction (Lund & Lloyd 1984). The differential diagnosis of the lesion may therefore be of sinus disease, an antro-choanal

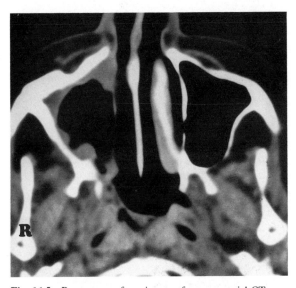

Fig. 16.5 Recurrence of carcinoma of antrum, axial CT scan. There is thickening of the postero-lateral wall and absence of the medial antro-lateral wall of the right antrum, indicative of previous surgery. Irregular soft tissue is seen adjacent to the remaining walls. Radiologically this cannot be distinguished from granulation tissue.

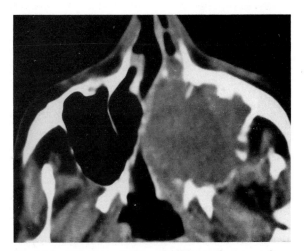

Fig. 16.6 Melanoma of nose, axial CT scan five years after removal of nasal melanoma. A soft tissue mass extends from the nose to the antrum, and is indistinguishable radiologically from an antral carcinoma.

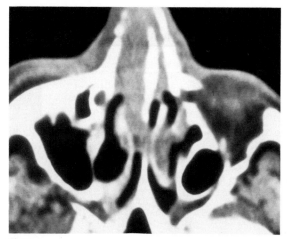

Fig. 16.7 Lymphoma of nose, axial CT scan. A soft tissue density is seen in the nasal cavity. The patient had no other evidence of lymphoma.

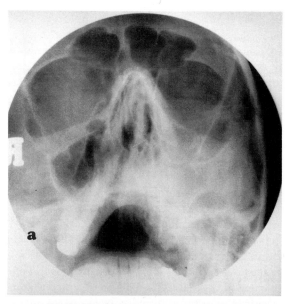

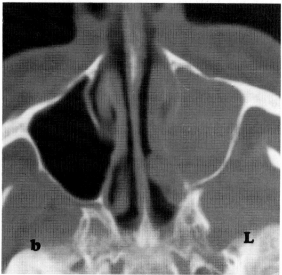

Fig. 16.8 Inverted papilloma, O.M. view (a) and axial CT section (b). A soft tissue mass is seen in the left antrum, extending into the adjacent nasal cavity. The medial wall of the antrum is thinned. This appearance may also be caused by a granuloma or a carcinoma.

polyp, or a carcinoma, depending on the signs present (Fig. 16.8). In all nasal tumours CT scans are needed to show the extent of the lesion before treatment; in order to show the nasal floor the scans should be in the coronal plane.

Treatment

Squamous carcinomas and plasmacytomas are generally treated by radiotherapy. Melanomas are treated by wide excision, but have a poor prognosis because they present late (Henk & Whittam 1982).

THE NASOPHARYNX AND RELATED REGIONS

Incidence and presentation

Tumours of the nasopharynx occur in the UK about half as frequently as those of the nose and sinuses. They are twice as common in males as in females and are seen in a wider age range, with anaplastic carcinomas sometimes occurring in patients in their twenties, and rhabdomyosarcomas being seen in young children. There is a marked racial variation, carcinomas of the nasopharynx accounting for 50% of all carcinomas in the Canton region of China. There is also an association with the Epstein–Barr virus, patients with nasopharyn-geal carcinomas often having high titres of antibody to the virus.

Presentation is most often with enlarged cervical lymph nodes or may be with nasal, auditory or neurological symptoms. Progressive cranial nerve involvement with altered sensation over the upper teeth and maxillary sinus, diplopia from VIth nerve involvement, and posterior spread affecting the IXth, Xth and XIth nerves may cause considerable difficulty in initial diagnosis. Investigation is indicated when typical lesions such as Bell's palsy or trigeminal neuralgia present atypically, or when progressive symptoms occur (Kalovidouris et al 1984).

Pathology and spread

The majority of nasopharyngeal tumours are malignant. Most are carcinomas and over 50% of these are anaplastic. Lymphomas, sarcomas, chordomas, myelomas and secondaries are also seen. Rhabdomyosarcomas may occur in small children. Any of the varieties of lymphoma may occur in the region, and difficulty in precise pathological diagnosis may be caused by the high proportion of lymphocytes often found in close relation to anaplastic carcinomas, and to their metastases (Friedmann & Osborn 1976). Antro-choanal polyps, juvenile angiofibromas and persistent adenoidal tissue may present with soft tissue masses in the nasopharynx in younger patients. Nasopharyngeal masses may also be caused by sellar tumours, sphenoid lesions and chordomas.

Tumour spread in the region may be local, along neurovascular bundles, or by lymphatics. Local spread is forwards into the pterygoid plates, pterygoid fossa, pterygo-maxillary fossa and infratemporal fossa, or upwards to the base of the skull and beyond, so that erosion of the petrous bone and even of the occipital condyle and lateral mass of the atlas may be seen. Lateral extension may occur into the Eustachian tube or levator palati muscle; into the parapharyngeal space and so to the carotid artery and jugular vein, with subsequent spread up to the cavernous sinus and the nerves lying there, or more posteriorly to the jugular canal and the nerves within it. Lymphatic spread is to the retropharyngeal, the upper deep cervical, jugulo-omohyoid, spinal accessory and inferior cervical glands.

Staging

Tumour confined to one area is T1. T2 tumours involve more than one site in the region of origin, and T3 lesions extend to the nasal cavity and/or the oropharynx. T4 lesions extend to the base of the skull and/or involve cranial nerves.

Radiology

Lateral and submento-vertical views are the only radiographs of any use in this area. We prefer lateral cephalometric films as giving a repeatable density at a standard magnification in a true lateral position. CT is preferred as the next investigation, although if it is not available conventional tomography and contrast nasopharyngography may be useful. Basal stereographic films can demonstrate the nasopharyngeal recess well, and can show early bone destruction in those patients with cervical glands from an unknown primary tumour. Magnetic resonance images may show a high signal intensity over the area of the tumour, depending on the pulse sequence.

On a lateral film a soft tissue mass is visible in about two-thirds of patients with symptoms suggestive of a nasopharyngeal mass. The most important sign is of a soft tissue density which is convex forwards arising from the postero-superior margin of the nasopharynx (Eller et al 1971). Normal adults have a forward concavity, with less soft tissue width in the roof than on the posterior wall, and any change in the shape or the proportions should be treated with suspicion in patients with symptoms (Fig. 16.9). Calcification may be present and when seen in association with a posterior mass and bone destruction in the region of the clivus is almost certainly due to a chordoma. Bone erosion may seen on the lateral view occasionally, but is more often seen on the submento-vertical view: two or three radiographs with slightly different angulations and centering points may be helpful, and bone erosion is often more obvious on submento-vertical films than on CT.

CT images should be interrogated and soft tissue and bone images produced. The soft tissue settings will show alterations in the normal outline of the air-filled nasopharynx, with rounding of the posterior angle and possible loss of the fat planes in the parapharyngeal area. If this sign is present contrast enhancement is needed to outline the vessels. Care should be taken in interpreting alterations in shape since there is often variable

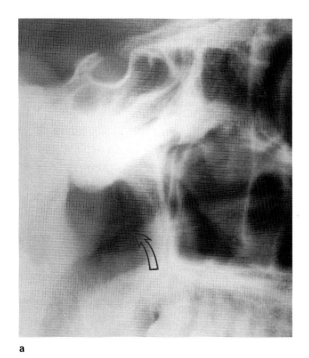

a

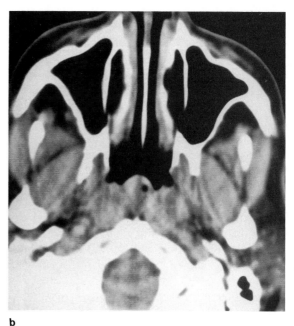

b

Fig. 16.9   Carcinoma of the nasopharynx, lateral film (a) and axial CT (b). A soft tissue mass with a forward convexity is seen in the posterior nasopharynx (arrow). On the axial view the soft tissues are symmetrical but much thicker than normal, reaching anteriorly to the Eustachian tube. The patient was a male aged 37, and at this age the shape is highly likely to be due to a tumour.

asymmetry in the shape of the nasopharynx depending on posture and relaxation of the musculature. Involvement of the mandibular branch of the Vth nerve will result in atrophy of the masticatory muscles (Silver et al 1983). Soft tissue parapharyngeal abnormalities should be investigated by MRI when this is available since it shows the tumour in three planes, demonstrates vessels without the use of contrast medium, and gives a better demonstration of soft tissue involvement of the base of the skull (Fig. 16.10) (Lloyd & Phelps 1986).

It may be surprisingly difficult to obtain a positive biopsy in a patient with a suspected nasopharyngeal tumour if the mucosa is intact, and CT may be very useful in indicating the site and depth from which the biopsy should be taken. Bone destruction in the base of the skull (Fig. 16.11) when present should be scanned during contrast infusion, and also if possible in the coronal plane. A chest X-ray should be taken since bone destruction could be from a primary

bronchial carcinoma, or a pulmonary metastasis may be present from a primary nasopharyngeal tumour. Distant metastases may be seen in bone or soft tissues as well as in the lung (Ghaffarian & Alaghehband 1980). Lesions affecting the skull base may be due to intracranial lesions growing downwards, intraosseous lesions, or infracranial lesions growing upwards (Whelan et al 1984) and the intracranial region should be examined carefully when destruction of the skull base is found.

Treatment

This is generally by radiotherapy, with block dissection of the neck for removal of spread to lymph nodes. The overall survival rate is in the region of 35% at 3 years, and there is a suggestion that chemotherapy using cisplatin may improve this (Khoury & Paterson 1987). The normal nasopharyngeal shape may remain distorted after radiotherapy, and biopsy will be needed to decide

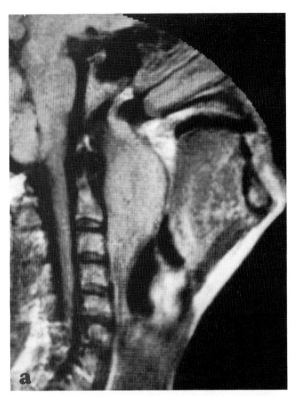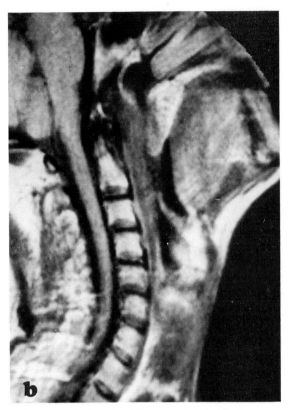

Fig. 16.10 Carcinoma of nasopharynx, before (a) and after (b) radiotherapy, sagittal section MRI scans. A high signal intensity mass is seen displacing the soft palate forwards. After treatment this has gone, leaving a poorly defined anterior border to the posterior soft tissues. (Spin echo SE 1100/40 images, reproduced by courtesy of Dr A. Leung of Mount Vernon Hospital.)

if there is recurrence should fresh symptoms occur (Fig. 16.12).

MOUTH, OROPHARYNX, SALIVARY GLANDS AND NECK

Incidence and presentation

Oral cancers account for some 2% of all malignant tumours in the UK; there has been a steady decline in the numbers found in males over the last four decades.

Presentation of intra-oral tumours is usually with a mass, which in the tongue is often on the lateral border of its middle third. About one quarter of cancers of the tougue occur at the base, and some 70% of these patients have cervical metastases present at presentation (Conley 1967). Tumours of the soft palate tend to present later,

and to metastasize earlier than lesions in the hard palate. The parotid is the salivary gland most often affected by tumours, followed by the sub-mandibular gland.

Pathology, site and spread

Almost 90% of the malignant tumours of the mouth and oropharynx are squamous carcinomas, and there is an association with smoking and drinking. Tumours are more common in men aged 50 and over and those of the base of the tongue tend to metastasize to regional nodes early and to have the worst prognosis. The potentially malignant salivary gland tumours have been called 'mixed tumours' but are now generally called pleomorphic adenomas. These comprise some 70% of all salivary gland masses. They tend to recur after enucleation, but if removed with an adequate

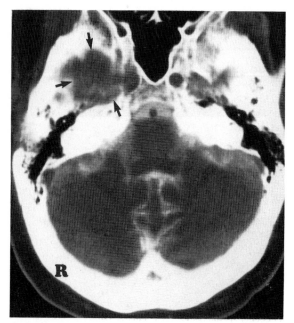

Fig. 16.11 Lymphoma of base of skull, axial CT. Contrast medium is present in the basal cisterns following myelography. There is erosion of the base of the skull in the middle fossa on the right side (arrows). The patient presented with sequential cranial nerve palsies. Successive biopsies, including one via a craniotomy, were normal. The diagnosis was eventually made when a lymphomatous deposit appeared in one humerus.

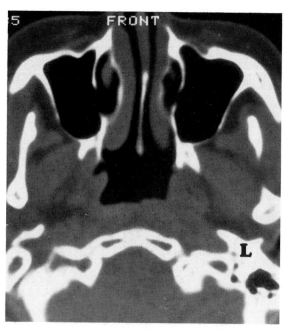

Fig. 16.12 Carcinoma of nasopharynx, axial CT two years after radiotherapy. The posterior angle on the left is blunted. The patient had recurrent nose bleeds, but repeated biopsies showed fibrosis only. The appearance cannot be distinguished radiologically from recurrence.

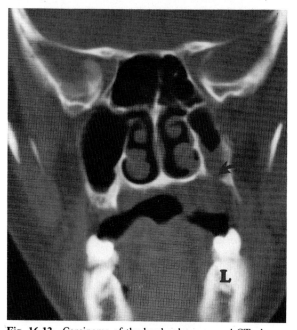

Fig. 16.13 Carcinoma of the hard palate, coronal CT. An increase in the soft tissue width below the hard palate is seen on the left, and this extends upwards into the inferior angle of the antrum (arrow), with erosion of the medial pterygoid plate.

margin of gland are cured. At any stage in their life history adenomas may start to grow rapidly and show both clinical and pathological evidence of malignancy (Lucas & Thackray 1976). Adenoid cystic carcinomas arise in the parotid and other salivary glands, and from mucosal glands of the nose, mouth, pharynx and respiratory tract. They are locally invasive and tend to recur unless excised with a wide margin. They show both haematogenous and lymphatic spread. These tumours have been called cylindromas, but the name is no longer used (Walter & Israel 1979).

Carcinoma and malignant lymphoma of the tonsil both tend to affect males more frequently; lymphoma is seen over a wider age range.

The lymphatic drainage of the mouth and oropharynx is to the superior deep cervical chain of nodes. Lymphatics from the lateral margins of the tongue drain to the nodes on the same side of the neck, whilst the central and basal parts drain to both sides.

Staging

Tumours of the oropharynx include the tongue posterior to the vallate papillae (the posterior third), tonsil and inferior surface of the soft palate; whilst the oral cavity includes the anterior two thirds of the tongue, the upper and lower alveolus, hard palate and floor of mouth. TNM classification is the same for both areas, with T1 tumours being 2 cm in diameter or less, T2, 2–4 cm and T3 over 4 cm. T4 tumours are those with extension to bone, muscle or antrum.

There is no TNM classification for salivary gland tumours, and the existing classifications are based on the diameter of the tumour.

Radiology

The oropharynx and oral cavity

Radiographs are of little help, but tomography may be useful in assessing bone changes in palatal tumours. CT is preferable, and since the palate runs in the axial plane, sections should be made at right angles to it, in the coronal plane. Both bone changes and the soft tissue mass may then be shown (Fig. 16.13). It has been noted that endoscopy and biopsy may produce oedema and changes in tissue planes shown on subsequent CT, making assessment of tumour extent difficult (Schaefer et al 1982). It is preferable for radiological assessment to precede biopsy.

Tonsillar tumours may show high signal intensity on some MRI sequences (Fig. 16.14), and cervical metastases may show as low density areas on CT, with distortion of tissue planes (Fig. 16.15). Tumours of the base of the tongue may be difficult to separate radiologically from those of the tonsil, and show similar high signal intensity on some MRI sequences (Fig. 16.16).

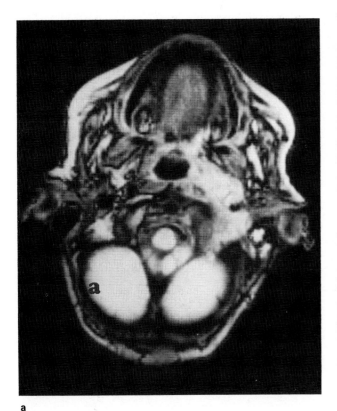

a

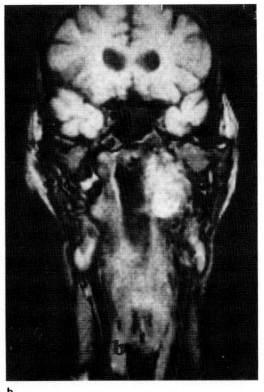

b

Fig. 16.14 Carcinoma of left tonsil, axial (a) and coronal (b) chemical shift MR images. High signal intensity is seen in the area of the tonsil, extending into the soft tissues adjacent to it. (MRI scans reproduced by courtesy of Dr A. Leung of Mount Vernon Hospital.)

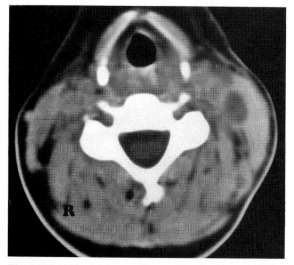

Fig. 16.15 Gland from carcinoma of tonsil, axial CT after contrast medium. A section at the level of the thyroid cartilage shows a low density area beneath the left sterno-mastoid, with distortion of the soft tissue planes.

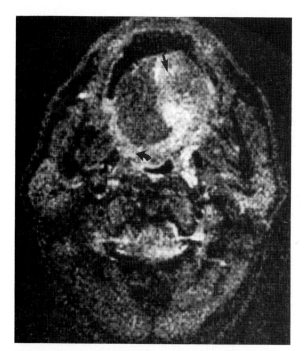

Fig. 16.16 Carcinoma of tongue, axial section MRI scan. High signal activity is shown in the left side of the tongue (straight arrow) extending into the left tonsil and across to the right side posteriorly (curved arrow). (Inversion recovery STIR 2200/130/40 images, reproduced by courtesy of Dr A. Leung of Mount Vernon Hospital.)

The salivary glands

Salivary gland tumours have in the past been shown by sialography, which shows the signs of displacement of the ducts by the mass within the gland. About 10% of tumours are in the deep lobe of the parotid gland, and investigation of this lobe is the principal indication for scanning the gland. The deep lobe is defined as the part of the gland lying beneath the facial nerve, adjacent to the masseter and ascending ramus of the mandible. Some tumours within it lie medial to the stylo-mandibular ligament and are then round in shape with little external evidence of swelling. Others grow through the tunnel between the ascending ramus of the mandible and the stylo-mandibular ligament to develop a 'dumb-bell' shape (Batsakis 1984), and spread can occur up to the base of the skull. With modern scanners there is no need to combine CT with sialography (McGahan et al 1984). Sections should be made during an infusion of 50–100 ml of contrast medium containing 300–350 mg of iodine per ml following a preliminary bolus of 50 ml, and will show the extent of the mass, with displacement of fat planes and adjacent structures (Fig. 16.17). Evidence of malignant be-

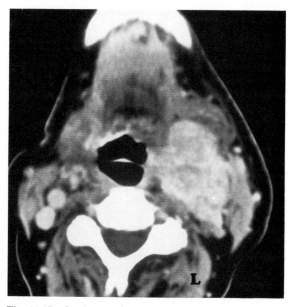

Fig. 16.17 Carcinoma of parotid, axial section after contrast medium. The carotid and jugular vein, seen clearly on the right, are involved in an enhancing mass on the left.

haviour is apparent when invasion of the carotid sheath or other defined structure or space is observed. Although MRI is said to be the preferred mode of investigation in the parapharyngeal region (Lloyd & Phelps 1986), there seems to be no major advance on the information provided by CT scanning in parotid tumours (Schaefer et al 1985).

The soft tissues of the neck

The neck is traditionally divided into two main anatomical compartments (Fig. 16.18). The anterior triangle is bounded anteriorly by the midline and posteriorly by the sternomastoid muscle, which is the anterior margin of the posterior triangle. The posterior border of this is the free edge of the trapezius. On transverse sections other potential spaces can be appreciated, and these are important in diagnosis since their loss or change in shape is an indication of an adjacent mass or invasion from the mass.

The parapharyngeal space (Fig. 16.19) has an inverted pyramidal shape with its base at the base of the skull and extends down to its apex at the level of the hyoid. Medially are the superior pharyngeal constrictor muscle and the fascia,

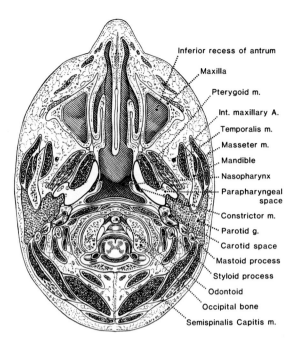

Fig. 16.19 Drawing in axial plane at level of parotid to show parapharyngeal space.

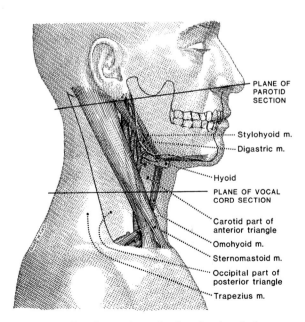

Fig. 16.18 Drawing to show triangles of neck and planes of sectional drawings in Figures 16.19 and 16.20.

forming the lateral wall of the nasopharynx. Laterally and anteriorly lie the pterygoid muscles, with the ramus of the mandible more laterally, and the deep lobe of the parotid indenting the outer margin of the space medial to the mandible. The maxillary artery lies further forward. Posterolaterally lies the carotid space with the internal carotid artery and jugular vein, the IX–XII cranial nerves, the cervical sympathetic nerves and some lymph nodes.

Malignant lesions within the parapharyngeal space are almost always parotid tumours or lymphatic metastases from the parotid, sinuses or pharynx (Shoss et al 1985). Patients may present with hoarseness from involvement of the tenth cranial nerve, paresis of the tongue from glossopharyngeal nerve involvement or Horner's syndrome (Unger & Chintapelli 1983).

Below the hyoid the carotid sheath (Fig. 16.20) lies in the space between the sternocleidomastoid antero-laterally and the anterior scalene muscle posteriorly (Silver et al 1984).

Although the cervical lymph nodes are usually clinically accessible there are patients in whom they are difficult to feel, and others in whom it is

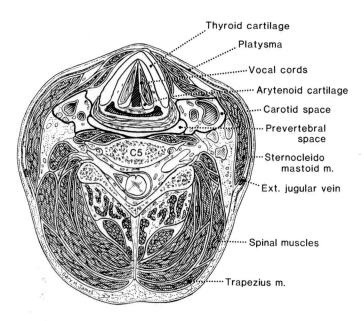

Fig. 16.20 Drawing in axial plane at level of vocal cords to show carotid and prevertebral space.

not certain whether there is a lymph node or another type of mass present. CT may then be helpful, and should be done during an infusion of contrast medium as detailed above. In patients in whom a pharyngeal tumour is suspected but has not been found the scan should always include the area up to the base of the skull. If a plane is visible between a nodal mass and the carotid artery or neck muscles it can be assumed that the mass is not fixed or adherent (Mancuso 1985).

Treatment

Radiotherapy is the treatment most used for oral and pharyngeal lesions, and there is some improvement in survival in patients with oro-pharyngeal tumours given methotrexate in addition to radiotherapy (Gupta et al 1987). Surgery is the preferred treatment for salivary gland tumours. About 50% of patients will have had at least one previous attempt at removal (Saunders et al 1986), reinforcing the need for an adequate margin at primary removal, with preservation of the facial nerve (Fig. 16.21). Parotid tumours are the least, and tonsillar tumours the most radiosensitive lesions in this area (Rafla 1982).

Parotid tumours may be difficult to remove completely and need follow-up; pulmonary metastases should also be looked for.

THE LARYNX AND HYPOPHARYNX

Incidence and presentation

Carcinoma of the larynx is the commonest tumour found in the head and neck, with some 1700 new cases and between 7 and 800 deaths being notified annually in England and Wales. Some 80% of cases occur in males, to give an annual incidence of newly diagnosed cases of 7/100 000 males aged 45–54, rising to 30/100 000 for males of 75 and over. The primary clinical symptom is hoarseness which occurs early in lesions affecting the vocal cords. Supraglottic lesions tend to present later and may have enlarged lymph nodes at presentation since the region is served by a large lymphatic network. Later there may be difficulty and pain on swallowing or pain referred to the ear.

The hypopharynx extends from the hyoid bone down to the lower border of the cricoid, and lies on the posterior and lateral borders of the larynx. Carcinoma of the pyriform fossa tends to occur in

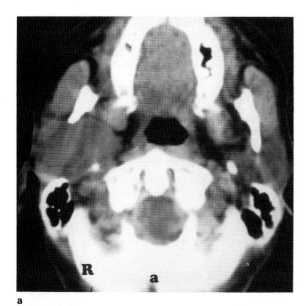

a

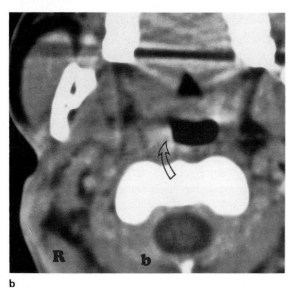

b

Fig. 16.21 Adenocystic carcinoma of parotid, axial CT. (a) A low density mass is seen extending deep to the mandible, with preservation of the parapharyngeal space. The tumour was then excised, for the third time. (b) Two years later a node is seen (arrow) indenting the margin of the nasopharynx, and on a separate section the mass had recurred.

men over 40 with a peak at 65, and tumours of the postcricoid space and posterior pharyngeal wall are more frequent in women between 40 and 60. They are associated with the Patterson–Kelly syndrome.

Pathology and spread

Most laryngeal tumours are well-differentiated squamous cell carcinomas with some being anaplastic. They may be topographically classified as follows:

1. Laryngopharyngeal carcinomas – those involving the piriform fossa or postcricoid region.

2. Supraglottic tumours, involving the posterior surface of the suprahyoid portion of the glottis, which includes the tip of the epiglottis, the aryepiglottic folds and the arytenoids; and the infrahyoid portion of the epiglottis, the vestibular folds and the ventricles.

3. Glottic tumours – those of the vocal folds and the anterior and posterior commissures.

4. Subglottic tumours.

Spread of laryngeal carcinoma is primarily by direct mucosal and submucosal extension. Upward and forward extension of supraglottic tumours may involve the posthyoid space. Glottic tumours involving the anterior commissure may penetrate the crico-thyroid ligament or the thyroid cartilage, and may reach the skin anteriorly. Areas of cartilage which have become ossified appear to be most readily invaded. This may be because tumour tends to spread along the collagen bundles which penetrate the internal perichondrium, and these are often the points at which ossification commences (Harrison 1984).

Both supra- and subglottic tumours metastasize to regional lymph glands early, are often more advanced at presentation than glottic tumours and have a worse prognosis. The lungs are the most frequent site for secondary tumours, which tend to be small and multiple (Fig. 16.22). Rarely bone metastases occur, producing either osteosclerosis or osteolysis (Loughran 1983).

Staging

Glottic tumours are classified as follows: T1 tumours are mobile tumours confined to the area, T1a being confined to one cord and T1b involving both cords. T2 tumours are confined to the larynx with extension to either the supraglottis or the subglottis, with either normal or impaired mobility. T3 lesions are confined to the larynx

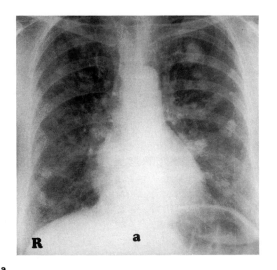

a

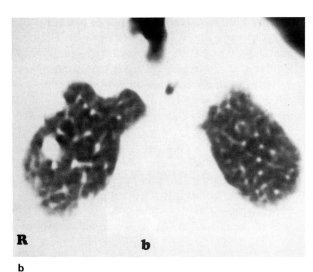

b

Fig. 16.22 Metastases from carcinoma of larynx, chest X-ray and axial CT. (a) Multiple rounded soft tissue densities of varying sizes are shown. (b) The CT section shows a metastasis in the right apex, extrapleural nodes indenting the pleura and a tracheostomy.

with fixation of one or both cords. T4 lesions have direct extension beyond the larynx.

Subglottic tumours are classified as follows: T1 lesions are confined to the area, in the subglottic area those confined to one side being T1a, and those with extension to both sides being T1b. T2 tumours are confined to the larynx, with extension to one or both cords with either normal or impaired mobility. T3 lesions are confined to the

larynx, with fixation of one or both cords. T4 tumours are those with destruction of cartilage with or without direct extension beyond the larynx.

In the supraglottic area T1a lesions are localized to one part of the area whilst T1b tumours are those involving the epiglottis and extending to the ventricular cavities or bands. T2 tumours extend to the glottis without fixation, T3 tumours show fixation and/or other evidence of deep infiltration, and T4 lesions show direct extension beyond the larynx.

Hypopharyngeal tumours are divided into those of the pyriform sinus, postcricoid area, and posterior pharyngeal wall, with T1 tumours being confined to the site of origin, T2 tumours extending into an adjacent area without fixation, and T3 tumours invading the larynx, laryngeal cartilages, prevertebral muscles or neighbouring structures.

Radiology

Lateral radiographs may show a mass outlined against the airfilled larynx (Fig. 16.23), and films taken during a Valsalva manoeuvre will distend the valleculae and pyriform fossae. Laryngograms can be used to outline abnormalities in the area but are now rarely done since they are less accurate in staging than CT (Archer et al 1981). CT is also more accurate in staging than direct inspection (Archer et al 1983) since at laryngoscopy there is difficulty in assessing subglottic tumours and extension into adjacent cartilage or soft tissues. Barium studies are often requested for hypopharyngeal lesions, but these present late, and the mass is usually obvious clinically. CT will demonstrate the mass and its extent (Fig. 16.24). Cancerous tissue is seen on T_1-weighted MR images (Fig. 16.25) as a homogeneous mass of intermediate signal intensity, that is of slightly higher intensity than the infrahyoid muscles (Castolijns et al 1987).

Conventional tomography in the coronal plane is still a useful method of demonstrating the upper and lower limits of tumours of the area, but if not available reconstruction CT scans may be helpful (Fig. 16.26). CT scans show the tumour (Fig. 16.27) together with its extension into adjacent cartilage or soft tissues (Lloyd et al 1981), and is

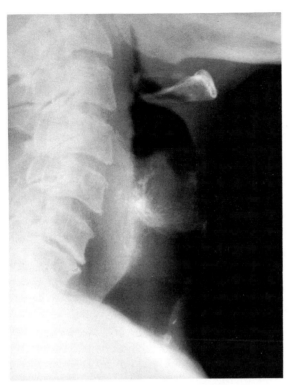

Fig. 16.23 Carcinoma of larynx, lateral film. There is irregular calcification of the thyroid cartilage, with a soft tissue mass above it.

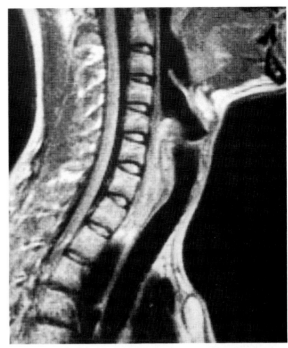

Fig. 16.25 Postcricoid carcinoma, sagittal MRI scan (SE 1100/40). An area of high signal intensity is seen in the postcricoid region in this 25-year-old man, indenting the larynx from behind. (MR image reproduced by courtesy of Dr A. Leung of Mount Vernon Hospital.)

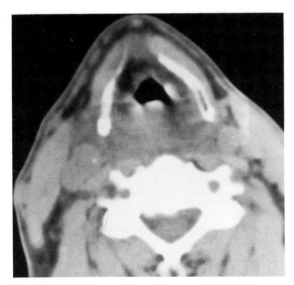

Fig. 16.24 Carcinoma of hypopharynx, axial CT. A large pharyngeal mass is shown behind the larynx, displacing it anteriorly.

useful in showing the tumour in relation to radiation treatment fields.

Technique

The patient's head is extended to 30° from the vertical and immobilized. A scout view will show the angulation of the larynx to the beam, and if necessary the gantry angle is adjusted so that the beam is at right angles to the anterior thyroid cartilage and parallel to the plane of the vocal cords. 4–6 mm thick sections are made from above the known limit of the lesion to 2–3 sections below it during quiet respiration. The regions of the vocal cords and any other region of interest should then be scanned using 2 mm thick slices during phonation of the letter 'E' (Gamsu et al 1981). This should be done using a low pitch to reduce vibration of the cords (Reid 1984). Phonation distends the lower end of the pyriform fossa by moving the arytenoids inwards, and helps in assessing cord mobility.

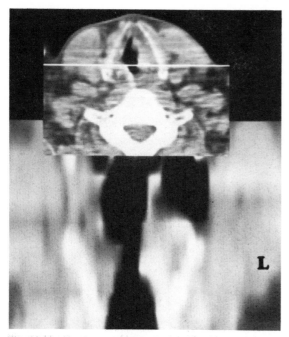

Fig. 16.26 Carcinoma of larynx, axial CT with coronal reconstruction. The section shows irregular enlargement of the left cord. Reconstruction shows the supraglottic mass extending upwards into the pyriform fossa, and down to blunt the infraglottic angle.

The radiological investigation should attempt to show:

1. The lowest point of extension of supraglottic tumours
2. The lateral extension of supraglottic masses into the pyriform fossa and upward extension to the vallecula
3. Extension laterally and anteriorly into the pre-epiglottic space
4. Involvement of the anterior commissure
5. Involvement of cartilage
6. Extent of subglottic extension
7. Enlargement of cervical nodes.

The signs which may be seen are listed in Table 16.2.

Difficulties in assessment may occur for a number of reasons. Ossification of cartilage is often irregular in normal people, and may mimic destruction. Enlarged glands adjacent to the larynx may appear on CT to be direct tumour extension. There may be a considerable amount of oedema in relation to the tumour, and this may cause rotation of the thyroid cartilage and widening of the thyro-arytenoid or cricothyroid space, and suggest a greater extension of tumour than is really present

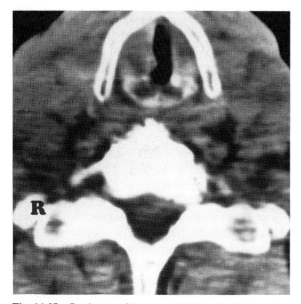

Fig. 16.27 Carcinoma of larynx, axial CT at level of vocal cords. The right cord is wider than the left, and there is a medial soft tissue mass outlined against the air between the cords.

Table 16.2 Radiological signs in carcinoma of the larynx

Radiographs
Soft tissue mass outlined against laryngeal air
Increased soft tissue width in region of thyroid cartilage, with loss of ventricular outline
Increased prevertebral soft tissue thickness
Loss of outline of epiglottis or valleculae

AP tomography
Rounding of the normally sharply angulated subglottic margin
Widening and increase in size of the false cord
Widening of the aryepiglottic fold
Loss of outline of the pyriform fossa

CT
The above signs and:
Extension of mass into low density pre-epiglottic space
Irregular loss of density of ossified region of cartilages
Overlapping of two thyroid alae anteriorly
Thickening of opposite cord (indicating tumour extension across midline)
Enlargement of cervical lymph nodes

MRI
Shows the mass with distortion of the normal planes, and there may be increased signal intensity on some sequences (Fig. 16.28)

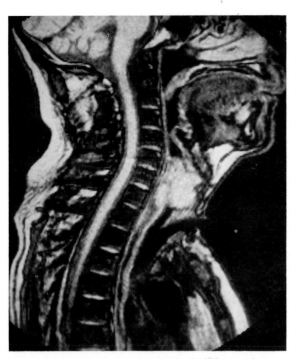

Fig. 16.28 Carcinoma of larynx, sagittal MRI scan. A tracheostomy tube is seen in situ, and high signal intensity is seen from the tumour on this chemical shift image. Less intensity was shown on the spin echo sequences. (Reproduced by courtesy of Dr A. Leung of Mount Vernon Hospital.)

(Reid 1984). Persistence of oedema for three months after the end of radiotherapy or returning after three months and not settling with antibiotics is strong evidence of persistence of tumour (Bahadur et al 1985). Distortion of normal structures by a large mass also causes overestimation of tumour size (Silverman et al 1984). CT does not demonstrate small foci of tumour in cartilage or soft tissue, so that early extension may be missed. Similar signs to those of laryngeal carcinoma on CT may be found in trauma, sarcoidosis, chronic inflammation of the vocal cords and laryngeal chondromas.

In patients having hemilaryngectomy (little practised in the United Kingdom) recurrence may be difficult to assess because of the distortion of tissues, but CT may show a mass distorting or narrowing the airway, or lying adjacent to the trachea (DiSantis et al 1984). MRI has also been found to be unreliable in patients with tumour recurrence

who had undergone previous radiation treatment (Castolijns et al 1987).

It is clear that radiological interpretation in this area may be difficult, and that evidence of tumour spread is often unreliable. This is particularly so after treatment, when oedema, infection and radionecrosis can all cause changes which are indistinguishable radiologically from tumour recurrence. When recurrence is suspected clinically, biopsy is necessary to decide if tumour is present.

Treatment

Carcinoma-in-situ of the vocal cords is treated by stripping of the cords, with radiotherapy given only if histological evidence of invasion is found (Henk & Whittam 1982). Radiotherapy is the treatment of choice for stage 1 and 2 cases, but some surgeons consider that cure rates are significantly lowered and morbidity increased if surgery is used to salvage radiation failures (Romm 1986). Survival is related to stage, and in a series treated mainly with ^{60}Co patients with stage 0 and 1 tumours had 100% survival at 5 years, with 90% survival for those in stage 2 and around 50% for patients in stages 3 and 4 (Jorgensen et al 1984).

The best treatment for carcinoma of the pyriform fossa is undecided since it has been claimed that radiotherapy actually diminished survival in patients with carcinoma of the pyriform fossa to 33% at 5 years, when surgery alone had a 55% survival rate (Yates & Crumley 1984). In surgery for hypopharyngeal cancer mortality is related to the N stage, with 30% survival at 5 years for N_0 and about 5% survival for stage N_3. It is also related to the type of operation, previous treatment, and the general condition of the patient (Stell et al 1983).

THE EYE

Presentation, pathology and incidence

Tumours of the eye and orbit present with proptosis, defective movement causing double vision, diminishing visual fields or loss of visual acuity, and the majority are diagnosed clinically. Although melanoma and lymphoma may be seen in the conjunctiva these are diagnosed clinically, and the principal areas in which radiology is of help is with tumours of the retina, the orbit and the lacrimal apparatus.

In children retinoblastoma is the most common primary intraocular tumour, and is the commonest eye tumour at all ages except for choroidal melanomas. It occurs in about 1 in 20 000 live births and both eyes are affected in about one-third of cases. Most cases are diagnosed at about 18 months and nearly all under the age of 3 years (Kanski 1984). Presentation is generally with a 'white lens', strabismus or proptosis. In most children both eyes are eventually affected, and the lesion is thought to be a developmental abnormality with a genetic tendency. The number of cases is increasing as more children survive. It may extend posteriorly into the optic nerve, and to the subarachnoid space with subsequent dissemination.

Staging is related to the size and position of the tumour. Stage 1 tumours are single or multiple tumours of less than 4 disc diameters at or behind the equator; stage 2 are those in the same region of 4–10 disc diameters in size; stage 3 are those anterior to the equator or a single tumour greater than 10 disc diameters at or behind the equator; and stages 4 and 5 involve larger tumours (Henk et al 1982).

The commonest orbital tumour in children is rhabdomyosarcoma. Neurofibromatosis is present in about half of the patients developing gliomas of the optic nerve. Metastases may be seen in the orbit from neuroblastomas, Ewing's sarcoma, Wilms' tumour, and in leukaemia.

In adults choroidal melanomas are the commonest intraocular tumours, mainly presenting in the fifth and sixth decades. These may present with a gradual unilateral change in vision, or may lift the retina, presenting more acutely with retinal detachment. Metastases and extension from sinus tumours are the most common malignant causes of orbital masses, which present with proptosis or localized swelling. Lymphoma may be seen as a localized lesion or as part of generalized disease, and myeloma may be seen in the orbit. Tumours of the lacrimal gland or lacrimal apparatus occur rarely. Proptosis may also be caused by dysthyroid

disease, vascular abnormalities such as haemangiomas and aneurysms, meningiomas, spread of infection from adjacent areas, granulomatous disease or 'pseudotumour' and intracranial lesions (Lloyd 1970).

Radiology

Postero-anterior, lateral, and occipito-mental views with both 45° and 35° angulations are taken as standard, with views of the optic foramina (Lloyd 1975). Tomography has generally been supplanted by CT scanning and MRI gives good images of the ocular and orbital soft tissues, with improved image detail if surface coils are used (Bilaniuk et al 1985). It has been suggested that it may become the primary method of investigation in orbital disease (Worthington et al 1986). Ultrasonography is another technique which is very useful in localizing intraocular and orbital lesions, and which is able to differentiate some tumours from other lesions on the basis of variations in echogenicity (Levine 1987).

Intraocular tumours are generally diagnosed without using radiological techniques, but these may be useful if the lens is opaque. Ultrasound is the primary method of investigation in this situation. CT and MRI can show intraocular masses but are rarely specific. However, the finding of calcification in an intraocular mass in a child under the age of 3 is highly suggestive of retinoblastoma, although over this age it may also be seen in Toxocara granulations, in vascular malformations and after haemorrhages (Mafee et al 1987).

In melanomas of the uveal tract blood-borne metastases occur in some 50% of cases, the mean time of appearance being four years after diagnosis, although some may not appear for 20 years. Most metastases appear in the liver, but are also seen in the chest, bone, skin and central nervous system.

The main rôle of radiology in the orbit is to differentiate the causes of proptosis. Plain films may show changes in the size of the orbit, optic canal and superior orbital fissure. Destruction of bone, hyperostosis or calcification may be seen. CT and MRI show the orbital muscles, optic nerve, superior orbital opthalmic vein and intraconal fat spaces as well as the intracranial soft tissues, whilst CT also shows bone detail and the adjacent sinuses.

The enlargement of orbital muscles in dysthyroid disease is generally easily seen. Changes in the optic nerve are clearly seen against the intraconal fat, and marked enhancement may be seen if a sheath meningioma is present. Abnormal soft tissue masses are clearly identified (Fig. 16.29), although there are rarely identifiable tissue characteristics. The extent of lacrimal apparatus tumours can also be shown on CT.

Treatment

In retinoblastoma stage 1 tumours may be treated by cryosurgery or light coagulation if suitably placed, by radioactive cobalt implants, or by lateral beam irradiation. For larger tumours irradiation to the whole eye is used, possibly followed by enucleation of the eye later. The treatment of melanomas depends on size and evidence of growth. Small lesions may be treated by photocoagulation, slightly larger lesions by radioactive cobalt or particle therapy, and larger lesions or those with local complications such as retinal detachment, pain or secondary glaucoma by enucleation.

Lymphoma and myeloma may be treated by local irradiation if there is no generalized disease, or by systemic treatment if this is present.

THE EAR

Tumours of the external and internal ears are uncommon and have similar symptoms. The majority of patients have had longstanding chronic suppurative otitis media, and may then develop bloodstaining of their discharge or pain. Most tumours are squamous cell carcinomas which may metastasize to cervical glands; less often in the external ear they may be basal cell carcinomas. Metastases to the temporal bone and middle ear may also occur. The principal differential diagnosis radiologically is cholesteatoma.

Bone destruction may be seen on plain radiographs, and the combination of soft tissue mass and bone destruction may be shown on CT (Fig. 16.30). Erosion of the articular fossa of the temporo-mandibular joint is nearly always due to carcinoma (Phelps & Lloyd 1984). Treatment may be by resection of the temporal bone, mastoidectomy accompanied by radiotherapy, or radiotherapy alone.

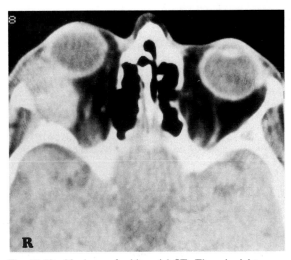

Fig. 16.29 Myeloma of orbit, axial CT. There is right-sided proptosis caused by a soft tissue mass postero-lateral to the eye. The optic nerve and superior ophthalmic vein are seen more medially.

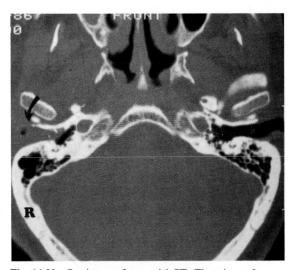

Fig. 16.30 Carcinoma of ear, axial CT. There is a soft tissue mass in the right external canal, with thinning of the anterior wall of the canal (arrow).

REFERENCES

Acheson E D, Hadfield E H, Macbeth R G 1967 Carcinoma of the nasal cavity and accessory sinuses in woodworkers. Lancet 1: 311–312

Archer C R, Sagel S S, Yeager V L, Martin S, Friedman W H 1981 Staging of carcinoma of the larynx: Comparative accuracy of CT and laryngography. American Journal of Roentgenology 136: 571–575

Archer C R, Yeager V L, Herbold D R 1983 Improved diagnostic accuracy in the TNM staging of laryngeal cancer using a new definition of regions based on computed tomography. Journal of Computer Assisted Tomography 7: 610–617

Bahadur S, Amatya R C, Kacker S K 1985 The enigma of post-radiation oedema and residual or recurrent carcinoma of the larynx and pyriform fossa. Journal of Laryngology and Otology 99: 763–765

Batsakis J G 1984 Deep lobe parotid gland tumours. Annals of Otology, Rhinology and Laryngology 93: 415–416

Bergeron R T, Osborn A G, Som P M 1984 Head and neck imaging excluding the brain. C V Mosby, St Louis

Bilaniuk L T, Schenck J F, Zimmerman R A et al 1985 Ocular and orbital lesions: surface coil MR imaging. Radiology 156: 669–674

Bryan G 1987 Diagnostic radiography, 4th edn. Churchill Livingstone, Edinburgh

Cable H R, Jeans W D, Cullen R J, Bull P O, Maw A R 1981 Computerised tomography of the Caldwell Luc cavity. Journal of Laryngology and Otology 95: 775–783

Castolijns J A, Kaiser M C, Gerritsen G J, van Haffum A H, Snow G B 1987 MR imaging of laryngeal cancer. Journal of Computer Assisted Tomography 11: 134–140

Castro E B, Lewis J S, Strong E W 1973 Plasmacytoma of paranasal sinuses and nasal cavity. Archives of Otolaryngology 97: 326–329

Conley J (ed) 1967 Cancer of the head and neck. Butterworths, Washington, p 271

DiSantis D J, Balfe D M, Hayden R, Sessions D, Sagel S S 1984 The neck after vertical hemilaryngectomy: computed tomographic study. Radiology 151: 683–687

Doll R 1967 Prevention of cancer. Nuffield Provincial Hospitals Trust, p 67

Eddleston B 1980 A simple approach to the investigation of malignant disease within the nasal and paranasal airways. In: Symington T, Williams A E, McVee J G (eds) Cancer – assessment and monitoring. Churchill Livingstone, Edinburgh, pp 177–187

Eddleston B, Johnson R J 1983 A comparison of conventional radiographic imaging and computed tomography in malignant disease of the paranasal sinuses and the postnasal space. Clinical Radiology 34: 161–172

Eller J L, Roberts J F, Ziter F M H 1971 Normal nasopharyngeal soft tissue in adults. American Journal of Roentgenology 112: 537–541

Forbes W St C, Fawcitt R A, Isherwood I, Webb R, Farrington T 1978 Computed tomography in the diagnosis of diseases of the paranasal sinuses. Clinical Radiology 29: 501–511

Freedman H M, DeSanto L W, Devine K D, Weiland L H 1973 Malignant melanoma of the nasal cavity and paranasal sinuses. Archives of Otolaryngology 97: 322–325

Friedmann I, Osborn D A 1976 Nose and nasal sinuses: nasopharynx: larynx. In: Symmers W St C (ed) Systemic pathology, 2nd edn. Churchill Livingstone, Edinburgh, pp 191–267

Gamsu G, Webb W R, Shallit J B, Moss A A 1981 CT in carcinoma of the larynx and pyriform sinus: value of phonation scans. American Journal of Roentgenology 136: 577–584

Gatenby R A, Mulhern C B, Strawitz J, Modofsky P J 1985 Comparison of clinical and computed tomographic staging of the head and neck tumors. American Journal of Neuroradiology 6: 399–401

Ghaffarian A, Alaghehband H 1980 Metastases from nasopharyngeal carcinoma in an unusual site. Clinical Radiology 31: 359–360

Glazer H S, Niemeyer J H, Balfe D M, Devineni V R 1986 Neck neoplasms: MR imaging. Part I. Initial evaluation. Radiology 160: 343–348

Gupta N K, Pointon R C S, Wilkinson P M 1987 A randomised clinical trial to contrast radiotherapy with radiotherapy and methotrexate given synchronously in head and neck cancer. Clinical Radiology 38: 575–581

Harmer M H (eds) 1978 TNM classification of malignant tumours. UICC, Geneva

Harrison D F N 1978 Critical look at the classification of maxillary sinus carcinomata. Annals of Otology, Rhinology and Laryngology 87: 3–9

Harrison D F N 1984 Significance and means by which laryngeal cancer invades thyroid cartilage. Annals of Otology, Rhinology and Laryngology 93: 293–296

Hasso A N 1984 CT of tumors and tumor-like conditions of the paranasal sinuses. Radiologic Clinics of North America 22: 119–130

Henk J M, Whittam D E 1982 Ear, nose and throat. In: Halnan K E (ed) Treatment of cancer. Chapman & Hall, London, pp 223–248

Henk J M, Wright J E, Sandland M R 1982 Eye and orbit. In: Halnan K E (ed) Treatment of cancer. Chapman & Hall, London, pp 171–189

Hordijk G J, Brons E N 1985 Carcinomas of the maxillary sinus: A retrospective survey. Clinical Otolaryngology 10: 285–288

Jeans W D 1984 The nose, paranasal sinuses and nasopharynx. In: du Boulay G H (ed) A textbook of radiological diagnosis, 5th edn, vol I. Lewis, London, pp 298–309

Jeans W D, Gilani S, Bullimore J 1982 The effect of CT scanning on staging tumours of the paranasal sinuses. Clinical Radiology 33: 173–179

Jorgensen K, Munk J, Andersen J E, Hjelm-Hansen M 1984 Carcinoma of the larynx. Acta Radiologica 23: 321–330

Kalovidouris A, Mancuso A A, Dillon W 1984 A CT-clinical approach to patients with symptoms related to the V, VII, IX–XII cranial nerves and cervical sympathetics. Radiology 151: 671-676

Kanski J J 1984 Clinical ophthalmology. Butterworths, London, pp 14.10–11

Khoury G G , Paterson I C M 1987 Nasopharyngeal carcinoma: a review of cases treated by radiotherapy and chemotherapy. Clinical Radiology 38: 17–20

Kolbenstvedt A, Wang Y, Larheim T A 1985 Unilateral demonstration of the atlas in ipsilateral maxillary alveolar bone destruction. Acta Radiologica 26: 173–176

Levine R A 1987 Orbital ultrasonography. Radiologic Clinics of North America 25: 447–469

Lloyd G A S 1970 The radiological investigation of proptosis. British Journal of Radiology 43: 1–18

Lloyd G A S 1975 Radiology of the orbit. Saunders, Philadelphia

Lloyd G A S, Phelps P D 1986 The demonstration of tumours of the parapharyngeal space by magnetic resonance imaging. British Journal of Radiology 59: 675–683

Lloyd G A S, Michaels L, Phelps P D 1981 The demonstration of cartilaginous involvement in laryngeal carcinoma by computerised tomography. Clinical Otolaryngology 6: 171–177

Loughran C F 1983 Bone metastases from squamous cell carcinoma of the larynx. Clinical Radiology 34: 447–450

Lucas R B, Thackray A C 1976 Mouth and salivary glands. In: Symmers W St C (ed) Systemic pathology. Churchill Livingstone, Edinburgh

Lund V J, Lloyd G A S 1984 Radiological changes associated with inverted papilloma of the nose and paranasal sinuses. British Journal of Radiology 57: 455–461

Lund V J, Howard D J, Lloyd G A S 1983 CT evaluation of paranasal sinus tumours for cranio-facial resection. British Journal of Radiology 56: 439–446

Mafee M F, Goldberg M F, Greenwald M J, Schulman J, Malmed A, Flanders A E 1987 Retinoblastoma and simulating lesions: role of CT and MR imaging. Radiologic Clinics of North America 25: 667–682

Mancuso A A 1985 Cervical node metastases. In: Bragg D G, Rubin P, Youker J E (eds) Oncologic imaging. Pergamon, New York, p 54

McGahan J P, Walter J P, Bernstein L 1984 Evaluation of the parotid gland. Radiology 152: 453–458

Morton R P, Sellars S L, Sealy R 1985 Computerised staging of cancer of the maxillary sinus. International Journal of BioMedical Computing 16: 191–199

Phelps P D, Lloyd G A S 1984 The ear and temporal bone. In: du Boulay G H (ed) A textbook of radiological diagnosis, 5th edn, vol 1. Lewis, London, p 363

Pointon R C S, Askill C, Hunter R D, Wilkinson P M 1983 Treatment of advanced head and neck cancer using synchronous therapy with methotrexate and irradiation. Clinical Radiology 34: 459–462

Rafla S 1982 Salivary glands. In: Halnan K E (ed) Treatment of cancer. Chapman & Hall, London, p 289

Reid M H 1984 Laryngeal carcinoma: high resolution computed tomography and thick anatomic sections. Radiology 151: 689–696

Romm S 1986 Cancer of the larynx: current concepts of diagnosis and treatment. Surgical Clinics of North America 66: 109–118

Samuel E, Lloyd G A S 1978 Clinical radiology of the ear, nose and throat, 2nd edn. Lewis, London

Saunders J R, Hirata R M, Jaques D A 1986 Salivary glands. Surgical Clinics of North America 66: 59–81

Schaefer S, Merkel M, Diehl J, Maravilla K, Anderson R 1982 Computed tomographic assessment of squamous cell carcinoma of oral and pharyngeal cavities. Archives of Otolaryngology 108: 688–692

Schaefer S D, Maravilla K R, Close L G, Burns D K, Merkel M A, Suss R A 1985 Evaluation of NMR versus CT for parotid masses: A preliminary report. Laryngoscope 95: 945–950

Shoss S M, Donovan D T, Alford B R 1985 Tumors of the parapharyngeal space. Archives of Otolaryngology 111: 753–757

Silver A J, Mawad M E, Hilal S K, Sane P, Ganti S R 1983 Computed tomography of the nasopharynx and related spaces. Part II: Pathology. Radiology 147: 733–738

Silver A J, Mawad M E, Hilal S K, Sane P, Ganti S R 1984 Computed tomography of the carotid space and related cervical spaces. Radiology 150: 723–728

Silverman P M, Bossen E H, Fisher S R, Cole T B, Korobkin M, Halvorsen R A 1984 Carcinoma of the larynx and hypopharynx: computed tomographic–histopathologic correlations. Radiology 151: 697–702

Stell P M, Missotten F, Singh S D, Ramadan M F, Morton R P 1983 Mortality after surgery for hypopharyngeal cancer. British Journal of Surgery 70: 713–718

Unger J M, Chintapelli K N 1983 Computed tomography of the parapharyngeal space. Journal of Computer Assisted Tomography 7: 605–609

Walter J B, Israel M S 1979 General pathology, 5th edn. Churchill Livingstone, Edinburgh, p 332

Whelan M A, Reede D L, Lin J P, Edwards J H 1984 The base of the skull. In: Bergeron R T, Osborn A G, Som P M (eds) Head and neck imaging. C V Mosby, St Louis

Worthington B S, Wright J E, Curati W L, Steiner R E, Rizk S 1986 The role of magnetic resonance imaging techniques in the evaluation of orbital and ocular disease. Clinical Radiology 37: 219–226

Yates A, Crumley R L 1984 Surgical treatment of pyriform sinus cancer. Laryngoscope 94: 1586–1590

Zizmor J, Noyek A M 1978 Calcifying and osteoblastic tumors of the nasal and paranasal cavities. Advances in Oto-Rhino-Laryngology 24: 115–142

17. The endocrine system

J. E. Adams

With a contribution on thyroid tumours by Dr B. Eddleston.

INTRODUCTION

The principal rôle of imaging in the management of functioning endocrine tumours is to localize and to define the size and extent of the tumour. Imaging techniques may also help to distinguish between functionally autonomous tumours and hyperplasia. In the case of malignant tumours, imaging techniques can provide information about the spread of the tumour, locally and to distant sites (lymph nodes, liver and bone). In the past, investigations to localize functional endocrine tumours were either imprecise (intravenous urography for adrenal tumours) or time consuming, potentially hazardous and technically difficult (arteriography, venography). The introduction of CT has had a profound effect on the diagnosis and localization of endocrine tumours, and as a result many of the invasive radiological investigations previously performed have become obsolete, or only necessary in occasional circumstances. CT has not only improved the preoperative accuracy of the diagnosis of such tumours (Hamberger et al 1982) but has also provided economic benefits. Few, if any, invasive procedures are now necessary and consequently the preoperative hospital stay of patients has been shortened (Newton et al 1983). In order to obtain the most useful diagnostic information from CT, it is essential to ensure that the optimum scanning technique is used, and that those interpreting the images are experienced in the field. With technological improvements, ultrasound has been increasingly applied to the localization of endocrine tumours in the neck and abdomen. Technical skill and expertise by those performing the scans are essential for the best results. Radionuclide scans can provide functional

and morphological information on endocrine tumours. Since the introduction of magnetic resonance imaging (MRI), this technique has been increasingly applied to anatomical sites previously examined only by CT. Technical developments which permit faster scanning and thinner sections to be obtained, and the use of surface coils which improve image quality in certain anatomical sites (e.g. the neck) make it likely that MR will be applied increasingly to the localization of endocrine tumours. Nonetheless, many endocrine tumours are small and unless thin sections or surface coil MR scanning is available, CT will remain the imaging technique of choice.

ADRENAL TUMOURS

Anatomy

There are two adrenal glands and both lie anteromedial to the upper poles of the kidneys. Each gland has a cortex and medulla, and is encased in a single capsule and surrounded by fat within Gerota's fascia. The cortex is of mesodermal origin and the medulla of ectodermal tissue. The right gland is triangular or pyramidal in shape; the left is semilunar in shape and usually slightly larger than the right. Each normal gland weighs about 5 g, is 2–3 cm in coronal width, 4–6 cm in craniocaudal length and 3–6 mm in anteroposterior diameter. During the first year of life the adrenals are relatively much larger than in an adult, being approximately one-third the size of the kidneys, whereas in adults the adrenals are about 1/30 the size of the kidneys. Congenital absence of an adrenal gland is rare, whereas accessory adrenal tissue is quite common and this may be composed of cortical or medullary tissue. These accessory remnants of cortical tissue, which are functionally active, are usually found in close proximity to the parent gland, occasionally embedded in the neighbouring kidney, or along the urogenital tract. The adrenal cortex is divided into three zones (glomerulosa, fasciculata, reticulata) which enclose the centrally placed medulla.

The adrenal cortex synthesizes and absorbs cholesterol which is then converted through a series of enzymatic steps to various steroid compounds and hormones. Aldosterone is secreted by the outer zone (glomerulosa) and cortisol and various sex hormones by the middle zone (fasciculata). The cells of the adrenal medulla arise from tissue of the neural crest. These medullary cells contain adrenaline and noradrenaline and consequently stain brown with chromic acid, which is why they are called chromaffin cells. The cells of the medulla synthesize and release catecholamines which have potent physiological and pathological effects. The adrenal glands have a rich vascular anastomosis arising from branches of the inferior phrenic artery, the aorta, and the renal artery. Venous drainage is into a single draining vein, the right entering the postero-lateral aspect of the inferior vena cava and the left draining into the left renal vein.

The normal adrenal gland secretes cortisol in response to ACTH which is secreted by the anterior pituitary gland. The major stimulus to aldosterone production is the renin/angiotensin system. Renin is an enzyme produced by the juxtaglomerular apparatus of the nephron, which cleaves a specific plasma globulin to form angiotensin I. This compound is further hydrolysed to angiotensin II, which acts directly on the adrenal cortex and stimulates aldosterone formation. This system is important in maintaining normal blood pressure (Liddle 1981).

Imaging techniques

In the past, techniques such as high dose intravenous urography with tomography, retroperitoneal air insufflation angiography and venous blood sampling were applied (Sutton 1975). The methods were either imprecise (intravenous urog-

raphy) or potentially hazardous, time consuming and called for considerable technical skills on the part of the radiologist (venous sampling and arteriography). Adrenal tumours are seldom large enough to cause displacement or distortion of the adjacent kidney (Fig. 17.1) and it is exceptional for calcification within a neoplasm to be visible on a plain radiograph of the abdomen. Invasive procedures such as angiography, venography and venous hormone sampling have been replaced by non-invasive techniques, principally CT (Moulton & Moulton 1988), abdominal ultrasound (Yeh 1988) and, more recently, magnetic resonance imaging (Egglin et al 1988).

CT is the most reliable imaging technique for identifying normal adrenal glands and adrenal tumours. On modern CT scanners, over 98% of normal adrenal glands are identified. Although the glands are small, there is a high contrast difference between them and the perinephric fat in which they lie within Gerota's fascia. The adrenals have two limbs, medial and lateral. The right adrenal has an inverted V configuration and lies between

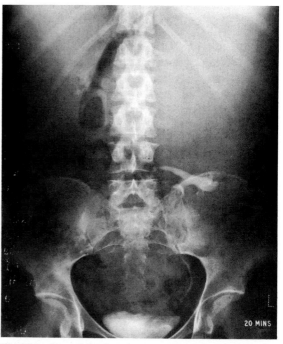

Fig. 17.1 Large left adrenal tumour which displaces the gas-filled stomach to the right and the left kidney inferiorly to the level of the iliac crest.

the right crus medially, the liver laterally and the inferior vena cava anteriorly (Fig. 17.2). The left gland has either an inverted V or Y configuration and lies between the left crus of the diaphragm medially, the upper pole of the left kidney postero-laterally and the tail of the pancreas antero-laterally (Fig. 17.2). There is considerable variation in the length and width of the limbs of normal glands (Brownlie & Kreel 1978) and the adrenals may become larger and irregular in outline in otherwise healthy elderly people (Dobbie 1969). Hyperplastic glands, although enlarged, tend to maintain the normal shape (Fig. 17.3). However, because of the wide variation in normal configuration, the judgement as to whether or not glands are hyperplastic is generally made on subjective assessment. Minor degrees of atrophy or hyperplasia of the adrenal glands may not be detectable by CT (Adams et al 1983). This precludes the use of CT as a screening procedure for adrenal disease in patients who do not have proven biochemical evidence of adrenal dysfunction. In a patient with biochemical evidence of adrenal hyperfunction, the finding of apparently normal glands on CT implies the presence of bilateral adrenal hyperplasia. The CT technique for examining the adrenal glands is 10 mm contiguous sections through the upper abdomen. If very small tumours are suspected, as is commonly

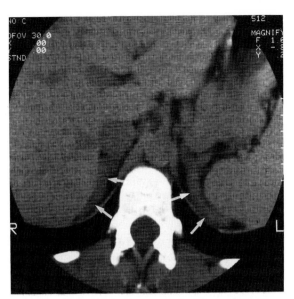

Fig. 17.3 Bilateral adrenal hyperplasia. The medial limbs of both adrenal glands are elongated and thickened (arrows) but the glands maintain their normal shape.

the case in primary aldosteronism, then 5 mm or even 3 mm sections may be required. The administration of preliminary oral and subsequent intravenous contrast medium for enhanced scanning helps to avoid other anatomical structures (gastric fundus, prominent splenic lobulation, renal or pancreatic masses, tortuous splenic vessels or porto-systemic shunts) being mistakenly diagnosed as adrenal tumours (Berliner et al 1982, Mitty et al 1983). Following the introduction and development of CT the accuracy of the preoperative localization of adrenal tumours increased substantially from 50% with other techniques to over 90% with CT (Hamberger et al 1982). CT is the method of choice for the detection of adrenal tumours.

Syndromes of adrenal dysfunction

Cushing's syndrome

Excessive production of cortisol from the adrenal cortex results in Cushing's syndrome. Clinically, this causes central obesity, cutaneous striae, muscular weakness, hypertension, diabetes mellitus, plethora, hirsutism, osteoporosis (30%) and renal

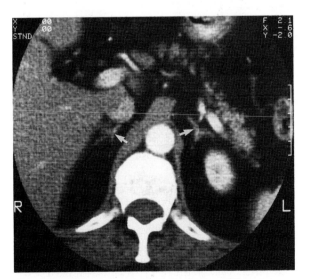

Fig. 17.2 Normal adrenal glands (arrows) on CT scan.

calculi (20%). The disease occurs in all races and both sexes, but is most common in adult women, usually between the ages of 20 and 60 years. The majority of cases (80%) are due to adrenal hyperplasia secondary to overproduction of ACTH by a basophil pituitary adenoma (Cushing's disease). The remainder result either from autonomous adrenal tumours (adenoma or carcinoma) or adrenal hyperplasia secondary to ectopic ACTH production. Adrenal carcinomas are usually large at clinical presentation and many (50%) are incompletely resectable; most metastasize to lymph nodes, the liver and lungs. Some (approximately 25%) may be completely resectable and curable. The clinical syndrome caused by ectopic ACTH production may be indistinguishable from hypercortisolism due to other causes (adrenal tumour or pituitary-dependent Cushing's disease), but the typical clinical features are often lacking; there may be severe wasting and weakness and features of progressive malignancy. Tumours which are ectopic sources of ACTH are most commonly located in the thorax. Oat cell carcinoma of the lung is the most common, followed by tumours of the thymus, pancreas and bronchus (including carcinoid tumours). More rarely phaeochromocytoma, paraganglionoma, ganglionoma and tumours of the thyroid, liver, prostate, ovary, breast, parotid gland and oesophagus have been reported (Liddle 1981). The diagnosis of Cushing's syndrome is based on biochemical grounds and is confirmed by a raised plasma cortisol level with loss of the normal diurnal variation, and raised urinary 17-hydroxycorticosteroids. The plasma ACTH is low in functionally autonomous adrenal tumours and high in Cushing's disease (pituitary-dependent and ectopic ACTH syndromes). The biochemical responses to the administration of metyrapone and varying doses of dexamethazone may also be helpful in differentiating between pituitary-dependent disease, autonomous adrenal tumour, and the ectopic ACTH syndrome. It is important that these diagnostic tests are performed before imaging is undertaken in order to ensure that the appropriate anatomical sites are examined.

Patients with Cushing's syndrome may present with osteoporosis and easy fracture. A common site for such fractures is the ribs, which may be seen on the chest radiograph, and which are often surrounded by profuse callus formation. There may be generalized osteopaenia and multiple wedge and crush fractures of the vertebral bodies. Once the diagnosis of adrenal cortical overactivity is confirmed on clinical and biochemical grounds,

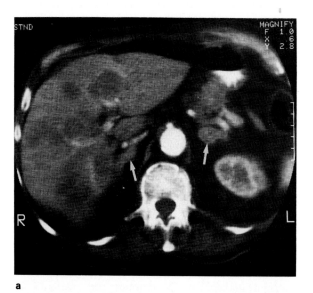

a

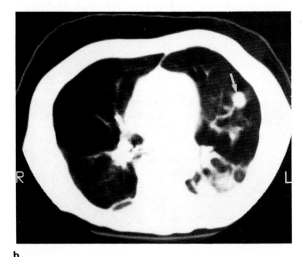

b

Fig. 17.4 Cushing's syndrome caused by ectopic ACTH production. (a) Hyperplasia of both adrenal glands (arrows), with multiple low attenuation metastases in the liver. (b) Scanning was continued through the thorax and a 1.5 cm soft tissue nodule (arrow) was identified in the left lung. This proved to be a bronchial carcinoid and was not visible on chest radiographs. (Acute inflammatory changes were present more posteriorly in the left lung at the time of the CT scan.)

imaging techniques are necessary to help define the adrenal pathology. Normal adrenals on CT or glands which are enlarged but retain a normal shape, confirm bilateral adrenal hyperplasia. In patients with Cushing's syndrome there is often an abundance of intra-abdominal and mediastinal fat. The majority of patients will have a pituitary adenoma producing ACTH and high resolution CT scanning of the pituitary would be appropriate. Less commonly, the ACTH stimulating the adrenals will be secreted from an ectopic tumour which may be identified by CT (Fig. 17.4). A patient with Cushing's disease who has no clinical or imaging evidence of a primary tumour, but who is found to have metastatic disease in conjunction with hyperplastic adrenal glands, should have the CT extended to include examination of the thorax at 1 cm intervals, since the primary tumour, not evident on the chest radiograph, may be indentified there (Fig. 17.4) (White et al 1982). Exceptionally, the source of ACTH may arise within an adrenal tumour (Jessop et al 1987). A soft tissue mass within one adrenal confirms an autonomous adrenal lesion as the cause of the Cushing's syndrome (Fig. 17.5). The opposite gland will appear either normal or atrophic, due to suppression of secretion of pituitary ACTH by the cortisol produced by the

tumour. Adrenocortical tumours account for about 18% of adults with Cushing's syndrome; adenoma and carcinoma occur with equal frequency. This contrasts with the findings in children where autonomous tumours are more common causes of the disease. In children with Cushing's syndrome most of these tumours (75%) are carcinomas (Fig. 17.6) (Jones et al 1985). Adrenal adenomas appear

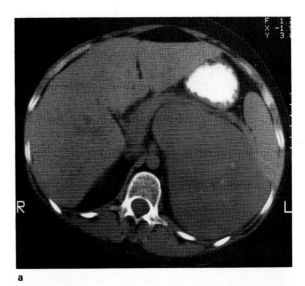

a

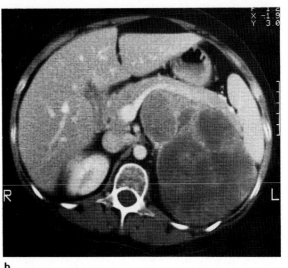

b

Fig. 17.6 Carcinoma left adrenal in a 14-year-old girl with Cushing's syndrome. (a) Large left adrenal tumour containing some calcification, and (b) showing heterogeneous enhancement after intravenous contrast medium, with low attenuation areas indicating necrosis. The mass displaces the tail of the pancreas, the splenic vein and spleen anteriorly.

Fig. 17.5 Cushing's syndrome caused by autonomous right adrenal tumour (arrow) lying between the upper pole of the right kidney posteriorly and the inferior vena cava anteriorly.

as well defined, round or oval masses which are generally between 2 and 5 cm in diameter (Fig. 7.5), but can be larger (Adams et al 1983, Moulton & Moulton 1988). Adenomas are usually homogeneous in attenuation and occasionally contain areas of calcification. When large, they can be heterogenous due to central necrosis, cyst formation or a high content of cholesterol. Adrenal carcinomas tend to be much larger than benign adenomas at first presentation, are often lobulated in outline and heterogenous in attenuation, and show marked postcontrast enhancement (Fig. 17.6). These attenuation and enhancement characteristics are helpful in differentiating between benign and malignant tumours (Adams et al 1983, Hussain et al 1985, Berland et al 1988). In carcinomas there may also be evidence of metastases in regional lymph nodes, the liver or the lungs. In occasional patients with bilateral adrenal hyperplasia a solitary mass lesion is seen in one gland, which raises the possibility of an autonomous nodule having developed as a consequence (Joffe & Brown 1983, Huebener & Treugut 1984, Smals et al 1984, Doppman et al 1988). It is important for the radiologist to comment on this because the finding could have an important bearing on treatment. The preferred method of treatment of pituitary-dependent Cushing's disease is now surgical removal or radiotherapy to the pituitary tumour, rather than bilateral adrenalectomy. However, should a functionally autonomous nodule have developed in a hyperplastic adrenal, pituitary adenomectomy would not cure the disease because the adrenal nodule will continue to produce cortisol unabated.

Primary aldosteronism (Conn's syndrome)

This condition results from the excessive production and secretion of the mineralo-corticoid, aldosterone, by the zona glomerulosa. Clinically patients present with hypertension, which typically responds to spironolactone, and symptoms caused by hypokalaemia (flaccid muscle weakness, tetany). In the majority of patients (80%) the condition is caused by a benign adenoma; the remainder have either idiopathic adrenocortical hyperplasia or, rarely, multiple adenoma. The rôle of imaging in primary aldosteronism is to differen-

tiate between an autonomous adrenal tumour and bilateral adrenal hyperplasia. This is an important differentiation to make because the treatment is different. Bilateral adrenal hyperplasia is treated medically, as patients respond poorly to bilateral adrenalectomy; autonomous localized tumours are treated surgically. Conn's tumours tend to be fairly small and may measure only 4–10 mm in size (Fig. 17.7) (Meek et al 1981). For their identification it is therefore essential that thinner (3 or 5 mm) contiguous sections are performed through the adrenals. A dynamic sequence of scans can be helpful, since variations in the phase of respiration in which the scans are performed will affect the position in which the adrenals lie in the scanning field. Aldosterone-secreting tumours are generally well defined and homogeneous in attenuation and show little enhancement after intravenous contrast medium. As with other adrenal tumours, their low attenuation reflects their high cholesterol content. This may account for the failure to detect some small tumours on CT (Schaner et al 1978). In hyperplasia, the glands may appear normal, symmetrically enlarged or nodular in outline (Adams et al 1983, Roberts et al 1985). Many aldosterone-secreting tumours are small and about

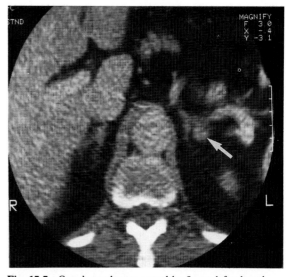

Fig. 17.7 Conn's syndrome caused by 8 mm left adrenal adenoma (arrow) arising from the lateral limb of the gland. The right adrenal is normal.

25% may be missed on CT. This means that in some patients adrenal venous sampling for aldosterone levels will be required to establish the precise location of the tumour (Dunnick et al 1982, Geisinger et al 1983).

Phaeochromocytoma

Phaeochromocytomas are tumours which arise from chromaffin cells and produce catecholamines (noradrenaline and adrenaline). The tumours mainly secrete noradrenaline with smaller quantities of adrenaline. The secretion of catecholamines may be episodic. Clinical symptoms include periodic headache and palpitations, and hypertension which may be intermittent or sustained. Approximately 90% of phaeochromocytomas arise from the adrenal medulla. The remaining 10% arise from chromaffin tissue in extra-adrenal sites, most commonly within the paravertebral sympathetic ganglion (Organ of Zuckerkandl) which lies near the aortic bifurcation, or in relation to the bladder. Tumours in the bladder result in the symptom of micturation syncope (Goldfien 1981). 10% of tumours are bilateral and about the same percentage are malignant. A higher proportion of tumours are malignant when they occur in children (30%) or arise in ectopic sites. The differentiation of benign from malignant tumours may be difficult or impossible on histological grounds. Local invasion or metastases demonstrated by imaging methods are therefore important features of malignancy.

Phaeochromocytomas occur in association with other endocrine tumours. In multiple endocrine neoplasia (MEN) type II (Sipple's syndrome) phaeochromocytoma occurs in association with primary hyperplasia of the parathyroid glands and medullary carcinoma of the thyroid (Keiser et al 1973). In MEN type IIb, phaeochromocytoma occurs in association with multiple mucosal neuromas, Marfanoid habitus and medullary carcinoma of the thyroid. In these familial disorders, the phaeochromocytomas are often bilateral and are more likely to be malignant. Patients with neurofibromatosis and von Hippel–Lindau syndrome are also at increased risk of developing phaeochromocytoma which may again be bilateral (Williams 1988). Rarely, adrenal phaeochromocytoma may be the source of ectopic ACTH production causing Cushing's syndrome and hyperplasia of the cortex of the opposite adrenal gland (Jessop et al 1987).

The diagnosis of phaeochromocytoma is confirmed biochemically by finding increased levels of urinary vanillylmandelic acid (VMA), normetadrenaline and elevated plasma concentrations of catecholamines. The plasma catecholamines are more reliable than the urinary catecholamine metabolites (VMA) in confirming the diagnosis of phaeochromocytoma (Bravo et al 1979). Before the CT scan is performed, a full bowel preparation should be given so that all the gastrointestinal tract is opacified. This is particularly important if ectopic abdominal tumours are to be detected. Sections (5 or 10 mm) are first performed through the adrenals. The finding of normal adrenals in a patient with unequivocal biochemical evidence of phaeochromocytoma suggests the presence of an ectopic tumour. In these circumstances scanning should then be continued through the abdomen and pelvis at contiguous or 2 cm intervals. This technique should demonstrate large ectopic tumour, particularly those in the Organ of Zuckerkandl. However, a normal CT scan through this anatomical region would not necessarily exclude the tumour being within the abdomen (Adams et al 1983). Phaeochromocytomas vary in size, are generally smooth in outline, but may be heterogenous with cystic components; some enhance quite dramatically with contrast medium because of their vascularity (Fig. 17.8) (Laursen & Damgaard-Pedersen 1980, Thomas et al 1980, Welsh et al 1983, Moulton & Moulton 1988).

Local invasion or metastatic spread to lymph nodes and bone are features of malignant tumours. Since ectopic tumours may develop anywhere along the chain of chromaffin cells which extends from the base of the skull to the symphysis pubis, alternative imaging techniques are required to localize those ectopic tumours not identified on abdominal CT. CT is not a good technique for surveying extensive anatomical areas because of the excessive number of CT sections required for such a study. At one time, selective venous sampling for plasma catecholamines was an important method for the localization of ectopic tumours (Allison et al 1983), but this is now seldom

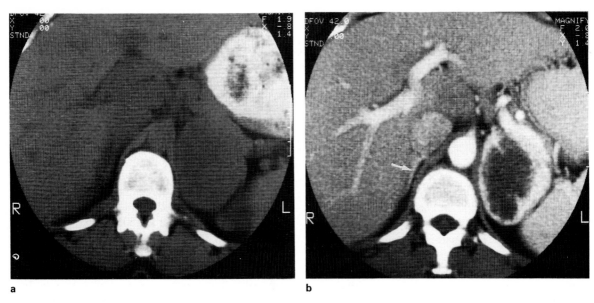

Fig. 17.8 Phaeochromocytoma. (a) Left adrenal tumour, with (b) marked contrast enhancement of its periphery and central low attenuation cystic components. The right adrenal is normal (arrow).

performed. Angiography in phaeochromocytomas carries increased morbidity with the possibility of inducing a hypertensive crisis; venography appears to be a safe procedure, as does the administration of intravenous contrast medium for CT scanning. The preferred technique for localizing ectopic tumours and metastases is radionuclide scanning, using [131]I- or ^{123}I-metaiodobenzylguanidine (MIBG) (Sisson et al 1981, Lancet Editorial 1984). ^{123}I-MIBG is now the preferred radionuclide as it has a short half-life (13.2 h), an optimum photon energy of 159 keV and provides better detection efficiency with a lower radiation dose than does ^{131}I-MIBG (Bomanji et al 1988). This radionuclide is taken up in chromaffin tissue synthesizing catecholamines. A phaeochromocytoma will appear as a localized 'hot spot' (Fig. 17.9) (Sisson et al 1981, Lancet Editorial 1984, Bomanji et al 1988). Should the site of the ectopic tumour be suggested from a radionuclide scan, CT scanning of the appropriate area should be performed to confirm the presence of a tumour and to demonstrate more clearly adjacent anatomy. Uptake of the radionuclide in metastases is helpful in the diagnosis and staging of malignant phaeochromocytoma (Fig. 17.9). ^{131}I-MIBG has therapeutic potential for tumour metastases if suf-

ficient of the radionuclide is taken up in the tumour sites. CT and ^{123}I-MIBG have complementary rôles in localizing phaeochromocytoma (Francis et al 1983, Bomanji et al 1988). Some advocate the routine use of MIBG scanning in patients with suspected phaeochromocytoma, followed by CT. An alternative and perhaps more economic approach might be to perform CT first, as outlined above, since in adults 90% of tumours will be single and located in an adrenal gland. CT is extremely reliable for identifying tumours situated in the adrenal gland, but less so in ectopic or metastatic sites (Bomanji et al 1988). ^{123}I-MIBG scanning could then be reserved for patients with normal adrenal glands on CT, in whom the tumour is likely to be ectopic (van Heerden et al 1982, Francis et al 1983).

Adrenogenital syndrome

These are rare disorders which result in virilization or feminization due to the respective excessive production of adrenal androgen and oestrogen. The most common aetiology is hydroxylase enzyme deficiencies which lead to congenital adrenal hyperplasia. In this condition the adrenals may appear normal or hyperplastic on CT. Other causes

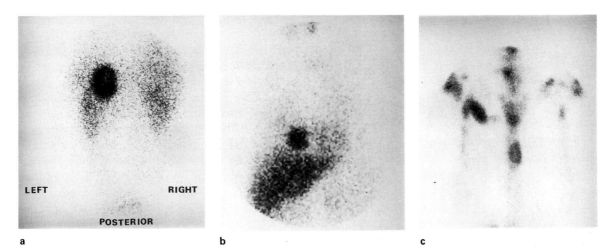

LEFT   RIGHT

POSTERIOR

a   b   c

Fig. 17.9 ^{123}I-MIBG radionuclide scan. (a) (posterior view), combined with a ^{123}I hippuran scan to demonstrate the kidneys, showing increased uptake in a large left phaeochromocytoma (same case as in Fig. 17.8. (b) Ectopic thoracic phaeochromocytoma lying above the liver (with permission from Dr M C Prescott, Department of Nuclear Medicine, Manchester Royal Infirmary). (c) Multiple skeletal metastases evident on ^{131}I-MIBG scan of thorax (with permission from Dr D M Ackery, Department of Nuclear Medicine, Southampton General Hospital).

of these syndromes include polycystic ovary disease, ovarian and autonomous adrenal tumours (adenoma or carcinoma), and it may be appropriate to extend the CT examination to include the pelvis.

Addison's disease

Clinically significant adrenocortical insufficiency can only develop when at least 90% of the adrenal cortex has been destroyed. In the past, the most common cause was bilateral adrenal tuberculosis, but now autoimmune disease is the most important cause of adrenal atrophy. On CT the adrenal glands may be normal or atrophic and may contain calcifications (Doppman et al 1982). In some patients with primary adrenal failure there is enlargement of the adrenal glands caused either by adrenal haemorrhage (Wolverson & Kannegiesser 1984), or, rarely, bilateral metastases.

Non-functioning adrenal tumours and masses

Since CT provides such an excellent technique for the demonstration of normal and abnormal adrenals, an increasing number of adrenal masses are now being identified in patients with no evidence of adrenal dysfunction (Glazer et al 1982, Prinz et al 1982, Copeland 1983, Mitnick et al 1983, Bernardino 1988). Single or multiple adenomas have been found in up to 9% of adrenal glands examined at autopsy (Hedeland et al 1968). These non-functioning lesions have the same appearances as functioning adrenal tumours. They are generally larger than 3 cm and may be 10 cm or more in diameter. Myelolipoma is a rare adrenal tumour which has a low CT attenuation because of its fat and bone marrow contents (Musante et al 1988). Occasionally, these tumours are bilateral. Adrenal cysts are uncommon but may be large; they are well-defined and of water attenuation on CT. Up to 15% may be bilateral (Moulton & Moulton 1988). The other causes of bilateral adrenal masses are haemorrhage (Wolverson & Kannegiesser 1984) and metastases (Fig. 17.10). Adrenal metastases may be found at autopsy in up to 27% of patients dying of malignant disease (Abrams et al 1950, Lump & McKenzie 1959). The most common tumours to metastasize to the adrenal are those which arise in lung and breast; others include carcinoma of the kidney, gastrointestinal tract, thyroid and pancreas and melanoma. The adrenal glands should therefore be included in the scanned areas in CT being performed as a staging procedure for these primary

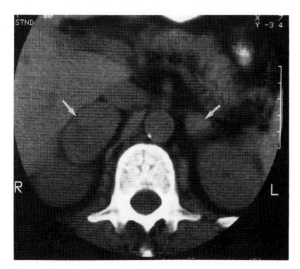

Fig. 17.10 Bilateral adrenal enlargement (arrows) due to metastases from bronchial carcinoma.

tumours. Primary lymphoma of the adrenal is rare (Vicks et al 1987), but the adrenals may be infiltrated in association with lymphomatous disease elsewhere in the abdomen, particularly retroperitoneal disease. Although adrenal metastases are common, not all adrenal masses occurring in patients with known carcinoma are necessarily indicative of metastatic disease (Ambrose et al 1980). Percutaneous aspiration biopsy, either using CT or ultrasound guidance, may be needed to establish the histological nature of the adrenal mass (Bernardino et al 1985, Koeniker et al 1988). Adrenal biopsy has proved to be an accurate and safe technique but is contraindicated in phaeochromocytoma, in which serious or even fatal complications may develop (Casola et al 1986). Other interventional radiological procedures have been less successful than needle biopsy. Remission of Conn's syndrome had previously been observed following adrenal venography (Fischer et al 1971). Consequently, adrenal ablation has been attempted by retrograde venous ethanol injection, but this proved an ineffective and dangerous procedure (Doppman & Girton 1984) and has been discarded.

Other imaging techniques

Ultrasound in the hands of an experienced operator may be usefully applied to the identification of adrenal masses, although CT remains the more sensitive imaging technique. A high resolution real time sector scanner is the equipment of choice and scans are performed in the transverse plane, using the liver as an acoustic window for the right adrenal and the spleen for the left adrenal (Sample 1978, Yeh 1988). Ultrasound may be particularly helpful in those patients in whom the adrenals are not well seen on CT. These are patients with little intra-abdominal fat, such as cachetic patients and the young (Abrams et al 1982). Ultrasound is also suitable for examining the adrenal glands for masses in staging primary malignant tumours known to metastasize to the adrenal. The anatomy of the adrenal glands is similar on ultrasound to that identified at CT. Adrenal tumours are usually hypoechoic in relation to the echogenic surrounding perinephric fat (Fig. 17.11). Small adrenal masses of less than 3 cm used to be difficult to identify with ultrasound, but with technical improvements in equipment the rate of detection of tumours in experienced hands is high (97%) (Yeh 1988). Ultrasound is helpful for guidance during biopsy techniques.

The rôle of ^{123}I-MIBG scanning in the localiz-

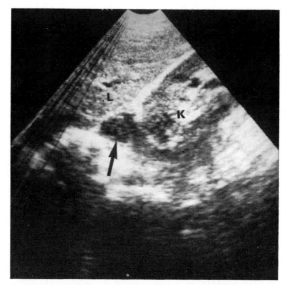

Fig. 17.11 Ultrasound (longitudinal) scan showing right adrenal tumour (arrow) lying above the right kidney (K) and below the liver (L).

ation of phaeochromocytoma, particularly if in an ectopic site, has already been discussed. Radio-labelled cholesterol techniques have been applied to the identification of adrenal cortical tumours and hyperplasia in both Cushing's and Conn's syndromes (Hawkins et al 1980). Such techniques can provide quantitative functional images and differentiate hyperplasia from a unilateral auto-nomous adrenal tumour. However, they are asso-ciated with fairly high doses of radiation, both to the adrenal and other structures. Scanning can only be performed after a number of days, whilst the radionuclide is incorporated into cholesterol synthesis. CT has made these techniques redun-dant in the majority of cases.

Magnetic resonance imaging has also been ap-plied to the identification of normal adrenal glands and adrenal tumours (Demas et al 1987, Egglin et al 1988). Most of the clinical experience has been reported using an intermediate magnetic field strength (0.3–0.6 T) and 10 mm thick sections. Normal adrenal tissue has an intermediate signal intensity on T_1-weighted images and a much lower signal than surrounding fat on T_2 pulse sequences. The ability for multiplanar imaging enables the delineation of normal adrenal glands and adrenal tumours. Imaging in these multiple planes may be helpful in identifying the organ of origin of large tumours which may otherwise be difficult to ascertain from CT. Ultrasound may also provide such information. Attempts have been made to characterize the MR signal from adrenal lesions to differentiate between adenomas, primary and secondary malignant neoplasms and phaeo-chromocytoma (Glazer et al 1986). Although some additional diagnostic information is derived from measurements of MR signal intensity, this is, as yet, inadequate for differentiating benign from malignant adrenal tumours (Egglin et al 1988).

PITUITARY TUMOURS

Introduction

Six main hormones are produced by the anterior pituitary gland. These are growth hormone (GH), prolactin (PRL), adenocorticotrophin (ACTH), thyrotrophin (TSH) and the gonadotrophins, fol-licle stimulating hormone (FSH) and luteinizing hormone (LH). GH and PRL are produced from acidophil cells, and ACTH from basophil cells. Hypothalamic stimulating factors, transported via the portal venous system of the gland, control the secretion of GH, ACTH, TSH and gonadotrophin. Their secrection is modified by negative feedback mechanisms. Prolactin secretion is under tonic in-hibition by dopamine (McNicol 1987). Adenomas of the pituitary are classified as microadenomas if their diameter is less than 10 mm and macro-adenomas if larger.

Prolactinomas are the commonest of the pituitary tumours. They cause amenorrhoea and infertility in young women, in whom they are generally microadenomas. However, when prolac-tinomas occur in older women and men, the tumours are larger and more aggressive (Daunt & Mowat 1985). The preferred treatment for prolac-tinomas is medical with bromocriptine, which is a dopamine agonist (Lancet Editorial 1982). With this treatment the secretion of prolactin falls and there is fairly rapid reduction in the size of the tumours, even in those which are large and extend outside the sella (Scotti et al 1982, Wass et al 1982). Although the secretion of prolactin tends to rise when treatment is stopped, there does not ap-pear to be a concomitant increase in the size of the tumour (Johnson et al 1984). Not all tumours respond to bromocriptine (Bonneville et al 1982), and in this case surgical adenomectomy is required, generally through a transphenoidal approach.

Tumours of somatatroph cells comprise ap-proximately 17% of pituitary tumours, and result in an increased circulating concentration of GH (Daughaday 1981). This increased secretion of GH leads to gigantism when the condition presents in childhood and to acromegaly in adult life. Up to 20% of acromegalics have hyperprolactinaemia. With the sophisticated immunohistochemistry which can now be performed on pituitary tissue, many tumours are recognized to be of mixed cell types, and to produce a variety of hormones, al-though usually one predominates to produce the characteristic clinical picture (McNicol 1987). In acromegaly there is progressive coarsening of facial features and an increase in the size of the soft tis-sues of the hands and feet. Hypertrophy of cartilages in the larynx causes the voice to become deep and husky. The proliferation of cartilage may cause the joint spaces to appear widened on radiographs and this is best seen at the metacarpophalangeal and metatarsophalangeal joints of the hands and feet. This hypertrophied cartilage fissures and predisposes to degenerative arthritis (Kellgren et al 1952). Acromegaly also results in hyperostosis with ossification at ligamentous insertions. Other radiological features of the condition are posterior vertebral scalloping and stenosis of the vertebral canal from new bone formation and degenerative arthritis at the apophyseal joints. The lateral skull shows prognathism with an increase in the angle of the mandible, thickening of the skull vault and prominence of the paranasal sinuses. The sella turcica is commonly expanded and eroded because the tumours are usually large at presentation. Bromocriptine has been used to treat patients with these tumours, but more often surgery is required. This is performed either through a transphenoidal approach or via a craniotomy. As these tumours are invasive, surgery seldom effects a complete cure and external irradiation therapy is often given to augment the treatment. Local implantation of radioactive isotopes (yttrium, gold and strontium) is now seldom performed because of the complications of rhinorrhea and meningitis (Daughaday 1981).

Corticotroph adenomas produce excess ACTH and cause Cushing's disease. These tumours are generally microadenomas and may be as small as 2 mm. They therefore seldom cause expansion of the sella turcica. Patients present with the characteristic clinical and biochemical features of hypercortisolism. There are high circulating concentrations of ACTH and cortisol (with loss of diurnal variation), and bilateral adrenal hyperplasia. In the past the condition was treated by bilateral adrenalectomy, and in 10% of these patients the pituitary tumour later increased in size in association with deepening pigmentation of the skin (Nelson's syndrome). The preferred treatment is now transphenoidal microsurgery, as was originally performed by Harvey Cushing in the 1920s (Teasdale 1983). The tumours, although small, may be locally invasive and postoperative external irradiation may also be required for cure.

Gonadotrophin tumours are rare, and account for only about 4% of pituitary adenomas. They occur in middle-aged men and present as large tumours with associated visual failure. Thyrotroph cell adenomas are rare (McNicol 1987).

Non-secretory pituitary tumours are generally chromophobe adenomas. However, with electron microscopy and histocytochemistry these tumours are often shown to contain secretory granules. These tumours may present incidentally through the unsuspected finding of an abnormal sella turcica on skull radiograph, or clinically because of hypopituitarism or parasellar symptoms and signs. Craniopharyngiomas are the most important non-pituitary tumours arising in the vicinity of the sella, with 20% arising within the sella and 80% in the suprasellar region. Craniopharyngiomas arise from remnants of Rathke's pouch and their composition varies from simple cysts to solid tumours. In the majority of cases (74%) the sella is enlarged and calcification is common (almost 70%). Other tumours (meningiomas, chordomas and metastases) and aneurysms may involve the sella and mimic non-functioning pituitary tumours in their clinical presentation.

In addition to their specific hormonal effects, large functionally active adenomas can also cause parasellar symptoms. Headaches are common and

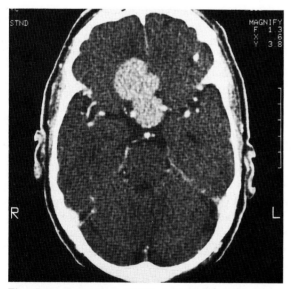

Fig. 17.12 Transverse axial CT of the pituitary. The scan shows large, enhancing, lobulated pituitary tumour extending into the suprasellar region and anterior cranial fossa.

involvement of the optic chiasma generally results in bitemporal hemianopia. Involvement of other cranial nerves is infrequent despite the close proximity of the third, fourth and sixth cranial nerves within the cavernous sinuses. Impaired function of the third nerve may occur, and involvement of olfactory nerves results in loss of the sense of smell.

Imaging in pituitary tumours

The rôle of imaging is to identify and define the extent of the pituitary tumour; this may have important implications for surgical management.

Skull radiography

Large tumours expand and erode the pituitary fossa. Asymmetrical erosion of the fossa causes the floor to slope downwards on one side in the coronal plane (PA 20° skull radiograph), resulting in a 'double floor' to the sella on the lateral skull view. The dorsum sella may be completely eroded and a soft tissue mass may be seen to extend into the sphenoid sinus. These abnormalities of the sella are generally seen in patients with acromegaly, craniopharyngiomas and non-functioning chromophobe adenomas. In other conditions the pituitary tumours are considerably smaller, and fewer than 5% of patients with Cushing's disease and about one-third of patients with prolactinomas have associated abnormalities of the sella. Plain radiography and tomography of the sella are of limited value in confirming the presence of a pituitary tumour unless there is gross expansion or erosion. Over one-third of normal sellae have a coronal slope to the floor of greater than 8° and there is poor correlation between asymmetry and thinning of the sellar floor and pituitary pathology (Burrow et al 1981, Wortzman & Rewcastle 1982). Linear, area and volume measurements of the sella can be made on radiographs, but as there is a wide variation in the normal range such measurements are seldom applied in practice (Di Chiro & Nelson 1962). For this reason, tomography of the sella has largely been abandoned because it provides little useful diagnostic information and incurs a high radiation dose. Other imaging techniques such as

air encephalography and cisternography have also become obsolete with the introduction of high resolution CT. This has resulted in considerable economic benefit in the diagnosis and management of patients with pituitary adenoma. Diagnosis is more accurate and few, if any, invasive imaging procedures are now necessary with consequent shortening of the preoperative in-patient hospital stay (Newton et al 1983).

For pituitary tissue to be visualized on CT, intravenous contrast medium must be used. Conventional 10 mm transverse axial sections through the brain are adequate for demonstrating large pituitary tumours with parasellar extension (Fig. 17.12). However, the ability to demonstrate normal pituitary anatomy and microadenomas wholly contained within the fossa has become possible only with technical developments in CT which allowed for thinner sections, reformatting of images and scanning in a direct coronal plane (Fig. 17.13) (Taylor 1982, Carr et al 1984). Preliminary 5 mm section may be performed before contrast medium is given. These thin (1–2 mm) contiguous sections are performed through the sellar and suprasellar regions during contrast medium infusion. If good quality reformatted images are to be generated from the CT sections obtained, it is imperative that the patient's head remains in an identical position throughout the scanning. An intravenous line should therefore be inserted before scanning commences and a non-ionic contrast medium should be used to avoid motion artefact. The contrast medium (100 ml) is injected by hand at a rate of 2 ml/s and scanning is commenced after 50 ml have been administered. For small children contrast medium is given in a dose of 2 ml per kg body weight, using the same technique as in adults. Generally the direct coronal scanning plane is preferred as this involves a lower dose of radiation to the lens of the eye. However, to obtain scans in this plane the patient lies supine, with the head hyperextended (Fig. 17.13). Some patients, particularly those with pituitary dysfunction such as Cushing's syndrome or acromegaly, may find this position difficult if not impossible to maintain. In such circumstances transverse axial sections may be obtained (Fig. 17.12) and from these, sagittal and coronal reformatted images can be generated by the computer. There is always some

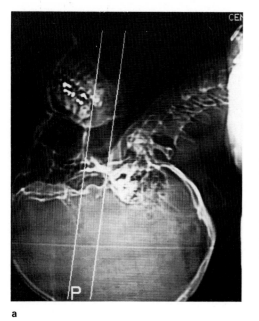
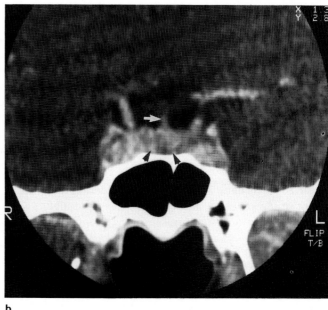

a   b

Fig. 17.13   Coronal CT of the pituitary. (a) Lateral scanned projection radiograph showing extended position of head. (b). 1.5 mm coronal section (postcontrast) through the normal pituitary gland (arrowheads) and infundibulum (arrow).

loss of spatial resolution in reformatted images. From the images obtained, the size and shape of the pituitary gland can be assessed and any non-enhancing area or region of abnormal enhancement identified. The normal vertical height of the

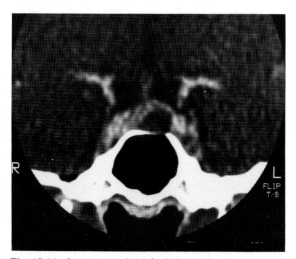

Fig. 17.14   Low attenuation left pituitary adenoma (postcontrast coronal CT) causing convexity of the upper margin of the gland, displacement of the infundibulum to the right and thinning of the adjacent sellar floor.

pituitary gland is about 5 mm ($\pm$1.5 mm) in males and a little larger, 7 mm ($\pm$1.5 mm), in females (Syvertsen et al 1979), with a flat or concave upper margin. Such measurements of pituitary size must always be performed using consistent viewing facilities (e.g. window width 250 HU; window level 50 HU). However, in women of childbearing age, the upper margin of the gland may be convex and the gland may be fairly bulky and measure up to 9.7 mm (Swartz et al 1983). The pituitary gland may be enlarged in patients with primary hypothyroidism. This hyperplasia regresses with treatment of the hypothyroidism (O'Kuno et al 1980, Silver et al 1981). The infundibulum also enhances and is generally seen throughout its length. It measures up to about 3 mm in diameter and, in coronal sections, normally lies vertically 1.5° $\pm$ 1.2° in the midline (Nakagawa et al 1984). Pituitary adenomas are usually demonstrated as low attenuation areas within the surrounding enhancing pituitary gland (Fig. 17.14) (Daniels et al 1981, Hendricks 1988). Depending on its size, the adenoma may cause convexity of the upper margin of the pituitary, with associated displacement of the infundibulum and erosion of the floor of the

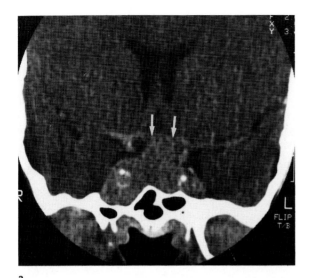

a

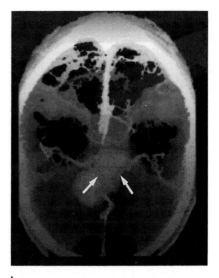

b

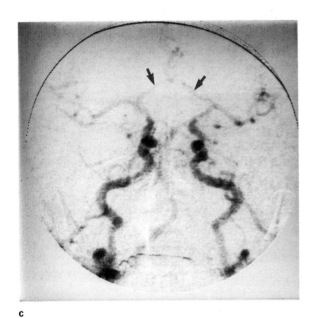

c

Fig. 17.15   Large pituitary tumours. (a) Coronal (postcontrast CT) showing extension of the tumour into the right middle cranial fossa and into the suprasellar region to abut the anterior cerebral vessels (arrows). (b) Reformation (supero-inferior view with part of cranium 'removed') from 1.5 mm contiguous CT sections (postcontrast) showing relation of anterior cerebral arteries (arrows) to large, lobulated pituitary tumour. (c) Digital subtraction intravenous angiogram on same patient, showing elevation of anterior cerebral arteries (arrows) by the tumour.

fossa (Fig. 17.14). Extension into the suprasellar region and adjacent cavernous sinus can also be identified. The relation of the suprasellar extension of the tumour to adjacent vessels can be determined but may be better appreciated by deriving 3D CT images from the high resolution CT study (Fig. 17.15) (Gholkar & Isherwood 1988). Extension into the cavernous sinus is important to note since this makes complete surgical removal of the

adenoma difficult or impossible. The presence of bony septa within the sphenoid sinus may make the transphenoidal operative approach more difficult, particularly if the septa lie in the midline. Such septa should be noted from the scan, as should the presence of any sinus infection. Dynamic sequential scanning through the same coronal section has been advocated to identify lateral displacement of the midline 'tuft sign' of the sinusoidal vessels which normally lie in the middle of the anterior lobe. Their displacement may be an additional helpful feature to indicate the presence and site of a microadenoma (Bonneville et al 1983). However, such dynamic scanning is not widely practiced. Adenomas are generally low in attenuation but may rarely be higher in attenuation than the surrounding pituitary gland (Gardeur et al 1981). While craniopharyngiomas are generally cystic, pituitary adenomas rarely are. The attenuation characteristics of an adenoma depend on the scanning technique and the interval between

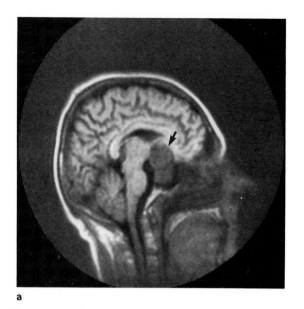
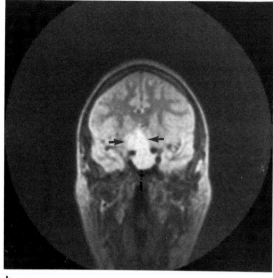

a   b

Fig. 17.16   Magnetic resonance scan of a pituitary tumour with suprasellar extension. (a) T_1-weighted sequence (IR 1500/500) in the mid-sagittal plane showing tumour (arrow) with intermediate signal intensity. (b) T_2-weighted sequence (SE 2000/80) in the coronal plane showing tumour with higher signal intensity than adjacent brain.

scanning and the administration of contrast medium. If scanning is delayed some time after the administration of contrast, adenomas which were originally hypodense may become isodense or even hyperdense in relation to the adjacent normal pituitary tissue (Hemminghytt et al 1983). Normal pituitary glands may appear heterogenous (Roppolo et al 1983) and this should not be mistakenly interpreted as indicating the site of an adenoma. A low attenuation area is not specific for a functioning adenoma. At autopsy, other lesions which would cause similar low attenuation areas are fairly frequently found; incidental micro-adenomas may occur in up to 20% of individuals, pars intermedia cysts in 13–20%, and in patients dying of disseminated malignancy, pituitary metastases or infarcts are present in 25% (Chambers et al 1982).

Studies which have correlated the CT diagnosis of the presence and site of adenomas and subsequent surgical findings have not unexpectedly revealed some inaccuracies on CT (Davies et al 1985, Teasdale et al 1986). Heterogeneity of the gland and convexity of the upper margin can be normal and should not be interpreted as evidence of an adenoma. A combination of abnormalities,

including displacement of the infundibulum and erosion of the adjacent fossa floor combined with a low attenuation area, makes the diagnosis and localization of pituitary adenoma by CT much more secure (Davis et al 1985). Accurate preoperative localization of adenoma is helpful to the surgeon, especially when considering transphenoidal microsurgery, which is being increasingly adopted as the surgical procedure of choice in appropriate patients with functioning pituitary adenoma (Teasdale 1983).

CT can also be used to assess the efficacy of medical treatment and quite dramatic reductions in the size of prolactinomas have been demonstrated within a month of starting treatment with bromocriptine, even when these are fairly large and extensive (Fig. 17.15) (Scotti et al 1982, Wass et al 1982, Chakera et al 1985). Not all tumours respond to bromocriptine; on treatment, the attenuation of the tumours may alter, becoming higher or lower than the pretreatment value (Bonneville et al 1982). In tumours with suprasellar extension, information can be obtained about the relation of the tumour to the carotid vessels using 3D CT (Gholkar & Isherwood 1988), but angiography may still be required to depict more clearly the parasellar vascular anatomy (Fig. 17.15) or to exclude other causes of the parasellar mass (e.g. meningioma or aneurysm) (Daniels et al 1981). Digital intravenous subtraction angiography is generally adequate for this purpose.

A number of artefacts may occur on CT. If there are dental fillings, a scan plane should be selected to avoid these since they cause streak artefact which degrades intrasellar detail on the direct coronal scan. On transverse scans, streaking between the high attenuation sphenoid and petrous ridges causes a cross artefact within the sella (Earnest et al 1981). This should not be mistakenly interpreted as an adenoma. Lesser degrees of enhancement in the posterior pituitary may cause an appearance resembling an apparent adenoma (Bonneville et al 1985) and on MRI, what was originally regarded as a posterior fat pad within the sella is probably the posterior pituitary (Mark et al 1984). If large pituitary tumours undergo spontaneous infarction, or are treated with radiotherapy, little pituitary tissue may remain and low attenuation cerebrospinal fluid (CSF) extends to fill the sella. This results in an 'empty sella' or 'partially empty sella', which may also be caused by herniation of CSF through a defective diaphragma sella. Minor degrees of herniation are frequent (Kaufman & Chamberlin 1972) as normal variants, and it is common to see some CSF extending into the fossa on high resolution CT. When there is an empty sella, the enhancing infundibulum extends down into the fossa and is surrounded by CSF, and should not be mistaken for an enhancing tumour nodule (Haughton et al 1981). The presence of a 'partially empty sella' does not preclude the coexistence of an adenoma (Smaltino et al 1980). A normal CT scan does not preclude the presence of an adenoma. To be identifiable on CT, pituitary adenomas have to be at least 2–3 mm in size, and in some patients with Cushing's syndrome the tumours may be smaller than this. For this reason, in occasional cases of Cushing's disease, simultaneous venous sampling for ACTH levels (basally or in response to the administration of corticotrophin releasing factor, CRF) from both inferior petrosal sinuses may be necessary to confirm and lateralize the presence of a pituitary adenoma (Landolt et al 1986). This technique may be helpful in differentiating pituitary-dependent disease from an ectopic ACTH syndrome when other evidence is lacking, and general venous sampling for ACTH levels may localize an occult ectopic ACTH tumour source (Findling & Tyrell 1986, Howlett et al 1986).

Magnetic resonance imaging has been applied to pituitary tumours (Hawkes et al 1983). In reports using medium (0.5 T) and high (1.5 T) magnetic field strengths with 7 mm thick slices, magnetic resonance has proved to be better than CT at defining the para- and suprasellar extent of large tumours (Fig. 17.16) (Glaser et al 1986). CT is more sensitive for focal lesions within the sella than MRI, at least at the present time, and CT remains the initial imaging technique of choice for suspected microadenoma (Davis et al 1987). However, thinner (3 mm) sections are now possible and with further improvements in technology, MR will probably also prove to be a sensitive way of identifying and localizing pituitary microadenoma. T_1-weighted sequences have been found to be most useful, with adenomas having a lower intensity signal than surrounding pituitary tissue. The T_2-weighted sequences are less helpful, since the tumour signal may be variable (Kucharczyk et al 1986).

PARATHYROID TUMOURS

Introduction

The parathyroid glands are derived from the endodermal germ layer and develop from a fold in the ventral wall of the pharynx during embryological differentiation. There are usually four glands in all, two upper and two lower glands. The upper glands develop from the fourth branchial pouch, are fairly consistent in position and related to the posterior aspect of the upper poles of the thyroid gland. Their blood supply is derived from the inferior thyroid artery. The lower glands arise from the third branchial pouch and, together with the thymus, migrate caudally and are consequently more variable in position than the upper glands. The inferior glands are usually related to the posterior aspect of the inferior lobes of the thyroid, but they may be located close to the carotid sheath and the thymus, in the anterior mediastinum or, more rarely, in the posterior mediastinum

(Doppman et al 1975). They may also be found in the pharyngeal submucosa when there is a failure to migrate, and rarely, actually within the thyroid gland (Spiegel et al 1975). The inferior glands are supplied by the inferior thyroid arteries, or the medial thoracic (internal mammary) artery if they are located in the mediastinum. In some people there may be five (8%) or even six (8%) parathyroid glands. The combined weight of all four glands is approximately 120 mg. Each normal gland is ellipsoid in shape and measures $6 \times 5 \times 2$ mm in size. These anatomical points are important when imaging techniques are performed for the preoperative localization of parathyroid tumours.

Parathyroid hormone (PTH) regulates, and is normally regulated by, the ionized serum calcium concentration which is maintained within narrow limits. Most parathyroid tumours are functionally active and lead to the clinical syndrome of primary hyperparathyroidism. The aetiology of the condition is uncertain, but genetic factors are relevant in a proportion of patients (familial hyperplasia, multiple endocrine neoplasia (MEN) syndrome). 'Secondary' hyperparathyroidism is induced by any condition or circumstances which cause the serum calcium to fall, as occurs in vitamin D deficiency, intestinal malabsorption of calcium, and in chronic renal failure (through lack of the active metabolite of vitamin D, 1,25-dihydroxy-cholecalciferol $(1,25-(OH)_2D)$ and retention of phosphorus). If this 'secondary' hyperparathyroidism is of sufficiently long standing, an autonomous adenoma may develop in the hyperplastic parathyroid glands, a condition referred to as 'tertiary' hyperparathyroidism (Aurbach et al 1981). This condition is usually associated with chronic renal disease but it has also been reported in patients with long-standing vitamin D deficiency and osteomalacia from other causes.

Primary hyperparathyroidism

PTH acts principally on the kidney and the skeleton, where it promotes the renal tubular reabsorption of calcium and the mobilization of calcium from bone. PTH also stimulates osteoclastic bone resorption, and increases the renal excretion of phosphorus. PTH stimulates the renal biosynthesis of the active metabolite of vitamin D, $1,25-(OH)_2D$, and thereby enhances the intestinal absorption of calcium. These various actions result in predictable biochemical changes typical of primary hyperparathyroidism: hypercalcaemia; normal or reduced serum phosphate and hypercalciuria. The diagnosis is confirmed by finding inappropriately normal or elevated levels of circulating PTH concentrations. Primary hyperparathyroidism has to be differentiated from other conditions which cause hypercalcaemia. These include malignant disease (with or without bone metastases), and less commonly vitamin D intoxication, sarcoidosis, the milk–alkali syndrome, thyrotoxicosis, and adrenal insufficiency. These conditions can usually be recognized on clinical grounds; serum PTH assay is helpful in diagnosis, as is the response of the serum calcium level to administration of corticosteroids. Glucocorticoids generally correct hypercalcaemia induced by factors other than PTH, but not in primary hyperparathyroidism. Differentiation of primary hyperparathyroidism from familial hypocalciuric hypercalcaemia (FHH) can be difficult. This condition is inherited as an autosomal dominant trait and has a biochemical profile similar to primary hyperparathyroidism, including circulating levels of PTH. A helpful differentiating feature is the lower renal clearance of filtered urinary calcium and magnesium in patients with FHH (Davies et al 1981). The differentiation from primary hyperparathyroidism is important because parathyroidectomy is usually of no benefit in FHH (Aurbach et al 1981).

Incidence

Primary hyperparathyroidism is relatively common and the incidence of the disease within the population is about 1 in 1000 (0.1%). Over the past 40 years the prevalence of the condition has increased some tenfold: this increase is due in large part to the detection by chance of hypercalcaemia in patients, many of whom are asymptomatic, through the routine use of multichannel autoanalysis of serum samples (Adams 1982).

Few patients now present with metabolic bone disease (osteitis fibrosa cystica). The most common clinical presentations are related to renal stones and nephrocalcinosis (25–35% of patients). The composition of the renal stones is usually calcium oxalate or calcium phosphate. The frequency of primary hyperparathyroidism among patients with calcium-containing renal stones is not great, probably about 5%. Hypertension is common, and is present in 40–60% of patients. Other clinical presentations of the disease include crystal arthropathy (pseudogout), chondrocalcinosis, osteoporosis, acute pancreatitis, peptic ulcer, depression, confusional states and proximal muscle weakness. Severe hypercalcaemia, which may be life threatening (parathyroid crisis) is, fortunately, rare. Most patients with primary hyperparathyroidism have mild disease and commonly have no symptoms (Adams 1982).

Surgical removal of the overactive parathyroid tissue is generally recommended and, in experienced hands, is successful in curing the condition in up to 95% of patients (Satava et al 1975). It is essential that surgery be performed by those experienced in the field. In 10–15% of patients, surgery may fail. to identify the parathyroid tumour (Aurbach et al 1981) and, even in experienced hands, complications of surgery occur and have proved fatal (Gough et al 1971). Such occurrences emphasize the importance of ensuring that the diagnosis of hyperparathyroidism is correct before neck exploration is undertaken and lends weight to the desirability for a sensitive and reliable technique for identifying the location of tumours before surgery is undertaken. The decision to operate, particularly in the elderly and those with asymptomatic disease, requires careful assessment. If conservative treatment is judged to be the management of choice, techniques for tumour localization are irrelevant, though renal function and blood pressure will need to be monitored at regular intervals. Although the majority (approximately 60%) of such asymptomatic patients treated conservatively show little change in serum calcium and renal function with time (Sampson et al 1987), some 20% will eventually require surgery (Purnell et al 1974).

The majority of patients (82%) with primary hyperparathyroidism have a single adenoma. This is generally of chief cell type or transitional between chief cell and oxyphil cells; pure oxyphil cell adenomas are rare. Chief cell hyperplasia of all the glands occurs in 14% of patients with hyperparathyroidism; the histological diagnosis is dependent on finding more than one affected parathyroid gland. For this reason, at least one apparently normal parathyroid gland must be identified at exploration of the neck, in addition to any tumour, and be examined by frozen section at the time of operation to identify the gland histology. The findings determine surgical management. If there is parathyroid hyperplasia, this will affect all four glands and subtotal parathyroidectomy (at least $3\frac{1}{2}$ glands) is indicated. Even then, hyperparathyroidism may recur, particularly in the multiple neoplasia syndromes. As subsequent neck explorations can be difficult and potentially hazardous (Wang 1977, Brennan et al 1978), some advocate the removal of all four hyperplastic glands from the outset, with a small portion of a gland then being re-implanted under the skin of the forearm, where it is more accessible should subsequent removal be required for recurrent disease (Wells et al 1976). It is generally agreed that chief cell hyperplasia is the histological lesion present in all the inherited forms of primary hyperparathyroidism. In multiple endocrine neoplasia (MEN) syndrome type I (Wermer's syndrome), which has an autosomal dominant mode of inheritance, hyperparathyroidism is the most common manifestation of the disease and occurs in 95% of cases. Other manifestations of the MEN (type I) syndrome include tumours which secrete gastrin (20–40%), insulin (2–10%) and other pancreatic islet cell peptides (glucagonoma, vipoma), and adenomas of the anterior pituitary which can secrete growth hormone, ACTH or prolactin.

Hyperparathyroidism occurs in 20–30% or more of patients with MEN type IIa (Sipple's syndrome). This condition has an autosomal dominant mode of inheritance and associated tumours include medullary ('C' cell) carcinoma of the thyroid (causing hypercalcitonaemia), and phaeochromocytoma (Keiser et al 1973). In MEN type IIb or III there is 'C' cell hyperplasia, associated with phaeochromocytoma, mucosal neuromas, ganglioneuromas and marfanoid features, but hyperparathyroidism is uncommon.

Carcinoma of the parathyroid is an infrequent cause of primary hyperparathyroidism (1–4%).

The tumour is slow growing but locally invasive. Cure may be obtained by adequate surgical excision and there is a 5-year survival of greater than 50%. However, recurrence is common (30%) and metastases occur late in 30% of patients, to regional lymph nodes, lung, liver and bone (Schwartz & Castleman 1973). Biochemical remission may rarely occur spontaneously, presumably due to infarction of the tumour (Klimiuk & Mainwaring 1980). This is, however, rare, since the parathyroid glands have a rich blood supply from both the inferior and superior thyroid arteries. Metastases, when solitary, may also be resected with benefit (Davies et al 1973a).

Imaging in parathyroid tumours

The role of imaging in primary hyperparathyroidism is firstly to confirm the presence of skeletal (subperiosteal erosions, bone cysts or chondrocalcinosis), renal (calculi, nephrocalcinosis) or other associated (e.g. acute pancreatitis) abnormalities consistent with or diagnostic of the disease, and secondly in preoperative localization of the tumour. Few patients (5–10%) show radiological evidence of osteitis fibrosa cystica. If skeletal abnormalities are present radiologically, subperiosteal erosions are most likely to be seen in the phalanges and skull; chondrocalcinosis occurs most frequently in the triangular ligament of the wrist, menisci and articular cartilage of the knees, and in the symphysis pubis. Selected radiographs of these areas may be performed (hands PA, lateral skull, AP knees), but extensive radiographic skeletal surveys are unrewarding. A plain AP abdominal radiograph should also be done to detect renal stones and nephrocalcinosis. Since no imaging technique thus far applied to the identification and localization of enlarged parathyroid glands has a specificity and sensitivity of 100%, such techniques can play no part in establishing or confirming the diagnosis of hyperparathyroidism, which ultimately rests on clinical and biochemical grounds. When surgical treatment of the disease is considered necessary, it may be appropriate to use imaging and other techniques to locate the parathyroid tumour preoperatively. Reliable and accurate preoperative localization of the tumour confers advantages at surgery. If the tumour is

confirmed to be in the predicted site and on frozen section is an adenoma, then only the other gland on the ipsilateral side need be identified and biopsied. If normal, the contralateral side need not be explored, so reducing operating time and morbidity.

Tumour localization

Parathyroid tumours are seldom large enough to be palpable or to cause any significant or detectable displacement or indentation of the trachea or oesophagus. Various localizing techniques have been applied in the past to the identification of parathyroid tumours. These included cine radiography, infusion of toluidine blue and radionuclide scanning using [75]selenomethionine. However, these have become obsolete as none was particularly successful and some were potentially hazardous (toluidine blue caused cardiac dysrhythmias and haemolytic anaemia). Before the introduction of non-invasive techniques for the localization of parathyroid tumours (ultrasound, CT and MRI), the most useful technique was a combination of arteriography and venography which would permit the correct localization of the tumour in about 95% of patients (Doppman 1976). These techniques are time consuming and potentially hazardous, and call for a great deal of skill and experience on the part of the radiologist, and they are now carried out infrequently. Venous sampling became possible with the development of reliable serum assays for parathyroid hormone. Samples of blood are taken for assay of parathyroid hormone from various veins in the neck and those draining the upper mediastinum. A careful record, or map, is made of the sites of sampling, and some advocate that each vessel from which a sample has been taken should be radiographically recorded (Shimkin et al 1972, Davies et al 1973b, Doppman 1976, Dunlop et al 1980). When a parathyroid adenoma is present the serum concentration of PTH in the vein draining the tumour is higher than that in the general circulation (hormone gradient). Such a localized gradient will not be present if all four glands are overactive, as occurs in primary parathyroid hyperplasia. Parathyroid adenomas can also be identified at angiography, and because they are fairly vascular they show a characteristic 'blush'. During angiography contrast medium is injected into the carotid and subclavian vessels, and selective injections can be made into the inferior thyroid and internal mammary arteries, and the thyrocervical trunk. Injection into the superior thyroid artery is generally omitted, as this causes considerable pain. Digital subtraction angiography (DSA) has also been applied to the localization of parathyroid tumours, and requires the injection of contrast medium only into the carotid and subclavian arteries bilaterally (Levy et al 1982, Obley et al 1984, Miller et al 1987b). In patients with recurrent hyperparathyroidism, the venous anatomy might be altered by the preceding surgery because some draining veins are often ligated at operation. In this setting, arteriography should precede parathyroid venous sampling in order to demonstrate venous drainage patterns (Doppman 1976). Some have advocated that intravenous DSA be used after parathyroid surgery (Clark et al 1985) but this technique is inadequate for demonstrating venous drainage patterns and intra-arterial DSA is required (Miller et al 1987b).

With the introduction of general purpose CT scanners in 1975, the technique was soon applied to the localization of parathyroid tumours. However, initial reports were disappointing and only large tumours could be identified and correctly localized (Adams et al 1981). These disappointing results were attributed to slow scanning time (20 s) which led to movement artefacts, relatively thick slices (13 mm) causing partial volume averaging and failure to identify small tumours, and the variable spatial orientation of parathyroid tumours. These tumours can be ellipsoid in shape with their long axis running parallel to the long axis of the body and closely applied to the thyroid gland. As a result, only a small diameter of the tumour can present on the transverse axial CT section. With advances in CT technology (thinner sections and rapid scanning) and the use of contrast enhancement, the anatomy of the neck can be demonstrated with greater precision and Doppman (1982) suggested that the application of CT to parathyroid tumour localization should be re-examined. With the use of contiguous 5 mm sections through the neck and upper mediastinum before and during contrast infusion, between 70% and 80% of tumours can be correctly localized (Som-

mer et al 1982). This technique involves in excess of 50 CT sections, and a satisfactory compromise is to perform 1 cm contiguous sections through the neck and upper mediastinum before giving contrast medium. If no abnormality is demonstrated in the mediastinum, thin (5 mm) sections can be reserved for postcontrast scans performed through the neck to the level of the thoracic inlet, since over 90% of tumours will be in close relationship to the thyroid gland. Using this technique, over 75% of tumours can be correctly localized (Kovarik et al 1981, Whitley et al 1981), although the success rate will clearly depend on the size of the tumour and the experience of those interpreting the images. Contrast medium is administered as an intravenous infusion (100 ml at a rate of 2 ml/s). The use of non-ionic contrast medium reduces degradation of scan quality by motion artefact. On precontrast scans, parathyroid tumours are generally seen as small, well-defined soft tissue masses, which have a lower attenuation (approximately 40 HU) than the adjacent iodine-containing thyroid tissue (attenuation: 90+ HU). After giving contrast medium, the parathyroid tumour enhances by much the same degree as thyroid tissue, although the absolute attenuation is generally lower in the parathyroid than in the thyroid gland (Fig. 17.17). Measurement of pre- and postcontrast attenuation values may therefore be helpful in differentiating thyroid from parathyroid tissue (unpublished observation). Parathyroid tumours are generally homogeneous, but some may have cystic components (Fig. 17.17). Some very large tumours undergo partial necrosis which shows as ill-defined centres of low attenuation.

Ultrasound has also been applied to the identification of parathyroid tumours (Sample et al 1978, Kalovidouris et al 1983, Krudy et al 1984, Butch et al 1985). Ultrasound examinations are best performed with either a 10 MHz 'near field', small parts transducer, or a 7.5 MHz 'near field' transducer, with the patient lying supine (Miller et al 1987a). The success rate for localization of tumours is around 70%. Parathyroid adenomas are usually small and round or oval in shape, with relatively low echogenicity when compared to the thyroid gland, but the echo patterns can vary (Fig. 17.18) (Graif et al 1987, Miller et al 1987a).

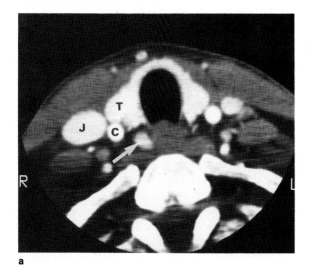

a

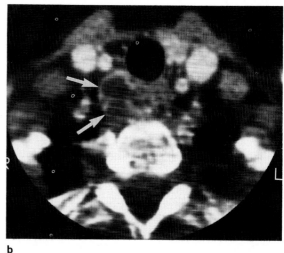

b

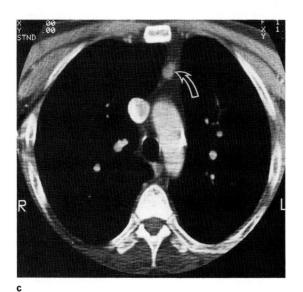

c

Fig. 17.17 Contrast enhanced CT scans. (a) Small right parathyroid adenoma (T = thyroid; J = internal jugular vein; C = carotid artery). (b) Large cystic right parathyroid tumour (arrow). (c) Ectopic parathyroid tumour in anterior mediastinum (arrow).

'hot' spot on the subtracted image (Fig. 17.19). Reports of the success of localization of tumours by this technique vary between 60% and 87% (Higgins & Auffermann 1988).

More recently, magnetic resonance imaging has

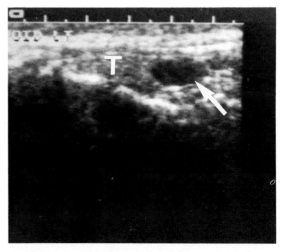

Fig. 17.18 Left lower parathyroid adenoma (arrow) lying adjacent to the inferior pole of the thyroid (T) on longitudinal ultrasound scan (with permission from Dr H Mamtora, Hope Hospital, Salford, Manchester).

Radionuclides are also used for the localization of parathyroid tumours and the best results are obtained with a subtraction technique. Initially, images of the thyroid are obtained after an intravenous injection of ^{99m}Tc pertechnetate. Thallium (^{102}T1) chloride, which is taken up in thyroid tissue and the parathyroid glands, is then given intravenously. By subtracting the thyroid (^{99m}Tc pertechnetate) image from the thyroid and parathyroid (thallium) image, a 'residual' thallium image remains (Ferlin et al 1983, Young et al 1983). A parathyroid tumour will give a localized

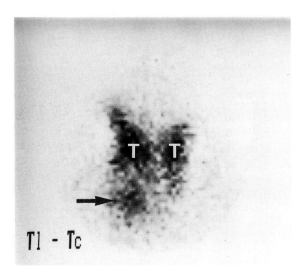

Fig. 17.19 Large right lower parathyroid tumour (arrow) on thallium subtraction radionuclide scan; same patient as Fig. 17.17 (a) (T = thyroid). (With permission from Dr M C Prescott, Department of Nuclear Medicine, Manchester Royal Infirmary.)

been used for the localization of tumours (Spritzer et al 1987). A success rate of between 64% and 79% has been reported, using both medium and high magnetic field strengths (Higgins & Auffermann 1988). Surface coils and various specially shaped coils for the neck have improved image quality (Kneeland et al 1987). Parathyroid adenomas usually have a low intensity signal on T_1-weighted images and a very high intensity signal on T_2-weighted images (Higgins & Fisher 1987), although the signal characteristics of tumours may vary.

In summary, all these non-invasive techniques have similar but variable success rates (60–90%) in localizing parathyroid tumours. In each, it is essential that optimum scanning technique is used and, in the case of ultrasound, that an experienced operator performs the scan. The same is true for the interpretation of all the techniques if the best results are to be obtained. Generally, a combination of two or more non-invasive techniques increases the success rate to over 85% (Higgins & Auffermann 1988). This may be important in patients who have had a previous neck exploration and have recurrent or persistent disease; re-exploration of the neck is technically difficult and potentially hazardous (Brennan et al 1978, Clark

et al 1985). The success rate with all imaging techniques is lower in patients who have had previous surgery than in those who have not, and yet accurate preoperative localization may be more important in this group. CT appears to be the most useful of the available non-invasive techniques in this setting, but again the use of several localizing techniques may improve upon successful localization rates. With the technical improvements in the image quality of non-invasive techniques, venography and angiography may only be required in exceptional cases. For tumours sited in the mediastinum, CT and MRI are the techniques of choice (Fig. 17.17); ultrasound is unhelpful and isotope imaging has limitations. A combination of techniques, perhaps including arteriography and venous sampling, may be required (Doppman et al 1975, Krudy et al 1981).

Although the incidence of thyroid abnormalities in the general population is 15%, there is a higher incidence (up to 40%) in association with parathyroid disease (Laing et al 1969). The coexistence of a goitre may make localization of a parathyroid tumour difficult or inaccurate by all imaging techniques. This has stimulated the development of the technique of percutaneous aspiration of apparent parathyroid tumours for histology or parathyroid hormone assays to confirm the precise origin of the tissue (Doppman et al 1983). Such interventional techniques have

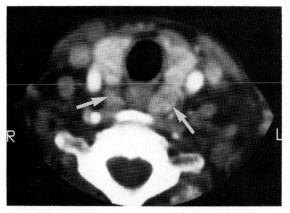

Fig. 17.20 Hyperparathyroidism secondary to renal failure with multiple parathyroid gland enlargement (arrows) indicating hyperplasia.

developed from diagnostic to therapeutic procedures and can be applied to patients with hyperparathyroidism in whom surgical treatment is not considered feasible. It has proved possible to infarct tumours at angiography (Doppman 1980) or to destroy tumours by instilling alcohol with ultrasound guidance (Karstrup et al 1987).

Secondary hyperparathyroidism and parathyroid hyperplasia

Preoperative localization of parathyroid tumours has been performed in patients with secondary hyperparathyroidism associated with chronic renal failure. Multiple gland enlargement can be identified (Fig. 17.20) (Takagi et al 1982). However, accurate preoperative localization has less impact on surgical management in secondary hyperparathyroidism because the surgeon is already committed to identify all four parathyroid glands and to perform a total or subtotal parathyroidectomy. In the inherited forms of primary hyperparathyroidism, localization techniques are likely to be less helpful, because the overactive parathyroid tissue is shared between all four (or more) hyperplastic glands rather than located in a single adenoma. Although hyperplastic, each affected gland may not be sufficiently enlarged to be identified by any imaging technique.

THYROID TUMOURS

Both benign and malignant tumours usually present as a visible and easily palpable neck mass of varying size. However, it should be remembered that metastases, commonly to lung or bone, may present before the primary thyroid lesion declares itself. Infrequently tumour may arise in ectopic thyroid tissue in the mediastinum or base of the tongue. So far as neck masses are concerned, the full extent of the lesion may be difficult to assess on clinical examination, because of its spread into surrounding musculature or extension behind the trachea or into the upper thorax. Frequently, the nature of a thyroid swelling may not be determined clinically, although suspicion of malignancy may be considered on the basis of a recent change in size of a goitre or a large, irregular, ill-defined mass producing compression of the trachea with associated stridor or hoarseness, and the presence of enlarged cervical lymph nodes.

Incidence

The number of cases of maligant neoplasm of the thyroid gland registered in England and Wales in the five years 1980–84 were 2921 females and 1054 males, a ratio of 2.77 to 1 (OPCS 1980–84). The highest incidence occurs in the middle-aged and elderly population.

Tumour types

Differentiated

Papillary. These may be seen at all ages, but are commoner in younger patients. They often have a tendency to remain localized in the neck, though may metastasize to regional lymph nodes. Distant metastases are less common than with other cancers, and the primary lesion may be delayed in presentation.

Follicular. These are more common in older patients, and more likely to produce metastases in distant sites, particularly bone and lung.

Undifferentiated (anaplastic)

This is commonly a rapidly growing tumour. Varying cell types may be identified e.g. spindle, giant, squamous and small round cell. Haematogenous dissemination is common with metastases in a variety of sites, but the clinical problems usually centre round an aggressive primary tumour.

Medullary carcinoma

This is a lesion arising from the parafollicular C cells. These secrete a distinctive tumour marker – calcitonin – and, not infrequently, have a slow rate of growth. Both familial and sporadic cases are recognized. They may be associated with other endocrine abnormalities such as parathyroid hyperplasia and phaeochromocytoma, as well as with Marfan's syndrome and mucosal fibromas (Keiser et al 1973).

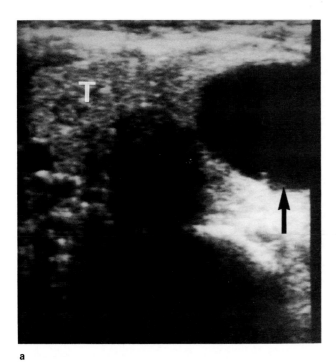

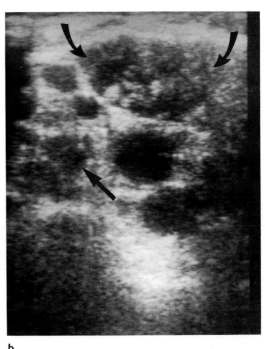

a   b

Fig. 17.21   Ultrasound scans (transverse plane) of the thyroid showing (a) anechoic cyst (arrow) in left lobe of the thyroid (T). (b) Carcinoma of the right lobe (curved arrows) with heterogenous echo pattern and lymphadenopathy (arrow). (With permission from Dr H Mamtora, Hope Hospital, Salford, Manchester.)

Malignant lymphoma

This is usually non-Hodgkin's lymphoma and can sometimes be difficult to distinguish from small round cell, undifferentiated carcinoma. Association with thyroiditis and circulating thyroid antibodies has been described (Hedley et al 1977, Williams et al 1977).

Rare malignancies

These include cases which are sometimes classified as sarcomas, though they may be undifferentiated carcinomas, squamous cell tumours or metastases from primary tumours in, for example, the lung.

Imaging

The rôle of imaging in thyroid tumours is to characterize a palpable thyroid mass (functioning or non-functioning, cystic or solid) and to define the extent of tumour, locally and in distant metastatic sites. The extent of radiological assessment of suspected or histologically confirmed thyroid cancer is determined by a number of factors including the nature of the presenting mass, the probability of metastases, of associated, related abnormalities and the complications which may arise from treatment. A wide variety of techniques is available.

Conventional radiology

Soft tissue views of the neck, with radiography of the thoracic inlet. These studies serve to demonstrate the presence of a tumour and its affect upon the trachea and extension into the upper thorax via the thoracic inlet. They may also demonstrate the presence of tumoral calcification which, though uncommon, can occur as fine stippling in papillary carcinoma, or as amorphous deposits in medullary carcinoma. The finding of calcification is not diagnostic of malignant disease, and ring calcifications are more likely to be associated with adenomata.

Chest radiography. This examination is useful

for establishing a baseline at the time of presentation. Clinically unsuspected metastases may be detected involving the lungs, pleura, rib cage or mediastinal lymph nodes. Classically, pulmonary metastases are round, discrete and well-defined. Sometimes, however, they may present as fine (1–2 mm) deposits, which, without high quality images, may not be perceived. Metastases in the pleura may not be identified if there is a coexisting pleural effusion or rib metastases.

Skeletal radiography. Metastases to the vertebral column, pelvis and long bones are commonly lytic in nature. They can be extremely destructive, e.g. within the blades of the ilia. A multilocular appearance, not unlike that of giant cell tumour, can occur, or the lesion may mimic the aggressive behaviour of the highly vascularized metastasis from a hypernephroma. Vertebral lesions can give rise to extradural compression, with resultant paraparesis/paraplegia, and myelography for identifying the site of obstruction is then indicated as treatment by decompression laminectomy, radiotherapy and/or radio-iodine treatment may be beneficial.

Post-treatment. In the examination of the treated patient, radiographic examination of the neck and upper thorax is of value in demonstrating reduction of the tumour following radiotherapy. Similarly, skeletal radiographs may be important in monitoring response to treatment, though there is seldom a very good restoration of bone architecture. Large defects may remain with formation of bony trabeculae and dense sclerosis around the edges of the lesion. The radiography of complications of therapy is largely concerned with the demonstration of mediastinal/pulmonary fibrosis from extended radiotherapy fields, or following high dose radioactive iodine therapy.

Ultrasound

In the past years this technology has assumed a distinctive rôle in the assessment of the nature of the thyroid nodule. Static B mode or real time scanning is used to:

1. Distinguish between a solid or cystic lesion (Fig. 17.21).
2. Identify homogeneous or heterogeneous echo patterns in a solid tumour.

3. Demonstrate papillary-like extensions into a cystic lesion from the surrounding wall.
4. Establish whether the lesion is clearly circumscribed or invasive.
5. Demonstrate whether a palpable abnormality is solitary or part of a multinodular process.
6. Identify cervical lymphadenopathy (Fig. 17.21).

The fact that a cyst contains solid material or there is heterogenicity of echo pattern within a lesion or there are both cystic and solid components present may make one suspect malignancy. However, ultrasonic appearances are not pathognomonic of benign or malignant lesions.

In this context the application of aspiration cytology has to be considered (Franklyn & Shepherd 1987). Previous use of a cutting needle (Wang et al 1976) has been supplanted by fine needle aspiration under ultrasound guidance, for both cystic and solid lesions. Cystic lesions have a lower malignancy rate than solid ones, though it must be remembered that some malignant tumours may undergo cystic degeneration or haemorrhage. Therefore, in the case of the solitary thyroid nodule, whether cystic, solid or of mixed echo pattern, there is a place for considering fine needle biopsy as a preliminary to surgical excision. Unfortunately, since the lesion in question may not show uniform involvement by malignant cells, a negative biopsy must not be allowed to engender a feeling of false diagnostic security.

Nuclear medicine

Radionuclide studies of the thyroid gland are now commonly undertaken in conjuction with ultrasound. 'Hot' nodules on radionuclide scanning are seldom found to be malignant (1–4%). The incidence of malignancy in 'cold' nodules is between 10 and 20%. It is also rare for a patient with thyroid malignancy to present with clinical thyrotoxicosis.

The application of nuclear medicine to thyroid malignancy is threefold:

1. Investigation before treatment
2. Assessment after treatment
3. Therapy.

Therapeutic applications have been dealt with elsewhere (Ch. 1). Radionuclide imaging before treatment is concerned with a. examination of the solitary nodule, b. the clinically or ultrasonically diagnosed multinodular goitre, c. elucidation of the cause of cervical node enlargement which is suspected to be malignant and where no other primary tumour can be found, and d. where the finding of pulmonary or bone metastases suggest the presence of a thyroid cancer, even though the gland itself may be normal to palpation. ^{99m}Tc pertechnetate is the commonly used radionuclide (Fig. 17.22). On occasion the results can be misleading, as uptake of ^{99m}Tc can occur in malignant tumours. The presence of a solitary thyroid nodule which appears functional ('hot') on the technetium scan, without evidence of thyrotoxicosis or of it being autonomous, is an indication for repeat scanning with radioiodine, when a malignant lesion will appear 'cold'. Either ^{123}I or ^{131}I may be used. ^{123}I is the better radionuclide, with a shorter half-life and lower radiation dose, but is more expensive and less readily available. Radioiodine studies are needed for detection of aberrant thyroid tissue, e.g. in the mediastinum. Almost 25% of the latter lie in the posterior mediastinum (Frazer & Pare 1979). A solitary 'cold' nodule should always be examined by ultrasound. The place of radionuclide imaging of the thyroid is predominantly related to tumours which are differentiated: there are distinct limitations in undifferentiated (anaplastic) lesions. Recently, there has been reference to 'specific' localization of medullary carcinoma by imaging with ^{99m}Tc pentavalent DMSA (Hoefnagel et al 1988).

Radionuclide imaging plays an important role in the investigation and management of treated patients, although this is dependent on the histology of the primary tumour. Functioning metastases may be demonstrated by scanning with ^{131}I but only if there has been total surgical removal of the primary tumour or ^{131}I ablation of residual functioning thyroid tissue. In some cases low level uptake in residual primary or metastatic disease can be increased by prior treatment with TSH. Recurrence at the primary site may also be demonstrated.

Bone imaging may be achieved by using a ^{99m}Tc diphosphanate, especially where the application of ^{131}I is not relevant. Thus the usual approach is to scan with ^{99m}Tc diphosphanate and use ^{131}I in those cases of well-differentiated primary tumour where the presence of functioning

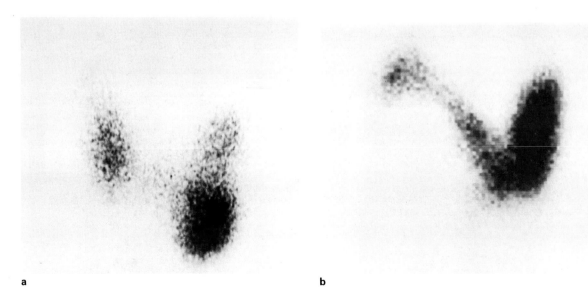

a   **b**

Fig. 17.22 ^{99m}Tc thyroid scans. (a) Functioning 'warm' nodule at the inferior pole of the left lobe. (b) Large non-functioning 'cold' nodule in the right lobe. (With permission from Dr M C Prescott, Department of Nuclear Medicine, Manchester Royal Infirmary.)

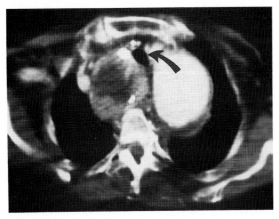

Fig. 17.23 Retrosternal goitre (postcontrast CT). The goitre on the right shows heterogeneous enhancement, and is displacing and compressing the trachea (arrow). There is also an aortic aneurysm.

metastases is suspected and radioiodine therapy is appropriate. Liver and brain metastases are usually identified by ultrasound and CT scanning respectively.

Computed tomography (CT)

Application of this technology can assist with:

1. Evaluation of the thyroid tumour in the neck or mediastinum and its effect on adjacent structures.

2. The identification of thyroid calcification.

3. The detection of metastases to the thorax.

4. Precise localization of the level of spinal cord compression as a substitute for, or an adjunct to, conventional myelography.

5. Staging in lymphoma.

6. The identification of adrenal tumours in association with medullary thyroid carcinoma.

On CT the thyroid is generally of higher attenuation (90 Hounsfield Units, HU) than other soft tissue (approximately 45 HU). Marked enhancement occurs with i.v. contrast medium. CT can demonstrate the presence of cysts, but it has distinct limitations in distinguishing between normal and abnormal (potentially malignant) tissue. The technique has not found an important rôle in the diagnosis and management of thyroid disease.

REFERENCES

Abrams H L, Spiro R, Goldstein N 1950 Metastases in carcinoma: Analysis of 1000 autopsied cases. Cancer 3: 74–85

Abrams H L, Siegelman S S, Adams D F et al 1982 Computed tomography versus ultrasound of the adrenal gland: a prospective study. Radiology 143: 121–128

Adams J E, Adams P H, Mamtora H, Isherwood I 1981 Computed tomography and the localisation of parathyroid tumours. Clinical Radiology 32: 251–254

Adams J E, Johnson R J, Rickards D, Isherwood I 1983 Computed tomography in adrenal disease. Clinical Radiology 34: 39–49

Adams P H 1982 Conservative management of primary hyperparathyroidism. Journal of The Royal College of Physicians of London 16: 184–190

Allison D J, Brown M J, Jones D H, Timmis J B 1983 Role of venous sampling in locating a phaeochromocytoma. British Medical Journal 286: 1122–1124

Ambrose M A, Bosniak M A, Lefleur R S, Mitty H A 1980 Adrenal adenoma associated with renal cell carcinoma. American Journal of Roentgenology 136: 81–84

Aurbach G D, Marx S J, Spiegal A M 1981 Parathyroid hormone, calcitonin and the calciferols. In: Williams R H (ed) Textbook of endocrinology. W B Saunders, London, pp 922–1031

Berland L L, Koslin D B, Kenney P J, Stanley R J, Lee J Y 1988 Differentiation between small benign adrenal masses with dynamic incremented CT. American Journal of Roentgenology 151: 95–101

Berliner L, Bosniak M A, Megibow A 1982 Adrenal

pseudotumours on computed tomography. Journal of Computer Assisted Tomography 6: 281–285

Bernardino M E 1988 Management of the asymptomatic patient with a unilateral adrenal mass. Radiology 166: 121–123

Bernardino M E, Walther M M, Phillips V M et al 1985 CT-guided adrenal biopsy: accuracy, safety and indications. American Journal of Roentgenology 144: 67–69

Bomanji J, Conroy B G, Britton K E, Reznek R H 1988 Imaging neural crest tumours with ^{123}I-metaiodobenzylguanidine and X-ray computed tomography: a comparative study. Clinical Radiology 39: 502–506

Bonneville J F, Poulignot D, Cattin F, Couturier M, Mollet E, Dietemann J L 1982 Computed tomographic demonstration of the effects of bromocriptine on pituitary microadenoma size. Radiology 143: 451–455

Bonneville J F, Cattin F, Moussa-Bacha K, Portha C 1983 Dynamic computed tomography of the pituitary gland: The 'tuft sign'. Radiology 149: 145–148

Bonneville J F, Cattin F, Portha C, Cuenin E, Clere P, Bartholomot B 1985 Computed tomographic demonstration of the posterior pituitary. American Journal of Neuroradiology 6: 889–892

Bravo E L, Taraz R C, Gifford R W, Stewart B H 1979 Circulating and urinary catecholamines in phaeochromocytoma. New England Journal of Medicine 301: 682–686

Brennan M F, Doppman J L, Marx S J, Spiegal A M, Brown E M, Aurbach G D 1978 Reoperative parathyroid surgery for persistent hyperparathyroidism. Surgery 83: 669–676

Brownlie K, Kreel L 1978 Computer assisted tomography of normal suprarenal glands. Journal of Computer Assisted Tomography 2: 1–10

Burrow G M, Wortzman G, Rewcastle N B, Holgate R C, Kovacs K 1981 Microadenomas of the pituitary and abnormal sellar tomograms in an unselected autopsy series. New England Journal of Medicine 304: 156–158

Butch R J, Simeone J F, Mueller P R 1985 Thyroid and parathyroid ultrasonography. Radiologic Clinics of North America 23: 57–71

Carr D H, Sandler L M, Joplin G F 1984 Computed tomography of sellar and paraseller lesions. Clinical Radiology 35: 281–286

Casola G, Nicolet V, Van Sonnenberg E et al 1986 Unsuspected phaeochromocytoma: risk of blood pressure alterations during percutaneous adrenal biopsy. Radiology 159: 733–735

Chakera T M H , Khangure M S, Pullen P 1985 Assessment by computed tomography of the response of pituitary macroadenomas to bromocryptine. Clinical Radiology 36: 223–226

Chambers E, Turski P, LaMasters D, Newton T 1982 Region of low density in the contrast enhanced pituitary gland; normal and pathological process. Radiology 144: 109–113

Clark O H, Okerlund M D, Moss A A et al 1985 Localisation studies in patients with persistent or recurrent hyperparathyroidism. Surgery 98: 1083–1094

Copeland P M 1983 The incidentally discovered adrenal mass. Annals of Internal Medicine 98: 940–945

Daniels DL, Williams A L, Thornton R S, Meyer G A, Cusick J F, Haughton V M 1981 Differential diagnosis of intrasellar tumours by computed tomography. Radiology 141: 697–701

Daughaday W H 1981 The adenohypophysis. In: Williams R H (ed) Textbook of endocrinology. W B Saunders, London, pp 73–116

Daunt N, Mowat P 1985 Computed tomographic appearances and clinical features of prolactin-secreting pituitary adenomas in young male patients. Clinical Radiology 36: 227–231

Davies D R, Dent C E, Ives D R 1973a Successful removal of single metastasis in recurrent parathyroid carcinoma. British Medical Journal 1: 397–398

Davies D R, Shaw D G, Ives D R, Thomas B M, Watson L 1973b Selective venous catheterisation and radioimmunoassay of parathyroid hormone in the diagnosis and localisation of parathyroid tumours. Lancet 1: 1097–1082

Davies M, Klimiuk P S, Adams P H, Lumb G A, Large D M, Anderson D C 1981 Familial hypocalciuric hypercalcaemia and acute pancreatitis. British Medical Journal 282: 1023–1025

Davis P C, Hoffman J C, Tindall G T, Braun IF 1985 Prolactin-secreting pituitary microadenomas: inaccuracy of high resolution CT imaging. American Journal of Roentgenology 144: 151–156

Davis P C, Hoffman J C, Spencer T, Tindall C T, Braun I F 1987 MR imaging of pituitary adenoma: CT, clinical and surgical correlation. American Journal of Roentgenology 148: 797–802

Demas B, Thurnher S, Hricak H 1987 The kidney, adrenal gland and retroperitoneum. In: Higgins C B, Hricak H (eds) Magnetic resonance imaging of the body. Raven Press, New York, pp 373–401

Di Chiro G, Nelson K B 1962 The volume of the sella turcica. American Journal of Radiology 87: 26–37

Dobbie J W 1969 Adrenocortical nodular hyperplasia: The aging adrenal. Journal of Pathology 99: 1–18

Doppman J L 1976 Parathyroid localisation; arteriography and venous sampling. Radiologic Clinics of North America 14: 163–188

Doppman J L 1980 The treatment of hyperparathyroidism by transcatheter techniques. Cardiovascular and Interventional Radiology 3: 268–276

Doppman J L 1982 CT localisation of cervical parathyroid glands: it deserves a second look. Journal of Computer Assisted Tomography 6: 519–520

Doppman J, Girton M 1984 Adrenal ablation by retrograde venous ethanol injection: an ineffective and dangerous procedure. Radiology 150: 667–672

Doppman J L, Mallette L E, Marx S J et al 1975 The localisation of abnormal mediastinal parathyroid glands. Radiology 115: 31–36

Doppman J L, Gill J R, Nienhuis A W, Earll J M, Long J A 1982 CT findings in Addison's disease. Journal of Computer Assisted Tomography 6: 757–761

Doppman J L, Adrian G K, Stephen J M et al 1983 Aspiration of enlarged parathyroid glands for parathyroid hormone assay. Radiology 148: 31–35

Doppman J L, Miller D L, Dwyer A J et al 1988 Macronodular hyperplasia in Cushing's disease. Radiology 166: 347–352

Dunlop D A B, Papapulos S E, Lodge R W, Fulton A J, Kendall B E, O'Riordan J L H 1980 Parathyroid venous sampling: anatomical considerations and results in 95 patients with primary hyperparathyroidism. British Journal of Radiology 53: 183–191

Dunnick N R, Doppman J L, Gill J R, Strott C A, Keiser H R, Brennan M F 1982 Localization of functional adrenal tumors by computed tomography and venous sampling. Radiology 142: 429–433

Earnest F, McCullough E C, Frank D A 1981 Fact or artifact: An analysis of artifact in high resolution computed tomographic scanning of the sella. Radiology 140: 109–113

Egglin T K, Hahn P F, Stark D D 1988 MRI of the adrenal glands. Seminars in Roentgenology 23: 280–287

Ferlin G, Borsato N, Camerani M, Conte N, Zotti D 1983 New perspectives in localising enlarged parathyroids by technetium–thallium subtraction scan. Journal of Nuclear Medicine 24: 438–441

Findling J S, Tyrell J B 1986 Occult ectopic secretion of corticotrophin. Archives of Internal Medicine 146: 929–933

Fischer C E, Turner F A, Horton R 1971 Remission of primary hyperaldosteronism after adrenal venography. New England Journal of Medicine 285: 334–336

Francis I R, Glazer C M, Shapiro B, Sisson J C, Gross B H 1983 Complementary roles of CT and ^{131}I MIBG scintigraphy in diagnosing phaeochromocytoma. American Journal of Roentgenology 141: 719–725

Franklyn J A, Shepherd M C 1987 Aspiration cytology of the thyroid. British Medical Journal 295: 510–511

Frazer R G, Pare J A P 1979 Diseases of the mediastinum – thyroid masses. In: Diagnosis of diseases of the chest. W B Saunders, London, pp 1824–1827

Gardeur D, Naidich T P, Metzger J 1981 CT analysis of intrasellar pituitary adenomas with emphasis on patterns of contrast enhancement. Neuroradiology 20: 241–247

Geisinger M A, Zelch M C, Bravo E L, Risius B F, O'Donovan P B, Borkowski G P 1983 Primary hyperaldosteronism: comparison of CT, adrenal venography and venous sampling. American Journal of Roentgenology 141: 299–302

Gholkar A, Isherwood I 1988 Three-dimensional computed tomographic reformations of intracranial vascular lesions. British Journal of Radiology 61: 1095–1099

Glaser B, Sheinfeld M, Benmair J, Kaplan N 1986 Magnetic resonance imaging of pituitary gland. Clinical Radiology 37: 9–14

Glazer G M, Woolsey E J, Borrello J et al 1986 Adrenal tissue characterisation using MR imaging. Radiology 158: 73–79

Glazer H S, Weyman P J, Sagel S S, Levitt R G, McClennan B L 1982 Non-functioning adrenal masses: incidental discovery on computed tomography. American Journal of Roentgenology 139: 81–85

Goldfien A 1981 Phaeochromocytoma. Clinics in Endocrinology and Metabolism 10: 607–630

Gough M H, Smith F, Bishop M C 1971 Parathyroidectomy for symptomless hyperparathyroidism: a surgical dilemma. Lancet 1: 1178

Graif M, Itzchak Y, Strauss S, Dolev E, Mohr R, Wolfstein I 1987 Parathyroid sonography: diagnostic accuracy related to shape, location and texture of the gland. British Journal of Radiology 60: 439–443

Hamberger B, Russell C F, Van Heerden J A et al 1982 Adrenal surgery: trends during the seventies. American Journal of Surgery 144: 523–526

Haughton V M, Rosenbaum A E, Williams A L, Drayer B 1981 Recognising the empty sella by CT: The infundibulum sign. American Journal of Roentgenology 136: 293–295

Hawkes R C, Holland G N, Moore W S, Corson R, Kean D M, Worthington B S 1983 The application of NMR imaging to the evaluation of pituitary and juxta-sellar tumors. American Journal of Neuroradiology 4: 221–222

Hawkins L A, Britton K E, Shapiro B 1980 Selenium-75 selenomethyl cholesterol: a new agent for quantitative functional scintigraphy of the adrenals: physical aspects. British Journal of Radiology 53: 883–889

Hedeland H, Ostergerg G, Hokfelt B 1968 On the prevelance of adrenocortical adenomas in autopsy material in relation to hypertension and diabetes. Acta Medica Scandinavica 184: 211–214

Hedley A J, Thjodliaffson B, Donald D et al 1977 Thyroid function in normal subjects in Iceland and North-east Scotland. Clinical Endocrinology 7: 377–382

Hemminghytt S, Kalkhoff R K, Daniels D L, Williams A L, Grogan J P, Haughton V M 1983 Computed tomographic study of hormone-secreting microadenomas. Radiology 146: 65–69

Hendricks M J 1988 Pituitary adenoma. In: Computed tomography of the pituitary gland – an anatomical and pathological study. Van Gorcum, Assen, The Netherlands, pp 77–106

Higgins C B, Auffermann W 1988 MR imaging of thyroid and parathyroid glands: a review of current status. American Journal of Radiology 151: 1095–1106

Higgins C B, Fisher M R 1987 The neck. In: Higgins C B, Hricak H (eds) Magnetic resonance imaging of the body. Raven Press, New York, pp 145–172

Hoefnagel C A, Delprat C C, Zanin D, van der Schoot J B 1988 New radionuclide tracers for the diagnosis and therapy of medullary thyroid carcinoma. Clinical Nuclear Medicine 13: 159–165

Howlett T A, Drury P L, Perry L, Doniach I, Rees L H, Besser G M 1986 Diagnosis and management of ACTH-dependent Cushing's syndrome: Comparison of the features in ectopic and pituitary ACTH production. Clinical Endocrinology 24: 699–713

Huebener K H, Treugut H 1984 Adrenal cortex dysfunction: CT findings. Radiology 150: 195–199

Hussain S, Belldegrun A, Seltzer S E, Richie J P, Gittes R F, Abrams H L 1985 Differentiation of malignant from benign adrenal masses: predictive indices on computed tomography. American Journal of Roentgenology 144: 61–65

Jessop D S, Cunnah D, Millar J G B et al 1987 A phaeochromocytoma presenting with Cushing's syndrome associated with increased concentrations of circulating corticotrophin-releasing factor. Journal of Endocrinology 113: 133–138

Joffe S N, Brown C 1983 Nodular adrenal hyperplasia and Cushing's syndrome. Surgery 94: 919–925

Johnson D G, Hall K, Kendall-Taylor P, Patrick D, Watson M, Cook D B 1984 Effect of dopamine agonist withdrawal after long term therapy in prolactinomas. Studies with high definition computerized tomography. Lancet 2: 187–192

Jones G S, Shah K J, Mann J R 1985 Adrenocortical carcinoma in infancy and childhood: a radiological report of ten cases. Clinical Radiology 36: 257–262

Kalovidouris A, Mancuso A, Sarti D 1983 Static Grey-scale parathyroid ultrasonography: is high resolution real time technique required? Clinical Radiology 34: 385–393

Karstrup S, Holm H H, Torp-Pedersen S, Hegedus L 1987 Ultrasonically guided percutaneous inactivation of parathyroid tumours. British Journal of Radiology 60: 667–670

Kaufman B, Chamberlin W B 1972 The ubiquitous 'empty' sella tucica. Acta Radiologica 13: 413–425

Keiser H R, Beaven M A, Doppman J, Wells S A, Buja L M 1973 Sipple's syndrome: medullary thyroid carcinoma, phaeochromocytoma and parathyroid disease. Annals of Internal Medicine 78: 561–579

Kellgren J H, Ball J, Tutton G K 1952 Articular and other changes in acromegaly: clinical and pathological study of 25 cases. Quarterly Journal of Medicine 21: 405–424

Klimiuk P S, Mainwaring A R 1980 Spontaneous biochemical remission in parathyroid carcinoma. British Medical Journal 281: 1394–1395

Kneeland J B, Krubsack A J, Lawson T L et al 1987 Enlarged parathyroid glands: high resolution local coil MR imaging. Radiology 162: 143–146

Koeniker R M, Mueller R R, Van Sonnenberg E 1988 Interventional radiology of the adrenal glands. Seminars in Roentgenology 23: 288–303

Kovarik J, Willvonseder R, Hofer R et al 1981 The value of computed tomography as a non-invasive method for preoperative localisation of parathyroid adenomas of the neck in primary hyperparathyroidism. Mineral and Electrolyte Metabolism 5: 228–232

Krudy A G, Doppman J L, Brennan M F et al 1981 The detection of mediastinal parathyroid glands by computed tomography, selective arteriography and venous sampling: an analysis of 17 cases. Radiology 140: 739–744

Krudy A G, Shawker T H, Doppman J L et al 1984

Ultrasonic parathyroid localisation in previously operated patients. Clinical Radiology 35: 113–118

Kucharczyk W, Davis D O, Kelly W M, Sze G, Norman D M, Newton T H 1986 Pituitary adenomas: high resolution MR imaging at 1.5 T. Radiology 161: 761–765

Laing V O, Frame B, Block M A 1969 Associated primary hyperparathyroidism and thyroid lesions. Archives of Surgery 98: 709–712

Lancet (Editorial) 1982 Prolactinomas: Bromocriptine rules OK? Lancet 1: 430–431

Lancet (Editorial) 1984 Iodobenzylguanidine for location and treatment of phaeochromocytoma. Lancet 2: 905–907

Landolt A M, Valavanis J G, Eberle A N 1986 Corticotrophin releasing factor test used with bilateral simultaneous inferior petrosal sinus blood sampling for the diagnosis of pituitary dependent Cushing's syndrome. Clinical Endocrinology 25: 687–696

Laursen K, Damgaard-Pedersen K 1980 CT for phaeochromocytoma diagnosis. American Journal of Roentgenology 134: 227–280

Levy J M, Hessel S J, Dippe S E, McFarland J O 1982 Digital subtraction angiography for localisation of parathyroid lesions. Annals of Internal Medicine 97: 710–712

Liddle G W 1981 The adrenals. In: Williams R H (ed) Textbook of endocrinology. W B Saunders, London, pp 249–292

Lump G, Mackenzie D H 1959 The incidence of metastases in adreanal glands and ovaries removed for carcinoma of the breast. Cancer 12: 521–526

McNicol A M 1987 Pituitary adenomas. Histopathology 11: 995–1011

Mark L, Pech P, Daniels D, Charles C, Williams A, Haughton V 1984 The pituitary fossa: a correlative anatomic and MR study. Radiology 153: 453–457

Meek D R, Duncan J G, McAreavey D 1981 Computed tomography in the localization of aldosterone-secreting adrenal adenomas. British Journal of Radiology 54: 1039–1043

Miller D L, Doppman J L, Shawker T H et al 1987a Localisation of parathyroid adenomas in patients who have undergone surgery. Part I non-invasive methods. Radiology 162: 133–137

Miller D L, Doppman J L, Shawker T H et al 1987b Localisation of parathyroid adenomas in patients who have undergone surgery. Part II invasive procedures. Radiology 162: 138–141

Mitnick J S, Bosniak M A, Megibow A, Naidich D P 1983 Non-functioning adrenal adenomas discovered incidentally on computed tomography. Radiology 148: 495–499

Mitty H A, Cohen B A, Sprayregen S, Schwartz K 1983 Adrenal pseudotumors on CT due to dilated portosystemic veins. American Journal of Roentgenology 141: 727–730

Moulton J S, Moulton J S 1988 CT of the adrenal glands. Seminars in Roentgenology 23: 288–303

Musante F, Derchi L E, Zappasodi F et al 1988 Myelolipoma of the adrenal gland: sonographic and CT features. American Journal of Roentgenology 151: 961–964

Nakagawa Y, Matsumoto K, Fukami T, Takase K 1984 Exploration of the pituitary stalk and gland by high resolution computed tomography. A comparative study of normal subjects and cases with microadenoma. Neuroradiology 26: 473–478

Newton D R, Witz S, Norman D, Newton T H 1983 Economic impact of CT scanning on the evaluation of pituitary adenomas. American Journal of Neuroradiology 4: 57–60

Obley D L, Winzelberg G G, Jarmolowski C R, Hydovitz J D, Danowski T S, Wholey M H 1984 Parathyroid adenomas studied by digital subtraction angiography. Radiology 153: 449–451

O'Kuno T, Sudo M, Momoi T et al 1980 Pituitary hyperplasia due to hypothyroidism. Journal of Computer Assisted Tomography 4: 600–602

Office of Population Censuses and Surveys (Cancer Statistics Registration) Series MBI Nos. 12–16, 1980–84. HMSO, London

Prinz R A, Brooks M H, Churchill R et al 1982 Incidental asymptomatic adrenal masses detected by computed tomographic scanning: is operation required? Journal of the American Medical Association 248: 701–704

Purnell D C, Scholz D A, Smith L H et al 1974 Treatment of primary hyperparathyroidism. American Journal of Medicine 56: 800–809

Roberts L R, Dunnick N R, Thompson W M et al 1985 Primary aldosteronism due to bilateral nodular hyperplasia: CT demonstration. Journal of Computer Assisted Tomography 9: 1125–1127

Roppolo H M N, Latchaw R E, Meyer J D, Curtin H D 1983 Normal pituitary gland: 1. Macroscopic anatomy – CT correlation. American Journal of Neurosurgery 4: 927–935

Sample W F 1978 Adrenal ultrasonography. Radiology 127: 461–466

Sample W F, Mitchell S P, Bledsoe R C 1978 Parathyroid ultrasonography. Radiology 127: 485–490

Sampson M J, Van't Hoff W, Bicknell E J 1987 The conservative management of primary hyperparathyroidism. Quarterly Journal of Medicine 248: 1009–1014

Satava R M, Beahrs O H, Scholz D A 1975 Success rate of cervical exploration for hyperparathyroidism. Archives of Surgery 110: 625–628

Schaner E G, Dunnick N R, Doppman J L, Stott C A, Gill J R, Javadpour N 1978 Adrenal cortical tumors with low attenuation coefficients: a pitfall in computed tomography diagnosis. Journal of Computer Assisted Tomography 2: 11–15

Schwartz A, Castleman B 1973 Parathyroid carcinoma: a study of 70 cases. Cancer 31: 600–605

Scotti G, Scialfa G, Pieralli S, Chiodini P G Spelta B, Dallabonzana D 1982 Macroprolactinomas: CT evaluation of reduction of tumour size after medical treatment. Neuroradiology 23: 123–126

Shimkin P M, Powell D, Doppman J L et al 1972 Parathyroid venous sampling. Radiology 104: 571–574

Silver B J, Kyner J L, Dick A R, Chang C H 1981 Primary hypothyroidism. Suprasellar pituitary enlargement and regression on computed tomographic scanning. Journal of the American Medical Association 246: 364–365

Sisson J C, Frager M S, Valk T W et al 1981 Scintigraphic localization of phaeochromocytoma. New England Journal of Medicine 305: 12–17

Smals A G H, Pieters G F, van Haelst U J G, Klopperborg P W 1984 Macronodular adrenocortical hyperplasia in long standing Cushing's disease. Journal of Clinical Endocrinology and Metabolism 58: 25–31

Smaltino F, Bernini F P, Muras I 1980 Computed tomography for diagnosis of empty sella associated with enchancing pituitary microadenoma. Journal of Computer Assisted Tomography 4: 592–599

Sommer B, Welter H F, Spelsberg F, Scherer U, Lissner J 1982 Computed tomography for localising enlarged parathyroid glands in primary hyperparathyroidism. Journal of Computer Assisted Tomography 6: 521–526

Spiegel A M, Marx S J, Doppman J L 1975 Intrathyroidal parathyroid adenoma or hyperplasia. An occasional overlooked cause of surgical failure in primary hyperparathyroidism. Journal of the American Medical Association 234: 1029–1033

Spritzer C E, Gefter W B, Hamilton R, Greenberg B M, Axel L, Kressel H Y 1987 Abnormal parathyroid glands: high resolution MR imaging. Radiology 162: 487–491

Sutton D 1975 The radiological diagnosis of adrenal tumours. British Journal of Radiology 48: 237–258

Swartz J D, Russell K B, Basile B A, O'Donnell P C, Popky G L 1983 High resolution computed tomographic appearances of the intrasellar contents in women of child-bearing age. Radiology 147: 115–117

Syvertsen A, Haughton V, Williams A L, Cusick J F 1979 The computed tomographic appearance of the normal pituitary gland and pituitary microadenoma. Radiology 133: 385–391

Takagi H, Tominaga Y, Uchida K et al 1982 Pre-operative diagnosis of secondary hyperparathyroidism using computed tomography. Journal of Computer Assisted Tomography 6: 527–528

Taylor S 1982 High resolution computed tomography of the sella. Radiologic Clinics of North America 20: 207–236

Teasdale E, Teasdale G, Mohsen F, MacPherson P 1986 High resolution computed tomography in pituitary microadenoma: is seeing believing? Clinical Radiology 37: 227–232

Teasdale G 1983 Surgical management of pituitary adenoma. In: Scanlon M (ed) Neuroendocrinology. Clinics in Endocrinology and Metabolism 12: 789–823. W B Saunders, London

Thomas J L, Bernardino M E, Samaan N A, Hickey R C 1980 CT of phaeochromocytoma. American Journal of Roentgenology 135: 477–482

van Heerden J A, Sheps S G, Hamberger B, Sheddy P F, Poston J G, Remine W H 1982 Phaeochromocytoma: current status and changing trends. Surgery 91: 367–373

Vicks B S, Perusek M, Johnson J, Tio F 1987 Primary

adrenal lymphoma: CT and sonographic appearances. Journal of Clinical Ultrasound 15: 135–139

Wang C A 1977 Parathyroid re-exploration. A clinical and pathological study of 112 cases. Annals of Surgery 186: 140–145

Wang C A, Vickery A L, Maloof F 1976 Needle biopsy of the thyroid. Surgical Gynaecology and Obstetrics 143: 365–368

Wass J A H, Williams J, Charlesworth M et al 1982 Bromocryptine in management of large pituitary tumours. British Medical Journal 284: 1908–1911

Wells S A, Ellis G J, Gunnells J C, Schneider A B, Sherwood L M 1976 Parathyroid autotransplantation in primary hyperparathyroid hyperplasia. New England Journal of Medicine 295: 57–62

Welsh T J, Sheedy P F, van Heerden J A, Sheps S G, Hattery R R, Stephens D H 1983 Phaeochromocytoma: value of computed tomography. Radiology 148: 501–503

White F E, White M C, Drury P L, Kelsey-Fry I 1982 Value of computed tomography of the abdomen and chest in investigation of Cushing's syndrome. British Medical Journal 284: 771–774

Whitley N O, Bohiman M, Conner T B, McCrea E S, Mason G R, Whitley J E 1981 Computed tomography for localisation of parathyroid adenomas. Journal of Computer Assisted Tomography 5: 812–817

Williams E D, Doniach I, Bjarnason O, Michie W 1977 Thyroid cancer in an iodide-rich area: a histopathological study. Cancer 39: 215–222

Williams T C 1988 Functional disorders of the adrenal glands: an overview. Seminars in Roentgenology 23: 304–313

Wolverson M K, Kannegiesser H 1984 CT of bilateral haemorrhage with acute adrenal insufficiency in the adult. American Journal of Radiology 142: 311–314

Wortzman G, Rewcastle N B 1982 Tomographic abnormalities simulating pituitary microadenomas. American Journal of Neuroradiology 3: 505–512

Yeh H C 1988 Ultrasonography of the adrenals. Seminars in Roentgenology 23: 250–258

Young A E, Gaunt J I, Croft D N, Collins R E, Wells C P, Coakley A J 1983 Location of parathyroid adenomas by thallium-201 and technetium-99m subtraction scanning. British Medical Journal 286: 1384–1386

18. Radiotherapy treatment planning

R. D. Hunter

INTRODUCTION

Using modern megavoltage radiotherapy equipment, a radiotherapist is able to treat any size or site of tumour and to treat anything from the whole body to a few cubic centimetres. Until recently the treatment volumes have been flat-sided or cylindrical but the latest technology now allows irregular three-dimensional volumes to be treated if required.

Modern megavoltage radiotherapy equipment, linear accelerators and telecobalt machines produce beams of ionizing radiation the quality of which is such that they do not produce satisfactory images on normal photographic film or on normal image intensifiers. This problem has resulted in the development of special equipment for treatment planning known as simulators. These devices are diagnostic X-ray machines mounted in the head of equipment which operates like a linear accelerator and allows different controlled source — skin distance positions, angled beams and isocentric rotations to be performed. The radiotherapist therefore uses a diagnostic image to confirm his therapy beam. It is at this point that a transfer of information from a diagnostic image to a therapy 'image' is potentially most fruitful and when the need for comparability of images is high.

PRINCIPLES

Radiotherapy treatment planning is based on the initial principle of defining the tumour volume in the patient. This may be achieved by direct observation, or may utilize information from clinical examination, endoscopy, and basic or sophisticated imaging investigations. The aim is initially to define the limits of disease. Once this tumour volume information is available a target volume can be defined. This involves allowing a margin of healthy tissue around the tumour with the aim of treating homogeneously the disease and the margins. The limits allowed depend on the type of tumour being treated and are a reflection of its radio-responsiveness and pattern of spread. Having defined the target volume the radiotherapist must create a treatment plan, the principal aim of which is to achieve a homogeneous dose distribution to the target volume with minimal irradiation of adjacent healthy tissues. Because of the need in most situations to use regular shaped fields, the resulting treatment volume may be larger and of a more regular shape than the true target volume. If the information used to create the treatment plan is incorrect then the tumour volume may not be inside the treatment volume. Such an error would result in a 'geographical miss' and failure of the treatment would be virtually certain. Treatment given with curative intent is defined as radical, whereas treatment aimed at improvement of symptoms or merely controlling the tumour temporarily is considered palliative.

Malignant tumours are a mixture of malignant cells and normal tissue. All radiotherapy treatments involve irradiating the normal tissues supporting the tumour and adjacent normal tissue. The nature and volume of normal tissue included in any treatment volume and its radiosensitivity help to dictate the limits of treatment possible. The aim of any radiological assessment prior to treatment is, therefore, to help to define the tumour volume, the normal tissue volume and the nature of the normal tissues involved in the treatment. In practice, radiological techniques are the most important adjunct to clinical examination in the planning exercise.

Many years ago malignant diseases were defined in terms of their responsiveness to ionizing radiation. Although this is a crude concept, it has stood the general test of time. Paterson defined tumours as being 'definitely radiosensitive', 'an intermediate group' and 'radioresistant' (Paterson 1936). In the first group are the lymphomas, leukaemias, seminomas of the testes and dysgerminomas of the ovary. In the second group are squamous cell carcinomas at any site, transitional cell carcinoma of the urinary tract and some types of adenocarcinoma, in particular adenocarcinoma of the breast. The resistant group of tumours includes adenocarcinomas at other sites, in particular the large bowel, sarcomatous and melanomatous tumours. The words radiosensitive, intermediate and resistant are not absolute but give a qualitative assessment of the ease with which the disease responds to ionizing radiation. In general terms, very sensitive tumours can be cured by relatively low absolute doses which do not sig-

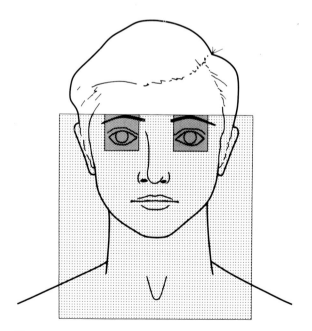

Fig. 18.1 Diagrammatic illustration of a typical wide field head and neck treatment applicable to patients with radiosensitive disease. The double hatched area over the eyes is shielded by placing blocks of lead on a tray in the megavoltage beam.

nificantly damage normal tissue. From a treatment planning point of view, this means that the tumour volume does not need to be defined very accurately and for many patients this means that standard large volume treatments, for example the head and neck or mantle techniques in Hodgkin's disease (Fig. 18.1), or whole abdominal radiation therapy in ovarian dysgerminoma, will be utilized no matter how extensive the disease is within the treatment volume. Even if standard treatments are not employed, treatment of nodal disease in Hodgkin's disease and non-Hodgkin's lymphoma with radiotherapy usually involves the use of large normal healthy tissue margins, for example 5 cm, around the areas of defined tumour. In these disease processes the radiotherapist needs to know which nodal areas are involved and to have a general idea of the volume of the nodes rather than an accurate assessment of tumour volume. This does not mean that the tumour volume within the primary site may not have an independent prognostic significance which may be of value in staging or defining what modality of treatment is used, but it is of less importance in the radiotherapy treatment planning. All that matters is to know which general areas are involved.

In the radical treatment of cancer the radiotherapist is principally involved in the management of the second group of tumours, and it is in these that target and volume definition are particularly important. They are numerically the most common group for radical radiotherapy techniques and in many cases small volume, high dose treatments taken to normal tissue tolerance are employed. The aim is always to keep the target volume as small as possible and to limit the normal tissues involved in the treatment volume by careful planning and shielding. This allows the delivery of the minimum volume homogeneous high dose treatment which can be delivered to the limits of normal supporting connective tissue tolerance. In all but the smallest primary carcinomas it is this attention to high dose, small volume treatment which will result in a significant proportion of these tumours being eradicated. This is the only way that cure without major radiation injury can be accomplished.

The third 'resistant' group of tumours may require consideration for radical radiotherapy: the problem is that they are unpredictable in their response to treatment. If they are small tumours which are not resectable then a carefully defined small volume, high dose treatment will eradicate a small but significant percentage. For the majority, treatment is only palliative because the tumours are advanced, recurrent or metastatic. In practice they may be treated using a large radiation field and given as much radiation as will be tolerable. This treatment will not normally approach normal tissue tolerance in the same way as for the more intermediate tumours.

Unfortunately, even moderately sensitive tumours are only curable by radiotherapy if they remain localized or have only spread to the immediate vicinity of the primary tumour. Widely metastatic though moderately sensitive tumour is incurable by radiotherapy, but may still be controlled by systemic chemotherapy or hormone therapy.

INDIVIDUAL TUMOURS

Head and neck

Many primary tumours of the head and neck region, particularly the mouth, oropharynx and larynx are very visible utilizing simple outpatient examination techniques and an idea of the tumour volume may be obtained in this way. This can be supplemented by digital examination of the mouth or pharynx and neck. Final information about the volume, particularly for nasopharyngeal, sinus and hypopharyngeal tumours, may require radiology.

There are a wide variety of important normal tissues in the head and neck region and inevitably some of these are close to the tumour volumes. They need careful definition prior to treatment planning.

Most head and neck tumours are carcinomas of squamous type but a variety of adenocarcinomas and sarcomatous tumours are seen in the nasopharyngeal region, parotid and minor salivary glands.

In modern practice patients are treated with small field radiation fields using high quality linear accelerator beams which offer the possibility of shielding sensitive normal tissues by introducing small shaped pieces of lead into the beam. This type of patient normally has a lightweight 'shell' made in the few days prior to starting treatment and the head position is controlled during treatment and on a day-to-day basis by the shell (Fig. 18.2). Most patients are treated lying supine on a flat couch; sometimes they require an inclined bed. Edentulous patients may need a bite block to stabilize the mandible during treatment and this can also be useful for unilateral mouth and palate tumours where the tongue may be moved outside the target volume by a suitably constructed bite block. All these manoeuvres may change the final position of the tumour relative to the bony skeleton, particularly in the floor of the mouth, tongue and buccal mucosa. It may therefore be helpful to insert inert markers, for example gold seeds, into the margins of the tumour under local anaesthetic shortly before the final treatment planning is undertaken. These can be visualized on radiographs taken on patients wearing their beam direction shells and their position relative to the markers on the shell easily defined (Fig. 18.3). This may be all that is required for planning treatment of mouth, tongue and palate lesions. In the larynx and hypopharynx AP tomography and/or CT scanning may supplement the clinical and endoscopic information about target volume. Soft tissue extension can be surprisingly great. It can also be very difficult to differentiate tumour from oedema in the larynx and the timing of treatment planning and CT scan relative to the biopsy should be known to avoid misinterpreting soft tissue swelling.

In suitable patients with small, non-metastatic radically treatable tumours a shell should be made, a lateral radiograph taken of the patient in their shell in the treatment position and a rough target volume defined utilizing information from clinical examination, radiology, endoscopy and any other imaging techniques. An optimal treatment plane can then be defined and the information transferred back onto the shell. With the patient in the treatment position CT scanning can be undertaken along the central plane of the treatment and a series of further CT scans taken on parallel planes at 1 cm intervals above and below the central plane. Information about the tumour volume and the important normal tissues can be defined on the images. This allows a target volume to be defined.

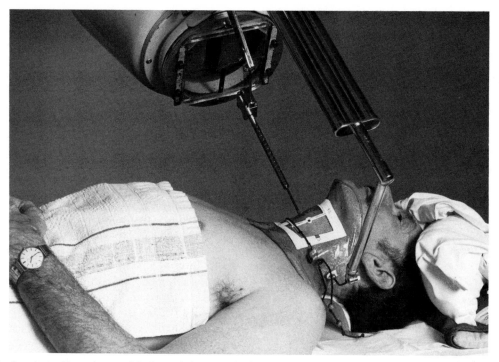

Fig. 18.2   A patient with carcinoma of the larynx being treated using a beam direction shell.

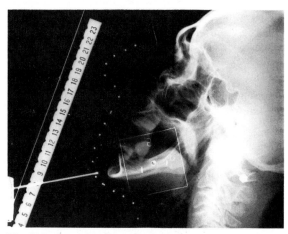

Fig. 18.3   Lateral radiograph of a patient with an alveolar squamous cell carcinoma. The patient is wearing a treatment shell. The limits of the carcinoma have been defined by tiny gold seed markers placed in the adjacent healthy tissue. One radiation field is simulated by the rectangular wire outlining the target volume.

Different treatment plans can be constructed and these can be tested by complete reconstruction of the dose distributions using a treatment planning computer (Fig. 18.4).

One difficult group of head and neck tumours uncommon in the UK but common in the Far East and one that the radiotherapist effectively faces alone is tumours of the nasopharynx. These are a motley collection of carcinomas with occasional lymphomas and sarcomas. Useful information from the history and clinical examination may be very limited and even after direct and endoscopic examination the disease may remain poorly defined. CT and MR scanning have easily surpassed the previously available imaging techniques in providing information about the site and volume of the primary tumour and the possibility of local metastatic spread. The particular problems for the radiotherapist are lateral extension into the retropharyngeal recesses and extension above the base of the skull. The former is important because it tended to be missed in small field treatments and the latter is important because it brings the tumour adjacent to the central nervous system and this may limit the dose of radiation which is possible.

Different philosophies can be adopted towards the normal tissues in the head and neck region depending on their sensitivity to radiation damage.

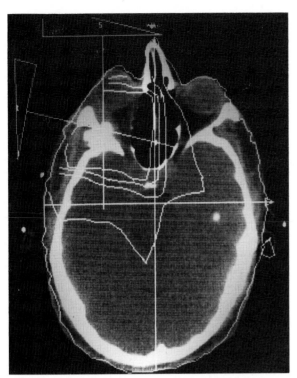

Fig. 18.4 CT treatment plan of a patient with a malignant tumour involving the right maxilla. A 2-field approach attempting to spare the anterior chamber of the left eye and to confine the radical treatment volume to the right orbit and retro-orbital tissues has been planned.

Certain tissues have to be included because of their close proximity to the tumour. Structures like the lens of the eye and the major salivary glands should be excluded if possible even from the exit beams of the fields, because they are so sensitive that even low doses will cause significant damage. The optic nerves, brain and brain stem should also be excluded if possible but may be included up to the limits of radiation tolerance and then excluded from the final part of the treatment. This approach involves the constant balancing of the therapeutic advantages of the higher dose of radiation against the problems of the type of damage which will result if radiation tolerance is exceeded. For example, the dose of radiation producing an identical level of tissue injury will infarct a temporal lobe, an optic nerve or the brain stem. The first will produce an injury that may be difficult to detect except by sophisticated psychological testing, the second will blind the eye and the

third will, in all probability, kill the patient. Considerations like these have to be balanced against the radiosensitivity of the disease to produce a final treatment plan.

Lung

The majority of patients in the UK presenting with carcinoma of the lung have advanced or metastatic disease at presentation. There is often a degree of collapse or consolidation of the lung which makes it difficult to define the tumour volume. In addition, most of these patients have been cigarette smokers and have chronic airways disease which will be significantly compromised by the use of large field radiation therapy, which normally destroys the function of healthy lung tissue included in the target volume. There is a need to keep the treatment volume as small as possible to mitigate this problem. For these patients chest radiographs and the bronchoscopic findings are all that is required to make a treatment decision. Many patients will not be treated and some will be offered simple treatment based on the information available. Some patients with significant lung collapse due to intraluminal disease of the main bronchi are treated by intraluminal laser or iridium-192 brachytherapy in an attempt to open up the airway and re-expand the lung to allow accurate staging.

Other patients have definable small volume primary tumours, usually peripherally sited without any overt evidence of metastases. These are normally squamous cell carcinomas or adenocarcinomas. The patients may be considered unsuitable for surgical resection for medical reasons including severe respiratory or cardiovascular disease. These primary tumours are usually easily defined on standard PA and lateral chest radiographs and the principal rôle of additional radiological investigations is in excluding metastatic disease, particularly hilar and mediastinal spread. These areas can be examined by AP or lateral tomography, transaxial tomography or CT scanning as defined in Chapter 4. Provided the radiotherapist is faced with a peripherally placed solitary malignant lesion without any evidence of metastatic spread a satisfactory radiation treatment can be planned.

The treatment position can be very variable and depends on the site of the primary tumour. This has to be defined before the last phase of the treatment planning exercise. Many patients may be planned supine but others will be planned lying prone with their hands above their heads or lying on the unaffected side with the arm held up and away from the chest. Whatever position is chosen the patient must be able to lie in it for about 10 minutes. In some situations this can be helped by the use of large chest shells to ensure that the treatment is reproducible on a day-to-day basis. Once the patient is comfortable in a treatment position, a series of CT scans is made through the midplane of the tumour and then contiguous 1 cm slices are obtained to a level above and below the limits of the tumour. Some system of satisfactorily defining the plane of section on the patient's skin is necessary and may involve the use of laser light beams on the CT scanner. It is common to apply a metal marker in the form of a cross (×) to the patient's skin. The position of the cross is marked on the skin with the patient in the treatment position, and the level of each CT slice relative to the cross can be calculated. The CT scan information can then be used in a treatment planning programme to define an optimum target volume and beam arrangement. This will also allow for the

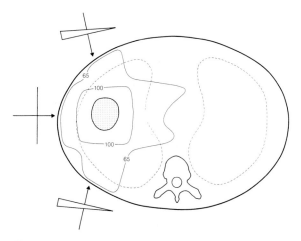

Fig. 18.5 Diagrammatic representation of a typical 3-field lung treatment for radical radiotherapy of carcinoma of the lung. Information about the site and size of the tumour and the volume of the lung are obtained from CT scanning. The target volume within the lung is hatched. The isodose lines for 100% and 65% of the intended dose are shown.

different attenuation of lung relative to soft tissue to be taken into consideration in the planning and will produce an accurate small volume high dose treatment (Fig. 18.5).

Oesophagus

This is usually a squamous cell carcinoma in the upper or middle third of the oesophagus. Occasionally these tumours are seen in the lower third or the radiotherapist may be attempting to control an adenocarcinoma at this site. Although the disease is relatively common, only a few patients are suitable for radical radiotherapy in spite of the histology. The site of the tumour is critically important in determining which radiotherapy technique can be used. In the lower neck and upper chest the oesophagus is very close to the spinal cord and lies at a varying angle relative to the skin surface of the neck and chest. This can create a very complex treatment planning problem.

An initial decision about the possibility of treatment is based on the site of the tumour in the oesophagus and the length affected. If the disease is greater than 5 cm in length the chance of control even with radical therapy is remote. In addition the degree of oesophageal narrowing, the functional effect on the patient's swallowing, the presence of any extra oesophageal soft tissue mass or a fistula to the trachea or bronchus all help the radiotherapist to make a judgement about suitability for treatment. Patients with metastases and fistulae and those in whom nutrition cannot be maintained both during and after treatment should not be irradiated. Most of this information can be obtained from chest radiography, barium swallow and endoscopic examination with biopsy.

In the presence of extensive or metastatic disease wide field X-ray techniques or the more modern intraluminal therapy using [60]cobalt, [137]caesium or [192]iridium may offer the patient considerable useful palliation (Fig. 18.6). These treatments can be planned without further radiological investigation. For patients with a potentially curable primary tumour, particularly in the cervical oesophagus and the upper thorax, further radiological investigation will aid treatment planning. Standard practice would be to try to re-

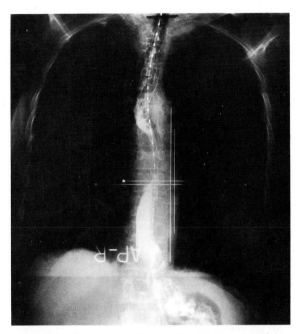

Fig. 18.6 AP radiograph of a patient with carcinoma of the oesophagus considered unsuitable for radical treatment. The mid-oesophageal carcinoma is identified by the use of contrast and a graduated intraluminal simulator wire has been passed through the oesophageal carcinoma in a nasogastric tube. The position of the tumour is related to the wire and a high intensity iridium source is passed down the tube during therapy.

late the malignant disease to the skin surface of the patient. Barium swallow radiographs taken with suitable skin markers can define the centre of the target volume in the AP and lateral views, and will give the depth of the tumour relative to the anterior chest wall and information about the plane of the part of the oesophagus containing the tumour and the site and plane of the spinal cord. Modern practice is to obtain CT scans of the patient in the treatment position, either prone or supine with hands either by the side or on the head. Using small volumes of oral contrast, CT scans should be performed through the centre of the lesion and then cranially and caudally at 1 cm intervals until the limits of the tumour and any associated soft tissue abnormality have been clearly defined. These scans will also allow the proximity of the spinal cord to the tumour to be defined at all levels. The most practical approach to these tumours, particularly in the lower or middle

oesophagus is the use of isocentric techniques in which the centre of the tumour is placed at the centre of the axis of rotation of the linear accelerator around the patient. To achieve this the central plane of the treatment field has to be clearly defined on the patient's skin and the distance from the skin surface to the centre of the tumour calculated and measured for each treatment field. The most common techniques involve irradiating the patient with lateral beams which pass through the lung and it is essential to calculate the thickness of lung that each individual beam will have to traverse. This can then be used in the calculations of tumour dosage to allow for the decreased attenuation of lung tissue. In practice, radiation therapy techniques for this disease involve the use of a minimum margin of 5 cm of healthy tissue above and below the defined limits of the primary disease which therefore means that treatments normally involve the use of long thin cylinders.

Upper oesophageal tumours remain difficult to plan and may require special beam direction devices to ensure homogeneity and a high dose without unnecessary damage to the spinal cord.

Bladder

The majority of patients treated by radical radiotherapy have T2 or T3 solitary transitional cell carcinomas of the bladder. Radiotherapy is a poor technique for widespread superficial disease which is best treated by surgery. Patients with locally advanced disease who would not tolerate radical radiotherapy or those with incurable T4 disease may have palliative X-ray therapy to relieve haematuria but here sophisticated techniques of tumour definition are unnecessary. The locally advanced T2 and T3 tumours often involve the lower posterior bladder wall. A special problem for the radiotherapist is the rarer involvement of the lateral, anterior or fundal walls. These latter surfaces move during the normal process of urine collection and micturition and the target volume is therefore potentially changing in shape and position. Radical bladder radiotherapy treatments are normally undertaken with the bladder as empty as possible, i.e. following micturition. Radiological assessment techniques often employ contrast to distend the bladder and therefore care must be taken when translating information from diagnostic images to planning.

The special problems in bladder cancer are to define the extent of the visible tumour at cystoscopy, to assess the depth of infiltration and to exclude overt pelvic metastases. It is helpful to know the number and position of the kidneys, their function in the presence of tumour and the residual volume of urine in the bladder following micturition. This information can help in the selection of patients for treatment and in the accurate definition of target volume.

Traditional radiotherapy planning techniques involve the use of small volumes of contrast, for example barium, instilled into the empty bladder with the patient supine. The hands are usually on the chest. AP and lateral radiographs are taken employing skin marker techniques and magnification rulers placed in both the AP and lateral beams (Fig. 18.7). These allow assessment of magnification and can help in the definition of the true site and size of the tumour. These techniques have, however, been recognized to be inaccurate particularly for lateral wall and fundal tumours, and significant numbers of geographical misses may occur. This is, of course, not surprising since the planning techniques are really defining the surface of the primary tumour rather than its true size. Ideally patients should have a CT scan while lying supine with their arms on the chest and a small amount, e.g. 20 ml, of contrast in the bladder. All the information available from cystoscopy and radiology, ultrasound, diagnostic CT and MR images should be used to define the primary tumour volume on the treatment planning scans. It is then normal to allow a minimum 1 cm margin of healthy tissue around the tumour volume and to use a 3-field or rotational technique to produce an accurate dose distribution to the tumour (Fig. 18.8). The most important normal tissue in this treatment is the rectum which in the male is immobile relative to the posterior bladder wall. In the female the vagina and uterus separate the bladder from the sigmoid and rectum. The position of the lower rectum can be defined by the introduction of a catheter or sponge containing radio-opaque material during the planning scans. The sigmoid colon and small bowel are also important but these latter structures may move relative to the target

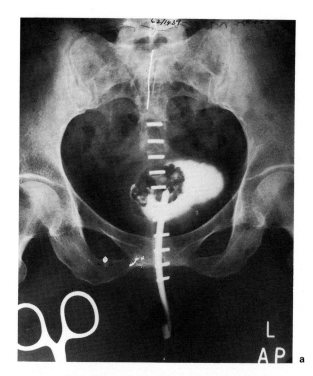

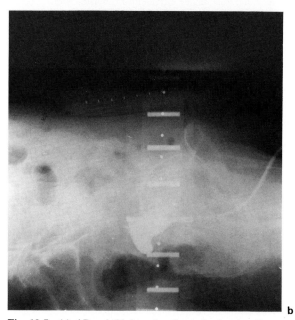

Fig. 18.7 (a) AP and (b) lateral radiograph planning films for a patient with carcinoma of the bladder. Contrast has been introduced through a urinary catheter. The anterior abdominal wall graduated marker overlies the tumour. On the lateral view the graduated markers placed on either side of the patient allow a mid-pelvic magnification factor to be worked out and the depth of the bladder relative to the skin to be calculated.

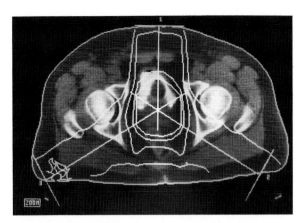

Fig 18.8 CT scan of the pelvis in a patient with stage II carcinoma of the bladder. The carcinoma is on the left lower lateral bladder wall. The isodose pattern from a possible 3-field treatment plan is shown.

volume during the course of treatment due to peristalsis. Successful radical radiotherapy depends on keeping this bowel component of the target volume as small as possible and relying on the peristaltic activity to reduce the effective normal tissue volume even further. Some radiotherapists employ techniques in which initially the whole of the true pelvis is irradiated through a standard large field 'sandwich' approach. The small volume techniques described above are then employed when the true pelvic tolerance has been reached but when there is considered to be further tolerance present in the primary tumour area. These boost or shrinking field techniques may involve the need to monitor the tumour during treatment and in particular to reassess the target volume by repeating the investigations discussed above.

Prostate

Carcinoma of the prostate is a disease of uncertain natural history. There is no agreement about the optimum treatment of early disease and ongoing trials are in progress internationally. In the last decade radical radiotherapy has become an acceptable alternative to radical prostatectomy or hormone therapy in patients with stage I or II disease, i.e. disease confined to the prostate. The radiological contribution to the treatment planning is less than in carcinoma of the bladder because

the tumour volume is more easily defined at the time of cystoscopy and EUA. Transrectal ultrasound may complement this examination and suggest periprostatic infiltration. The volume of the tumours accepted for treatment tend to be small relative to bladder carcinomas and their position is relatively fixed in relation to the base of the bladder and the rectum. The principal problem facing the radiotherapist is that by the time any satisfactory margin is placed on the primary tumour volume it is inevitable that this target volume will contain a significant amount of rectal tissue. Treatment plans involve small 3-field or rotational techniques very similar to those used in carcinoma of the bladder. The planning exercise is effectively identical to that employed for carcinoma of the bladder although the target volume is less. The exercise can be accomplished using a urinary catheter, bladder contrast, skin markers and magnification rulers in association with AP and lateral radiographs. Ideally CT scanning should be employed. This site of primary disease is of particular interest to radiotherapists who are involved in sophisticated three-dimensional treatment planning exercises because of the perceived need to limit the volume of rectal mucosa and other bowel tissues in the treatment volume.

Three-dimensional reconstruction of the prostate in the treatment position reveals that it can be considered as a small pyramid lying on its side with the base towards the bladder. Standard treatment planning allows generous margins distally and narrow margins around the base of the bladder and the seminal vesicles. An ideal plan should involve an even margin around the tumour volume, an exercise which does not necessarily reduce the final treatment volume but does ensure that the treatment volume and the target volume are as close to each other as possible.

Some European and North American centres favour the use of interstitial techniques in which the radiation is placed within the tissues of the tumour and the surrounding normal tissue in the form of small permanent seeds of [125]iodine or temporary implants of radioactive materials like [192]iridium. The information required for these latter techniques is not significantly different from that used for external beam techniques and there is not a lot of evidence to suggest that the results in terms of tumour control are any different. The latter techniques do allow a smaller effective tumour volume to be irradiated and therefore can reduce the risks of morbidity, particularly to the rectal mucosa.

Gynaecological cancer

In modern practice radiotherapy has a major rôle to play in the management of cervical and vaginal carcinoma, a supporting rôle in endometrial cancer and a very limited rôle in ovarian and vulval cancer.

Cervix

Radical radiotherapy remains the normal approach to more than 80% of patients with primary disease of the cervix and vagina, and particularly for patients with stage II disease and beyond. These patients are normally treated with a combination of external beam therapy and intracavitary therapy utilizing radioactive sources in the uterus and vagina. There are very special problems from a treatment planning point of view. The true pelvis is occupied by the lower urinary, genital and gastrointestinal tracts; the latter often includes small and large bowel. The tissues are adjacent to, vary in position from and are capable of individual movement relative to each other throughout the course of treatment. To compound the problem the intracavitary techniques produce inhomogeneous dose distributions with high dose rates close to the sources and a rapidly falling dose gradient out into the adjacent tissue. Initial treatment planning in carcinoma of the cervix is usually based on the findings at EUA, the IVU and lymphangiography if available. CT scanning is usually unhelpful unless enlarged iliac or para-aortic nodes are present. Most centres start therapy utilizing a target volume including the whole of the true pelvis, which may extend up to the L4/5 junction or even into the para-aortic area. Sometimes the lower central pelvic tissues are shielded initially by placing lead blocks in the appropriate parts of the field.

It is obvious that fine details of the tumour volume are relatively unimportant at this stage provided that the fields encompass the disease. X-ray therapy is given for 3–5 weeks until the normal general pelvic tolerance begins to limit the dosage (Fig. 18.9). At this point intracavitary therapy can be given. There are a variety of techniques but all involve the introduction of radioactive sources in applicators into the uterus and vagina. The high dose rates close to the sources mean that normal tissues like the bladder, rectum and sigmoid colon can easily be over-treated if they lie close to the sources during the treatment period. Modern treatment planning attempts to define dosimetry points in normal tissues to guide the radiotherapist in prescribing dosage. Some of these techniques are described in ICRU Report 38 (1985) which addresses the problem of expressing dose in intracavitary therapy. Modern imaging techniques including ultrasound and CT scanning can contribute by helping to define the position, shape and distance of important tissues from the sources

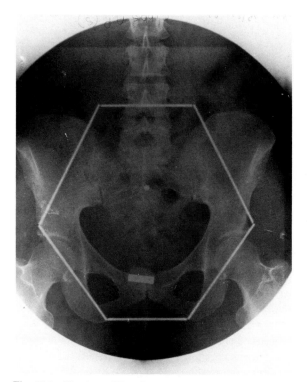

Fig. 18.9 Simulator AP radiograph of the pelvis in a patient with carcinoma of the cervix. A typical wide field radiotherapy treatment is outlined by the hexagonal wire. The marker overlying the pubis is in the vaginal vault.

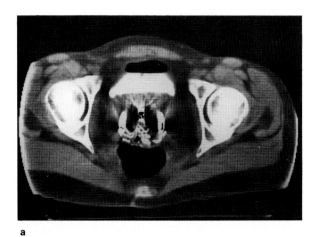

a

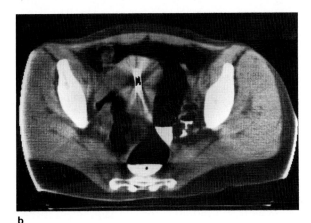

b

Fig. 18.10 CT scans through the pelvis of a patient undergoing intracavitary therapy. Standard applicators have been placed in the uterus and vagina. (a) CT scan through the upper vagina at the level of the vaginal sources. The position of the sources in the vagina, the packing separating them from the rectum, and the bladder are all visible. (b) CT scan through the pelvis at the level of the uterus. The central uterine applicator is separated from the surrounding bowel by the thick muscle of the uterus.

(Fig. 18.10). Their regular use demonstrates a wide range of normal anatomical variation between patients being treated with standard techniques. These variations of anatomy are a major and important contributory cause of radiation-induced morbidity. Further attempts to develop simple non-invasive imaging techniques for use in each patient at the time of treatment are to be encouraged. At the present moment CT is the most useful technique but ultrasound, if it could be developed more fully, would be more practical.

If CT images are generated in patients undergoing intracavitary therapy then dose distributions can be computed and the impact of variations of dose distribution studied (Fig. 18.11).

Endometrium

With the exception of a small number of patients with localized carcinoma of the endometrium who are unfit for pelvic surgery, the majority of patients for radiotherapy treatment have been staged by their total abdominal hysterectomy and BSO. Patients with high grade, locally invasive or locally metastatic carcinomas may benefit from adjuvant postoperative radiotherapy to the whole pelvis. This is normally done using standard techniques and does not require any special imaging. An exception to the standard techniques might be the patient with evidence of vaginal vault recurrence after apparently successful surgery. In this patient imaging techniques to investigate the integrity of the lower urinary tract and to define the extent of the vault recurrence and any evidence of nodal disease in the pelvis and para-aortic region would help to define an individual treatment plan.

Ovary

The majority of patients present with advanced disease unsuitable for radiotherapy and they are

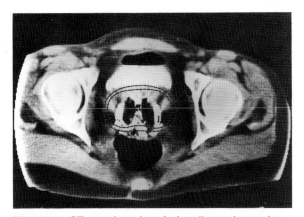

Fig. 18.11 CT scan through vaginal applicators in a patient undergoing intracavitary therapy. The relevant isodose distribution around the sources has been plotted. The outer line shown receives only 50% of the dose of the inner line, emphasizing the steep gradient of dosage in these treatments.

treated by chemotherapy, normally achieving high grade palliation at the best. The small number of patients with early stage disease (I and II) are normally treated primarily by surgery and offered postoperative radiotherapy or chemotherapy depending on the experience of the treating staff. The radiotherapy techniques used involve treating the whole pelvis or whole abdomen and the radiological input is normally only to define the position of the diaphragms in a supine patient and the number, size and position of the kidneys to allow the former to be included in the treatment field and the latter to be excluded towards the end of the treatment to prevent radiation nephropathy.

The central nervous system

The majority of tumours in adults within the central nervous system are metastases which are normally multiple. The commonest primary tumours are gliomas. Neither group has ever been shown to benefit from sophisticated pretreatment assessment. Metastases are normally treated by large latterly-placed treatment fields which take the anterior, middle and posterior fossae into the same treatment volume. Even apparently solitary metastatic deposits are radiotherapeutically probably best treated in this manner. Gliomas are by nature solitary and non-metastatic but they are highly infiltrative and large normal tissue margins continue to be used in practice. The only new factor which may, in time, influence this situation is the use of MR imaging. The images provide higher contrast resolution than CT scans and may allow more focused treatment to be undertaken. This is the subject of clinical trial.

Radiotherapists are also asked to treat unresectable or malignant meningiomatous and angiomatous tumours and some troublesome AV malformations. In these situations the three-dimensional definition of the abnormality, its site within the CNS and the proximity of adjacent vital tissues are important in planning treatment.

Another special CNS site is the pituitary gland and the unusual, often unresectable tumours of the surrounding tissues. The accurate definition of the intracranial and extracranial components of these tumours and their relationship to the optic chiasma, hypothalamus and optic nerves in the postoperative situation can aid the production of a satisfactory treatment plan.

Bone and soft tissue

Radiotherapeutic treatment of this group, with the exception of Ewing's sarcoma, is normally palliative and as a result the margins used in any treatments are often generous and defined as much in terms of the likely spread in the bone or compartment as they are in terms of actual disease. With bone tumours skip lesions and extra-osseous extension must be included to effect palliation.

Soft tissue tumours are sometimes tackled as radically as possible if alternative therapy is not available. Many are relatively superficial in limbs or on the trunk and sophisticated radiology may add little to clinical examination and a knowledge of the anatomy of the region and the behaviour of the different tumours in planning the necessary large fields. The most important information comes from identification of extra-compartmental spread.

CONCLUSION

Radiology plays an important rôle in the assessment of different tumours for radiotherapy. There is a need for a close working relationship between radiologist and radiotherapist. The problem is that if information generated from initial diagnostic techniques does not fulfil the requirements of treatment planning then the patient will have to undergo further pretreatment studies. That may not be so important when only radiographs are involved, but when more sophisticated radiological techniques like CT scanning or MR imaging are being used, it becomes wasteful and inefficient. Investigations which generate information for both diagnostic and therapeutic purposes must, therefore, be the aim of everyone involved. In some situations this may be possible using the same images, or for example by taking more CT sections with the bladder drained in patients with vesical cancer. In other situations the need for treatment planning in unconventional positions or the use of added beam direction devices may require specific verification studies. Preliminary discussion and an understanding of the different needs is in everyone's interests, most of all the patients.

REFERENCES

ICRU 1985 Report 38: Dose and volume specification for reporting intracavitary therapy in gynaecology, section 3.3.11

Paterson R 1948 The treatment of malignant disease by radium and X-rays, Ch. 1. Edward Arnold, London, pp 23–25

Suggested background reading

Easson E, Pointon R (eds) 1985 The radiotherapy of malignant disease, 3rd edn. Springer-Verlag, Berlin

Hopestone H (ed) 1986 Radiotherapy in clinical practice. Butterworths, London

Dobbs J, Barrett A (eds) 1985 Practical radiotherapy planning. Edward Arnold, London

Appendix 1   Parathyroid imaging using Thallium ^{201}Tl and Technetium ^{99m}Tc

Insert butterfly needle into an arm vein.

Position patient, using a head support and head band to limit patient movement.

Set up energy windows for both principal thallium energies e.g. 55–91 and 155–184 keV.

Inject ^{201}Tl 75 MBq.

Use console to centre and magnify thallium 'thyroid' image × 2.5.

Collect data for 20 min, e.g. 4 × 5 min.

Sum as appropriate for a single view.

Change to ^{99m}Tc window.

Inject ^{99m}Tc pertechnetate 20 MBq.

Collect the data for 15 min as 3 × 5 min.

Use 10–15 min image for subtraction.

Display thallium and petechnetate images.

Define a contour around the pertechnetate thyroid image.

Perform Goris interpolative background subtraction on the thallium image to reduce contribution from underlying tissues.

Perform incremental subtraction of increasing fractions of the pretechnetate thyroid image until zero areas appear in the thallium image.

Check hot spots on the subtracted thallium image against the pertechnetate image to exclude thyroid adenoma.

Display optimized thallium image hot spots in the pertechnetate thyroid contour.

Arrange hard copy of the three images.

Index